TOWARDS NEW THERAPIES FOR PARKINSON'S DISEASE

Edited by **David I. Finkelstein**

Towards New Therapies for Parkinson's Disease
Edited by David I. Finkelstein

Published by InTech

Janeza Trdine 9, 51000 Rijeka, Croatia

Publishing Process Manager Silvia Vlase

Technical Editor Teodora Smiljanic

Cover Designer InTech Design Team

Additional hard copies can be obtained from orders@intechopen.com

Towards New Therapies for Parkinson's Disease, Edited by David I. Finkelstein
p. cm.
ISBN 978-953-307-463-4

For EU product safety concerns:
IN TECH d.o.o., Prolaz Marije Krucifikse Kozulić 3, 51000 Rijeka, Croatia, info@intechopen.com or visit our website at intechopen.com.

Meet the editor

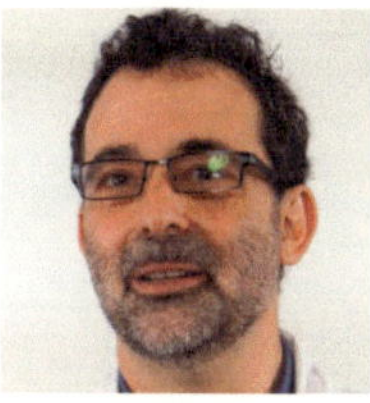

Dr. David I. Finkelstein received a BSc (1979 LaTrobe University, Melbourne Australia), MSc (1986) and PhD in Physiology (1991) from Monash University, Australia. He is a full time researcher that gives specialist undergraduate and postgraduate lectures in neurobiology and anatomy to science, medical and physiotherapy students. His research investigates the neurobiology on neurodegeneration with particular emphasis on the processes that occur during Parkinson's Disease. He has produced around 100 publications in refereed journals as well as numerous book chapters and international conference presentations. He is a scientific consultant for two biotechnology companies producing and developing novel small molecules for the treatment of neurodegenerative diseases (Parkinson's, Alzheimer's and Huntington's Diseases). He is an editor and a reviewer for many international journals and granting bodies.

Contents

Preface

The current research investigating new ways to treat Parkinson's disease (PD) is taking many directions. Current therapies successfully ameliorate the symptoms of the disease but the course of the disease appears to be unperturbed. This book is intended for the clinician or scientist looking towards the future. The brief outline of the book is as follows.

Chapter 1 explores the issues surrounding the application of subthalamic nucleus deep brain stimulation (STN-DBS), for PD has been shown to induce dramatic and stable long-term improvement of patients' motor symptoms. However some of the motor symptoms, and most of the non-motor symptoms, may not be improved by STN-DBS, and may even deteriorate after surgery. Even after the successful introduction of STN-DBS as a treatment for PD, controversy still exists and this chapter examines a variety of issues: patient selection criteria, the anatomical target, imaging, targeting methods, microelectrode recordings, and anesthetic procedures.

Chapter 2 discusses the economic burden of PD. The cost of therapies has become and will increasingly become a very important topic for governments and the health industry. From the perspective of a general neurologist, health economics can appear not be a priority, however it is a growing topic in most modern healthcare systems. Additional demands are being made by health policy decision makers, who can influence medical decisions through coverage and reimbursement policies. Physicians and other professional caregivers increasingly must consider the economic implications of their decisions.

Chapter 3, proposes that infusion of apomorphine is a good therapeutic option, rapidly stimulating receptors, thereby assisting in the management of motor fluctuations in the advanced phase of the disease. Apomorphine has the added advantage as it is effective as a rescue therapy that can be administered with a penject.

Chapter 4 examines the role of alpha-synuclein and the Immune Response in PD. This chapter proposes mechanisms through which alpha-synuclein might be affecting the immune system that appear not to be just a consequence of disease progression, but to actively contribute to the delicate balance between neuroprotection and neurotoxicity that ultimately underlies a given stage of disease.

Chapter 5 describes the investigations of Joseph Knoll in the early 1960's that resulted in the development deprenyl a monoamine oxidase (MAO-B) inhibitor. The chapter reviews extensive studies and potential uses of the MAO-B inhibitors. The author proposes that the concept of the prophylactic use of deprenyl proposed by Knoll, may decrease the prevalence of neurodegenerative diseases, such as, Parkinson's and Alzheimer's diseases.

In Chapter 6 the authors review and describe the use of organotypic cultures as a model to study molecular mechanisms of PD as well as the use as a tool for preclinical studies of pharmacological and cell therapy treatment. It is proposed that disease can be modelled by application of drugs, toxins or by various transfection systems. Various treatment options can also be explored in this versatile system.

In Chapter 7 the authors present the view that polyphenols may meet the challenge for novel molecules that could simultaneously target multiple PD pathways without significant side-effects, be non-toxic at higher concentrations and have the ability to cross the blood-brain. Polyphenols are derived from various plant sources.

Chapter 8: microtubule-associated protein tau has risk alleles for PD, and mutations that cause brain degenerative diseases termed tauopathies. Aggregated phosphorylated tau forms neurofibrillary tangles in these pathologies. This chapter identifies the inhibition of Tau phosphorylation as a potential strategy in treating PD.

Chapter 9: The subcortical nuclei of the basal ganglia are of great importance in initiation of normal body motor activities. Excitatory amino acids play an important role in these normal activities of these nuclei but dysfunction of the transmitter system has been implicated in some neurodegenerative diseases. In this chapter the authors pre-treat animals with glutamate metabotropic receptor agonists prevent the development 6-OHDA induced Parkinsonian movements. The authors suggest that the glutamate is potential target for investigations into new therapies for PD.

Chapter 10: Glial cell line-derived neurotrophic factor (GDNF) is considered a strong survival factor for dopaminergic neurons. This has led to the proposed use of GDNF as a potential therapy to slow down or even reverse neurodegeneration in PD. In this chapter the authors explore less common perspectives and alternative therapeutic approaches in PD. They believe that this chapter may draw attention to new directions of GDNF research.

The authors of Chapter 11 express the views that despite the recent disappointing results in clinical trials, there remains an optimism that neurotrophic factors will prove to be useful in PD therapy. Optimisation of delivery methods is needed, and vital information is being gleaned from studies in animal models of PD. For future clinical trials, optimisation of surgical and infusion protocols, as well as careful patient selection, will be critical to advance this promising therapeutic approach.

Chapters 12 and 13 consider gene therapy to be one of the most promising approaches to develop an effective treatment for PD. The existence of blood brain barrier and the ability to control gene expression are currently limitations of this technology. Studies in animals studies have been developing the technologies to regulate gene expression and to deliver the materials in the periphery and have the product expressed in the neurons. These chapters consider viral and non viral ways of delivering the genes to the brain.

In Chapter 14 the authors propose the use of S-adenosylmethionine (SAM, a methyl group donor molecule necessary for DNA methylation) as an epigenetic tool to increase the expression of adenosine A2A receptors in PD. It has been proposed that the inactivation of A2A receptor enhances the affinity of D2R for dopamine, this being the probable mechanism underlying the dopaminergic like effect of A2AR antagonists in some patients.

Chapters 15 and 16 investigate the prospects of implantation of dopaminergic neurons as a therapy that may reverse some of the central symptoms of PD. Over the last decades, approximately 400 PD patients have been grafted, with substantial motor improvements being reported particularly in younger patients. In these chapters the authors examine the historical approaches and what has been learnt from those as well as the current status. They discuss crucial issues that remain to be resolved to develop cell replacement into an effective and safe therapy.

Once the technology for transplantation of tissues into people with PD, there will be a need to resolve the regulatory issues. Chapter 17 examines the technologies involved in the transplantation of foetal ventral mesencephalic grafts in people with PD and then goes on to examine the new regulatory challenges.

This book is intended for researchers and clinicians interested in developing new and innovative therapies for Parkinson's Disease. The editor would like to thank all the authors for their contributions in the book. Finally, gratitude should be expressed also to the team at InTech for the initiative and help in publishing this book.

Assoc. Prof. David I. Finkelstein
The Mental Health Research Institute, The University of Melbourne
Australia

Part 1

Issues Regarding Current Human Therapies

1

Controversial Issues in Deep Brain Stimulation in Parkinson's Disease

Shin-Yuan Chen[1,2], Sheng-Tzung Tsai[2] and Sheng-Huang Lin[3]
[1]*Division of Functional Neuroscience,*
[2]*Department of Neurosurgery*
[3]*Neurology, Neuro-Medical Scientific Center*
Tzu Chi General Hospital / Tzu Chi University, Hualien
Taiwan

1. Introduction

Since 1992, the application of subthalamic nucleus deep brain stimulation (STN-DBS) for Parkinson's disease (PD) has been shown to induce dramatic and stable long-term improvement of patients' motor symptoms. However, some of the motor symptoms, and most of the non-motor symptoms, may not be improved by STN-DBS; in fact, they may deteriorate after surgery. Even after the successful introduction of STN-DBS as a treatment for PD, controversy still exists over a variety of issues: patient selection criteria, the anatomical target such as STN or globus pallidus (GPi), targeting methods (MRI alone, CT scan with image fusion, or ventriculography), microelectrode recordings (yes/no), and anesthetic procedures (awake with sedative or under general anesthesia). In this chapter we will discuss these controversial issues by integrating our experience with a review of the literature.

2. Patient selection for deep brain stimulation (DBS)

A successful DBS surgery may involve several surgical procedures, but patient selection is always a key issue to address because it contributes to whether there is a good surgical outcome. In 1992, a common evaluation protocol for PD was suggested by the the Core Assessment Program for Intracerebral Transplantations(CAPIT) committee, which allowed for comparisons between different study groups. For example, they defined "off-medication" and "on-medication" status. The core assessment methodologies of this protocol include the following: Unified Parkinson's Disease Rating Scale (UPDRS), Hoehn and Yahr Staging, Dyskinesia Rating Scale, Self-reporting diary, and timed test for bradykinesia [1]. In 1996, the Network for European CNS Transplantation and Restoration (NECTAR), developed a new Core Assessment Program for Surgical Interventional Therapies in PD (CAPSIT-PD) and gave advice to add evaluations for cognitive function and quality of life [2]. Since then, thousands of papers have been published in the fields of PD and DBS, and clinicians and researchers have paid attention to the issue of patient selection in order to ensure a good outcome [3-9].

In 2009, Australia offered a referral guideline for neurologists to establish methods for enrolling ideal PD candidates for DBS. In 2010, consensus was reached for DBS in PD. With respect to patient selection, these experts stated that, "...Best results have been reported in patients with advanced PD and (1) levodopa response, (2) younger age, (3) no or few axial non–LD-responsive motor symptoms, (4) no or very mild cognitive impairment, and (5) absence of or well controlled psychiatric disease" [10]. The ideal candidate has all of the above components; however, even with these guidelines, pitfalls and controversy still exist.

Diagnosis

It is important to differentiate PD from atypical parkinsonism to ensure a good long-term outcome of STN-DBS, but it can be hard to discriminate between them because they share clinical features such as bradykinesia, rigidity and tremor. It is especially difficult when the disease is in its early stage and l-dopa responsiveness is moderate. Poor prognostic factors for STN-DBS can be the following: a poor response to l-dopa, the additional presence of pyramidal or cerebellar signs (e.g., ataxia), an early presentation of posture instability and autonomic failure (e.g., hypotension), within 5 years of onset, a non-tremor dominant presentation, and persistent unilateral disease [11-12]. The UK Brain Bank Diagnostic Criteria for PD is recommended for assessing all surgical candidates, although it should be noted that the early symptoms of PD, such as hyposmia, REM sleep behavioral disorders, constipation and depression may precede the obvious motor symptoms and are not included on the list [13]. The use of Hoehn and Yahr (H&Y) staging and the Unified Parkinson's Disease Rating Scale (UPDRS) is a basic requirement for evaluating patients before starting any PD intervention. In 2007, the revising process for the UPDRS was started by a task force of the Movement Disorder Society (MDS), which is aimed at incorporating more detail on non-motor symptoms, but it has not yet been published [14-17].

Age at time of surgery

Age is a confounding factor and has a negative correlation with STN-DBS outcome. A trend for greater long-term STN-DBS improvements on the UPDRS part II and part III measures in younger patients has been shown; however, it is also effective in elderly patients, though the benefits may persist for only a short period of time [18]. Most studies also have shown a negative correlation with motor outcome, non-motor outcome (e.g., apathy and depression) and quality of life upon long-term follow-up [18-22]. While the cut-off age proposed by most studies is 70 years old, the benefits and risks of surgery should be weighed to meet the expectations of the patient and the care giver.

Disease duration and severity

Advanced PD patients with obvious medication side effects of motor fluctuation and/or dyskinesia would be good candidates for DBS. However, an H&Y Stage 1 patient with tremor dominant symptoms who is within 5 years of onset can also be a good candidate for DBS and show a substantial benefit, as can a bed-ridden Stage 5 patient. Because there have been no proven neuroprotective effects of DBS, the recommendation for an earlier intervention is based on quality of life, which will improve substantially in domains related to movement disorders and general health [23]. Though some authors postulate that disease severity may be correlated with STN-DBS outcome, a study of ours found that the outcome was not correlated with H&Y staging or disease duration [18].

Levodopa (LD) responsiveness

LD responsiveness, as measured by the UPDRS part III, may predict the motor outcome of STN-DBS in a PD patient with disabling motor fluctuations and dyskinesia. In fact, this is true for all cardinal symptoms (except LD refractory tremor) that can be well controlled by STN-DBS. Pre-operative LD responsiveness may only lead to consistent UPDRS part III improvement from STN-DBS at 3 months, and its predictive value may not be valid for long-term follow-up due to co-morbid non-motor symptoms. The pre-operative LD responsiveness of tremor and axial symptoms are stable predictors for the long-term effect of DBS [18].

Cognitive, psychiatric, and other non-motor symptoms

Non-motor symptoms in PD patients are a significant source of disability and impairment in the performance of activities of daily living. The non-motor symptoms of PD include dementia, sleep disorders, and dysautonomia along with neuropsychiatric and sensory complaints. Most centers exclude PD patients with dementia and neuropsychiatric symptoms from STN-DBS. As for sleep disorders and sensory complaints, some reports have shown improvement after treatment when these symptoms are present. More generally, normal pre-operative cognitive functioning is positively correlated with post-operative improvement in UPDRS part III at a long-term follow-up [18]. STN-DBS may still lead to a decline in cognitive and executive function even with strict inclusion criteria [24]; however, it has been suggested that sub-optimal contact stimulation (caused by the small volume of STN) is more strongly correlated with post-operative psychiatric events. Although there are still debates about post-operative psychiatric events, the possibility of increased depression and suicide risk prompts us to evaluate the patient's psychological function in detail prior to the operation.

3. STN-DBS versus GPi-DBS: Which target is better for PD patients?

STN-DBS is the current gold-standard surgical treatment in PD, but a high occurrence of adverse effects and neuropsychological problems following STN-DBS stimulation cause some centers to study alternative surgical targets, such as the GPi. The issues to consider when choosing a target for DBS include the following: a different set of patient selection criteria, the amount of levodopa being used, the extent of levodopa-related dyskinesia, battery life and surgeon preference.

In randomized trials, DBS has been demonstrated to be superior to the best known-medical treatment for advanced PD. Under most circumstances, STN is the chosen target rather than GPi. Although several reports have shown that the efficacy of pallidal stimulation decreases over the long-term follow up [25], others have demonstrated a persistent benefit from pallidal stimulation for up to 3 years [26]. In 2005, the first randomized trial was published by Anderson and colleagues, and their patients showed a similar improvement in motor function from subthalamic and pallidal stimulation [27]. Still, deciding which target is best is a topic still subject to debate, and several points of view need to be considered.

The effect of target on motor function

PD is characterized by disabling motor symptoms. Previous reports seem to have concluded that STN-DBS improves more than GPi-DBS in UPDRS part III (motor) [26-28]. However, a recent large randomized trial showed a similar improvement from either STN or GPi stimulation [29]. It should be noted that the follow-up duration in this study was only 24 months and GPi might show less of a benefit after a longer period of time [25, 30].

The effect of target on non-motor symptoms

Non-motor symptoms of PD have received more attention in recent years and seem to play a pivotal role in the change in quality of life caused by the amelioration of motor disabilities through medical or surgical treatment [31]. An increased percentage of post-stimulation behavioral and cognitive complications is still a major concern for STN-DBS [27, 32-33] as it is not conclusively known whether DBS causes a change in these non-motor symptoms. Although a recent randomized trial comparing PD patients undergoing STN stimulation to those who only received the best medication-based treatment showed no significant differences [34], a second study comparing STN stimulation with GPi did show that depression was worse in those who received STN-DBS [29]. This finding reminds us that non-motor symptoms should be considered during target selection for patients who plan to receive electrode implantation.

The effect of target on reducing medication dosages

One of the main reasons that pallidal stimulation has not become popular may be that it limits the amount one can decrease medication dosages. Most studies have shown that patients who undergo STN stimulation require a lower dose of dopaminergic medication than those who undergo GPi stimulation [28-29]. This effect is probably due to different mechanisms of action underlying the STN and GPi response to electrical current. It has been suggested that STN stimulation reverses the sensitization phenomenon that underpins levodopa induced dyskinesia (LID) [35]. In fact, STN stimulation per se cannot ameliorate LID without decreasing dopaminergic medication[36]. Contrary to this, GPi stimulation may itself decrease the severity of LID [37]. The interaction between STN and GPi activity has been suggested to play a major role in the pathogenesis of dyskinesia, and the amelioration of stimulation-related dyskinesia through proximal contact (i.e., stimulating pallido-subthalamic fibers) shown in previous reports and our own young onset PD (YOPD) patients suggests a more beneficial effect of GPi than STN in ameliorating treatment-related dyskinesia. Overall, most comparative studies showed that the daily dosage of levodopa can be reduced only in an STN-DBS group [26].

The effect of target on battery life

The stimulation amplitude within the implantable pulse generator (IPG) is one significant determinant of battery life. In a multicenter study, Rodriguez-Oroz and colleagues found a similar amplitude for patients undergoing STN and GPi stimulation for 3 to 4 years [26]. However, most studies (including one large randomized trial) have shown that STN stimulation requires significantly less electrical power around 0.7~0.8 V and a pulse width of 20 µsec [38]. These parameters allow patients to receive STN stimulation for a longer period of time between pulse-generator replacements as compared to GPi stimulation. Most cost-effectiveness studies also have confirmed this benefit of STN stimulation over solely medication-based treatment for advanced PD. For countries where DBS devices are not reimbursed by health insurance, such as Taiwan, the replacement of the IPG will be a large burden for most patients. Larger amplitudes and pulse widths for GPi stimulation may lead to more frequent battery replacement and more device-related complications [30]. Improving future IPG technology may alleviate this economic consideration.

Adverse effects of target

Adverse effects of stimulation in general include cognitive decline, verbal fluency deterioration, gait disorders and mood instability (in the form of compulsiveness or depression). Most studies show that the adverse effects of stimulation are more common in STN-DBS [27, 29]. In the COMPARE trial, which was a prospective randomized trial, it was shown that under optimal conditions there was no significant difference in the incidence of mood or cognitive alteration following DBS implantation. However, a sub-scale analysis of the Visual Analogue Mood Scale showed that there was more "anger" after STN-DBS. Another randomized trial also has suggested that depression may be worse after subthalamic stimulation but improved after pallidal stimulation.

The volume of the STN (~158 mm^3) is much smaller than the GPi (~478 mm^3) nucleus. Moreover, the sub-territory within the STN nucleus and surrounding fibers involve motor, associative and limbic circuitry that are more compact and close together. Therefore, a sub-optimal electrode placement or electrical-current perturbation is more often going to be associated with STN stimulation, which may lead to mood changes and verbal fluency dysfunction.

Although a randomized control trial has shown a comparable benefit for GPi stimulation compared to STN stimulation, longer follow-up studies are needed to decide which target is preferable for each patient. We have made a comparison of the targets in Table 1. Clinical trials are ongoing for alternative targets in the pedunculopontine nucleus, radiation prelemniscalis, and caudal zona incerta, and stimulation on these targets may improve symptoms that are currently unresponsive to treatment with either levodopa or STN stimulation.

	STN stimulation	GPi stimulation
Motor improvement	50~60%, coherent [29, 34]	27~50%, variable in long-term [29, 72]
Mood effect	higher, esp. suboptimal contact	seems unchanged
LEDD reduction	greater reduction (31.5%)	less reduction (17.8%)
Battery life	lower amplitude	higher amplitude
General adverse effect	56%	51%

Table 1. Comparison of STN and GPi stimulation

4. Targeting methods in DBS: MRI alone versus CT scan fused with MRI and/or ventriculography

There are a number of targeting methods used in DBS. Which method is used depends on the facilities of the institution and the familiarity of the surgeon with a given procedure. Most practicing centers use magnetic resonance imaging (MRI) as the only tool for targeting, but others use image fusion techniques to co-register MRI and computed tomography (CT) images, or intra-operative ventriculography, which is the traditional targeting method, for determining targeting accuracy. Below we compare these methods on acquisition time, procedure complexity, and ultimate accuracy.

The size of the STN is extremely small and it has an ovoid shape and oblique orientation [39]. The accuracy of DBS targeting may be one of the most important factor in surgical outcome because the position of the electrode determines the area across which the electrical current diffuses. Given that there are very few evidence-based studies that have directly compared the safety and effectiveness of the various imaging techniques, the best targeting method remains under debate. The methods include MRI, CT, ventriculography and various combinations thereof.

Stereotactic targeting with ventriculography is the traditional method for stereotactic functional neurosurgery that has been in use for decades. While it is still used by some teams, there are concerns over its invasiveness and serious complications, such as CSF leakage and intracranial hemorrhage, which are major obstacles for most functional neurosurgeons [40]. The method involves injecting a contrast medium into the right frontal horn and acquiring representative images to determine the location of the anterior commissure and posterior commissure, which then can be used to calculate various target coordinates [41]. Compared with targeting methods that may have higher accuracy (e.g., ventriculography), targeting with MRI can be affected by the anterior displacement of the anterior commissure (AC), which elongates anterior commissure - posterior commissure (AC-PC) length [40]. A magnetic field can cause this nonlinear distortion, especially in the anterior-posterior and medial-lateral axis.

Most centers only use MRI for targeting while others use image fusion techniques to co-register MRI and CT scans. MRI-directed targeting for STN-DBS has proven to be a simple yet accurate method in most DBS practicing centers; it has been a standard procedure in our hospital since 2002 [42]. The advantages of MRI includes better demarcation of deep nuclei (e.g., the red and subthalamic nucleus) as references for targeting, better visualization of critical structures that can prevent inadvertent injury (e.g., lateral ventricles and vasculatures within sulci) and a clear delineation of simulating trajectory for electrode.

There are three current strategies to localize the coordinates of targets on stereotactic MRI. In direct targeting, the STN is located on MRI without any references, which is inherently prone to errors. The vague configuration of the STN makes determining the STN boundaries on a T2-weighted MR image rely on the subjective visual impression of the neurosurgeon. An indirect method of targeting uses the AC and PC as reference points, thereby avoiding bias when differentiating the border between the STN and substantia nigra, which has been shown to be more accurate than direct targeting. Targeting based on the red nucleus (RN) has not only the same accuracy as indirect targeting but also less variance, which indicates greater precision across subjects (Fig. 1) [43]. Although MRI-based targeting is becoming more popular, the potential distortion of the STN that a nonlinear magnetic field can induce is still a major concern. To counter this, some groups still use ventriculography which reliably identifies the AC-PC for indirect targeting methods using intraventricular landmarks.

Although the AC-PC and the target itself (e.g., the STN) are poorly visualized on CT, MRI fused to stereotactic CT are believed to combine the advantages of both modalities, thereby increasing the spatial validity of the image and ensuring a more accurate localization, which continues to improve as fusion technology improves [44]. In our experience, stereotactic CT fused to MRI during DBS surgery can allow for a longer microelectrode recording length of STN and fewer recording tracts (Fig. 2). This indirectly demonstrates that stereotactic CT may have a better pre-operative targeting ability leading to the stimulation of optimal anatomical sites. It should be noted that it may be difficult for advanced PD patients to

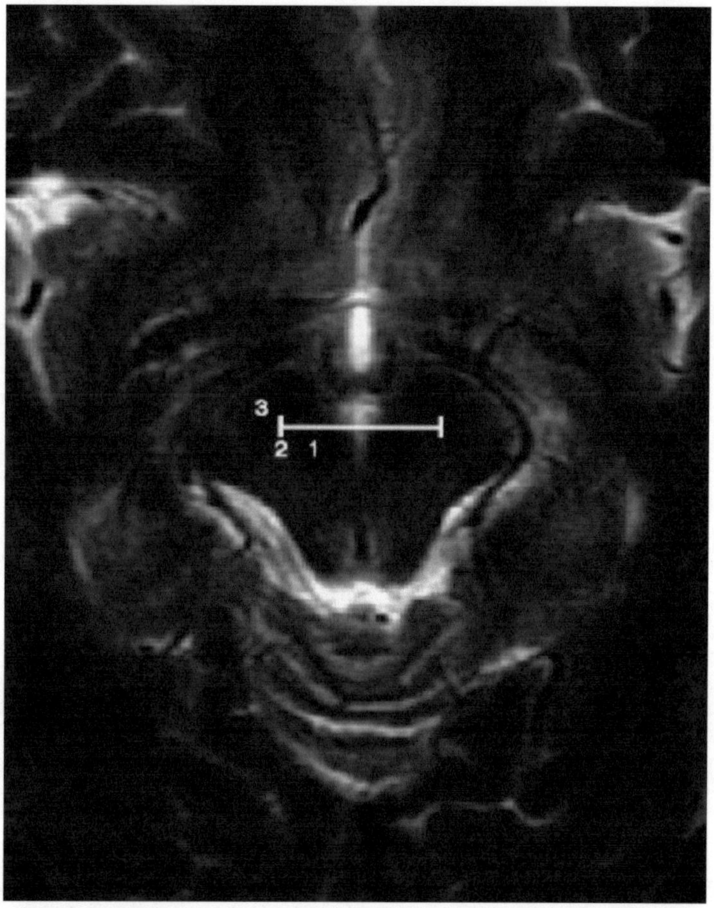

Fig. 1. Direct targeting using MR images is depicted. The target coordinates for the tip of the permanent implantable electrode are at the intersection of the perpendicular lines. The horizontal line is located along the anterior border of the red nucleus. The longitudinal lines are at 2-mm intervals from the lateral border of the red nucleus. Axial section taken at the level of the superior colliculus, just below the lowest border of the STN (4.5 mm below the mid-commissural point). 1= red nucleus; 2=substantia nigra reticulata; 3=crus cerebri.

undergo MRI with a stereotactic frame, especially in an un-medicated state where obvious tremors or severe stoop posture will be present. There is a risk for these patients when sedated in the MRI suite in an attempt to quell the severe tremor because the scanning time for MRI may take more than 20 minutes. For this reason, some centers use a specific protocol for direct visualization of the STN in stereotactic MRI, which saves time [45]. At our institution, a stereotactic CT scan takes about 3 minutes, which is far below the average MRI acquisition time of 20-25 minutes for most protocols.

With advances in imaging technology, we may be able to define the border of the STN directly using MRI in the future and eliminate the inherent error of nonlinear MRI distortion.

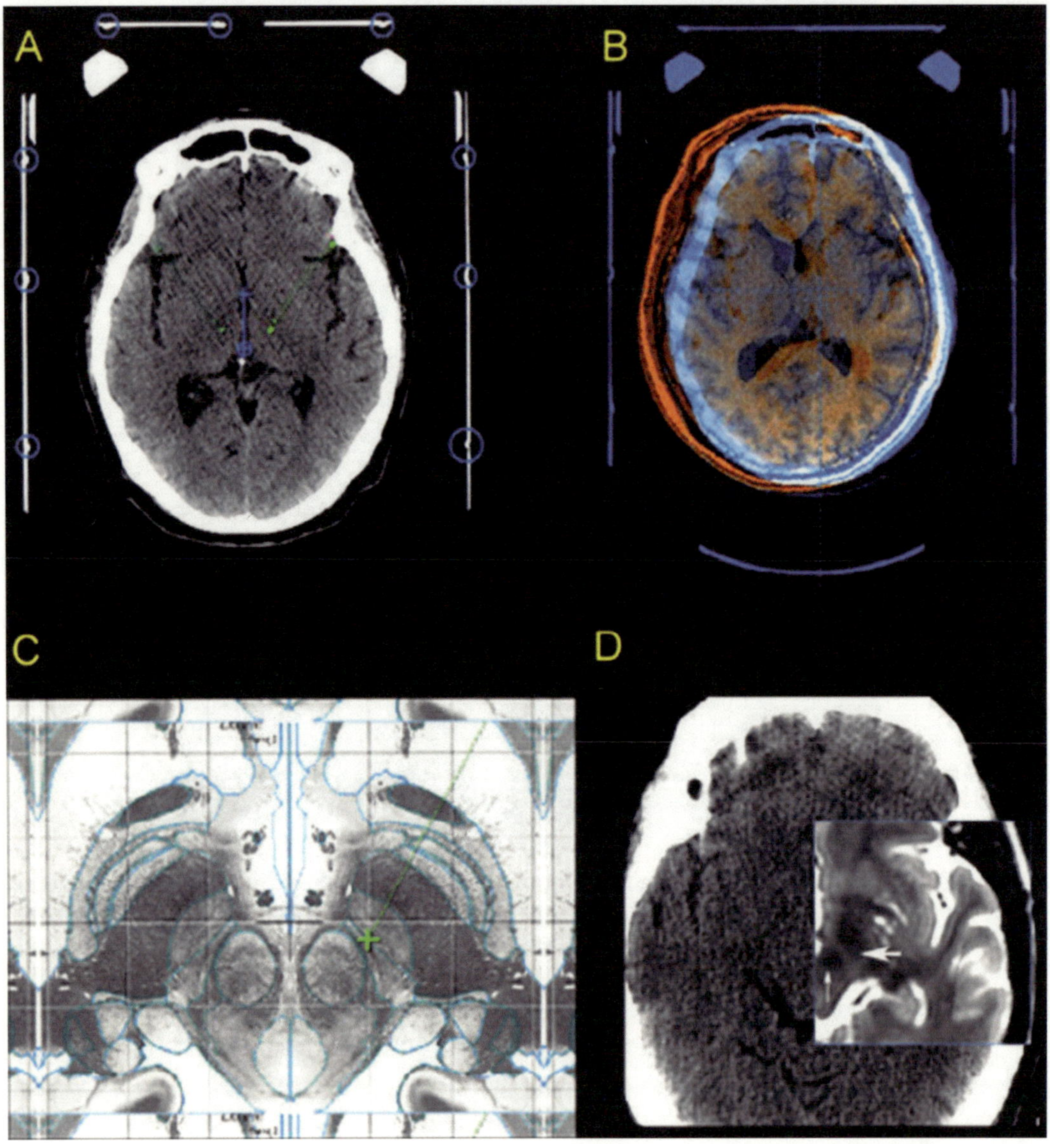

Fig. 2. (A) Stereotactic axial computed tomography (CT) images for fiducial registration. (B) Nonfused axial magnetic resonance image (MRI) T1 images and stereotactic CT images. (C) Co-registered Schaltenbran-Wahren atlas for red nucleus and subthalamic nucleus (STN) target planning simulation. (D) Fused axial MRI T2 and CT images, spyglass with visualization of red nucleus (thin arrow) and STN (thick arrow).

5. The necessity of microelectrode recording in STN-DBS surgery

Precise results in DBS surgery are traditionally achieved by MRI targeting followed by electrophysiological confirmation with microelectrode recording (MER) [46]. MRI scans are not always of sufficient quality to identify the target structure and are always susceptible to image distortion. MER can localize the target with more precision when MRI targeting is not precise enough. MER is used in DBS surgery to identify the target's structural border, the subdivisions of the targeted structure and the outlines of its three-dimensional shape. MRI and MER are complementary in DBS surgery [47]; however, there are disadvantages of MER in DBS surgery, including the following: 1) it is time consuming, 2) it may increase the risk of a hemorrhage complication and 3) it is not always useful, for example when the target is located in white matter or has a large and distinct boundary that can be easily visualized with MRI. Here we will focus on whether MER is necessary in STN-DBS surgery for treating PD.

Direct MRI targeting without MER is possible in STN-DBS surgery with the recent advances in high-resolution MRI (field strength of 3-Tesla or more) and advanced image processing techniques. However, there is a paucity of publications that report on the use of stereotactic MRI for direct visualization in STN-DBS surgery without MER [48]. Recently, a large series of STN-DBS without MER has been published by Foltynie et al. [49]. We compared their results with those of Krack et al [50], who performed STN-DBS with MER which recruited from a single center. Table 2 compares the demographic data of the studies' patients, effect of DBS and complications of surgery. The baseline data of the patients are comparable except that Krack's sample size is less than Foltynie's. However, we should note that Krack's report is designed for long term follow-up (5 years later) and they recruited the first 49 STN-DBS patients from their center. The effect of STN-DBS at a one-year follow-up was similar in the two studies. The DBS effect is better in Krack's study but not significantly so. In terms of surgery-related adverse events, Krack showed greater transient confusion and intracerebral hemorrhage in their patients. Foltynie showed less transient confusion and no hemorrhage events.

The risk of intracerebral hemorrhage inevitably increases with a greater number of micro- or DBS electrode penetration events [51-52]. Post-operative transient confusion in DBS surgery is common. The incidence of transient confusion in STN-DBS surgery is 15.6% [53]. This phenomenon is often attributed to a mild pneumocephalus that occurs during surgery. It is not a precisely understood phenomenon, but it occurs more frequently in older and cognitively disabled patients. The risk for and volume of pneumocephalus positively correlates with the amount of time the skull is open during surgery. MER may therefore increase the risk of pneumocephalus because it is time consuming.

Based on the above comparison, the same therapeutic effect for patients can be achieved in STN-DBS with and without MER, but MER has more surgery-related adverse events. Others have reported that the use of MER improves the outcome of STN-DBS [42]. With the advancement of MRI technology and imaging processing, MRI-guided STN-DBS without MER may be an alternative surgical method for advanced PD patients. The reports of MRI-guided STN-DBS are sparse; therefore, we cannot conclude that this surgical method is better than STN-DBS with MER. Overall, the necessity of MER in STN-DBS surgery remains controversial.

	With MER (Krack et al)			Without MER (Foltynie et al)		
Demographic data	Mean	±	SD	Mean	±	SD
Sex (no. of patients)	24 men	/	25 women	49 men	/	30 women
Age at surgery	55.0	±	7.5 (34-68)	57.3	±	7.7 (34.5-70.2)
Duration of disease	14.6	±	5.0	13.4	±	7.0
L-dopa equivalent dose	1409.0	±	605.0	1620.0	±	641.0
Effect of STN DBS						
UPDRS III motor scores Baseline off-medication	55.7	±	11.9	51.5	±	14.9
UPDRS III motor scores One year after operation on-stimulation, off-medication	19.0	±	11.1	23.8	±	11.2
UPDRS III motor scores One year after operation on-stimulation, on-medication	11.4	±	8.9	14.5	±	8.3
Adverse events related to procedure						
Intracerebral hemorrhage	2			0		
Transient confusion	12			7		
Seizures	2			2		

Table 2. Comparison between DBS with and without MER

6. Anesthetic considerations in DBS: Awake versus general anesthesia

Traditionally, DBS is an awake surgical procedure in order to allow electrophysiological mapping and stimulation testing to assess motor responses and potential side effects. However, PD patients with obvious "off-medication" symptoms of anxiety, painful dystonia, and respiratory distress may not be good candidates for the lengthy tolerating the surgical procedures while awake [54-57]. In this section, we will report our own experience with general anesthesia during DBS surgery with MER and compare it with data from awake procedures (see Table 3).

Operation procedures:	Awake DBS	General Anesthetic DBS
Patient's condition	communicative and cooperative; Can tolerate severe off-symptoms	Anxious; Cannot tolerate severe off-symptoms, such as: pain, dystonia and/or respiratory difficulties
Anesthetic agents	None	Desflurane (Patient intubated under regular induction and muscle relaxant, keep Mac around 0.8~1.0) [54]
Sedative agents	propofol / remifentanil (intermittent use, e.g. during trephination)	None
MER signals	Yes	Yes
Passive movement-related MER signals	Yes	Yes
Test stimulation	Yes	No
Motor outcome	Good	Good
Surgical complication	Comparable	Comparable
Stimulation side effect	Lower	May be higher
Risk period	During surgery	Induction and extubation
Patient monitoring by anesthesiologist	Yes	Yes

Mac: minimum alveolar concentration

Table 3. Comparison between awake DBS and general anesthetic DBS procedures

Awake DBS procedures

Most DBS centers prefer that their PD patients receive electrode implantation procedures in an awake state in order to retrieve sound electrophysiological signals from MER and to perform test stimulation. Time is crucial for a patient to tolerate the procedure while awake. Patel et al tried an MRI direct-targeting method with macro-stimulation alone. They conclude that without MER the procedure is more efficient and safe but still has a good outcome [58-59]. In the awake state, macro-stimulation is beneficial because it excludes the side effect from electrode stimulation [59]. Sedative agents are inevitable during awake procedures, especially during trephination. Propofol is popular during DBS procedures as a brief general anesthetic agent, but it may require full-time surveillance of the patient's airway and vital signs by an anesthesiologist. The function of the patient's airway can be a severe problem in an advanced PD patient's "off" state.

MER has been shown to perform properly and without affecting the surgical outcome only when remifentanil was completely stopped and the dose of propofol was carefully monitored [52, 58, 60-61]. Duque et al reported a case with these same anesthetic agents using Bispectral Analysis of the Electroencephalogram (BIS) to monitor cortical activity in order to titrate the hypnotics, which may interfere with MER procedures. While this technique may be useful, it is not convenient [62].

General anesthetic DBS procedures

A detailed MER mapping within the STN may lead to an optimal placement of DBS electrodes, but the drawbacks are the length of the procedure and that the patient must be kept awake during the procedure. Some patients with severe "off-medication" PD symptoms, such as major anxiety, poorly tolerated off-medication dystonia, or respiratory difficulties may refuse DBS or may be poor candidates for DBS in an awake state [55, 57]. STN-DBS during a state of general anesthesia may be another choice for those patients with advanced PD for whom symptoms are difficult to control with medication only.

In patients with advanced PD who undergo STN-DBS while awake, test stimulation after the permanent electrode is implanted is helpful to confirm the electrode position. The test stimulation verifies the maximal clinical effects intraoperatively as well as the side effects of low voltage in the case that the electrode position was sub-optimal. Test stimulation in patients receiving a general anesthetic is controversial. Hertel et al. performed test stimulation to verify possible capsular effects when using low-voltage electrode stimulation, and the voltage causing the capsular effects may be incorrectly estimated if the excitability of the capsule has been decreased by general anesthesia. In our study, we did not perform test stimulation, but no patient suffered post-operative capsular effects because our selection criteria for the trajectory of electrode implantation chose the most appropriate track [54].

The knowledge of STN topography is crucial in general anesthesia DBS surgery; therefore, MER must be used as it is the only intra-operative tool to identify the STN, map its boundaries, and map its sensorimotor component through the detection of movement-related neuronal firing [61, 63-65].

The role of anesthesiologist in DBS surgery

Most anesthesiologists are treating intubated patients under general anesthesia and in awake procedures like DBS, it can be challenging to ensure neuronal firing on the one hand and monitor patient safety the other. Avoiding medications that may interfere with MER can negatively affect patient safety, especially when the patient is agitated by a prolonged DBS procedure. However, it also is difficult to maintain a secure airway if the patient is too deeply unconscious [66-67]. In hypertensive patients, the alpha-2 agonist dexmedetomidine has been suggested as an effective sedative agent that may provide the patient comfort and good blood-pressure control and yet still allow satisfactory MER mapping by the neurophysiologist [67]. Complications may still occur during awake DBS procedures. Deoganokar reported a case of venous air embolism in an elderly PD patient with a myocardial infarction [68]. Glossop and Dobbs also report two cases of coronary artery vasospasm during electrode implantation. Though these patients recovered, the authors suggest full monitoring by an anesthesiologist throughout the surgical procedures [69].

The effect of the anesthetic agent desflurane

Desflurane (2,2,2-trifluoro-1-fluoroethyl-difluoromethyl ether) is a highly fluorinated methylethyl ether used for maintenance of a general anesthetic. It has the most rapid onset and offset of all of the volatile anesthetic drugs used for general anesthesia because of its low solubility in blood. It also is popular in neurosurgery because it can allow early extubation and facilitate early neurological evaluation [70-71]. MER also can be performed well at an anesthetic level of 0.8±0.2 minimum alveolar concentration (MAC) [54].

7. Conclusion

The subthalamic nucleus plays an important role in the functional control of motor activity in the indirect dopaminergic pathway of the basal ganglia. Twenty years after the first introduction of DBS to treat PD, it remains as an important alternative treatment to l-dopa, especially in the patient with motor fluctuation and obvious l-dopa related complication. Centers performing DBS may have different protocol according to their experiences and facilities. Controversial points exist inevitably, however, through proper patient selections, cooperation between multidisciplinary teams, and refine surgical techniques we can ensure a good outcome for DBS candidate.

8. Acknowledgment

This work was supported by Master Cheng Yen, President of the Tzu-Chi Foundation, and Tzu-Chi General Hospital grant TCSP 0104.

9. References

[1] Langston J, Widner H, Goetz C, Brooks D, Fahn S, Freeman T, Watts R. Core assessment program for intracerebral transplantations (CAPIT). Mov Disord 1992;7(1):2-13.

[2] Defer G, Widner H, Marie R, Remy P, Levivier M. Core assessment program for surgical interventional therapies in Parkinson's disease (CAPSIT-PD). Mov Disord 1999;14(4):572-84.

[3] Moro E, Allert N, Eleopra R, Houeto J, Phan T, Stoevelaar H. A decision tool to support appropriate referral for deep brain stimulation in Parkinson's disease. J Neurol 2009;256(1):83-8.

[4] Yoshida F, Miyagi Y, Kishimoto J, Morioka T, Murakami N, Hashiguchi K, Samura K, Sakae N, Yamasaki R, Kawaguchi M, Sasaki T. Subthalamic nucleus stimulation does not cause deterioration of preexisting hallucinations in Parkinson's disease patients. Stereotact Funct Neurosurg 2009;87(1):45-9.

[5] Okun MS, Fernandez HH, Rodriguez RL, Foote KD. Identifying candidates for deep brain stimulation in Parkinson's disease: the role of the primary care physician. Geriatrics 2007;62(5):18-24.

[6] Okun MS, Fernandez HH, Pedraza O, Misra M, Lyons KE, Pahwa R, Tarsy D, Scollins L, Corapi K, Friehs GM, Grace J, Romrell J, Foote KD. Development and initial validation of a screening tool for Parkinson disease surgical candidates. Neurology 2004;63(1):161-3.

[7] Amick M, Grace J. Deep brain stimulation surgery for Parkinson's disease: the role of neuropsychological assessment. Med Health R I 2006;89(4):130-3.

[8] Chang V, Chou K. Deep brain stimulation for Parkinson's disease: patient selection and motor outcomes. Med Health R I 2006;89(4):142-4.

[9] Lang AE, Widner H. Deep brain stimulation for Parkinson's disease: Patient selection and evaluation. Movement Disorders 2002;17(S3):S94-S101.

[10] Bronstein JM, Tagliati M, Alterman RL, Lozano AM, Volkmann J, Stefani A, Horak FB, Okun MS, Foote KD, Krack P, Pahwa R, Henderson JM, Hariz MI, Bakay RA, Rezai A, Marks WJ, Jr, Moro E, Vitek JL, Weaver FM, Gross RE, DeLong MR. Deep Brain Stimulation for Parkinson Disease: An Expert Consensus and Review of Key Issues. Arch Neurol 2010:archneurol.2010.260.

[11] Williams DR, Warren JD, Lees AJ. Using the presence of visual hallucinations to differentiate Parkinson's disease from atypical parkinsonism. Journal of Neurology, Neurosurgery & Psychiatry 2008;79(6):652-5.

[12] Kollensperger M, Geser F, Seppi K, Stampfer-Kountche... M, Sawires M, Scherfler C, Boesch S, Mueller J, Koukouni V, Quinn N, Pellecchia M, Barone P, Schimke N, Dodel R, Oertel W, Dupont E, Ostergaard K, Daniels C, Deuschl G, Gurevich T, Giladi N, Coelho M, Sampaio C, Nilsson C, Widner H, Sorbo F, Albanese A, Cardozo A, Tolosa E, Abele M, Klockgether T, Kamm C, Gasser T, Djaldetti R, Colosimo C, Meco G, Schrag A, Poewe W, Wenning G. Red flags for multiple system atrophy. Mov Disord 2008;23(8):1093-9.

[13] Reichmann H. Clinical criteria for the diagnosis of Parkinson's disease. Neurodegener Dis 2010;7(5):284-90.

[14] Zhao Y, Wee H, Chan Y, Seah S, Au W, Lau P, Pica E, Li S, Luo N, Tan L. Progression of Parkinson's disease as evaluated by Hoehn and Yahr stage transition times. Mov Disord 2010;25(6):702-8.

[15] Goetz C, Poewe W, Rascol O, Sampaio C, Stebbins G, Counsell C, Giladi N, Holloway R, Moore C, Wenning G, Yahr M, Seidl L. Movement Disorder Society Task Force report on the Hoehn and Yahr staging scale: status and recommendations. Mov Disord 2004;19(9):1020-8.

[16] The Unified Parkinson's Disease Rating Scale (UPDRS): status and recommendations. Mov Disord 2003;18(7):738-50.

[17] Goetz C, Fahn S, Martinez-Martin P, Poewe W, Sampaio C, Stebbins G, Stern M, Tilley B, Dodel R, Dubois B, Holloway R, Jankovic J, Kulisevsky J, Lang A, Lees A, Leurgans S, LeWitt P, Nyenhuis D, Olanow C, Rascol O, Schrag A, Teresi J, Van Hilten J, LaPelle N. Movement Disorder Society-sponsored revision of the Unified Parkinson's Disease Rating Scale (MDS-UPDRS): Process, format, and clinimetric testing plan. Mov Disord 2007;22(1):41-7.

[18] Tsai S, Lin S, Chou Y, Pan Y, Hung H, Li C, Lin S, Chen S. Prognostic factors of subthalamic stimulation in Parkinson's disease: a comparative study between short- and long-term effects. Stereotact Funct Neurosurg 2009;87(4):241-8.

[19] Romito L, Contarino M, Vanacore N, Bentivoglio A, Scerrati M, Albanese A. Replacement of dopaminergic medication with subthalamic nucleus stimulation in Parkinson's disease: long-term observation. Mov Disord 2009;24(4):557-63.

[20] Ory-Magne F, Brefel-Courbon C, Simonetta-Moreau M, Fabre N, Lotterie J, Chaynes P, Berry I, Lazorthes Y, Rascol O. Does ageing influence deep brain stimulation outcomes in Parkinson's disease? Mov Disord 2007;22(10):1457-63.

[21] Derost P-P, Ouchchane L, Morand D, Ulla M, Llorca P-M, Barget M, Debilly B, Lemaire J-J, Durif F. Is STN-DBS appropriate to treat severe Parkinson disease in an elderly population? Neurology 2007;68(17):1345-55.

[22] Vesper J, Haak S, Ostertag C, Nikkhah G. Subthalamic nucleus deep brain stimulation in elderly patients--analysis of outcome and complications. BMC Neurol 2007;7:7.

[23] Ferrara J, Diamond A, Hunter C, Davidson A, Almaguer M, Jankovic J. Impact of STN-DBS on life and health satisfaction in patients with Parkinson's disease. Journal of Neurology, Neurosurgery & Psychiatry 2010;81(3):315-9.

[24] York MK, Dulay M, Macias A, Levin HS, Grossman R, Simpson R, Jankovic J. Cognitive declines following bilateral subthalamic nucleus deep brain stimulation for the treatment of Parkinson's disease. Journal of Neurology, Neurosurgery & Psychiatry 2008;79(7):789-95.

[25] Houeto JL, Bejjani PB, Damier P, Staedler C, Bonnet AM, Pidoux B, Dormont D, Cornu P, Agid Y. Failure of long-term pallidal stimulation corrected by subthalamic stimulation in PD. Neurology 2000;55(5):728-30.

[26] Rodriguez-Oroz MC, Obeso JA, Lang AE, Houeto J-L, Pollak P, Rehncrona S, Kulisevsky J, Albanese A, Volkmann J, Hariz MI, Quinn NP, Speelman JD, Guridi J, Zamarbide I, Gironell A, Molet J, Pascual-Sedano B, Pidoux B, Bonnet AM, Agid Y, Xie J, Benabid A-L, Lozano AM, Saint-Cyr J, Romito L, Contarino MF, Scerrati M, Fraix V, Van Blercom N. Bilateral deep brain stimulation in Parkinson's disease: a multicentre study with 4 years follow-up. Brain 2005;128(10):2240-9.

[27] Anderson VC, Burchiel KJ, Hogarth P, Favre J, Hammerstad JP. Pallidal vs Subthalamic Nucleus Deep Brain Stimulation in Parkinson Disease. Arch Neurol 2005;62(4):554-60.

[28] Moro E, Lozano A, Pollak P, Agid Y, Rehncrona S, Volkmann J, Kulisevsky J, Obeso J, Albanese A, Hariz M, Quinn N, Speelman J, Benabid A, Fraix V, Mendes A, Welter M, Houeto J, Cornu P, Dormont D, Tornqvist A, Ekberg R, Schnitzler A, Timmermann L, Wojtecki L, Gironell A, Rodriguez-Oroz M, Guridi J, Bentivoglio A, Contarino M, Romito L, Scerrati M, Janssens M, Lang A. Long-term results of a multicenter study on subthalamic and pallidal stimulation in Parkinson's disease. Mov Disord 2010;25(5):578-86.

[29] Follett K, Weaver F, Stern M, Hur K, Harris C, Luo P, Marks W, Rothlind J, Sagher O, Moy C, Pahwa R, Burchiel K, Hogarth P, Lai E, Duda J, Holloway K, Samii A, Horn S, Bronstein J, Stoner G, Starr P, Simpson R, Baltuch G, De Salles A, Huang G, Reda D. Pallidal versus subthalamic deep-brain stimulation for Parkinson's disease. N Engl J Med 2010;362(22):2077-91.

[30] Volkmann J, Allert N, Voges J, Sturm V, Schnitzler A, Freund H. Long-term results of bilateral pallidal stimulation in Parkinson's disease. Ann Neurol 2004;55(6):871-5.

[31] Schupbach M, Gargiulo M, Welter ML, Mallet L, Behar C, Houeto JL, Maltete D, Mesnage V, Agid Y. Neurosurgery in Parkinson disease: a distressed mind in a repaired body? Neurology 2006;66(12):1811-6.

[32] Voon V, Fernagut P, Wickens J, Baunez C, Rodriguez M, Pavon N, Juncos J, Obeso J, Bezard E. Chronic dopaminergic stimulation in Parkinson's disease: from dyskinesias to impulse control disorders. Lancet Neurol 2009;8(12):1140-9.

[33] Voon V, Krack P, Lang AE, Lozano AM, Dujardin K, Schüpbach M, D'Ambrosia J, Thobois S, Tamma F, Herzog J, Speelman JD, Samanta J, Kubu C, Rossignol H,

Poon Y-Y, Saint-Cyr JA, Ardouin C, Moro E. A multicentre study on suicide outcomes following subthalamic stimulation for Parkinson's disease. Brain 2008;131(10):2720-8.
[34] Deuschl G, Schade-Brittinger C, Krack P, Volkmann J, Schafer H, Botzel K, Daniels C, Deutschlander A, Dillmann U, Eisner W, Gruber D, Hamel W, Herzog J, Hilker R, Klebe S, Kloss M, Koy J, Krause M, Kupsch A, Lorenz D, Lorenzl S, Mehdorn H, Moringlane J, Oertel W, Pinsker M, Reichmann H, Reuss A, Schneider G, Schnitzler A, Steude U, Sturm V, Timmermann L, Tronnier V, Trottenberg T, Wojtecki L, Wolf E, Poewe W, Voges J. A randomized trial of deep-brain stimulation for Parkinson's disease. N Engl J Med 2006;355(9):896-908.
[35] Bejjani B, Arnulf I, Demeret S, Damier P, Bonnet A, Houeto J, Agid Y. Levodopa-induced dyskinesias in Parkinson's disease: is sensitization reversible? Ann Neurol 2000;47(5):655-8.
[36] Nutt JG, Rufener SL, Carter JH, Anderson VC, Pahwa R, Hammerstad JP, Burchiel KJ. Interactions between deep brain stimulation and levodopa in Parkinson's disease. Neurology 2001;57(10):1835-42.
[37] Bejjani B, Damier P, Arnulf I, Bonnet AM, Vidailhet M, Dormont D, Pidoux B, Cornu P, Marsault C, Agid Y. Pallidal stimulation for Parkinson's disease. Two targets? Neurology 1997;49(6):1564-9.
[38] Volkmann J, Allert N, Voges J, Weiss PH, Freund H-J, Sturm V. Safety and efficacy of pallidal or subthalamic nucleus stimulation in advanced PD. Neurology 2001;56(4):548-51.
[39] Hamani C, Saint-Cyr JA, Fraser J, Kaplitt M, Lozano AM. The subthalamic nucleus in the context of movement disorders. Brain 2004;127(1):4-20.
[40] Breit S, LeBas J, Koudsie A, Schulz J, Benazzouz A, Pollak P, Benabid A. Pretargeting for the implantation of stimulation electrodes into the subthalamic nucleus: a comparative study of magnetic resonance imaging and ventriculography. Neurosurgery 2006;58(1 Suppl):ONS83-95.
[41] Cuny E, Guehl D, Burbaud P, Gross C, Dousset V, Rougier A. Lack of agreement between direct magnetic resonance imaging and statistical determination of a subthalamic target: the role of electrophysiological guidance. J Neurosurg 2002;97(3):591-7.
[42] Chen S, Lee C, Lin S, Hsin Y, Lee T, Yen P, Chou Y, Lee C, Annie Hsieh W, Su C, Lin S. Microelectrode recording can be a good adjunct in magnetic resonance image-directed subthalamic nucleus deep brain stimulation for parkinsonism. Surg Neurol 2006;65(3):253-60; discussion 60-1.
[43] Andrade-Souza Y, Schwalb J, Hamani C, Eltahawy H, Hoque T, Saint-Cyr J, Lozano A. Comparison of three methods of targeting the subthalamic nucleus for chronic stimulation in Parkinson's disease. Neurosurgery 2005;56(2 Suppl):360-8; discussion -8.
[44] Aziz TZ, Nandi D, Parkin S, Liu X, Giladi N, Bain P, Gregory RG, Joint C, Scott RB, Stein JF. Targeting the subthalamic nucleus. Stereotact Funct Neurosurg 2001;77(1-4):87-90.
[45] Hariz M, Krack P, Melvill R, Jorgensen J, Hamel W, Hirabayashi H, Lenders M, Wesslen N, Tengvar M, Yousry T. A quick and universal method for stereotactic

visualization of the subthalamic nucleus before and after implantation of deep brain stimulation electrodes. Stereotact Funct Neurosurg 2003;80(1-4):96-101.
[46] Vitek JL, Bakay RA, Hashimoto T, Kaneoke Y, Mewes K, Zhang JY, Rye D, Starr P, Baron M, Turner R, DeLong MR. Microelectrode-guided pallidotomy: technical approach and its application in medically intractable Parkinson's disease. J Neurosurg 1998;88(6):1027-43.
[47] Starr PA, Vitek JL, Bakay RA. Deep brain stimulation for movement disorders. Neurosurg Clin N Am 1998;9(2):381-402.
[48] Patel NK, Plaha P, Gill SS. Magnetic resonance imaging-directed method for functional neurosurgery using implantable guide tubes. Neurosurgery 2007;61(5 Suppl 2):358-65; discussion 65-6.
[49] Foltynie T, Zrinzo L, Martinez-Torres I, Tripoliti E, Petersen E, Holl E, Aviles-Olmos I, Jahanshahi M, Hariz M, Limousin P. MRI-guided STN DBS in Parkinson's disease without microelectrode recording: efficacy and safety. J Neurol Neurosurg Psychiatry 2010.
[50] Krack P, Batir A, Van Blercom N, Chabardes S, Fraix V, Ardouin C, Koudsie A, Limousin PD, Benazzouz A, LeBas JF, Benabid AL, Pollak P. Five-year follow-up of bilateral stimulation of the subthalamic nucleus in advanced Parkinson's disease. N Engl J Med 2003;349(20):1925-34.
[51] Ben-Haim S, Asaad WF, Gale JT, Eskandar EN. Risk factors for hemorrhage during microelectrode-guided deep brain stimulation and the introduction of an improved microelectrode design. Neurosurgery 2009;64(4):754-62; discussion 62-3.
[52] Binder DK, Rau GM, Starr PA. Risk factors for hemorrhage during microelectrode-guided deep brain stimulator implantation for movement disorders. Neurosurgery 2005;56(4):722-32; discussion -32.
[53] Kleiner-Fisman G, Herzog J, Fisman DN, Tamma F, Lyons KE, Pahwa R, Lang AE, Deuschl G. Subthalamic nucleus deep brain stimulation: summary and meta-analysis of outcomes. Mov Disord 2006;21 Suppl 14:S290-304.
[54] Lin S, Chen T, Lin S, Shyr M, Chou Y, Hsieh W, Tsai S, Chen S. Subthalamic deep brain stimulation after anesthetic inhalation in Parkinson disease: a preliminary study. J Neurosurg 2008;109(2):238-44.
[55] Hertel F, Zuchner M, Weimar I, Gemmar P, Noll B, Bettag M, Decker C. Implantation of electrodes for deep brain stimulation of the subthalamic nucleus in advanced Parkinson's disease with the aid of intraoperative microrecording under general anesthesia. Neurosurgery 2006;59(5):E1138; discussion E.
[56] Yamada K, Goto S, Kuratsu J, Matsuzaki K, Tamura T, Nagahiro S, Murase N, Shimazu H, Kaji R. Stereotactic surgery for subthalamic nucleus stimulation under general anesthesia: a retrospective evaluation of Japanese patients with Parkinson's disease. Parkinsonism Relat Disord 2007;13(2):101-7.
[57] Maltete D, Navarro S, Welter M-L, Roche S, Bonnet A-M, Houeto J-L, Mesnage V, Pidoux B, Dormont D, Cornu P, Agid Y. Subthalamic Stimulation in Parkinson Disease: With or Without Anesthesia? Arch Neurol 2004;61(3):390-2.
[58] Patel NK, Plaha P, O'Sullivan K, McCarter R, Heywood P, Gill SS. MRI directed bilateral stimulation of the subthalamic nucleus in patients with Parkinson's disease. Journal of Neurology, Neurosurgery & Psychiatry 2003;74(12):1631-7.

[59] Tabbal S, Revilla F, Mink J, Schneider-Gibson P, Wernle A, de Erausquin G, Perlmutter J, Rich K, Dowling J. Safety and efficacy of subthalamic nucleus deep brain stimulation performed with limited intraoperative mapping for treatment of Parkinson's disease. Neurosurgery 2007;61(3 Suppl):119-27; discussion 27-9.
[60] Amirnovin R, Williams Z, Cosgrove G, Eskandar E. Experience with microelectrode guided subthalamic nucleus deep brain stimulation. Neurosurgery 2006;58(1 Suppl):ONS96-102; discussion ONS96-.
[61] Hariz M, Blomstedt P, Limousin P. The myth of microelectrode recording in ensuring a precise location of the DBS electrode within the sensorimotor part of the subthalamic nucleus. Mov Disord 2004;19(7):863-4.
[62] Duque P, Mateo O, Ruiz F, de Viloria J, Contreras A, Grandas F. Intraoperative microrecording under general anaesthesia with bispectral analysis monitoring in a case of deep brain stimulation surgery for Parkinson's disease. Eur J Neurol 2008;15(8):e76-7.
[63] Romanelli P, Heit G, Hill B, Kraus A, Hastie T, Bronte-Stewart H. Microelectrode recording revealing a somatotopic body map in the subthalamic nucleus in humans with Parkinson disease. J Neurosurg 2004;100(4):611-8.
[64] Mandat T, Hurwitz T, Honey C. Hypomania as an adverse effect of subthalamic nucleus stimulation: report of two cases. Acta Neurochir (Wien) 2006;148(8):895-7; discussion 8.
[65] Tsai S, Lin S, Lin S, Chen J, Lee C, Chen S. Neuropsychological effects after chronic subthalamic stimulation and the topography of the nucleus in Parkinson's disease. Neurosurgery 2007;61(5):E1024-9; discussion E9-30.
[66] Kalenka A, Schwarz A. Anaesthesia and Parkinson's disease: how to manage with new therapies? Curr Opin Anesthesiol 2009;22(3):419-24.
[67] Rozet I, Muangman S, Vavilala MS, Lee LA, Souter MJ, Domino KJ, Slimp JC, Goodkin R, Lam AM. Clinical Experience with Dexmedetomidine for Implantation of Deep Brain Stimulators in Parkinson's Disease. Anesthesia & Analgesia 2006;103(5):1224-8.
[68] Deogaonkar A, Avitsian R, Henderson J, Schubert A. Venous air embolism during deep brain stimulation surgery in an awake supine patient. Stereotact Funct Neurosurg 2005;83(1):32-5.
[69] Glossop A, Dobbs P. Coronary artery vasospasm during awake deep brain stimulation surgery. British Journal of Anaesthesia 2008;101(2):222-4.
[70] Magni G, Rosa IL, Melillo G, Savio A, Rosa G. A Comparison Between Sevoflurane and Desflurane Anesthesia in Patients Undergoing Craniotomy for Supratentorial Intracranial Surgery. Anesthesia & Analgesia 2009;109(2):567-71.
[71] Bilotta F, Doronzio A, Cuzzone V, Caramia R, Rosa G. Early postoperative cognitive recovery and gas exchange patterns after balanced anesthesia with sevoflurane or desflurane in overweight and obese patients undergoing craniotomy: a prospective randomized trial. J Neurosurg Anesthesiol 2009;21(3):207-13.
[72] Kumar R, Lozano AM, Montgomery E, Lang AE. Pallidotomy and deep brain stimulation of the pallidum and subthalamic nucleus in advanced Parkinson's disease. Mov Disord 1998;13 Suppl 1:73-82.

2

Cost and Efficacy of Therapies for Advanced Parkinson's Disease

Francesc Valldeoriola
Institut de Neurociències, Hospital Clínic, Universitat de Barcelona, Barcelona, Spain

1. Introduction

The economic burden of Parkinson's disease (PD) has become a very important health topic. From the perspective of a general neurologist, health economics can appear as not prioritary; however, it is a growing topic in most modern healthcare systems; consequently health professionals should have at least a minimal understanding of how health economic information is derived. It has become important that payers and providers consider the significant impact the disease has on quality of life and how resource utilisation is directed to improve PD related clinical problems. Such measures are determinant in assessing the value of drug therapy, particularly for chronic conditions such as PD, and in determining the appropriate placement of medications on plan formularies. In the past, a comprehensive examination of a clinical condition would focus almost exclusively on areas considered relevant to patient management, such as diagnosis, etiology, treatment, and prognosis. Now, however, additional demands are being made by health policy decision makers, who can influence medical decisions through coverage and reimbursement policies. Physicians and other professional caregivers increasingly must consider the economic implications of their decisions, which has led to increased demand for disease-specific cost information.

2. Economic burden of Parkinson disease

PD is a progressive neurodegenerative disorder of the central nervous system with motor, cognitive, behavioural and autonomic symptoms. PD has a significant economic burden from all perspectives: society, health system, and individual patient and relatives. This is due to the high prevalence of the disease, 6.3 million people around the world (European Parkinson's disease Association [EPDA], 2008), the nature of the symptoms and the fact that no cure exists and treatments are only aimed at relieving the effects of the disease and to improve patients' quality of life.

In Spain, taking into account a population of around 47 million people (Spanish National Institute of Statistics, 2010), and considering the different incidence and prevalence rates published (Abasolo-Osionaga et al., 2006; Benito-León et al., 2003; Bergareche et al., 2004; Claveria et al., 2002), the average incidence has been estimated at around 6,400 new cases per year, and the average prevalence at 150,000 people (European Parkinson's Disease Association [EPDA], 2008) with PD. It is estimated that 30% of these patients are in an advanced stage of the disease (Kulisevsky, 2005). The economic impact of PD is mainly driven by in-patient care and nursing home costs caused by motor and non-motor symptoms that lead patients of PD to progressive disability. In addition, the cost of illness increases dramatically with severity as patients at the advanced stages are bedridden, wheelchair bound or institutionalized.

According to the most recent version of the World Health Organisation (WHO) report on Global Burden of Disease, published in 2008 (Mathers et al., 2008), neuropsychiatric conditions are responsible for 22% of global disability adjusted life years (DALYs) for women aged 15–59 years, the largest cause group in all regions outside Africa. The DALY is used as a measure to quantify the burden of the disease and consists on the years of life lived in less than full health or lost from premature death. It is also important to consider that these costs will increase along with the prevalence of these diseases due to the aging of the population in Europe.

Several studies have been performed to date in different countries to analyze the economic and social burden of PD. According to this literature, the main drivers of the total direct cost of PD are hospitalization and drug costs (Keranen et al., 2003; O'Brien et al., 2009) and the main drivers of total indirect cost are nursing care and productivity loss (Dengler et al., 2006; Hagell et al., 2002; O'Brien et al., 2009).

In the United States, the annual economic impact of PD was estimated in 2007 at $10.78 billion, being 58% of this amount related to direct medical costs ($6.22 billion) (O'Brien et al., 2009). Nursing home care ($2.6 billion) and PD-related medications ($1.47 billion) accounted for 63% of direct medical costs. Regarding indirect costs, annual lost productivity for persons with PD was estimated at $1 billion and caregivers cost at $2.36 billion. When considering the individual economic data, annual cost per patient was $21,626 (direct cost: $12,491).

Another study published in the United States (Huse et al., 2005) in 2005 quantified direct medical care costs for individual patients with PD and compared them with the costs obtained in a control group of persons without PD. Total annual direct cots were $23,101 per patient with PD versus $11,247 for controls. According to the study and based on annual data, PD patients spent approximately 2 more days in the hospital, 43 more days in long-term care institutions, and required more than 20 additional prescriptions than controls. These differences led to an increment of total annual health care costs of approximately $12,000 in PD patients. Around 50% of this excess cost was for long-term care, 24% for outpatient services, 15% for hospitalization and 14% for pharmacological treatment. The study projected the total cost of PD for the United States to be around $23 billion annually.

In an Australian study (Cordato et al., 2006) the total direct health-care cost of PD for patients with Hoehn and Yahr stage 3 was found to be four times higher than that of an age- and sex-matched control group of patients without PD. The estimated annual cost was Australian $7,020 per patient. Medication was the most costly component for both groups, being significantly higher for PD patients. Within the PD group, the health care costs attributable to PD were significantly higher than health care costs not related to PD (for a 3 month period, A$1,202 versus A$553).

As concerns European data, no Pan-European survey of the economic cost of PD has been performed to date. However, several studies from different countries are available in the literature. Some of the most representative ones have been considered for this chapter.

A review of the literature on the economic impact of PD in UK (Findley, 2007) reported an estimated total cost of PD in the UK between £449 million and £3.3 billion annually, depending on the methodology and prevalence rate considered in each individual analysis.

In another study in 2003, service use and costs for PD patients in the UK (McCrone et al., 2007) were measured. The annual costs were £13,804 per patient. Formal care costs accounted for 20% of this amount, while informal care was related to the 80% of the burden. Predictors of higher costs were identified, being male gender, level of disability and depression the more significant ones.

A study published in 2003 (Zecchinelli et al., 2003) assessed health care costs associated with PD in Italy. Patients and results were classified using the Hoehn and Yahr scale. Annual direct health costs were €4,320 for mild stage (1-2), €4,748 for moderate stage (2.5-3) and €6,175 for severe stage (4-5). The average was estimated at €4,808. These results were identified as lower than the real cost, as they didn't consider the societal perspective and neither informal care nor health care costs incurred in the private sector were included.

In Germany a 3-year prospective study of the economic cost of PD (Dengler et al., 2006) was performed in 2006. The average annual cost per patient was estimated at €12,091, of which 55,9% accounted for direct costs. Drugs took up the major share of direct costs, €5,763 per year. Indirect costs accounted for €4,851 per patient per year. Within this, 76% of the costs were related to nursing care and the loss of productivity.

In Sweden resource use and costs in patients with PD were collected from medical records of a cohort of 127 patients (Hagell et al., 2002) in 1996 (year 2000 costs). Direct health care costs averaged approximately €3,200 per patient per year, of which drugs were the most costly component. Non-medical direct costs were higher, €4,800 per patient per year, and costs due to lost productivity were around €5,800 per patient per year. The average total annual cost for PD was therefore estimated at €13,800 per patient.

Costs of PD illness were studied in a Russian Cohort of 100 patients (year 2008 costs) (Winter et al., 2009). From the societal perspective, total annual costs per patient amounted to €5,240 per patient, with direct costs accounting for 67% and indirect costs for 33% of the total. The main drivers of the burden were informal care and drugs. Global costs for the nation were estimated at €1.1 billion per year.

One of the most recent European studies, published in 2010, was performed in a cohort of 100 Czech patients with idiopathic PD to evaluate direct and indirect costs and to identify cost-driving factors (Winter et al., 2010b). Results were assessed for a 6-month period and have been projected to annual costs. Total annual costs for PD were €11,020 per patient. Direct costs accounted for 60% of the total costs and indirect for 40%. Independent cost-driving factors included disease severity, motor complications, psychosis and age.

The degenerative nature of PD leads to an increase of resource consumption in its advance stages. In fact, disease severity has been identified as a strong cost-predictor in several of the studies already mentioned. Motor complications (fluctuations, dyskinesias, dystonia) have been identified as factors increasing PD-related costs (Dowding et al., 2006; McCrone et al., 2007; Winter et al., 2010a; Winter et al., 2010b; Zecchinelli et al., 2003).

In a 6-month observational study of PD in France, Germany and the UK, patients with different degrees of motor complications, measured using the Unified Parkinson Disease Rating Scale (UPDRS), and its effects on health care costs were examined (Péchevis et al., 2005). Dyskinesia (UPDRS part IVa) was associated with significant increases in total health care costs. Each unit increase in dyskinesia score lead to €562 additional costs per patient over a 6-month period.

A 2007 published study developed in the UK (Thanvi et al., 2007) showed that Levodopa induced dyskinesia increased health care costs. Relationship between increasing cost of care and severity of the disease as measured by Hoehn and Yahr stage was proven to be statistically significant. A correlation was also found between the severity of the disease, patient's age and the use of Social Services.

If we focus on advanced PD (APD) treatment costs, a systematic review of the available economic evidence of deep brain stimulation (DBS) for APD was performed in 2009 (Puig-Junoy & Puig, 2009). Ten studies were identified, five of them being simple cost analyses and the other five, full economic evaluations.

The cost studies included were: one description of costs of the treatment with DBS (McIntosh et al., 2003) and four comparative analyses (Charles et al., 2004; D'Ausilio et al., 2003; Fraix et al., 2006; Gerzeli et al., 2002) of DBS versus conservative pharmacological treatment. In the comparative analyses, a significant difference was observed when annual average pharmacological cost was compared between conservative treatment and DBS. The independent average cost of the DBS intervention was specified in four of the five cost studies. These results showed some variability from €20.033 (Gerzeli et al., 2002) to -€33.220 (McIntosh et al., 2003), explained mainly by differences in resources utilization, which was highly driven by surgeons' level of experience. The intervention duration and costs decreased along with the increase of professional experience on DBS.

It was also observed that pharmacological treatment costs were lower in patients after DBS intervention than in patients that remained in conservative pharmacological treatment. Regarding costs distribution, the higher resource consumption for DBS was experienced during the first year of the therapy. The comparison of DBS costs to conventional pharmacological alternative is sensitive to the inclusion of non-health related costs. When productivity loss and informal care costs were considered (Gerzeli et al., 2002), the cost of the DBS alternative was lower to the cost of the conventional pharmacological treatment.

3. Cost-effectiveness of bilateral subthalamic stimulation in advanced Parkinson's disease

Levodopa combined with adjunct medical therapy is the standard medical treatment for individuals with PD. However, prolonged use of levodopa can cause disabling motor fluctuations and dyskinesias. When medication is no longer effective or produces unacceptable side effects, surgical treatments may be a possible alternative. Ablative surgery and DBS are the main surgical treatments for advanced refractory PD. Ablative surgery includes pallidotomy, thalamotomy and subthalamotomy, which destroy the globus pallidus (GPi), thalamic nucleus and subthalamic nucleus (STN), respectively. Once the suitable target tissue has been located, it is destroyed by a radio frequency or thermocoagulation method. Expert opinion suggests nowadays that ablative procedures are rarely performed in Western countries although such procedures are still available as a treatment option for individuals in developing countries. Ablative surgery has largely been replaced by DBS, in part because DBS is potentially reversible and is perceived to be associated with improved safety and effectiveness and, in part, because ablative surgery is irreversible and regarded as having limited effectiveness and significant safety concerns. In patients with inadequate control of parkinsonian symptoms by medical treatments, bilateral subthalamic nucleus deep brain stimulation (STN-DBS) has emerged as a surgical choice for APD and has been shown to improve motor function, motor fluctuations, and health related quality of life (HRQoL) and to reduce medication usage and drug induced dyskinesia (Deuschl et al., 2006; Krack et al., 2003; Martínez-Martín et al., 2002; Rodríguez-Oroz et al., 2005; Siderowf et al., 2006; Schupbach et al., 2005; Valldeoriola et al., 2002). DBS was approved by the Food and Drug Administration (FDA) and the European Agency for the Evaluation of Medical Products (EMEA) for the treatment of APD, but it is still considered a relatively expensive therapy. Authorities are concerned because of the increased health expenses and are taking containment measures based on the principle that the distribution of resources must be supported by the efficiency and not exclusively by the direct clinical benefit (Greenberg et al., 1999; Weinstein et al., 2001).

The DBS procedure is generally performed in two separate steps, implantation of leads followed by implantation of the neurostimulator to which the leads are connected. Patients need to be tested initially for their responsiveness to therapy. This is accomplished by implanting a lead at the relevant site using a combination of stereotactic techniques such as image-guided stereotactic localisation and physiological techniques such as microelectrode mapping or macrostimulation. The implantation procedure is generally performed under local anaesthetic. The placement of the electrode at a particular site is determined by the patient's response to stimulation, involving physical evaluation of the lower limbs and face muscles, and interpretation of the microelectrode recording data. Once the target that elicits the best response has been localised, the testing electrodes are removed and replaced with permanent leads.

Although DBS is non-ablative, the procedure may give rise to complications and side effects, some of which are neither reversible nor adaptable. The complications from DBS can arise before surgery, during surgery, in the immediate post-operative period, and after surgery. Data available on adverse events are derived from case series. Findings from these studies indicated the risk associated with DBS but did not allow quantisation of those risks compared with the Best Medical Treatment (BMT). A systematic review of case series to assess the safety and effectiveness of bilateral STN-DBS for the symptoms of PD in a total of 537 individuals has been performed (Amani et al., 2005). The authors reported the mortality rate, adverse events related to stimulation, general neurological and surgical complications and hardware-related complications. Mortality occurred at a rate of 0.4 per cent.

The adverse events related to stimulation (and rates of occurrence) were: hypophonia (5.8%), eyelid apraxia (4.6%), increased libido (0.8%), sialorrhea (0.9%) and decreased memory (1.1%). Other stimulation-related adverse events included dystonia, paraesthesias, diplopia, dyskinesias and dysarthria; however these events were not reported in the studies or were underestimated. The adverse events related to general neurological and surgical complications (and rates of occurrence) were: depression (4.7%), mania/hypomania (2.0%), peri-operative confusion (13.7%), cerebrospinal fluid leak (0.1%), meningitis (0.1%), venous phlebitis (0.7%), pneumonia (0.4%), urinary tract infections (0.3%), pulmonary embolism (0.5%), seizures (0.9%), haemorrhage (2.8%). Weight gain was also considered to fall into this category, but was reported to be under-quantified in the studies. The adverse events from hardware-related complications (and rates of occurrence) were: lead problems including lead migration, breakage and repositioning (4.5%), and infections of the hardware (3.4%).

The results shown n the literature review indicated that DBS allowed the maintenance of abilities to perform activities and increased motor function in the absence of effective medical treatment. In the absence of a comparator group, it is not possible to quantify the effect attributable to DBS; however, the worsening of akinesia, speech, postural stability, freezing of gait and cognitive function is consistent with the natural history of PD over time (Krack et al., 2003).

The effectiveness of DBS for the treatment of symptoms of PD has been assessed from one double-blind crossover and three case-control studies. DBS appears to be effective for the treatment of PD symptoms, with statistically significant changes observed between case and control participants in UPDRS and PDQ-39SI scores. These results therefore show that DBS can ameliorate the symptoms of PD (as measured by the UPDRS ADL and Motor sections) and reduce the antiparkinsonian medication required to maintain control of the symptoms of PD. Patients experienced up to a 90 per cent reduction at 24 months following surgery in the daily OFF rate. However, the assessment of the effectiveness of DBS for the treatment of symptoms is generally limited by the number of individuals analysed; significant losses to follow-up in some studies; and follow-up of the participants to a maximum of only 48 months.

The reduction in antiparkinsonian medication after DBS may also significantly reduce some of the side effects of high-dose levodopa treatment over a long time (Charles et al., 2004; Mínguez-Castellanos et al., 2005; Molinuevo et al., 2000).

Most of the studies on cost-effectiveness in STN-DBS have been designed in the absence of a control group of similar characteristics receiving conventional oral medication supposed to be the BMT possible. In some of the studies, the costs of expensive therapies such as apomorphine pump infusions were also considered within the concept of BMT.

A cost-effectiveness study has been published with the aim of assessing the long term cost-effectiveness of DBS versus BMT (Tomaszewski & Holloway, 2001) using modelling techniques to predict long term clinical and economical consequences of using DBS and BMT in advanced PD patients, showing that DBS may be an efficient therapy to treat PD patients. Such mathematical models can be useful to predict long-term cost-effectiveness, considering that long-term studies are difficult to perform in clinical practice. It is likely that such positive cost-effectiveness results would extend at least to the next two or three years after the intervention. This possibility was suggested in a survey which showed a 32% increase in total costs during the first year after surgery but a reduction of 54% for the second year, when compared to preoperative values (Charles et al., 2004). Other studies have shown similar results: a retrospective cost-effectiveness study of DBS in Germany in 46 parkinsonian patients (Meissner et al., 2005) showed an estimated Incremental Cost Effectiveness Ratio (ICER) of €979 for one point improvement of the UPDRS-III in one year; in this survey the annual pharmacological expenses were of €11,230 one year before the implantation while of only €4,449 two years after surgery. A multicentric French survey (Fraix et al., 2006) observed similar improvement of UPDRS scores and decrement of PD costs. In another survey, a prospective analysis, the incremental cost per total UPDRS unit improvement turned out to be €920 (Spottke et al., 2002). Some studies have included the cost of the battery replacement after five years of use (D'Ausilio et al., 2003; McIntosh et al., 2003; Tomaszewski & Holloway, 2001).

Only a few studies considered a social perspective by showing costs derived from the losses and gains of productivity of both the patient and the caregiver before and after the intervention. Most of studies, however, are based in a retrospective design, with a short number of patients and follow-up and the absence of a control group of patients of similar clinical characteristics.

Due to the absence of prospective studies comparing cost-efficacy of STN-DBS with control patients, we designed an open, prospective longitudinal study comparative of the cost, effectiveness and HRQoL between the treatment with STN-DBS and BMT in patients with

APD (Valldeoriola et al., 2007). Twenty-nine patients were enrolled in the study. All were included in a waiting list for STN-DBS at our centre. All participating patients signed an informed consent form. Among the patients in the waiting list for STN-DBS, the first consecutive fourteen patients were enrolled in the treatment group and the last consecutive fifteen patients were enrolled in the control group. The treatment group was assigned to STN-DBS; the control group was assigned to BMT. Both groups (STN-DBS and BMT) were largely comparable in their clinical and demographic variables including mean levodopa equivalent doses. The study estimated only direct costs. We divided them into two categories: direct medical costs, related to costs for goods and services used in the prevention, diagnosis, treatment and rehabilitation of the illness (for example costs for medical visits, hospitalization and pharmaceuticals); and direct non-medical costs, generally assumed by the patient, including expenses related to the disease (for example transportation, social services, adaptation of accommodation and any kind of special equipment, facilities or orthopaedic material). Our results showed that the ICER needed to obtain an additional improvement of one unit in the total UPDRS score was €239.8. Current management of APD includes combinations of expensive drugs and therefore savings after STN-DBS were mainly attributable to the reduction of pharmacological expenses. The incremental cost-effectiveness was of €34,389 per QALY. The quality-adjusted life year (QALY) is a measure of disease burden, including both the quality and the quantity of life lived. It is used in assessing the value for money of a medical intervention. The QALY model requires utility independent, risk neutral, and constant proportional trade-off behaviour. The QALY is based on the number of years of life that would be added by the intervention. Each year in perfect health is assigned the value of 1.0 down to a value of 0.0 for death.

We also performed sensitivity analyses under different situations. When we excluded the BMT patient group patient who had a prolonged hospitalisation from the analysis, the incremental cost per QALY was of €44,078 (X1.3). In this study, two patients in the BMT group were treated with Continuous Subcutaneous Infusion of Apomorphine (CSIA), a therapy that is also considered to be expensive. Consequently we also calculated the cost-effectiveness of STN-DBS when excluding these patients, obtaining a result of €62,148 per QALY (X1.8). This study showed STN-DBS anti-parkinsonian clinical efficacy and that cost-effectiveness is directly related to clinical improvement in parkinsonism and to the reduction of pharmacological expenses after the intervention. As shown by others (Charles et al., 2004; Fraix et al., 2006; Meissner et al., 2005; Spottke et al., 2002), this survey in the Spanish setting showed that STN-DBS is within the adequate limits to be considered as an efficient therapy. Considering the published data available in the literature assessing DBS for APD, it can be considered safe, effective and cost-effective compared with BMT. There is sufficient evidence of safety and effectiveness, and robust information on cost-effectiveness is unlikely to emerge but the total cost is acceptable for patients in whom other therapies are insufficient.

The insertion of a DBS system incurs upfront costs but may result in cost savings from its effect of controlling the motor symptoms of PD as disease progresses, allowing patients to live in more functional health states for longer periods of time with improved QoL. To date, there appears to be no evidence that DBS delays the progression of PD or affects the mortality rate, although it may be argued that mortality due to falling, for example, may decrease with improvements in motor skills. These savings could be realised through a reduced demand for services or a lower expenditure on certain examinations.

4. Cost analysis of DBS, CSIA and CDLCI in advanced Parkinson's disease: The SCOPE Study

For physicians in general and for neurologists in special, it becomes quite challenging to achieve an antiparkinsonian medication regimen that keeps the patient mobile while at the same time does not create side effects that outweigh the benefits of treatment, impacting patient's quality of life (Adler, 2002). In these APD patients, refractory to pharmacological treatment, three treatments may be recommended such as DBS, Continuous Duodenal Levodopa–Carbidopa Infusion (CDLCI), and CSIA. These therapies are not recommended for all patients with APD and an adequate patient selection allows the optimization of results obtained with the three therapeutic options.

Additionally, the three treatments have no clear positioning in the treatment pathway of APD patients, which leaves the decision about the eligibility of APD patients for one therapy or another to neurologists. Such decision can therefore be subjective and largely depends on the patient's clinical status, patients' and physicians' preferences, as well as previous hospital experience, availability of these treatments or economic constraints.

To date, as it has been described, no economic evaluation has been published comparing the costs-effectiveness profile of these three therapeutic options that exist for APD. The main reason could be the lack of published direct clinical evidence comparing at least two of the three therapies. In these cases, a modelling method can be done as a simulation of the cost-effectiveness results (Stahl , 2008).

A healthcare costs compqarison considering all the costs in the medium and long term (not only the acquisition costs) associated with the treatments and their consequences of chronic diseases management like PD is a valuable tool both for payers and physicians, offering useful information to support their decision making in the treatment of this patient population (Mycka et al., 2010).

In order to address this evidence gap, the first cost study worldwide has already been submitted (Valldeoriola et al., 2011). The SCOPE study[1] is a descriptive, quantitative and economic analysis that tried to compare the healthcare costs associated with these three alternative treatments for a 5-years, period in patients with APD in the perspective of the Spanish Healthcare System.

One DBS battery replacement was included in the analysis, as the average battery life of a non-rechargeable neurostimulator has seem to oscillate between four to five years (Bin-Mahfoodh et al., 2003; Krack et al., 2003). The costs of the devices and components of CDLCI and CSIA (infusion pump, catheters, etc.) were not included; thus it was assumed that they were provided free of charge by the supplier, and therefore their cost to the healthcare system was zero. Once all the health resources associated with the therapies were identified and quantified, its cost per unit or 'price` was obtained from the Spanish health resources database (Spanish Cost Database, e-salud (Spanish Cost Database, e-salud, 2010). Finally,

[1] SCOPE: eStudio COstes Parkinson Enfermedad. The SCOPE Study was evaluated and approved by the Ethics Committee of Clinical Research of the Hospital Clinic i Provincial, Barcelona.

the average total cost for each of the three therapies per patient was then obtained for the 5-years, period. In order to test the statistical differences of mean costs, the data analysis was carried out with the SPSS 15.0 software package for Windows and comparisons among the three therapies (non-parametric Kruskal–Wallis one-way analysis of variance by ranks multiple comparisons) and between the two therapies with the lower average total costs, DBS vs CSIA (Hollander & Wolf, 1999).

Due to the higher APD costs in the first six months, when patients consume more health resources (extra visits, hospitalization, dose adjustments, etc.) (D'Ausilio at al., 2003; McIntosh et al., 2003; Tomaszewski & Holloway, 2001), it was decided to divide the HQR in four sections, or phases.

In Table 1, the average cost per patient associated with the three alternative therapies in the baseline scenario for different phases are shown.

Phases	**Average Costs**		
	DBS	**CDLCI**	**CSIA**
1. Pre-treatment period to hospitalization	1,141 ± 411	1,705 ± 357	1,231 ± 267
2. Hospitalization period to discharge (includes Procedure or Treatment Administration)	27,236 ± 3,105 *	3,165 ± 501 *	785 ± 197 *
3. Discharge from hospital to 6 months post-op	4,768 ± 918 * #	25,521 ± 2,381 *	12,094 ± 2,158 * #
4. From month 6 to year 5	54,869 ± 4,190 * #	203,596 ± 8,737 *	127,284 ± 9,184 * #
Total cost per 5 years	88,014 ± 2,580 * #	233,986 ± 10,552 *	141,393 ± 9,945 * #
Average Cost per year	17,603±516 * #	46,797 ±2,110 *	28,279 ±1,989 * #

(*) Comparison of the three therapies (p<0.05). (#) DBS vs. CSIA comparison (p<0.05).

Table 1. Results of the baseline scenario expressed as an average ± standard error. Costs per patient (€, 2010).

As observed, during the pre-treatment phase, costs are similar for the three alternative therapies. In phase 2, DBS is associated with higher costs due to the therapy acquisition cost. However, starting from discharge to 5 years follow-up, DBS is the least costly therapy compared to CDLCI and CSIA. Differences are statistically significant in the comparison of the three therapies ($p<0.0001$) and for the DBS vs. CSIA comparison ($p=0.023$ and $p<0.0001$, respectively for phases 3, discharge from hospital to 6 months and 4, from month 6 to year 5). This suggests that in the long term DBS is a cost-minimizing therapy versus CDLCI and CSIA. The yearly average cost of DBS was €17,603 compared to €46,797 ($p=0.001$) for CDLCI and €28,279 for CSIA ($p=0.008$), indicating that for every patient treated during one year with CDLCI, two patients could be treated with DBS (or €29,194 could be saved) and for every patient treated during one year with CSIA, €10,676 could be saved if DBS would be chosen. Figure 1 describes Cumulative annual costs for the three therapies for the 5-year period. Results show that starting from year two, DBS is the therapy associated with the lowest cumulative costs compared with CDLCI and CSIA. All the differences were statistically significant (p<0.0001) for multiple comparisons (among the three therapies) and starting from year two, the difference in costs between DBS and CSIA was statistically significant for the DBS vs. CSIA comparison (p=0.008).

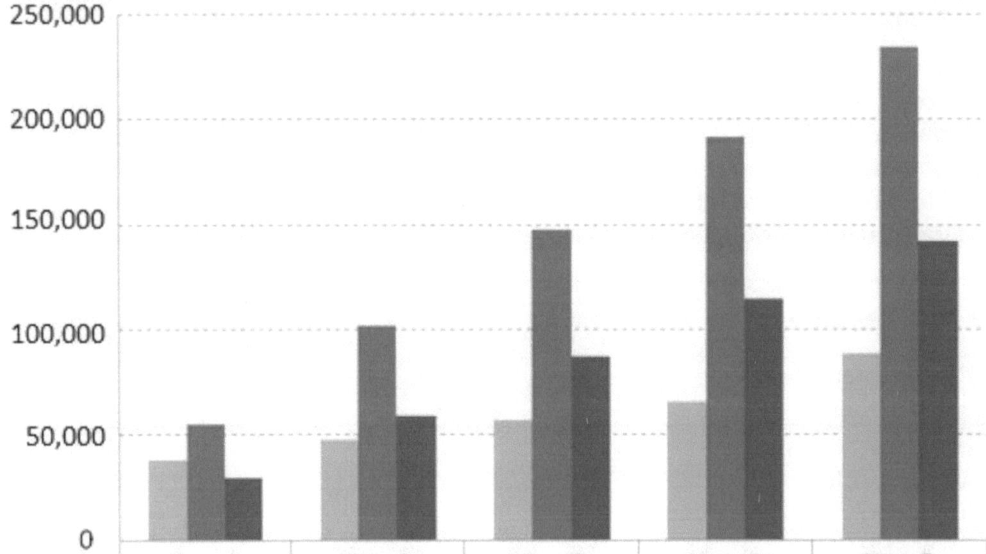

	Year 1	Year 2	Year 3	Year 4	Year 5
DBS	37,983*	47,377*	56,498*	65,352*	88,014*
CDLCI	54,530*	101,402*	146,910*	191,092*	233,986*
CSIA	29,201*	58,504*	86,955*	114,576*	141,393*

(*) All differences became statistically significant (p<0.05) for multiple comparisons (among the three therapies) and for the DBS vs. CSIA comparison (p<0.05).

Fig. 1. Cumulative annual costs for DBS, CDLCI and CSIA (€, 2010)

At year 5, mean cumulative costs per patient associated with DBS amount to €88,014±2,580, €141,393±9,945 for CSIA and €233,986±10,552 with CDLCI (p<0.0001) (see Figure 1). For DBS, the high initial investment required during the first two phases (pre-treatment period to discharge; 32.2% of the total 5-year cost) is offset by decreases in antiparkinsonian pharmacological treatment and follow-up costs. The majority of the DBS costs are incurred before the initial sixth month. As explained, these results were obtained considering one battery replacement in the 5-years period and without including acquisition costs for CDLCI and CSIA devices and components (infusion pump, catheters, etc; only drug costs): consequently, if these costs were included, results would probably have been more favourable for DBS.

During the total 5-year period, with the amount necessary to treat one patient with CDLCI, two patients could be treated if DBS is chosen (or €145,972 could be saved) and €53,379 could be saved with CSIA.

Around 95% of the total 5-years cost of CDLCI and CSIA is related to constant pharmacological costs, mainly driven by Levodopa–Carbidopa intestinal gel cartridges and

Apomorphine ampoules acquisition costs (84.4% for CDLCI and 65.7% for CSIA), while for DBS, antiparkinsonian drugs represent only 43% of the total (see Figure 2).

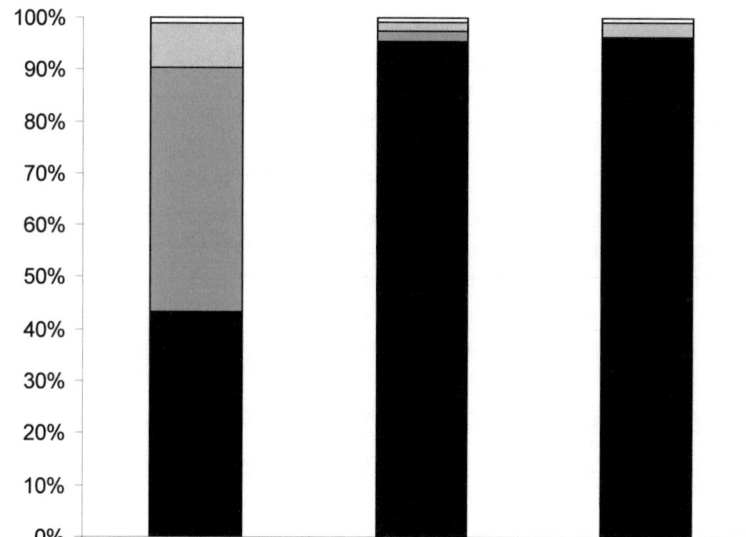

	DBS	CDLCI	CSIA
□ Adverse Events	1%	1%	1%
□ Follow-up	8%	2%	3%
■ Implant / Admin.	47%	2%	0%
■ Pharmacological	43%	95%	96%

■ Pharmacological ■ Implant / Admin. □ Follow-up □ Adverse Events

Fig. 2. Costs Distribution of each therapy in the 5 years (€, 2010)

Several alternative scenarios were tested in the sensitivity analysis: e.g., a second replacement in DBS therapy and a reduction of CDLCI and Apomorphine pharmacological costs. In all different the scenarios DBS remained the lowest costly therapy, even with the most unfavourable assumptions ($p<0.05$).

Due to the complexity and variability in the treatment of APD, the decision was taken to apply the Panel approach. This may be the main limitation of the study described. However, a Panel of Experts can contribute to mapping complex treatment processes, and to provide estimates of health care resources (Simoens, 2006). It is worth mentioning that the eleven experts of the Panel can be considered representative of the clinical practice of APD in Spain, as both neurologists and neurosurgeons from nine centres located in five different Spanish regions were involved, with experience on at least two of the three alternative therapies evaluated in this analysis.

Other published studies that estimated healthcare costs at least with one of the therapies to check if similar results are obtained. Only one Swedish study from 2008 estimated the annual cost of CDLCI (Sydow, 2008). Cost estimates oscillated between €40,000 and €80,000 according to the dosage used. These results corroborated the results of the SCOPE study, as

it was observed an average drug cost of €44,839 per patient per year and the intestinal gel cartridges of CDLCI represented an 84.4% of this total drug costs.
For DBS, as it was described, several published international economic evaluations were conducted in other countries, as presented in the review by Puig-Junoy et al (Puig-Junoy & Puig, 2009). Alike our study, five cost studies and five complete economic evaluations of DBS showed a reduction in medication costs associated with DBS.
From this survey, it can be concluded that despite DBS is perceived as a costly therapy, the initial investment for the implant is offset by a reduction in the consumption of other healthcare resources by patients over the years. For every patient yearly treated with CDLCI, two patients could be treated with DBS (€29,194 saved) and for every patient treated with CSIA; €10,676 could be saved if DBS would be chosen. On the other hand, CDLCI and CSIA are shown to require a constant use of relatively similar health resources, with pharmacological costs being the main source. Based on the results of this study, DBS seems to be the less costly therapy under the Spanish NHS perspective, compared to CDLCI and CSIA when applied to the adequate candidates.

5. Modelling interventions for advanced Parkinson's disease

Parkinson's disease is a complex illness, encompassing many different symptoms and costs, which makes undertaking an economic evaluation challenging. Numerous cost-effectiveness analyses have been published over the last 10-15 years, with significantly different approaches used to represent the progression of the disease, the effect of treatment upon symptoms and other outcomes, and the duration of treatment effect. Furthermore, there is currently an absence of an analysis which directly compares all relevant treatment options for patients with advanced PD. Outlined below are some of the key aspects for consideration in future economic evaluations of interventions for advanced PD.

5.1 Treatment comparisons

There are multiple interventions available for the management of patients with APD. For example, DBS, CDLCI, CSIA and BMT are all options for patients at this stage of thedisease, and although there may be specific reasons for choosing one therapy over another, it is appropriate to consider the full range of interventions available. To date, economic evaluations have focused on comparing a limited number of interventions, rather than addressing the relative cost-effectiveness of each of the interventions listed above.
An analysis which considers a wide range of interventions would be beneficial, both in terms of helping payers to understand the value of each intervention, and in helping clinicians to make informed treatment decisions for their patients.

5.2 Disease indicators

PD is a complex disease which has many different aspects affecting management costs and health outcomes. When attempting to model the disease and the impact of different interventions, it is important to capture both the natural progression of the disease and the changes in disease indicators which occur over time. Previous models have dealt with disease progression in different ways: some have used UPDRS scores as the basis for measuring disease progression, whilst others have used the Hoehn and Yahr scale.
The majority of cost-effectiveness models (across all therapeutic areas) use a Markovian approach, in which patients are categorised into one of a finite number of health states. Data

are then used to estimate the movement of patients between these states over time, to reflect changes in disease status (this could include events such as disease progression and Mortality). In PD, the Hoehn and Yahr scale offers a logical way of splitting patients up into a relatively small number of categories. Trial data could then be used to determine how quickly patients move between these states e.g. from Hoehn and Yahr 2 to Hoehn and Yahr 3, and also to inform how mortality differs between the various stages. The UPDRS scale is less amenable to this approach, since there is no natural way of partitioning patients into categories according to their score. Since the Hoehn and Yahr class in the 'OFF' periods represents the status of the underlying disease, this is the most appropriate way of defining which Hoehn and Yahr class a patient is in at a given point in time.

There are other aspects of advanced PD which are relevant to both costs and health outcomes. For example, the amount of 'OFF' time is a key outcome, whilst outcomes such as non-motor symptoms and dyskinesias are also relevant endpoints to consider within a cost-effectiveness model. Each intervention impacts upon these aspects of the disease in different ways, and representing these differences is key to a comparative assessment of cost-effectiveness.

5.3 Quality of life

PD is a debilitating condition which can have a significant impact upon patients' quality of life (QoL). Some of the aspects of the disease which influence QoL include:

- The proportion of time the patient spends in the 'OFF' state;
- The severity of the 'OFF' periods;
- The predictability of the 'OFF' stages;
- Disease progression (e.g. in terms of Hoehn and Yahr stage).

Previous cost-effectiveness analyses have focused solely on the impact of motor fluctuations; however, there is a growing view that non-motor symptoms are also important determinants of QoL. Such symptoms may include depression, pain and sleep problems, and whilst the effect of these outcomes may be captured inherently within QoL assessments made routinely during trials, it is important that the effect of interventions upon these outcomes is addressed.

A standard approach to accounting for quality of life is to assign a health state utility to each health state within a model (e.g. one utility for Hoehn and Yahr 3, and a separate utility for Hoehn and Yahr 4). However, given that interventions for PD are focused on symptoms rather than underlying disease progression, such an approach may not be sufficiently sensitive to detect important treatment differences e.g. to represent the impact of an intervention which reduces the amount of 'OFF' time. In order to capture effects such as these, one approach would be to separate patients within each Hoehn and Yahr class into different levels of 'OFF' time, or to evaluate the change in their level of 'OFF' time compared with the baseline level.

Numerous tools have been used to assess patients' QoL during treatment, including generic and disease-specific questionnaires. Typical examples of generic tools include the EQ-5D and the SF-36, which can be readily converted into estimates of utility for the purposes of carrying out cost-utility analysis. The key disease-specific instrument for the measurement of QoL is the PDQ-39. However, to date, no mapping algorithm has been developed to allow the results of this tool to be mapped to health state utilities and so its use in cost-effectiveness modelling is currently limited.

A final issue relating to QoL is the impact of the disease upon patients' carers and families. Whilst this effect has been little-studied, it is a relevant outcome to consider owing to the burden which advanced PD can have upon these individuals. It is, however, a difficult endpoint to quantify, and this probably explains its omission from previous economic evaluations.

5.4 Costs

Advanced PD is associated with a wide range of costs for health systems, patients and their carers. Accurately representing the costs associated with the disease, and the impact of each intervention upon these costs, has a large bearing upon the cost-effectiveness outputs of a model. In general, a disease model which closely reflects the true natural history of the disease and incorporates its key aspects makes the process of assigning costs much simpler. Some examples of costs which should be included in a cost-effectiveness analysis include:

- Device acquisition and implantation;
- Management of device-related adverse events e.g. infections;
- Pump infections (for patients on CDLCI);
- Device explantation;
- Battery replacement;
- Ongoing drug costs;
- Nursing home care for patients with very severe disease;
- Inpatient care;
- Routine follow-up appointments.

This list focuses on costs falling on the health services; however, there are also wider costs associated with PD which are relevant. For example, some patients are forced to take early retirement due to the debilitating nature of the disease, and this has an impact upon society in terms of lost productivity of the workforce. This societal cost impact also extends to patients' families, who sometimes have to give up work.

5.5 Long-term outcomes

The majority of existing economic evaluations in the field of advanced PD have used a relatively short time horizon for assessing cost-effectiveness (between five and ten years), primarily due to the absence of robust trial data to populate long-term outcomes. This is a sensible approach, since any extrapolation of the trial data to predict long-term outcomes is inherently subject to considerable uncertainty. However, given that the impact of interventions may be expected to continue in the long-term, assessing the relative cost-effectiveness of different interventions over a longer time horizon may be beneficial. Many economic models in other fields (e.g. oncology) use a lifetime horizon in which patients are followed until death; such an approach would allow scenarios to be explored under assumptions of different levels of long-term treatment effect.

6. Conclusion

Disease management requires constant evaluation in regard of the quality of treatment as well as of cost-effectiveness. We have reviewed the issue of cost-effectiveness in PD and we think it is demonstrated that there is a need for formal and informal care of patients suffering from chronic progressive diseases which is major challenge for health and social care systems in the years to come. However, more research is necessary to evaluate the full burden of PD and to explore efficacy and effectiveness of the disease management. At the present moment, giving the scarce evidence that we have found and the lack of direct prospective comparisons, it seems that DBS is the most cost-effective therapy for APD.

7. Acknowledgment

I thank Dr. Pablo Martínez-Martín for his valuable contribution to this chapter.

8. References

Abasolo-Osionaga, E.; Abecia-Inchaurregui, L.C.; Fernández-Díaz, E., et al. (2006). Prevalencia y coste farmacológico de la enfermedad del Parkinson en España. *Revista de neurología*, Vol.43, No.11, pp.641-645, ISSN 0210-0010

Adler, CH. (2002). Relevance of motor complications in Parkinson's disease. *Neurology*, Vol.58, No.4, Suppl.1, pp.51-56, ISSN 0028-3878

Benito-León, J.; Bermejo-Pareja, F.; Rodriguez, J., et al. (2003). Neurological Disorders in Central Spain (NEDICES) Study Group. Prevalence of PD and other types of parkinsonism in three elderly populations of central Spain. *Movement Disorders*, Vol.18, No.4, pp.267-274, ISSN 1531-8257

Bergareche, A.; De La Puente, E.; López de Munain, A., et al. (2004). Prevalence of Parkinson's disease and other types of Parkinsonism. A door-to-door survey in Bidasoa, Spain. *Journal of Neurology*, Vol.251, No.3, pp.340-345, ISSN 0340-5354

Bin-Mahfoodh, M.; Hamani, C.; Sime, E., et al. (2003). Longevity of batteries in internal pulse generators used for deep brain stimulation. *Stereotactic and functional neurosurgery*, Vol.80, No.1-4, pp.56-60, ISSN 1011-6125

Charles, P.D.; Padaliya, B.B.; Newman, A.J., et al. (2004). Deep brain stimulation of the subthalamic nucleus reduces antiparkinsonian medication costs. *Parkinsonism & Related Disorders*, Vol.10, No.8, pp.475-479, ISSN 1353-8020

Claveria, L.E.; Duarte, J.; Sevillano, M.D., et al. (2002). Prevalence of Parkinson's disease in Cantalejo, Spain: a door-to-door survey. *Movement Disorders*, Vol.17, No.2, pp.242-249, ISSN 1531-8257

Cordato, D.J.; Schwartz, R.; Abbott, E., et al. (2006). A comparison of health-care costs involved in treating people with and without Parkinson's disease in Southern Sydney, New South Wales, Australia. *Journal of clinical neuroscience*, Vol.13, No.6, pp.655-658, ISSN 0967 -5868

D'Ausilio, A.; Marconi, S.; Antonini, A., et al. (2003). Cost analysis in Italy of various strategies for the treatment of Parkinson disease in the advanced phase. *Recenti progressi in medicina*, Vol.94, No.11, pp.484-493, ISSN 0034-1193

Dengler, I. ; Leukel, N.; Meuser, T., et al. (2006). Prospective study of the direct and indirect costs of idiopathic Parkinson's disease. *Nervenarz*, Vol.77, No.10, pp.1204-1209, ISSN 0028- 2804

Deuschl, G.; Schade-Brittinger, C.; Krack, P., et al. (2006). A randomised trial of deep-brain stimulation for Parkinson's disease. *The New England Journal of Medicine*, Vol.355, No.9, pp.896-908, ISSN 1533-4406

Dowding, C.H.; Shenton, C.L. & Salek, S.S. (2006). A review of the health-related quality of life and economic impact of Parkinson's disease. *Drugs & Aging*, Vol.23, No.9, pp.693-721, ISSN 1170-229X

European Parkinson's Disease Association, EPDA. (2008). Life with Parkinson's, 31.01.2011, Available from: <http://www.parkinsonsawareness.eu.com/campaign-literature/what-is-parkinsons-disease>

Findley, L.J. (2007). The economic impact of Parkinson's disease. *Parkinsonism and Related Disorders*, Vol.13, Suppl., pp.S8-S12, ISSN 1353-8020

Fraix, V.; Houeto, J.L.; Lagrange, C., et al. (2006). SPARK Study Group. Clinical and economic results of bilateral subthalamic nucleus stimulation in Parkinson's disease. *Journal of Neurology, Neurosurgery & Psychiatry*, Vol.77, No.4, pp.443-449, ISSN 0022-3050

Gerzeli, S.; Cavallo, M.C.; Caprari, F., et al. Gruppo di Studio DBS. (2002). Analysis of deep brain stimulation (DBS) costs: an observational study on Italian patients. *Pharmacoeconomics-Italian Research Articles*, Vol.4, pp.66-79, ISSN 2035-6137

Greenberg, P.E.; Arcelus, A.; Birnbaum, H.G., et al. (1999). Pharmacoeconomics and health policy. Current applications and prospects for the future. *PharmacoEconomics*, Vol.16, No.5, pp.425-432, ISSN 1170-7690

Hagell, P.; Nordling, S.; Reimer, J., et al. (2002). Resource utilisation and costs in a Swedish Cohort of patients with Parkinson's disease. *Movement Disorders*, Vol.17, No.6, pp.1213-1220, ISSN 1531-8257

Hamani, C.; Richter, E.; Schwalb J.L., et al,. (2005). Bilateral subthalamic nucleus stimulation for Parkinson's disease: a systematic review of the clinical literature. *Neurosurgery*, Vol.56, No.6, pp.1313-1321, ISSN 0148-396X

Hollander, M. & Wolfe, D. A. (1999). *Nonparametric Statistical Methods* (2nd Ed.), Wiley-interscience, ISBN: 0471190454, New York

Huse, D.M.; Schulman, M.A.; Orsini, L. et al. (2005). Burden of Illness in Parkinson´s Disease. *Movement Disorders*, Vol.20, No.11, pp.1449-1454, ISSN 1531-8257

Keranen, T.; Kaakkola, S.; Sotaniemi, K., et al. (2003). Economic burden and quality of life impairment increase with severity of PD. *Parkinsonism and Related Disorders*, Vol.9, No.3, pp.163 -168, ISSN 1353-8020

Krack, P.; Batir, A.; Van Blercom, N. et al. (2003). Five-year follow-up of bilateral stimulation of the subthalamic nucleus in advanced Parkinson's disease. *The New England Journal of Medicine*, Vol.349, No.20, pp.1925-1934, ISSN 1533-4406

Kulisevsky, J. (2005). *Estimulación cerebral profunda en el tratamiento de la enfermedad de Parkinson: programa de actualización*. Profármaco.2 Editions, Barcelona

Martínez-Martín, P.; Valldeoriola, F.; Tolosa, E., et al. (2002). Bilateral subthalamic nucleus stimulation and quality of life in advanced Parkinson's disease. *Movement Disorders*, Vol.17, No.2, pp.372-377, ISSN 1531-8257

Mathers, C.; Boerma, T.; Fat, D.M. et al. (2008) World Health Organisation: The Global Burden of Disease: 2004 update, 08.02.2011, Available from: <http://www.who.int/healthinfo/global_burden_disease/GBD_report_2004update_full.pdf>

McCrone, P.; Allcock, L.M. & Burn, D.J. (2007). Predicting the cost of Parkinson's disease. *Movement Disorders*, Vol.22, No.6, pp.804 -812, ISSN 1531-8257

McIntosh, E.; Gray, A. & Aziz, T. (2003). Estimating the costs of surgical innovations: the case for subthalamic nucleus stimulation in the treatment of advanced Parkinson's disease. *Movement Disorders*, Vol.18, No.9, pp.993 -999, ISSN 1531-8257

Meissner, W.; Schreiter, D.; Volkmann, J., et al. (2005). Deep brain stimulation in late stage Parkinson's disease: a retrospective cost analysis in Germany. *Journal of Neurology*, Vol.252, No.2, pp.218-223, ISSN 0340-5354

Minguez-Castellanos, A.; Escamilla-Sevilla, F.; Katati, M.J., et al. (2005). Different patterns of medication change after subthalamic or pallidal stimulation for Parkinson's disease: target related effect or selection bias?. *Journal of Neurology Neurosurgery and Psychiatry*, Vol.76, No.1, pp. 34-99, ISSN 1560-7992

Molinuevo, J.L.; Valldeoriola, F.; Tolosa, E., et al. (2000). Levodopa withdrawal after bilateral subthalamic nucleus stimulation in advanced Parkinson disease. *Archives of Neurolog,y* Vol.57, No.7, pp. 983-988, ISSN 1089-1980

Mycka, J.M.; Dellamano, R.; Kolassa, E.M., et al. (2010). Good Research Practices for Measuring Drug Costs in Cost Effectiveness Analyses:An Industry Perspective: The ISPOR Drug Cost Task Force Report—Part V. *Value in Health*, Vol.13, No.1, pp.25-27, ISSN 1524-4733

O'Brien, J.A. ; Ward, A. ; Michels, S.L. , et al. (2009). Economic burden associated with Parkinson´s disease. *Drug Benefit Trends*, Vol.21, No.6, pp.179-190, ISSN 1080-5826

Péchevis, M. ; Clarke, C.E. ; Vieregge, P., et al. (2005). Trial Study Group. Effects of dyskinesias in Parkinson's disease on quality of life and health-related costs: a prospective European study. *European Journal of Neurology*, Vol.12, No.12, pp.956-963, ISSN 1468-1331

Puig-Junoy, J. & Puig, R. (2009). Review of the economic evidence on the use of deep brain stimulation in late stage Parkinson's disease. *Neurologia*, Vol.24, No.4, pp.220-229, ISSN 0210-0010

Rodríguez-Oroz, M.C.; Obeso, J.A.; Lang, A.E., et al. (2005). Bilateral deep brain stimulation in Parkinson's disease: a multicentre study with 4 years follow-up. *Brain*, Vol.128, pp.2240-2249, ISSN 0006-8950

Schupbach, W.M.; Chastan, N.; Welter, M.L., et al. (2005). Stimulation of the subthalamic nucleus in Parkinson's disease: a 5 year follow up. *Journal of Neurology, Neurosurgery & Psychiatry*, Vol.76, No.12, pp.1640-1644, ISSN 0022-3050

Siderowf, A.; Jaggi, J.L.; Xie, S.X., et al. (2006). Long-term effects of bilateral subthalamic nucleus stimulation on health-related quality of life in advanced Parkinson's disease. *Movement Disorders*, Vol.21, No.6, pp.746 -753, ISSN 1531-8257

Simoens, S. (2006). Using the Delphi technique in economic evaluation: time to revisit the oracle?. *Journal of Clinical Pharmacy and Therapeutics*, Vol.31, No.3, pp.519-522, ISSN 1365-2710

Oblikue Consulting. (2010). Spanish Cost Database, e-salud, 08.02.2011, Available from: <. http://www.oblikue.com/bddcostes/>

Spanish National Institute of Statistics. (2010). Estimaciones de la población actual, In: Cifras de población y Censos demográficos, 31.01.2011, Available from: <http://www.ine.es/inebmenu/mnu_cifraspob.htm>

Spottke, E.A.; Volkmann, J.; Lorenz, D., et al. (2002). Evaluation of healthcare utilization and health status of patients with Parkinson's disease treated with deep brain stimulation of the subthalamic nucleus. *Journal of Neurology*, Vol.249, No.6, pp.759 - 766, ISSN 0340-5354

Stahl, J.E. (2008). Modelling Methods for Pharmacoeconomics and Health Technology Assessment. An Overview and Guide. *Pharmacoeconomics*, Vol.26, No.2, pp.131-148, ISSN 1170-7690

Sydow, O. (2008). Parkinson's disease: recent development in therapies for advanced disease with a focus on deep brain stimulation (DBS) and duodenal levodopa infusion. *Federation of European Biochemical Societies Journal*, Vol.275, No.7, pp.1370-1376, ISSN 0014-5793

Thanvi, B.; Lo, N. & Robinson, T. (2007). Levodopa-induced dyskinesia in Parkinson's disease: clinical features, pathogenesis, prevention and treatment. *Postgraduate Medical Journal*, Vol.83, Vol.980, pp.384-388, ISSN 1469-0756

Tomaszewski, K.J. & Holloway, R.G. (2001). Deep-brain stimulation in the treatment of Parkinson's disease: a cost-effectiveness analysis. *Neurology*, Vol.57, No.4, pp.663-671, ISSN 0028-3878

Valldeoriola, F.; Morsi, O.; Tolosa, E., et al. (2007). Prospective comparative study on cost-effectiveness of subthalamic stimulation and best medical treatment in advanced Parkinson's disease. *Movement Disorders*, Vol.22, No.15, pp.2183 -2191, ISSN 1531-8257

Valldeoriola, F.; Pilleri, M.; Tolosa, E., et al. (2002). Bilateral subthalamic stimulation monotherapy in advanced Parkinson's disease: long term follow-up of patients. *Movement Disorders*, Vol.17, No.1, pp.125 -132, ISSN 1531-8257

Valldeoriola, F.; Puig-Junoy, J.; Puig-Peiró,R., et al. Workgroup of the SCOPE Study. (2011) Cost analysis of Deep Brain Stimulation, Apomorphine Infusion Pumps and Continuous Duodenal Levodopa-Carbidopa Infusion in Patients with Advanced Parkinson's Disease in Spain: SCOPE Study. Submitted to *Movement Disorders*. n.d.

Weinstein, M.C.; Toy, E.L.; Sandberg, E.A, et al. (2001). Modeling for health care and other policy decisions: uses, roles, and validity. *Value in Health,* Vol.4, No.5, pp.348 -361, ISSN 1524-4733

Winter, Y.; Balzer-Geldsetzer, M.; von Campenhausen S., et al. (2010a). Trends in resource utilization for Parkinson´s disease in Germany. *Journal of the Neurological Sciences* , Vol.294, No.1-2 , pp.18-22, ISSN 0022-510X

Winter, Y.; von Campenhausen, S.; Brozova, H., et al. (2010b). Costs of Parkinson´s disease in Easern Europe: A Czech cohort study. *Parkinsonism and Related Disorders,* Vol.16, No.1, pp.51 -56, ISSN 1353-8020

Winter, Y.; von Campenhausen, S.; Popov, G., et al. (2009). Cost of Illness in a Russian Cohort of Patients with Parkinson's Disease. *Pharmacoeconomics,* Vol.27, No.7, pp.571-584, ISSN 1170-7690

Zecchinelli, A.; Cprari, F.; Ponzi, P., et al. (2003). Social costs of Parkinson's disease in Italy, *6th ISPOR Annual European Congress,* Barcelona, November 2003

3

Botulinum A Toxin Intravesical Injections in the Treatment of Refractory Overactive Bladder in Patients with Parkinson's Disease

Antonella Giannantoni, Silvia Proietti, Antonella Conte,
Massimo Porena and Alfredo Berardelli
Department of Urology and Andrology, University of Perugia
Department of Neurology and Psychiatry, Sapienza, University of Rome and IRCCS Neuromed Institute
Italy

1. Introduction

In Parkinson's disease (PD) non-motor symptoms including urinary disorders have been recognized as important features of the disease (Emre, 2003; Hely et al., 2005; Mathias, 2002; Pfeiffer, 2003; Rojo et al., 2003; Senard et al., 1997; Winge et al., 2003; Lang & Obeso, 2004). In this chapter we will review the clinical features, the pathophysiology and the treatment of urinary disturbances in PD. We will also discuss recent data on the use of intradetrusorial botulinum A toxin injections (BoNT/A) (Giannantoni et al., 2009; Giannantoni et al., 2011).

2. Parkinson's disease and neurogenic bladder

2.1 Prevalence of urinary symptoms

Earlier studies suggested that the prevalence of urinary symptoms in patients with PD ranges from 38% to 71% (Andersen 1985; Berger et al., 1987; Hald & We, 1982; Hattori et al., 1992; Porter et al., 1971) however in a number of these studies the clinical distinction between PD and other parkinsonisms, including multiple-system atrophy (MSA) was not addressed. Furthermore, some studies were based on patients presenting to urology clinics with urinary symptoms. (Berger et al., 1987; Hattori et al., 1992; Pavlakis et al., 1983). More recent studies in PD using validated questionnaires showed that the prevalence of urinary symptoms varied between 27% (Araki & Kuno, 2000a) to 39% (Campos-Sousa et al., 2003) and using a non validated questionnaire was greater than 40% (Sakakibara et al., 2001). Additionally Araki and Kuno (2000a) found a correlation between urinary disturbances and neurological disability and between severity of urinary disturbances and stages of the disease (Sakakibara et al., 2001), suggesting a relationship between dopaminergic degeneration and voiding dysfunction (Sakakibara et al., 2001).

2.2 Clinical features of urinary symptoms

Nocturia is the most prevalent lower urinary tract symptom (LUTS) reported by PD patients (>60%) (Campos-Sousa et al., 2003). Patients complain also of urgency (33%–54%)

(Araki & Kuno, 2000a; Campos Sousa et al., 2003) and frequency (16%–36%) (Araki & Kuno, 2000a; Campos Sousa et al., 2003), and urge urinary incontinence, particularly if poor mobility complicates their bladder disorder (Araki & Kuno 2000a; Campos Sousa et al., 2003; Lemack et al., 2000). Men with PD often have a coexisting benign prostatic hyperplasia worsening detrusor overactivity. In female patients overactive (urgency, frequency, urge incontinence) and obstructive (hesitancy, poor flow, dribbling) symptoms may also coexist. Evidence of bladder dysfunction in genetically determined Parkinsonism is controversial. In one study at least three cases of PARK1 α-synuclein-positive individuals were incontinent (Spira et al., 2001), while in another none of 17 patients with autosomal-recessive–type juvenile PD had bladder dysfunction (Ishikawa & Tsuji, 1996).

2.3 Neurogenic causes of bladder symptoms and voiding dysfunction in PD

There are several neurogenic causes of bladder symptoms in PD. Some Authors have suggested that an impaired relaxation or bradykinesia of the urethral sphincter can result in voiding dysfunction (Christmas et al., 1988; Galloway 1983) due to bladder outflow obstruction and, therefore, to detrusor overactivity. Studies using cystometry, however, have shown that obstructive voiding patterns are not common in PD patients (Araki et al., 2000b; Dmochowski, 1999) indicating that other mechanisms play a significant role.

3. Normal nervous control of the micturition reflex

Urinary storing and micturition rely on the interplay of a number of neural structures in the brain, spinal cord and peripheral ganglia. The complex relationship between central and peripheral pathways makes lower urinary tract (LUT) susceptible to a variety of neurologic disorders.

3.1 The role of Central Nervous System (CNS) in the control of the micturition reflex

The normal micturition reflex in the adult is mediated by a spino-bulbo-spinal pathway, which passes through relay centers in the brain. Micturition occurs in response to afferent signals from the lower urinary tract, and the distension of the bladder wall is considered the primary stimulus (de Groat et al., 1999; de Groat & Yoshimura, 2001).

During bladder filling, once threshold tension is achieved, afferent impulses, conveyed mainly by the pelvic nerve, reach the CNS. Afferent neurons send information to the periaqueductal gray, and relay with the pontine tegmentum, where two different regions involved in micturition control have been described acting independently (Blok & Holstege, 1999a, Griffiths et al., 1990). One is a dorsomedially located M-region, corresponding to Barrington's nucleus or the pontine micturition center (PMC). A more laterally located L-region may serve as a pontine urine storage center, and likely suppress bladder contraction by regulating the activity of the striated musculature of the bladder outlet during urine storage. Centers rostral to the pons control the beginning of micturition. The forebrain, therefore, even though not essential for the basic micturition reflex plays a role in determining when and where micturition should take place (Blok & Holstege, 1999b). Recent positron emission tomography studies gave further information on the brain structures involved in urine storage and voiding (Athwal et al., 2001; Blok et al., 1997; Matsuura et al., 2002; Nour et al., 2000).

3.2 Neurotransmitters mainly involved in voiding dysfunction due to Parkinson's disease

The micturition reflexes use several transmitter systems that may be targets for drugs aimed at control of micturition. Among these, dopamine and GABA pathways are fully involved in the control of micturition reflex and depletion of dopamine and GABA has been observed in Parkinson's disease.

3.2.1 Dopamine

Central dopaminergic pathways can have both facilitatory and inhibitory effects on micturition by actions on D1-like (D1 or D5) and D2-like (D2, D3, or D4) dopaminergic receptors. Patients with PD often have neurogenic detrusor over activity and voiding dysfunction (Berger et al., 1987), possibly as a consequence of nigrostriatal dopamine depletion and failure to activate inhibitory D1-like receptors (Yoshimura et al., 1993). Micturition, however, can be activated via D2-like receptors involving brainstem and spinal cord circuits. Microinjection of dopamine into the pontine micturition center reduced bladder capacity and facilitated the micturition reflex in cats (de Groat et al., 1993). Apomorphine, which stimulates both D1- and D2-like receptors, induced bladder overactivity in anesthetized rats (Sillén et al., 1981). In female rats, the role of dopamine D1 and D2 receptors in the volume induced micturition reflex, was investigated cystometrically (Seki et al., 2001) and the results, which are in agreement with previously data (de Groat & Yoshimura, 2001), suggested that D1 receptors tonically inhibit and D2 receptors facilitate the micturition reflex. In conclusion central dopaminergic pathways exhibit different effects on micturition via multiple receptors at different sites in the central nervous system.

3.2.2 GABA

GABA pathways are also involved in voiding dysfunction due to Parkinson's disease. GABA (γ-amino butyric acid) has been identified as an inhibitory transmitter at both spinal and supraspinal synapses in the mammalian CNS. At least in some species, the supraspinal micturition reflex pathway is under a tonic GABAergic inhibitory control (de Groat et al., 1993, 1999). GABA functions appear to be triggered by binding of GABA to its ionotropic receptors, GABA-A and GABA-C, which are ligand-gated chloride channels, and its metabotropic receptor, GABA-B (Chebib & Johnston, 1999). Since blockade of GABA-A and GABA-B receptors in the spinal cord (Igawa et al., 1993; Pehrson et al., 2002) and brain (Maggi et al., 1987; Pehrson et al., 2002) stimulated rat micturition, an endogenous activation of GABA-A and GABA-B receptors may be responsible for continuous inhibition of the micturition reflex within the CNS. In the spinal cord, GABA-A receptors are more numerous than GABA-B receptors, except for the dorsal horn where GABA-B receptors predominate (Malcangio and Bowery, 1996; Coggeshall and Carlton, 1997). It is well known that stimulation of the PMC results in an immediate relaxation of the external striated sphincter and a contraction of the detrusor muscle of the bladder. Blok et al. (Block et al., 1997) demonstrated in cats a direct pathway from the PMC to the dorsal gray commissure of the sacral cord. It was suggested that the pathway produced relaxation of the external striated sphincter during micturition via GABA -mediated inhibitory modulation on the urethral sphincter motoneurons in the Onuf nucleus.

4. The pathophysiology of voiding dysfunction in Parkinson's disease

The hypothesis most widely accepted is that in healthy individuals basal ganglia output has an overall inhibitory effect on the micturition reflex. In PD animal models depletion of dopaminergic neurones induces overactive bladder, (Yoshimura et al., 1993, 1998, 2003) and D1 receptor agonists produce inhibition of the micturition reflex in a dose-dependent manner while D2 receptor stimulation facilitates micturition. In PD degeneration of dopaminergic neurons in the substantia nigra leads to detrusor hyperactivity, through an inability to activate the D1-mediated tonic inhibition. A parallel mechanism may be that in PD, the inhibitory dopaminergic neurons originating in the substantia nigra may be more damaged than the excitatory dopaminergic neurons originating in the VTA, thereby inducing urgency and frequency.

Patients with PD and bladder symptoms have less uptake of [123I]-2ß-carbomethoxy-3 ß-(4-iodophenyl) tropane (ß-CIT) in the striatum than patients with PD but without bladder dysfunction, indicating a correlation between urinary dysfunction and degeneration of the nigrostriatal dopaminergic cells (Sakakibara et al., 2001). Winge and colleagues (Winge et al., 2005) recently demonstrated that the presence of bladder symptoms correlate with the decrease in the total number of dopaminergic neurones in the striatum and that the degeneration of the caudate correlates with severity of bladder symptoms. It is also possible that anti-parkinsonian medications may affect bladder function, but the results on the effects of levodopa or apomorphine are controversial. In one study, detrusor overactivity improved after administration of apomorphine and, to a lesser extent, after levodopa (Aranda & Cramer, 1993), but in patients showing on–off phenomena, detrusor overactivity improved with levodopa in some patients and worsened in others (Fitzmaurice et al., 1985). A recent study suggested that in advanced PD, levodopa exacerbates detrusor overactivity in the filling phase, but also improves bladder emptying through increased detrusor contractility (Uchiyama et al., 2003). The unpredictable effect of medication is not related to stage of disease, age, or whether the patient had symptoms of bladder dysfunction (Winge et al., 2002). In the study of Winge and colleagues (Winge et al., 2004), the authors suggested that the effects of medication are mediated through cortical mechanisms, as the ability to separate and integrate sensory input measured using urodynamics is influenced by medication.

5. Management of urinary symptoms in Parkinson's Disease

Questionnaires including "bother" scores identify LUTS in PD with higher specificity than questionnaires without "bother" scores (Winge et al., 2003). When addressing bladder problems in patients with Parkinsonism in daily clinical work, systematic interview is needed. Addressing nocturia, urgency, frequency feeling of incomplete emptying and (urge) incontinence often provides the needed information for initiating treatment. It is important to address how these symptoms affect the daily life of the patients, as symptoms of overactive bladder may be particularly unpleasant in a patient with an akinetic rigid syndrome with postural instability.

Neurogenic bladder symptoms are generally treated with anticholinergics (Andersson, 2000; Appell, 1997) including oxybutynin chloride, tolterodine tartrate, and trospium chloride and possibly also solifenacin. No placebo control double-blind or randomized studies, however, have been performed in PD. Anticholinergics can be used in PD patients with urgency and frequency since they reduce the parasympathetic effect on the bladder. Patients generally tolerate anticholinergic drugs and benefit from their use. A study in patients without neurological diseases showed that the extended release tolterodine produces less side effects than oxybutinin (Sussman & Garely, 2002; Todorova et al., 2001). Anticholinergics usually provide only modest clinical improvement and in more than 60% of treated patients they induce adverse effects such as dry mouth and constipation (Di Stasi, 2001; Winge & Fowler, 2006). Another disadvantage is that anticholinergics may induce or worsen cognitive impairment (Kay & Ebinger, 2008; Winge & Fowler, 2006). There are no studies, however, addressing the issue of possible worsening of cognitive impairment using anticholinergics in patients with PD.

6. Botulinum A toxin as second line treatment for refractory detrusor over activity and over active bladder symptoms

To date when urinary incontinence persists and patients become severely disabled a long-term indwelling catheter remains the only option for avoiding urinary incontinence. Botulinum A toxin has been successfully introduced for the treatment of intractable detrusor overactivity (Schurch et al., 2000) and it is now widely used for a number of neurological conditions characterized by muscle hyperactivity (Jankovic, 2004; Ward et al., 2006). Intravesical injections of BoNT/A provide satisfactory long-term results, and are now considered as second line-therapy in neurogenic patients who do not respond to standard anticholinergics. The use of botulinum neurotoxins in the lower urinary tract (LUT) was pioneered as early as 20 yr ago with injections into the urethral sphincter (Dykstra et al., 1988) reducing bladder-voiding pressures, urethral pressures, and post void residual (PVR) urine.

BoNT/A consists of a light chain attached to a heavy chain via a disulfide bond with an associated zinc atom. It is synthesised as a single-chain polypeptide with a molecular weight of 150 kDa, which is then cleft into its active dichain polypeptide form. The heavy chain (about 100 kDa) allows for binding to the neuron and internalisation of the toxin, whereas the light chain (about 50 kDa) actively cleaves SNAP25 (synaptosomal-associated protein with a molecular weight 25 kDa) on the protein complex that is responsible for docking and releasing vesicles containing neurotransmitters (Dolly, 2003).

In neurogenic detrusor overactivity as well as in patients with idiopathic detrusor overactivity, the post-treatment reduction in detrusor pressures during both phasic involuntary contractions and on voiding (Popat et al., 2005; Reitz et al., 2004; Schurch et al., 2005) suggests an effect of BoNT/A on the motor innervation of the detrusor, although the neurological deficit which additionally affects voiding efficiency in the NDO group may partly explain the high rate of posttreatment clean intermittent self-catheterisations (CISC). Patients, however, also report a rapid reduction in their sensations of urgency, which are associated with involuntary detrusor overactivity (Rapp et al., 2004; Schmid et al., 2006). Although the exact nature and cause of urgency remains to be elucidated, abnormal afferent activity is thought to be a significant cause of spinal NDO (Yoshimura, 1999), and much less is known about the role of afferents in IDO. In both neural and bladder tissue, BoNT/A affected the release of numerous sensory transmitters other than ACh, including adenosine triphosphate (ATP), substance P, calcitonin gene related peptide (CGRP), and glutamate. BoNT/A may also interfere with vesicle trafficking (Apostolidis et al., 2006), expression of sensory receptors (Apostolidis et al., 2005) and nerve growth factor (NGF) in the bladder wall (Giannantoni et al., 2006). It is therefore likely that in addition to a direct effect on detrusor motor innervation, BoNT/A also modulates intrinsic bladder reflexes through a multimodal effect on sensory pathways.

In neurogenic patients it has been demonstrated that BoNT/A decrease symptoms of neurogenic detrusor overactivity. The majority of treated patients had spinal neurogenic detrusor overactivity due to spinal cord injury or multiple sclerosis. Despite heterogeneous designs, almost all single-injection published studies showed significant improvements in outcomes measures including frequency of incontinence episodes, maximum cystometric capacity and maximum detrusor pressure. In spinal NDO patients the mean percentage of those who became fully continent was 56.6% (range: 30–87%) whereas the rate of full return to continence was only 8% in patients with NDO due to cerebrovascular accident. After a rapid onset of effect (Kalsi et al., 2008), the mean duration of efficacy in single-injection studies was 8 months (range: 12–36 wk). Repeated treatments showed sustained clinical benefits in open-label studies using up to five injections of Botox or seven injections of Dysport (Del Popolo et al., 2008; Grosse et al., 2005; Karsenty et al., 2006, Reitz et al., 2007).

7. Botulinum A toxin in the treatment of refractory detrusor overactivity and overactive bladder symptoms due to Parkinson's disease

Since 2000 we have been using BoNT/A as second line therapy for refractory overactive bladder symptoms and detrusor overactivity (DO) of both neurogenic and non-neurogenic origin. Here we review the results of our open label, prospective, non randomized study on the use of BoNT/A in patients with Parkinson's disease affected by intractable overactive bladder (OAB) symptoms and DO (Giannantoni et al., 2009, Giannatoni et al., 2011).

7.1 Patients and methods

Seventeen patients diagnosed with PD according to United Kingdom Brain Bank criteria and affected by overactive bladder symptoms and DO were enrolled in a prospective study. They were all refractory to standard anticholinergic therapy. Disease severity was assessed with the Unified Parkinson's Disease Rating Scale and Hoehn-Yahr stages 1 to 5. All patients had moderate-severe disability. Patients were studied while they were on their usual drug regimens for PD. Exclusion criteria were urogenital prolapsed in females, bladder outlet obstruction due to benign prostatic hyperplasia in men and recurrent urinary tract infections. No patients were on anticoagulant therapy or drugs interfering with neuromuscular transmission. The study was approved by the local ethics committee and patients provided informed consent. Patients unwilling or unable to perform intermittent catheterization, were excluded from the study. We used 150 ml as a cutoff residual volume for starting intermittent bladder catheterization.

7.2 Preliminary urological assessment

History, physical examination, serum laboratory tests, urinalysis, urine culture and urinary tract imaging by ultrasound were performed before commencing the study. The daily frequency of urinary symptoms was assessed with a voiding diary that patients completed for 30 days before the study. Patients were also asked to complete a standardized QoL questionnaire on urinary incontinence (I-QoL). Patients underwent urodynamics, including pressure flow studies and the recording of the electromyographic activity of pelvic floor muscle and external urethral sphincter, according to International Continence Society

Standards. During cystometry first volume and maximum pressure of uninhibited detrusor contractions (UDC) and maximum cystometric capacity were recorded. On pressure flow study detrusor pressure at maximum flow rate (pDetQmax), maximum flow rate (Qmax) and postvoid residual volume were monitored. All patients received a single treatment with BoNT/A (Botox, Allergan, Irvine-CA, USA) diluted in normal saline injected into the detrusor muscle. The trigone, the posterior and lateral walls of the bladder have been injected during cystoscopy, under short lasting general anaesthesia. Six out of the seventeen patients received 200 UI of BoNT/A, whereas eleven of the seventeen PD patients received 100 UI of BoNT/A. Primary outcome measures were: changes in day-time and night-time urinary frequency and frequency of daily urinary incontinence episodes and in I-QoL questionnaire; secondary outcomes were changes on the impact of urinary symptoms in daily life activities was evaluated with VAS scores and in urodynamic parameters. Clinical, urodynamic and I-QoL and VAS were performed before, one, three and six months after BoNT/A injection. Urinalysis and culture were performed also at the same time intervals.

7.3 Statistical analysis

Friedman's repeated measures ANOVA was used to evaluate changes in the clinical scores and urodynamic findings of PD patients. Wilcoxon's test was performed for the post-hoc analysis. Pearson's correlation coefficient was also applied and Holm's correction for multiple comparisons was used to disclose false significance. $P<0.05$ was considered to indicate statistical significance.

7.4 Clinical results

Before treatment all seventeen patients complained of increased daytime (9.29±0.3 episodes/day) and night-time urinary frequency (4.11±0.6 episodes/night) and daily episodes of urinary incontinence (5.05±0.2 episodes/day). They also had urgency and low I-QoL scores (22.8±2) and VAS scores (3.3±0.1). After BoNT/A treatment daytime and night-time urinary frequency and the number of daily episodes of urinary incontinence were significantly reduced (daytime urinary frequency: $p<0.0001$; night-time urinary frequency: $p=0.002$; daily urinary incontinence episodes: $p=0.001$) (Fig.1) at one, three and six months follow up. Six out seventeen patients achieved a complete urinary continence at one and 3-mos follow up. After BoNT/A treatment there was also a significant improvement in the I-QoL and VAS scores after BoNT/A (I-QoL: $p<0.0001$; VAS: $p<0.0002$) at one, three and six months. Finally, we did not find any significant difference between the improvement observed in daytime and night-time urinary frequency, in the number of episodes of daily urinary incontinence and in the I-QoL and VAS scores in PD patients who received 100 UI with that obtained in patients treated with 200 UI of BoNT/A ($p>0.05$). Clinical results are showed in Fig.1.

7.5 Urodynamic results

Baseline: all the patients showed detrusor overactivity; mean values of UDC-first volume UDC-p max and maximum cystometric capacity were 219±20ml, 30±2cmH20 and 265±16ml, respectively. On pressure-flow studies, mean values of pDetQmax and Qmax were 22.3±2 cmH_2O and 18.3±1.5ml/sec, respectively. All patients completely emptied their bladders.
After BoNT/A treatment, we observed a significant decrease in the first volume and the maximum pressure of uninhibited detrusor contractions and a significant increase in

maximum cystometric capacity at one, three and six months after treatment. Changes in these parameters were similar in both groups of PD patients (Fig.2). With regards to post-void residual volume, it was similar in PD patients receiving 100 and 200 UI of BoNT/A at one month, whereas it returned to baseline values only in PD patients receiving 100 UI at three and six months after BoNT/A injection. Overall, three patients needed to perform intermittent catheterization twice daily for 3 months due to a high increase in post void residual volume after BoNT/A injection.

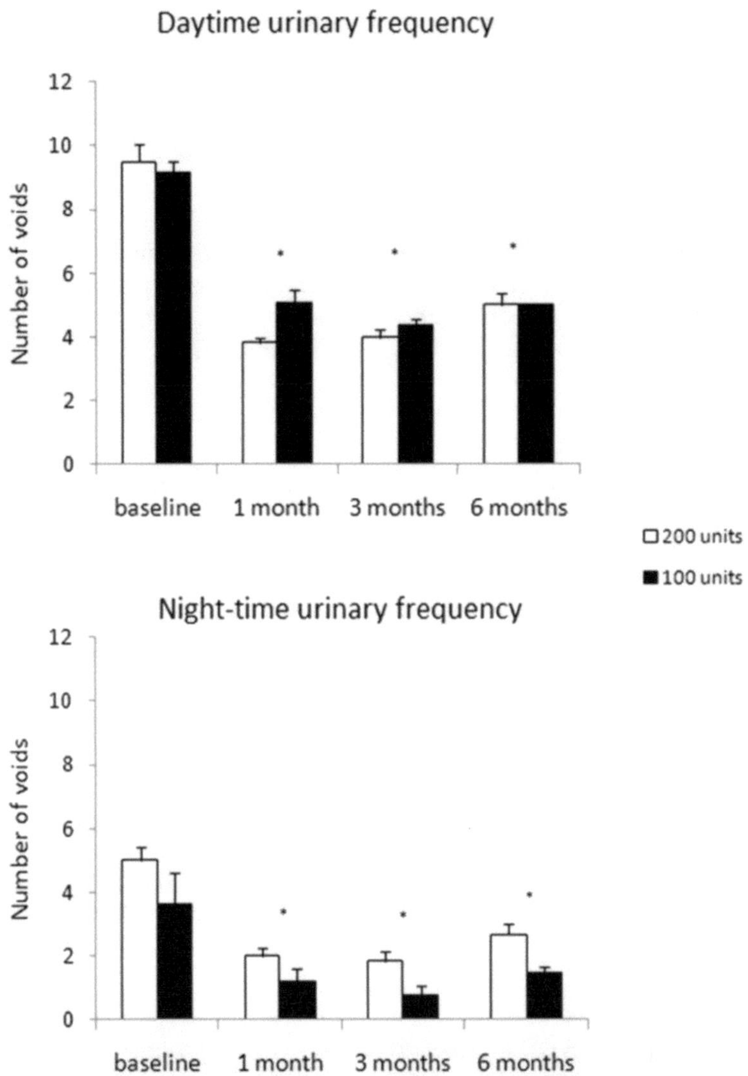

Fig. 1. Daytime urinary frequency (upper panel) and night-time urinary frequency (lower panel) in patients with Parkinson's disease at baseline, one, three and six months after BoNT/A injection. Open bars represent mean data ±SE in patients injected with 200 units, closed bars data in patients injected with 100 units. Asterisks indicate statistical significance

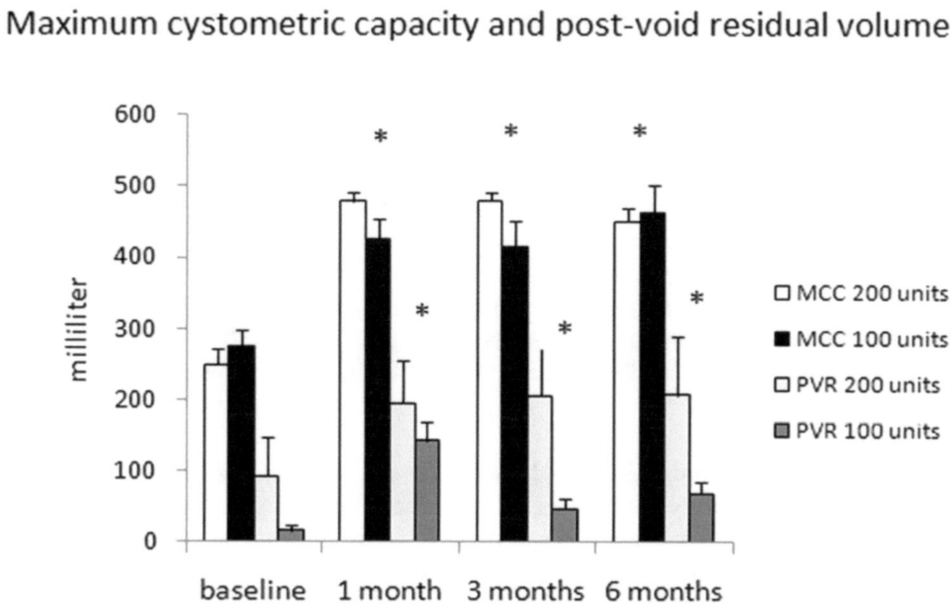

Fig. 2. Maximum cystometric capacity and post-void residual volume in patients with Parkinson's disease at baseline, one, three and six months after BoNT/A injection. Each bar represents mean data ±SE in patients injected with 200 units and 100 units. Asterisks indicate statistical significance.

7.6 Correlations between clinical and urodynamic variables

Changes in the I-QoL significantly correlated with daytime urinary frequency ($r=-0.69$, $p=0.002$) in all the PD patients.

7.7 Discussion

In our PD patients, BoNT/A intradetrusorial injection induced a significant reduction in daytime and night-time urinary frequency and in the frequency of urinary incontinence, an increase in the quality of life scores and a significant amelioration in urodynamic parameters. The follow-up assessment extends our previous findings at three months (Giannantoni et al., 2009) by showing that the BoNT/A-induced clinical and urodynamic improvement lasts at least six months (Giannantoni et al., 2011). We also noted that clinical and urodynamic amelioration was similar when comparing patients treated with 100 UI of BoNT/A with those treated with 200 UI. Worth of noting, incomplete voiding symptoms were unrelated to the BoNT/A dosage used. Also patients with multiple sclerosis treated with 100 Units and patients with idiopathic overactive bladder treated with 200 and 300 units of BoNT/A showed an increase in post-void residual volume (Flynn et al., 2009; Mehnert et al., 2010; Sahai et al., 2009). Our results on post-void residual volume are in contrast with those reported by Kulaksizoglu and Parman (Kulaksizoglu & Parman, 2010) who treated parkinsonian patients with Dysport 500 Units. In their series none of the patients studied needed intermittent catheterization. Despite of the presence of post-void residual volume in our PD patients, we did not observe a significant reduction in other parameters accounting for detrusor muscle strength (PdetQmax, Qmax). It is well known that BoNT/A induces striated muscle denervation and weakness lasting about 3-4 months (Hamjian et al., 1994; Schiavo et al., 1994). In striated muscle it has been observed that the neurotoxin not only modulates extra-fusal component but also influences the altered muscle spindle afferent input (Abbruzzese et al., 2006; Currà & Berardelli, 2009; Rosales & Dressler, 2010; Trompetto et al., 2008). In detrusor smooth muscle the effects of BoNT/A injection last longer than in striated muscle. In vitro and in vivo experimental studies suggest that the long-lasting effect of the BoNT/A injection in the detrusor muscle could be attributed to the lack of axonal sprouting, as observed in detrusor biopsies after toxin injection (Haferkamp et al., 2004). Studies on biopsies from patients with neurogenic overactive bladder who receive an intradetrusor BoNT/A injection (Apostolidis et al., 2006; Giannantoni et al., 2006), however, have shown decreased levels of sensory receptors P2X3, TRPV1 and NGF, thereby suggesting that BoNT/A may act by reducing the afferent nervous transmission.

7.8 Conclusions

PD patients with OAB symptoms and detrusor overactivity refractory to standard treatments can be successfully treated with intravesical injections of BoNT/A. Low doses (100 U BoNT/A) induces similar clinical and urodynamic efficacy as higher doses of the neurotoxin. The reported increase in post void residual volume is present only in some patients and lasts for a limited time. Low doses of BoNT/A can be used as second-line treatment for OAB symptoms and DO also in patients with PD.

8. References

Abbruzzese, G. & Berardelli, A.(2006). Neurophysiological effects of botulinum toxin type A. Neurotox Res,Vol. 9, pp. 109-114.

Andersen, JT. (1985). Disturbances of bladder and urethral function in Parkinson's disease. Int Urol Nephrol, Vol. 17, pp. 35- 41.

Andersson, KE. (2000). Treatment of overactive bladder: other drug mechanisms. Urology, Vol. 55, pp. 51–57.

Andersson, KE. (2002). Bladder activation: afferent mechanisms. Urology, Vol. 59, Suppl. 1, pp. 43-50.

Apostolidis, A.; Popat, R.; Yiangou, Y., Cockayne, D.; Ford, A.P.; Davis, J.B.; Dasgupta; P.; Fowler, J.C. & Anand, P. (2005). Decreased sensory receptors P2x3 and Trpv1 in suburothelial nerve fibers following intradetrusor injections of botulinum toxin for human detrusor overactivity. J Urol, Vol. 174, pp. 977–83.

Apostolidis, A.; Dasgupta, P. & Fowler, C.J. (2006). Proposed mechanism for the efficacy of injected botulinum toxin in the treatment of human detrusor overactivity. Eur Urol, Vol 49, pp.644–50.

Appell, R.A. (1997). Clinical efficacy and safety of tolterodine in the treatment of overactive bladder: a pooled analysis. Urology, Vol 50, pp. 90– 96.

Araki, I. & Kuno, S. (2000a). Assessment of voiding dysfunction in Parkinson's disease by the international prostate symptom score. J Neurol Neurosurg Psychiatry, Vol 68, pp. 429–433.

Araki, I.; Kitahara, M.; Oida, T. & Kuno, S. (2000b). Voiding dysfunction and parkinson's disease: urodynamic abnormalities and urinary symptoms. J Urol, Vol 164, pp. 1640 –1643.

Aranda, B.; Perrigot, M.; Mazieres, L.& Pierrot-Deseilligny, E. (1983). Bladder sphincter disorders in Parkinson's disease. Rev Neurol, Vol 139, pp. 283–288.

Aranda, B.& Cramer, P. (1993). Effects of apomorphine and L-dopa on the parkinsonian bladder. Neurourol Urodyn, Vol 12, pp. 203–209.

Athwal, B.S.; Berkley, K.J.; Hussain, I.; Brennan, A.; Craggs, M.; Sakakibara, R., Frackowiak, R.S.& Fowler, C.J. (2001). Brain responses to changes in bladder volume and urge to void in healthy men. Brain, Vol 124, pp. 369–377.

Berger, .Y; Blaivas, J.G.; DeLaRocha, E.R.& Salinas, J.M. (1987). Urodynamic findings in Parkinson's disease. J Urol, Vol 138,pp.836–838.

Birder, L.A. & De Groat, W.C. (1992) The effect of glutamate antagonists on c-fos expression induced in spinal neurons by irritation of the lower urinary tract. Brain Res, Vol 580, pp.115–120.

Blok, B.F. & Holstege, G. (1999) Two pontine micturition centers in the cat are not interconnected directly: implications for the central organization of micturition. J Comp Neurol, Vol 403, pp.209–218.

Blok, B.F. & Holstege, G. (1999b) The central control of micturition and continence: implications for urology. BJU Int,Vol 83,Suppl 2, pp. 1–6

Blok, B.F., De Weerd H.& Holstege, G. (1997a). The pontine micturition centre projects to sacral cord GABA immunoreactive neurons in the cat. Neurosci Lett, Vol 233, pp.109–112.-

Blok, B.F., Willemsen, A.T., & Holstege, G. (1997b). A PET study on brain control of micturition in humans. Brain, Vol 120, pp. 111–121.

Campos-Sousa, R.N.; Quagliato, E.; Da Silva, B.B.; De CR, J.R.; Ribeiro, S.C.& De Carvalho, D.F. (2003). Urinary symptoms in Parkinson's disease: prevalence and associated factors. Arq Neuropsiquiatr, Vol 61, pp.359–363.

Chebib, M. & Johnston, G.A.R. (1999). The 'ABC' of GABA receptors: a brief review. Clin Exp Pharmacol Physiol, Vol 26, pp.937–940.

Christmas, T.J.; Kempster, P.A.; Chapple, C.R.; Frankel, J.P.; Lees, A.J.; Stern, G.M. & Milroy, E.J.(1988). Role of subcutaneous apomorphine in parkinsonian voiding dysfunction. Lancet, Vol 2, pp. 1451–1453.

Coggeshall, R.E.& Carlton, S.M. (1997). Receptor localization in the mammalian dorsal horn and primary afferent neurons. Brain Res Brain Res Rev, Vol 24, pp. 28–66.

Currà, A. & Berardelli, A. (2009). Do the unintended actions of botulinum toxin at distant sites have clinical implications? Neurology, Vol 72, pp. 1095-9.

de Groat, W.C. & Yoshimura, N. (2001). Pharmacology of the lower urinary tract. Annu Rev Pharmacol Toxicol, Vol 41, pp. 691–721.

Del Popolo, G.; Filocamo M.T.; Li Marzi, V.; Macchiarella, A.; Cecconi, F.; Lombardi, G. & Nicita, G. (2008). Neurogenic detrusor overactivity treated with English botulinum toxin A: 8-year experience of one single centre. Eur Urol, Vol. 53, pp.1013–1020.

Di Stasi, S.M.; Giannantoni, A.; Vespasiani, G.; Navarra, P.; Capelli, G.; Massoud, R.& Stephen, R.L.(2001).Intravesical electromotive administration of oxybutynin in patients with detrusor hyperreflexia unresponsive to standard anticholinergic regimens. J Urol, Vol 165, pp. 491-.498

Dmochowski, R.R.(1999) Female voiding dysfunction and movement disorders. Int Urogynecol J Pelvic Floor Dysfunct Vol 10, pp. 144–151.

Dolly, O. (2003). Synaptic transmission: inhibition of neurotransmitter release by botulinum toxins. Headache, Vol 43, Suppl. 1, pp. 16-24.

Dykstra, D.D.; Sidi, A.A.; Scott, A.B.; Pagel, J.M. & Goldish, G.D.(1988). Effects of botulinum A toxin on detrusor-sphincter dyssynergia in spinal cord injury patients. J Urol, Vol 139, pp.919–922.

Emre, M.(2003). Dementia associated with Parkinson's disease. Lancet Neurol Vol 2, pp. 229 –237.

Fitzmaurice, H.; Fowler, C.J.; Rickards, D.; Kirby, R.S. ; Quinn, N.P. ; Marsden, C.D. ; Milroy, E.J. & Turner-Warwick, R.T. (1985). Micturition disturbance in Parkinson's disease. Br J Urol, Vol 57, pp. 652– 656.

Fowler, C.J.(2007) Update of the neurology of Parkinson's disease. Neurourol Urodyn, Vol 26, pp.103-109.

Flynn, M.K.; Amundsen, C.L.; Perevich, M.; Liu, F. & Webster, G.D. (2009). Outcome of a randomized, double-blind, placebo controlled trial of botulinum A toxin for refractory overactive bladder. J Urol, Vol. 181, pp. 2608-2615.

Gray, R.; Stern, G.& Malone-Lee, J. (1995). Lower urinary tract dysfunction in Parkinson's disease: changes relate to age and not disease. Age Ageing, Vol. 24, pp.499 –504.

Galloway NT. (1983). Urethral sphincter abnormalities in parkinsonism. Br J Urol, Vol. 55, pp. 691– 693.

Griffiths, D.; Holstege, G.; Dalm, X. & De Wall, H. (1990). Control and coordination of bladder and urethral function in the brainstem of the cat. Neurourol Urodyn,Vol. 9, pp.63–82.

Giannantoni, A.; Di Stasi, S.M.; Nardicchi, V.; Zucchi, A.; Macchioni, L.; Bini, V.; Goracci, G.& Porena, M.(2006). Botulinum-A toxin injections into the detrusor muscle decrease nerve growth factor bladder tissue levels in patients with neurogenic detrusor overactivity. J Urol, Vol. 175, pp. 2341–2344.

Giannantoni, A.; Rossi, A.; Mearini, E.; Del Zingaro, M.; Porena, M. & Berardelli, A. (2009). Botulinum toxin A for overactive bladder and detrusor muscle overactivity in patients with Parkinson's disease and multiple system atrophy. J Urol, Vol.182, pp. 1453-1457.

Giannantoni, A.; Conte, A.; Proietti, S.; Giovannozzi, S.; Rossi, A.; Fabbrini, G.; Porena, M. & Berardelli, A. (2011) Botulinum Toxin Type A in Patients With Parkinson's Disease and Refractory Overactive Bladder. J Urol, 2011 Jul 24 [Epub ahead of print]

Grosse, J.; Kramer, G. & Stöhrer, M. (2005). Success of repeat detrusor injections of botulinum A toxin in patients with severe neurogenic detrusor overactivity and incontinence. Eur Urol, Vol. 47, pp. 653–659.

Haferkamp, A.; Schurch, B.; Reitz, A.; Krengel, U.; Grosse, J.; Kramer, G.; Schumacher, S.; Bastian, P.J.; Büttner, R. & Müller, S.C. (2004). Lack of ultrastructural detrusor changes following endoscopic injection of botulinum toxin type A in overactive neurogenic bladder. Eur Urol, Vol. 46, 784-791.

Hald, T. & WE, B. (1982). The urinary bladder, neurology and dynamics. Baltimore, MD: Williams and Wilkins

Hattori, T.; Yasuda, K.; Kita, K.& Hirayama, K. (1992). Voiding dysfunction in Parkinson's disease. Jpn J Psychiatry Neurol, Vol. 46, pp. 181–186.

Hamjian, J.A.& Walker, F.O.(1994) Serial neurophysiological studies of intramuscular botulinum-A toxin in humans. Muscle Nerve, Vol. 17, pp. 1385-1392.

Hely, M.A.; Morris, J.G.; Reid, W.G.& Trafficante, R. (2005). Sydney multicenter study of Parkinson's disease: non—L-dopa–responsive problems dominate at 15 years. Mov Disord, Vol. 20, pp. 190 –199.

Hughes, A.J.; Daniel, S.E.; Kilford, L. & Lees, A.J. (1992). Accuracy of clinical diagnosis of idiopathic Parkinson's disease: a clinico-pathological study of 100 cases. J Neurol Neurosurg Psychiatry, Vol. 55, pp. 181-184.

Igawa, Y.; Mattiasson, A.& Andersson, K.E. (1993). Effects of GABA-receptor stimulation and blockade on micturition in normal rats and rats with bladder outflow obstruction. J Urol, Vol. 150, pp. 537–542.

Ishikawa, A. & Tsuji, S. (1996). Clinical analysis of 17 patients in 12 Japanese families with autosomal-recessive type juvenile parkinsonism. Neurology, Vol. 47, pp. 160 –166.

Jankovic, J. (2004). Botulinum toxin in clinical practice. J Neurol Neurosurg Psychiatry, Vol 7, pp. 951-957

Kalsi, V.; Apostolidis, A.; Gonzales ,G.; Elneil, S.; Dasgupta, P. & Fowler, C.J. (2008). Early effect on the overactive bladder symptoms following botulinum neurotoxin type A injections for detrusor overactivity. Eur Urol, Vol.54, pp.181–187.

Karsenty, G.; Reitz, A.; Lindemann, G.; Boy, S. & Schurch, B. (2006). Persistence of therapeutic effect after repeated injections of botulinum toxin type A to treat incontinence due to neurogenic detrusor overactivity. Urology, Vol. 68, pp. 1193–1197.

Kay, G.G. & Ebinger, U. (2008). Preserving cognitive function for patients with overactive bladder: evidence for a differential effect with darifenacin. Int J Clin Pract, Vol 62, pp. 1792-1800.

Kulaksizoglu, H. & Parman, Y.(2010). Use of botulinum toxin-A for the treatment of overactive bladder symptoms in patients with Parkinson's disease. Parkinsonism Relat Disord, Vol.16, pp. 531-534.

Lang, A.E. & Obeso, J.A. (2004). Challenges in Parkinson's disease: restoration of the nigrostriatal dopamine system is not enough. Lancet Neurol, Vol 3, pp.309 –316.

Lemack, G.E.; Dewey, R.B.; Roehrborn, C.G.; O'Suilleabhain, P.E. & Zimmern, P.E. (2000). Questionnaire-based assessment of bladder dysfunction in patients with mild to moderate Parkinson's disease.Urology, Vol. 56, pp.250 –254.

Maggi, C.A.; Furio, M.; Santicioli, P.; Conte, B & Meli, A. (1987). Spinal and supraspinal components of GABAergic inhibition of the micturition reflex in rats. J Pharmacol Exp Ther, Vol 240, pp. 998–1005.

Malcangio, M. & Bowery, N.G. (1996). GABA and its receptors in the spinal cord. Trends Pharmacol Sci 17:457–462.

Mathias, C.J. (2002). Neurodegeneration, parkinsonian syndromes and autonomic failure. Auton Neurosci, Vol. 96, pp.50 –58.

Matsuura, S.; Kakizaki, H.; Mitsui, T.; Shiga, T.; Tamaki, N. & Koyanagi, T. (2002). Human brain region response to distention or cold stimulation of the bladder: a positron emission tomography study. J Urol, Vol. 168, pp. 2035–2039.

Mehnert, U.; Birzele, J.; Reuter, K. & Schurch, B. (2010). The effect of botulinum toxin type A on overactive bladder symptoms in patients with multiple sclerosis: a pilot study. J Urol, Vol 184, pp.1011-1016.

Nour, S.; Svarer, C.; Kristensen, J.K.; Paulson, O.B. & Law, I.(2000). Cerebral activation during micturition in normal men. Brain, Vol 123, pp. 781–789

O'Donnell, P.D. (1990). Central actions of bethanechol on the urinary bladder in dogs.J Urol, Vol 143, pp. 634–637.

Pavlakis, A.J.; Siroky, M.B.; Goldstein, I. & Krane, R.J. (1983). Neurourologic findings in Parkinson's disease. J Urol, Vol. 129, pp. 80–83.

Pehrson, R.; Lehmann, A.& Andersson, K.E. (2002) Effects of gamma-aminobutyrate B receptor modulation on normal micturition and oxyhemoglobin induced detrusor overactivity in female rats. J Urol, Vol.168, pp. 2700–2705.

Pfeiffer, R.F. (2003). Gastrointestinal dysfunction in Parkinson's disease. Lancet Neurol, Vol. 2, pp.107–116.

Popat, R.; Apostolidis, A.; Kalsi, V.; Gonzales, G.; Fowler, C.J. & Dasgupta, P. (2005). A comparison between the response of patients with idiopathic detrusor overactivity and neurogenic detrusor overactivity to the first intradetrusor injection of botulinum-A toxin. J Urol, Vol.174, pp.984–988.

Porter, R.W. & Bors, E. (1971) Neurogenic bladder in parkinsonism: effect of thalamotomy. J Neurosurg, Vol. 34, pp. 27–32.

Rapp, D.E.; Lucioni, A.; Katz, E.E.; O'Connor, R.C.; Gerber, G.S. & Bales, G.T. (2004). Use of botulinum-A toxin for the treatment of refractory overactive bladder symptoms: an initial experience. Urology, Vol 63, pp. 1071–1075.

Reitz, A.; Stö hrer, M.; Kramer, G.; Del Popolo, G.; Chartier-Kastler, E.; Panneck, J.; Burgdörfer, H.; Göcking K.; Madersbacher, H.; Schumacher, S.; Richter, R.; von Tobel, J. & Schurch, B. (2004).European experience of 200 cases treated with botulinum-A toxin injections into the detrusor muscle for urinary incontinence due to neurogenic detrusor overactivity. Eur Urol, Vol. 45, pp.510–515.

Reitz, A.; Denys, P.; Fermanian, C.; Schurch, B.; Comperat, E. & Chartier-Kastler, E. (2007). Do repeat intradetrusor botulinum toxin type A injections yield valuable results? Clinical and urodynamic results after five injections in patients with neurogenic detrusor overactivity. Eur Urol, Vol. 52, pp. 1729–35.

Rojo, A.; Aguilar, M.; Garolera, M.T.; Cubo, E.; Navas, I. & Quintana, S. (2003). Depression in Parkinson's disease: clinical correlates and outcome.Parkinsonism Relat Disord, Vol. 10, pp. 23–28.

Rosales, R.L. & Dressler, D. (2010). On muscle spindles, dystonia and botulinum toxin. Eur J Neurol, Vol. 17, pp. 71-80.

Sahai, A.; Dowson, C.; Khan, M.S.& Dasgupta, P. (2009). Improvement in quality of life after botulinum toxin-A injections for idiopathic detrusor overactivity: results from a randomized double-blind placebo-controlled trial. BJU Int, Vol. 103, pp. 1509-1515.

Sakakibara, R.; Shinotoh, H.; Uchiyama, T.; Yoshiyama, M.; Hattori, T. & Yamanishi, T. (2001). SPECT imaging of the dopamine transporter with [(123)I]-beta-CIT reveals marked decline of nigrostriatal dopaminergic function in Parkinson's disease with urinary dysfunction. J Neurol Sci, Vol 187, pp. 55 -59.

Sakakibara, R.; Shinotoh, H.; Uchiyama, T.; Sakuma, M.; Kashiwado, M.; Yoshiyama, M. & Hattori, T. (2001). Questionnaire-based assessment of pelvic organ dysfunction in Parkinson's disease. Auton Neurosci, Vol. 92, pp. 76-85.

Schiavo, G.; Rossetto, O.; Benfenati, F.; Poulain, B. & Montecucco, C. (1994). Tetanus and botulinum neurotoxins are zinc proteases specific for components of the neuroexocytosis apparatus. Ann NY Acad Sci, Vol. 710, pp. 65-75.

Schurch, B.; Stohrer, M.; Kramer, G.; Schmid, D.M.; Gaul, G. & Hauri, D. (2000). Botulinum-A toxin for treating detrusor hyperreflexia in spinal cord injured patients: a new alternative to anticholinergic drugs? Preliminary results. J Urol, Vol. 164, pp. 692–697.

Schurch, B.; de Sèze, M.; Denys, P.; Chartier-Kastler, E.; Haab, F.; Everaert, K.; Plante, P.; Perrouin-Verbe, B.; Kumar, C.; Fraczek, S. & Brin, M.F. (2005). Botulinum toxin type A is a safe and effective treatment for neurogenic urinary incontinence: results of a single treatment, randomized, placebo controlled 6-mo study. J Urol, Vol. 174, pp. 196–200.

Schmid, D.M.; Sauermann, P.; Werner, M.; Schuessler, B.; Blick, N.; Muentener, M.; Strebel, R.T.; Perucchini, D.; Scheiner, D.; Schaer, G.; John, H.; Reitz, A.; Hauri, D.& Schurch, B. (2006). Experience with 100 cases treated with botulinum-A toxin injections in the detrusor muscle for idiopathic overactive bladder syndrome refractory to anticholinergics. J Urol, Vol 176, pp. 177–185.

Seki, S.; Igawa, Y.; Kaidoh, K.; Ishizuka, O.; Nishizawa, O. & Andersson, K.E. (2001). Role of dopamine D1 and D2 receptors in the micturition reflex in conscious rats. Neurourol Urodyn, Vol. 20, pp.105–113.

Senard, J.M.; Rai, S.; Lapeyre-Mestre, M.; Brefel, C.; Rascol, O.; Rascol, A. & Montastruc, J.L. (1997). Prevalence of orthostatic hypotension in Parkinson's disease. J Neurol Neurosurg Psychiatry, Vol 63, pp. 584–589.

Sille´n, U.; Rubenson, A. & Hja¨lmås, K. (1981). On the localization and mediation of the centrally induced hyperactive urinary bladder response to L-dopa in the rat. Acta Physiol Scand, Vol 112, pp. 137–140

Spira, P.J.; Sharpe, D.M.; Halliday, G.; Cavanagh, J. & Nicholson, G.A. (2001). Clinical and pathological features of a parkinsonian syndrome in a family with an Ala53Thr alpha-synuclein mutation. Ann Neurol, Vol. 49, pp. 313–319.

Stöhrer, M.; Goepel, M.; Kondo, A.; Kramer, G.; Madersbacher, H.; Millard, R.; Rossier, A & Wyndaele, J.J. (1999).The standardization of terminology in neurogenic lower urinary tract dysfunction: with suggestions for diagnostic procedures. International Continence Society Standardization Committee. Neurourol Urodyn, Vol 18, pp.139-158.

Sussman, D. & Garely, A. (2002). Treatment of overactive bladder with once-daily extended-release tolterodine or oxybutynin: the antimuscarinic clinical effectiveness trial (ACET). Curr Med Res Opin, Vol. 18, pp. 177–184.

Todorova, A.; Vonderheid-Guth, B. & Dimpfel, W. (2001). Effects of tolterodine, trospium chloride, and oxybutynin on the central nervous system. J Clin Pharmacol, Vol. 41, pp.636–644.

Trompetto, C.; Currà, A.; Buccolieri, A.; Suppa, A.; Abbruzzese, A. & Berardelli, A. (2006). Botulinum toxin changes intrafusal feedback in dystonia: a study with the tonic vibration reflex. Mov Disord, Vol. 21, pp. 777-782.

Trompetto, C.; Bove, M.; Avanzino, L.; Francavilla, G.; Berardelli, A. & Abbruzzese G. (2008). Intrafusal effects of botulinum toxin in post-stroke upper limb spasticity. Eur J Neurol, Vol 15, pp.367-370.

Uchiyama, T.; Sakakibara, R.; Hattori, T.; Yamanishi, T. (2003). Short-term effect of a single levodopa dose on micturition disturbance in Parkinson's disease patients with the wearing-off phenomenon. Mov Disord, Vol 18, pp. 573–578.

Wagner, T.H.; Patrick, D.L.; Bavendam, T.G. et al. (1996). Quality of life of persons with urinary incontinence: development of a new measure. Urology, Vol 47, pp. 67-71.

Ward, A.B.; Molenaers, G.; Colosimo, C. & Berardelli, A. (2006). Clinical value of botulinum toxin in neurological indications. Eur J Neurol, Vol. 13, Suppl. 4, pp. 20-26.

Winge, K.; Werdelin, L.M.; Krøyer, K. & Stimpel, H. (2002). Bladder dysfunction in young patients with Parkinson's disease. Mov Disord, Vol 17, Suppl. 5, S 218.

Winge K.; Rasmussen, D.; Werdelin, L.M..(2003). Constipation in neurological diseases. J Neurol Neurosurg Psychiatry, Vol 74, pp. 13–19.

Winge, K.; Werdelin, L.M.; Nielsen, K.K & Stimpel, H. (2004). Effects of dopaminergic treatment on bladder function in Parkinson's disease. Neurourol Urodyn, Vol. 23, pp. 689–696.

Winge, K.; Friberg, L.; Werdelin, L.; Nielsen, K.K. & Stimpel, H. (2005). Relationship between nigrostriatal dopaminergic degeneration, urinary symptoms, and bladder control in Parkinson's disease. Eur J Neurol, Vol 12, pp. 842– 850

Winge, K. & Fowler, C.J. (2006). Bladder dysfunction in Parkinsonism: mechanism, prevalence, symptoms and management. Mov Disord, Vo 21, pp 737-745.

Yoshimura, N.; Mizuta, E.; Kuno, S.; Sasa, M.& Yoshida, O. (1993). The dopamine D1 receptor agonist SKF 38393 suppresses detrusor hyperreflexia in the monkey with parkinsonism induced by 1-methyl-4- phenyl-1,2,3,6-tetrahydropyridine (MPTP). Neuropharmacology, Vol 32, pp. 315–321.

Yoshimura, N. ; Mizuta, E. ; Yoshida, O. & Kuno, S. (1998). Therapeutic effects of dopamine D1/D2 receptor agonists on detrusor hyperreflexia in 1-methyl-4-phenyl-1,2,3,6-tetrahydropyridine-lesioned parkinsonian cynomolgus monkeys. J Pharmacol Exp Ther, Vol 286, pp. 228–233.

Yoshimura, N. (1999). Bladder afferent pathway and spinal cord injury: possible mechanisms inducing hyperreflexia of the urinary bladder. Prog Neurobiol, Vol. 57, pp. 583–606.

Yoshimura, N.; Kuno, S.; Chancellor, M.B.; de Groat, W.C. & Seki, S. (2003). Dopaminergic mechanisms underlying bladder hyperactivity in rats with a unilateral 6-hydroxydopamine (6-OHDA) lesion of the nigrostriatal pathway. Br J Pharmacol, Vol 139, pp. 1425–1432.

Part 2

Models of Disease

Alpha-Synuclein and the Immune Response in Parkinson's Disease

Cintia Roodveldt[1], Adahir Labrador-Garrido[1], Guillermo Izquierdo[2] and David Pozo[1]
[1]*CABIMER-Andalusian Center for Molecular Biology & Regenerative Medicine CSIC-University of Seville-UPO-Junta de Andalucía, Seville*
[2] *Clinical Neurosciences Management Unit, Virgen Macarena University Hospital, University of Seville Medical School, Seville*
Spain

1. Introduction

In the last few years, it has become evident that the immunological component is of central importance in Parkinson's Disease (PD) pathogenesis and progression. This can also certainly be said about the prominent role that the protein α-synuclein (αSyn) is currently believed to play in the pathobiology of this neurodegenerative disorder. Moreover, the multiple mechanisms through which αSyn might be affecting the immune system appear not to be just a consequence of disease progression, but to actively contribute to the delicate balance between neuroprotection and neurotoxicity that ultimately underlies a given stage of disease.

PD is a proteinopathy, whose pathological hallmark is the presence of deposits of aggregated αSyn in intracellular fibrillar inclusions in neurons of the *substantia nigra pars compacta* (SN) of the brain, known as Lewy bodies (LB) (Croisier et al., 2005; Spillantini et al., 1998), and the loss of dopaminergic neurons (Braak et al., 2003). Three missense mutations, A53T, A30P and E46K, as well as multiple copies of the wild-type (Wt) αSyn gene, are linked to early-onset, familial PD (Gasser, 2005; Kruger et al., 1998; Polymeropoulos et al., 1997; Zarranz et al., 2004). Given that αSyn is the major component of LB in both familial and sporadic PD cases (Spillantini et al., 1998), αSyn is considered a critical factor in PD aetiology. Currently, the cellular and molecular mechanisms underlying the pathological actions of αSyn are poorly understood, and the factors contributing to sporadic PD, representing the vast majority of PD cases, are not known.

αSyn, together with β- and γ-synucleins, belong to the family of synucleins, a group of closely related, brain-enriched proteins. This 140 aa-residue protein is largely located in neuronal presynaptic terminals (Kim et al., 2004b) and in the nucleus (Yu et al., 2007). In particular, it is found in the neocortex, hippocampus and SN (Kim et al., 2004b), and in other brain regions, as well as within astrocytes, microglia and oligodendroglia (Austin et al., 2006; Mori et al., 2002; Richter-Landsberg et al., 2000). It is known to interact with a variety of proteins (Jenco et al., 1998; Peng et al., 2005) and lipid membranes (Jo et al., 2000). The physiological functions of αSyn are still being established, but its interaction with presynaptic membranes and lipids suggests a role in the regulation of synaptic vesicle pools including dopamine release control (Perez & Hastings, 2004) and in lipid metabolism (Cabin et al., 2002; Castagnet et al., 2005; Golovko et al., 2009).

Both *in vitro* and *in vivo* in LB, αSyn can self-assemble to form ordered fibrillar aggregates, characterized by a cross β-sheet structure, that are morphologically similar to the amyloid fibrils found in neuritic plaques in Alzheimer´s disease (AD) as well as in deposits associated with other amyloidogenic processes (Chiti & Dobson, 2006). The initial phase of the aggregation process is thought to involve the formation of intermediate oligomers and protofibrillar species which, according to accumulating experimental evidence, can be more toxic to cells than the mature fibrils into which they develop (Bucciantini et al., 2002; Stefani & Dobson, 2003). These and other findings suggest a common structure-linked toxicity among pre-fibrillar species, and propose similar mechanisms contributing to pathogenesis for this group of diseases (Baglioni et al., 2006; Bucciantini et al., 2004). Overall, different hypotheses have been proposed that postulate that αSyn induces a 'gain of toxic function' upon aggregation (Bennett, 2005).

While αSyn is typically considered as an intracellular protein, it has also been found to be normally present in extracellular biological fluids, including human cerebrospinal fluid (CSF) and blood plasma (Borghi et al., 2000; El-Agnaf et al., 2003; El-Agnaf et al., 2006; Lee et al., 2006; Tokuda et al., 2006). However, αSyn levels have been found to be elevated in plasma from PD and multiple system atrophy (MSA) patients relative to age-matched controls (Lee et al., 2006), while lower levels than normal have been detected in CSF from PD patients (Tokuda et al., 2006). On the other hand, two studies by El-Agnaf and colleagues showed an elevated content of oligomeric αSyn spedies present in plasma (El-Agnaf et al., 2006) and post mortem CSF (Tokuda et al., 2010) from PD patients, compared to controls, indicating that changes in the levels and characteristics of extracellular αSyn are associated with the disease (Lee, 2008). Even though membrane permeability from dying cells could be one contributing factor, it has been suggested that vesicle-mediated exocytosis from normal cells is probably the main source of extracellular αSyn (Lee, 2008). By using brain homogenates and neuronal cell cultures, Lee and colleagues (Lee et al., 2005) have shown that both monomeric and aggregated αSyn can be secreted by an unconventional secretory pathway. On the other hand, extracellular αSyn has been shown to be taken up by neuronal and microglial cells in culture, although the nature of the mechanism involved is still controversial (Lee, 2008). In addition, two recent studies have provided strong evidence for a neuron-to-neuron and neuron-to-non-neuronal cell transmission of αSyn aggregates and their associated cytotoxicity, in cellular and mouse models of PD (Danzer et al., 2011; Desplats et al., 2009), highlighting the importance of extracellular αSyn in the pathogenic mechanism of α-synucleinopathies.

2. Neuroinflammation in PD

Another prominent pathological feature of PD brains is the presence of a robust inflammatory response mediated by activated microglia and reactive astrocytes in affected areas of the SN (Glass et al., 2010). Inflammation is the first response of the immune system to pathogens or irritation. In acute conditions, it protects tissue against invading agents and promotes healing. However, a chronic inflammatory state can turn harmful towards the host´s own tissue (Gao & Hong, 2008; Kim & Joh, 2006). Microglia are the resident immunocompetent cells in the brain (Aloisi, 2001), capable of antigen presentation to lymphocytes (Kreutzberg, 1996) and rapid activation in response to immune insults and invading of PD pathogenesis in the central nervous system (CNS) (Kim & Joh, 2006). As a result of pathogen invasion or tissue damage, microglia switch to an activated phenotype and thereby promote an inflammatory response that serves to further engage the immune system by recruiting other cells to the site of brain lesion, and initiate tissue repair (Glass et al., 2010). However, uncontrolled inflammation may result in production of neurotoxic factors that can be highly detrimental (Gao & Hong, 2008; Glass et al., 2010). Indeed, inflammation in the CNS and sustained overactivation of microglia, i.e. reactive microgliosis, are currently believed to be actively involved in the pathogenesis of various neurodegenerative diseases including PD, AD, multiple sclerosis (MS), and amyotrophic lateral sclerosis (ALS) (Gao & Hong, 2008; Glass et al., 2010; Kim & Joh, 2006; Long-Smith et al., 2009).

At present, whether microglial activation ultimately protects or actually exacerbates neuronal loss in the context of PD and other related diseases is still under debate (Delgado & Ganea, 2003; Gao & Hong, 2008; Halliday & Stevens, 2011; Sanchez-Pernaute et al., 2004; Vila et al., 2001; Wu et al., 2002; Wyss-Coray & Mucke, 2002), although the current view favours the second hypothesis. Evidence of microglial attack in PD is supported by findings from epidemiological studies, animal models, and cell culture experiments (McGeer & McGeer, 2008). Epidemiological studies have revealed that taking ibuprofen anti-inflammatory agent regularly is associated with a 35% lower risk of PD (Chen et al., 2005; Chen et al., 2003), supporting the concept that inflammatory attack is contributing to dopaminergic neuronal loss. On the other hand, *in vivo* studies show that the specific early up-regulation of SN microglia in PD correlates with disease severity and dopamine terminal loss (Orr et al., 2005; Ouchi et al., 2005). Overall, studies based on animal models and *in vitro* cell culture, indicate that dopaminergic cells are highly sensitive to inflammatory attack (Castano et al., 1998; Fernagut & Chesselet, 2004) and that microglial cells can be strongly activated to mount such an inflammatory response (Austin et al., 2006). Moreover, it has been recently reported that treatment with CSF from PD patients strongly affects cultured microglial cells, resulting in reduced cell growth, morphological changes, as well as increased content and aggregation of αSyn (Schiess et al., 2010). This illustrates how microglia itself, and not only dopaminergic neurons, can be highly affected by the medium in a PD scenario.

3. αSyn-induced microglial activation

The results gathered thus far using the different PD animal models have substantially increased our understanding of PD's pathogenesis by usually providing different but probably complementary information. Thus, while the MPTP mouse model of PD indicates that inflammation in the SN can be self-propagating and leads to progressive neurodegeneration, the αSyn transgenic animal model demonstrates that overexpression of this endogenous protein can certainly provide a powerful source of inflammation (McGeer & McGeer, 2008). Whether microglial activation is essentially caused by the release of aberrant αSyn species to the extracellular space, (Reynolds et al., 2008b; Wersinger & Sidhu, 2006; Zhang et al., 2005), or otherwise, that neuronal death itself drives microglial immune responses in an αSyn-independent manner (Giasson et al., 2000; Mandel et al., 2005; Przedborski et al., 2001), is still under debate. However, there is ample accumulated evidence pointing at αSyn as the main trigger of microglial activation in PD (Roodveldt et al., 2008). For example, several studies have demonstrated that extracellular and nigral αSyn- containing aggregates are often surrounded by activated microglia or inflammatory mediators in PD brains (McGeer et al., 1988; Yamada et al., 1992), similarly to what has been described for amyloid plaques in AD (Griffin et al., 2006). Moreover, the extent of microglial activation in the SN from PD patients has been found to be correlated with the degree of αSyn accumulation (Croisier et al., 2005) and with increased αSyn levels as evidenced by in vitro (Kim et al., 2009; Klegeris et al., 2008) and in vivo (Lee et al., 2009a) studies, strongly supporting the view that the protein has a major role in phenotypic changes of microglia. Up to this point, a considerable number of *in vivo* studies with animal models of PD that directly link αSyn with microglial activation have been reported. It has been demonstrated in mice that overexpression of αSyn alone (by using adeno-associated virus, AAV) is sufficient to trigger neuroinflammation, involving not only classical microglial activation but also stimulation of adaptive immunity, preceding the appearance of overt neurodegeneration signs (Theodore et al., 2008). In line with this finding, a rat AAV-based model for overexpressing the A53T αSyn variant in the SN revealed dramatic changes in cytoskeletal protein levels and activated microglia-mediated neuroinflammation in the striatum (with increased release levels of IL-1β, IFN-γ, and TNF-α proinflammatory cytokines), well before neuronal loss was evident (Chung et al., 2009). Another recent study using a AAV rat PD model showed that overexpression of Wt αSyn in the SN not only leads to persistent microglia activation, but that depending on the degree of αSyn-induced neurophatology that models either the onset or the late stages of the disease, different microglial responses will occur: upon lower αSyn expression levels where only neurodegeneration occurs, microglia with antigen-presenting capabilities predominate, whereas levels that can induce neuronal cell death correlate with long-term induction of macrophagic microglia (Sanchez-Guajardo et al., 2010), suggesting that microglia may play different roles during disease progression (Sanchez-Guajardo et al., 2010).

Two recent studies have explored the link between neuroinflammation and αSyn dysfunction by lipopolysacharide (LPS) injection in rat (Choi et al., 2010) or mice (Gao et al., 2011), to trigger systemic and brain inflammation. In the first study, the authors observed increased microglia activation and secretion of proinflammatory cytokines as well as greater nitration of proteins including αSyn, in elderly rats, suggesting that an exaggerated neuroinflammatory response that occurs naturally with aging might contribute to αSyn aggregation and dopaminergic neurodegeneration in PD (Choi et al., 2010). In the second study, the authors evaluated dopaminergic neurodegeneration, αSyn pathology and neuroinflammation in Wt and transgenic A53T αSyn-overexpressing mice (Gao et al., 2011). They observed that, while both models initially displayed acute neuroinflammation, only the latter developed persistent neuroinflammation together with chronic progressive degeneration of nigrostriatal dopamine pathway, accumulation of aggregated, nitrated αSyn, and formation of LB (Gao et al., 2011), suggesting that genetic factors and environmental exposures act synergistically to precipitate the development of PD. On the other hand, microglial cells from αSyn-knockout mice have been shown to exhibit a remarkably different morphology compared to Wt cells (Austin et al., 2006), displaying elevated levels of secreted pro-inflammatory cytokines such as TNF-α and IL-6 after activation, indicating that αSyn plays a critical role in modulating the microglial activation state. More recently, the authors have found that microglial activation in this model is accompanied by increased protein levels of three enzymes involved in lipid-mediated signalling, which suggests a broader function for αSyn in brain physiology beyond synapsis control (Austin et al., 2011).

In the last few years, several *in vitro* studies have focused on the effects of extracellular αSyn on microglial activation. Zhang *et al.* (Zhang et al., 2005) first reported that exogeneous, aggregated αSyn cause activation of microglial cells, which then become toxic towards cultured dopaminergic neurons. Their results indicate that microglial phagocytosis of αSyn and activation of NADPH oxidase, are critical in αSyn-induced microglial activation and neurotoxicity. This finding is highly relevant considering that aggregated αSyn has been shown to be secreted by exocytosis from neuroblastoma and primary neuronal cells (Danzer et al., 2011; Lee et al., 2005), and by stressed neurons (Klegeris et al., 2008). Moreover, following the discovery that αSyn aggregates can be released from neurons and transmitted to neighbouring cells (Desplats et al., 2009), a study has recently shown that αSyn release by SH-SY5Y neuroglioma cells, especially when treated with MPP^+ neurotoxin, are able to activate the inflammatory response in a microglial cell line (Alvarez-Erviti et al., 2011).

Up to this point, research on αSyn-mediated cell response has focused primarily on the effects on neuroinflammation (Benner et al., 2008) or microglial activation (Cookson, 2009; Reynolds et al., 2008a; Thomas et al., 2007; Zhang et al., 2007; Zhang et al., 2005) of αSyn in its aggregated form. Interestingly, Reynolds and coworkers (Reynolds et al., 2008b) have found that nitrated, aggregated αSyn (N-αSyn) has a stronger stimulating effect on microglia than that of nitrated but non-aggregated αSyn. In addition, several investigations have found that N-αSyn, which has been detected in LB of human brains with PD (Giasson et al., 2000) and has been linked to neurodegeneration in PD mouse models (Benner et al., 2008; Gao et al., 2008), induces a neurotoxic inflammatory microglial phenotype that accelerates dopaminergic neuronal loss (Biasini et al., 2004; Thomas et al., 2007; Zhang et al., 2005; Zhou et al., 2005). By integrating genomic and proteomic techniques, Gendelman and colleagues created a fingerprint of microglial cell activation following its interactions with aggregated N-αSyn in cell culture (Reynolds et al., 2008a), indicating that the activation, which was found to be capable of mediating dopaminergic neurotoxicity, is mainly mediated by the NF-κB pathway (Reynolds et al., 2008a). However, whether extracellular αSyn contains the same modifications than the protein found in LB (Anderson et al., 2006; Giasson et al., 2000; Hodara et al., 2004), which is a typically pro-oxidative environment, is still uncertain (Lee, 2008).

Over the last few years, certain differential functions for non-aggregated, extracellular aSyn in glia have been reported. It has been observed that, in contrast to the aggregated form, monomeric αSyn enhances microglial phagocytosis (Park et al., 2008). A few investigations that explore the effects of non-aggregated αSyn on the cytokine release profile of potentially relevant cells have been recently done using monocytic (Klegeris et al., 2008) or macrophage (Lee et al., 2009b) cell lines, and primary astrocyte (Klegeris et al., 2006) or microglial (Roodveldt et al., 2010; Su et al., 2009; Su et al., 2008) cultures. Indeed, we have observed a strong innate immune response in primary glial and microglial cell cultures elicited by exogenous, non-aggregated αSyn (Roodveldt et al., 2010). Interestingly, a comparative study using unmodified aSyn has recently shown that exogenous non-aggregated αSyn induces higher TNF-α, IL-1β and ROS release levels than aggregated αSyn in microglia (Lee et al.,

2010). These and other recent findings point at the importance of exploring the effects on the immune response of aggregated as well as non-aggregated αSyn.

Even though a study using monocytic THP-1 cell line (Klegeris et al., 2008) had shown modest increases in IL-1β and TNF-α secretion levels after stimulation with A30P, A53T, or E46K αSyn mutants compared to the Wt protein, there is a lack of a comprehensive study of the effect exerted by non-aggregated αSyn, performed with primary cell cultures. With this in mind, we analysed the cytokine release profile of primary microglial cultures —which represesnts a more comparable physiological environment— after stimulation with Wt or the PD-linked αSyn mutants (Roodveldt et al., 2010). Indeed, we found remarkable differences between the αSyn variants in the interleukin and chemokine release profiles and significant effects on the microglial phagocytic capacity (Roodveldt et al., 2010). In particular, we observed marked differences in IL-6 and IL-1β pro-inflammtory cytokines, IL-10 immunoregulatory cytokine, as well as IP-10/CXCL10, RANTES/CCL5, MCP-1/CCL2 and MIP-1α/CCL3 chemokines release levels. Our results indicate that extracellular, non-aggregated Wt αSyn produces a moderate to low pro-inflammatory response in glia, together with a reduction of the immunoregulatory response, and a moderate stimulation of Th1 chemokine secretion. The A30P and E46K pathological variants, on the other hand, can induce strong pro-inflammatory and immunoregulatory responses, together with marked increases in chemokine release levels. This exacerbated innate immune response might explain the earlier onset and more rapid evolution of these two genetic cases of PD as compared to the sporadic kind. Intriguingly, our results from the pathologically-linked A53T variant showed not to provoke a significant innate immune response, which might suggest that other neurodegeneration mechanisms contributing to the pathogenesis of PD, probably involving the adaptive immune response, might exist in this case. Combined with the effect on microglial phagocytosis, our results indicate that these αSyn-induced phenotypes might reflect either a classical (A30P and E36K) or an alternative (A53T) microglial activation state, or a hybrid phenotype (Wt), which could probably explain the different disease progression modes that can occur in PD. Alternative activation of macrophages and microglia is a response to tissue injury that is thought to be involved in tissue repair and restoration (Ponomarev et al., 2007), and has been suggested to play a role in repair and extracellular matrix remodelling in AD (Colton et al., 2006). Currently, there is no other indication that such an activation mode could be operating in the context of PD.

Upon activation, microglia and astrocytes start secreting inflammatory cytokines in order to communicate and mount the immune response to counteract disease or injury. The cytokines TNF-α, IL-1β, IL-2, IL-4, IL-6, TGF-α, TGF-β1, TGF-β2 have all been reported to be increased in the nigrostriatal region and CSF of patients with PD or DLB (Croisier & Graeber, 2006). As a result of αSyn-induced activation of microglia *in vitro*, a few cytokines and metabolites have been shown to be significantly up-regulated (reviewed in (Roodveldt et al., 2008)): IL-6, IL-1β, ICAM-1, TNF-α, IFN-γ, MCP-1, O_2^-, iROS, and PEG_2, glutamate, and iCys. In general, disease-linked αSyn variants show a stronger effect on cytokines release than does the Wt protein. Interestingly, analysis of the microglia transcriptome by Gendelman and coworkers (Reynolds et al., 2008a) after stimulation with aggregated N-αSyn, revealed a significant up-regulation of the toll-like receptor 2 (TLR-2) gene. TLRs are known to sense the molecular signatures of microbial pathogens, and play a fundamental role in innate immune responses, inducing the expression of diverse inflammatory genes

(Kawai & Akira, 2007). Therefore, it seems plausible that cells challenged with αSyn, or with certain forms of αSyn, could become hyper-responsive to inflammatory signals.

Activated microglia can also produce substantial amounts of superoxide radicals, which may be the major source of the oxidative stress thought to be largely responsible for dopaminergic cell death in PD. The generation of ROS by microglia activated by αSyn (Thomas et al., 2007) can result in oxidation and nitration of proteins, DNA modifications, and lipid peroxidation, leading to neurotoxicity (Zhang et al., 2005). Oxidation (Ko et al., 2000; Souza et al., 2000) and nitration (Giasson et al., 2000; Souza et al., 2000) of αSyn, in turn, can lead to the formation of more aggregates, which could result in increased cytotoxic effects. Consistent with this, Kelly *et al.* have shown that high levels of oxidized cholesterol metabolites in brains from PD and dementia with LB patients, accelerate αSyn fibrillation (Bosco et al., 2006). On the other hand, McGeer and colleagues (Klegeris et al., 2007a) have reported that αSyn-stimulated microglia, in combination with IFN-γ, produce and increase in the toxicity on human monocytic cells exerted by neurotoxic secretions (Klegeris et al., 2007a). Interestingly, this toxicity can be diminished with specific ligands for ryanodine receptors (Klegeris et al., 2007a), which are known to help mediate the efflux of Ca^{2+} ions from intracellular stores and avoid uncontrolled increases in $[Ca^{2+}]_i$ that may lead to cell death (Giorgi et al., 2008).

Further insight into the mechanism of pathogenesis might derive from the findings that several proteins which are thought to be linked to PD are up-regulated as a result of αSyn-induced microglial activation. Gendelman and co-workers, by determining the activated microglia proteome profile (Reynolds et al., 2008a), found that aggregated N-αSyn activation of microglia results in differential expression of several proteins. These range from proteins involved in oxidative stress, cell adhesion, glycolysis, growth control, and migration, to cytoskeletal proteins. It is worth noting that two of those proteins found to be most up-regulated, calmodulin and ubiquitin, have been shown to interact with αSyn with possible functional consequences. Calmodulin has been shown, *in vitro*, to bind to αSyn in a Ca^{2+}-dependent manner (Lee et al., 2002) and to inhibit αSyn fibrillation (Martinez et al., 2003). On the other hand, a fraction of αSyn found in LB is mono-ubiquitinated (Hasegawa et al., 2002; Tofaris et al., 2003), but the role of this modification remains unclear. Recently, it has been demonstrated that the ubiquitin-protein isopeptide ligase, seven in absentia homolog (SIAH), directly interacts with and monoubiquitinates αSyn, promoting its aggregation (Lee et al., 2008; Rott et al., 2008) and apoptosis (Lee et al., 2008). In addition, there is also evidence implicating a role for the ubiquitin-proteasome system (UPS) in PD (reviewed in (Lim & Tan, 2007)). Also of interest are the elevated levels of Hsp70 observed upon microglial activation. This central chaperone has been demonstrated to inhibit αSyn aggregation *in vitro* (Dedmon et al., 2005; Huang et al., 2006; Roodveldt et al., 2009), in neuroglioma cells (Klucken et al., 2004) as well as in fly (Auluck et al., 2002) and mouse (Klucken et al., 2004) models of PD, protecting cells from the cytotoxic effects of aggregates.

4. Links between αSyn and astrocytes and oligodendrocytes

Together with microglial cells, astrocytes and oligodendrocytes are part of glia, which normally serve neuroprotective functions but, given adverse stimulation as discussed before, they may contribute to develop chronic neuroinflammation (Halliday & Stevens, 2011; McGeer & McGeer, 2008). Compared to microglia, the functions of astrocytes are poorly understood. Because they have been shown to produce both pro-inflammatory and anti-inflammatory agents, these cells are thought to have a dual role (McGeer & McGeer, 2008). Many ICAM-1-positive astrocytes are seen in the SN of PD brains and this may attract reactive microglia to the area since microglia carry the counter receptor LFA-1 (Miklossy et al., 2006). Indeed, αSyn has been shown to be capable of both of activating microglia and stimulating astrocytes to produce IL-6 and ICAM-1 (Klegeris et al., 2006). On the other hand, astrocytes have been shown to secrete a number of neurotrophic factors that protect dopaminergic neurons in some models of PD (McGeer & McGeer, 2008), but the mechanisms underlying most of these functions are not yet known. Astrocytes have been shown to express αSyn (Tanji et al., 2001). Interestingly, the presence of αSyn-containing inclusion bodies in astrocytes of sporadic PD brains has been observed (Braak et al., 2007; Terada et al., 2003; Wakabayashi et al., 2000). Finally, a recent study showed that astrocyte expression of A53T αSyn leads to the development of progressed paralysis, strong microglial activation, and neurodegeneration (Gu et al., 2010).

There is still little data on the role of oligodendrocytes in PD. αSyn-containing inclusions have been detected in this cell type in MSA, in DLB, and in PD (Campbell et al., 2001; Wakabayashi et al., 2000). McGeer and colleagues have reported the presence of complement-activated oligodendrocytes in the SN of PD cases (Yamada et al., 1992). Intriguingly, transgenic mice overexpressing Wt αSyn in oligodendrocytes have been observed to develop severe neurological alterations and neurodegeneration (Shults et al., 2005; Yazawa et al., 2005), drawing the attention to a possible role of these glial cells in PD.

5. Expression of αSyn by immunocompetent cells

Given that αSyn expression has been reported also in non-neuronal cells, it is currently thought to play a role besides dopamine release control. While searching for a link between the CNS and peripheral immune system in PD, Kim *et al.* (Kim et al., 2004a) found that αSyn was up-regulated in peripheral blood mononuclear cells (PBMC) at the gene level, in idiopathic PD *vs.* non-PD controls. Moreover, by *in vitro* transfection with Wt, A30P and A53T αSyn genes, they found that αSyn expression is correlated to glucocorticoid-sensitive apoptosis, possibly caused by the enhanced expression of glucocorticoid receptor (GR), caspase activation, CD95 (Fas) up-regulation, and ROS production. However, the increase in ROS production by overexpression of the αSyn mutants was markedly greater than for Wt αSyn. αSyn expression has also been found in cultured human macrophages (Tanji et al., 2002) and its expression levels have been reported to increase by stimulation with pro-inflammatory cytokine IL-1β or LPS (Tanji et al., 2002), further supporting a role for αSyn in the inflammatory process. Finally, expression of αSyn in cultured human T cells, B cells, natural killer (NK) cells and in monocytes/macrophages, have been reported (Shin et al., 2000). Currently, it is not known whether expression or aggregation, of αSyn in T cells can be regulated by ligand activation of the T cell. This may be relevant as it could represent a key link between regulation of the adaptive immunity and □Syn expression levels.

6. αSyn and the adaptive immune response in PD

In the last few years, mounting evidence has pointed at a possible participation of the adaptive immune system in PD pathogenesis. However, whether this immune response actually contributes to neurodegeneration, and in that case by which mechanism, remains unknown. The initial observations in PD patients that a small amount of CD8+ T-lymphocytes occur in proximity to degenerating nigral neurons (McGeer et al., 1988), and the occurrence in LB of components of the classical or antibody-triggered complement cascade (Yamada et al., 1992) had suggested a possible involvement of the adaptive immunity in the PD process. More recently, the finding of accumulated IgG in the SN of PD patients and increased expression of IgG-binding receptors on activated microglia (Orr et al., 2005), and the detection of anti-αSyn autoantibodies (AAb) in blood serum of PD patients (Papachroni et al., 2007), suggest that the pathological process may involve adaptive immune-mediated mechanisms. In addition, the observation that humoral immune mechanisms can trigger microglial-mediated neuronal injury in animal models of PD (He et al., 2002), and the finding by Standaert and colleagues of IgG deposition in mouse brains following AAV-mediated αSyn overexpression in the SN (Theodore et al., 2008), further support a role of the adaptive immune system in disease progression.

A possible consequence of the initial microglial activation in the affected regions of PD brains is the local permeabilization of the blood-brain barrier (BBB), leading to infiltration to the affected regions by B- and/or T-lymphocytes (Racke et al., 2000). Indeed, a remarkable T- and B-cell infiltration into the SN linked to αSyn overexpression was observed at the early stages, i.e. before the appearance of significant dopaminergic neuronal loss, reaching levels in the SN of up to 10-fold and 5-fold compared to controls (Theodore et al., 2008). A recent study by Hunot and colleagues (Brochard et al., 2009) has shown that CD8+ and CD4+ T-cells, but not B-cells, had invaded the brain in PD patients and in MPTP-treated mice during the course of neural degeneration. Furthermore, based on these results the authors propose that T-cell dependant toxicity is essentially mediated by CD4+ T-cells and requires the expression of FasL (Brochard et al., 2009). Given that the FasL pathway had been shown to produce proinflammatory cytokine responses in macrophages (Park et al., 2003), the authors speculate that the CD4+ Th FasL-mediated activation of microglia could participate in neuroinflammation and neurodegeneration processes in PD (Brochard et al., 2009).

Based on results obtained with an MPTP murine model of the disease, Gendelman and colleagues (Reynolds et al., 2010) have suggested that the αSyn-specific regulatory T-cells (Treg cells), which are regulatory components of the adaptive immunity, might be able to counteract the autoaggresive effector T-cell responses that exacerbate neuroinflammation (Benner et al., 2008), and therefore contribute to attenuate neurodegeneration in PD. Indeed, the same group has reported that microglial cells stimulated with N-αSyn are susceptible of essentially opposing immune regulatory responses by Treg cells (CD4+, CD245+) and effector T-cells (CD4+, CD25-) in culture (Reynolds et al., 2009a). By analysing an array of cytokines released by treated microglia, the authors found that, while the effector T-cell subset exacerbates microglial-mediated inflammation and may induce neurotoxic responses, Treg cells are able to suppress N-αSyn microglial-induced reactive-oxygen species (ROS) and NF-κB activation and are proposed to be neuroprotective (Reynolds et al., 2009a). Furthermore, the study indicates that Treg cells can regulate microglial inflammation by inducing Fas-FasL-mediated apoptosis of N-αSyn-stimulated microglial cells (Reynolds et al., 2009a). By using a proteomic analysis, the authors further showed that these Treg cells can significantly alter the microglial protein expression profile for certain proteins linked to cell metabolism, migration, protein transport and degradation, redox biology, and cytoskeletal and bioenergetic metabolism, to presumably attenuate the neurotoxic phenotype caused by N-αSyn stimulation (Reynolds et al., 2009b).

Thus far, accumulated data demonstrate that in the MPTP model of PD, misfolded and aggregated αSyn are secreted from neurons, which promotes pro-inflammatory M1-type microglia and cytotoxic T-cells, therefore amplifying neuronal damage. In sporadic human PD, it is currently unkown which factor triggers disease onset, but it has been proposed that under certain circumstances, a similar set of temporal and mechanistic events could transform neuroprotective microglia and T cells into cytotoxic cells, thereby accelerating disease progression (Appel et al., 2010). This way, activated microglia and the cytokine milieu that they generate might promote T-cell differentiation into different cell subsets in the context of PD (Appel et al., 2010). Indeed, it has been shown that M1 (pro-inflammatory) cells promote, whereas M2 (non-inflammatory) cells reduce, $CD4^+$ Th1 cell proliferation and function (Verreck et al., 2004), but also that, conversely, T-cells can dictate microglial pro- or anti-inflammatory phenotypes (Giuliani et al., 2003; Kebir et al., 2007; Mount et al., 2007). Whether microglia dictate the specific T-cell phenotype or otherwise, that T-cells dictate the specific microglial phenotype (i.e. M1 *vs.* M2), is still unknown (Appel et al., 2010). But overall, the communication established between microglia, T cells and neurons seem to indicate that the immune response is not only a consequence of injury, but that it actively contributes to the balance between neuroprotection and neurotoxicity (Appel et al., 2010; Stone et al., 2009).

To analyse the possibility that humoral immunity may play a role in initiating or regulating inflammation, Orr *et al.* (Orr et al., 2005) analysed the association between nigral degeneration and humoral immune markers in brain tissue of patients with idiopathic or genetic PD and controls. All the patients with PD revealed IgG, but not IgM, binding on dopamine neurons. Moreover, the proportion of IgG-immunopositive neurons showed a negative correlation with the degree of cell loss in the SN, and positive correlation with the number of activated microglia. IgG was found to be concentrated at the cell surface of neurons, but also on their LB, and was shown to co-localize with αSyn. These results, in combination with their finding that activated microglia express high-affinity IgG receptors (FcγRI) in both idiopathic and genetic forms of PD, might suggest that the activation of microglia may be induced by neuronal IgG (Orr et al., 2005).

The question regarding the functional importance of antibodies against antigen-specific, disease-associated neuronal proteins still needs to be addressed. It has been demonstrated that an IgG fraction purified from serum of PD patients causes death of dopaminergic neurons *in vivo* following stereotaxic injection in the SN of experimental animals (Chen et al., 1998), and the presence of immunoglobulins in PD brain tissue have been proposed to lead to the targeting of dopaminergic nigral neurons for destruction (Orr et al., 2005). Currently, it remains unknown whether these anti-αSyn AAb are neurotoxic, or on the contrary, they actually have a neuroprotective role, as has been shown in a human αSyn transgenic mouse model of PD (Masliah et al., 2005).

A recent study has assessed the presence of auto-antibodies (AAb) against all three synucleins in the peripheral blood serum of PD patients and healthy controls (Papachroni et al., 2007). While the presence of AAb against β- and γ-Syn showed no association with PD, multi-epitopic AAb against αSyn were detected in 65% of all patients, with a strong correlation with the inherited mode of the disease. In addition, a recent study based on measuring AAb levels against monomeric, oligomeric, and fibrillar αSyn in serum from PD patients (Gruden et al., 2011), showed that all three AAb specificities reached the highest values after 5-year of disease duration, and subsided in 10-year sufferers. Intriguingly, there was a ca. 15-fold increase in AAb titre values relative to monomeric αSyn (72% of patients), and a ca. 4-fold increase for αSyn oligomers (56% of patients). Moreover, the authors also found a decline in $CD3^+$, $CD4^+$ and CD8+ T-lymphocyte and B-lymphocyte subsets. Based on these results, they suggest that αSyn toxicity elimination by AAb in early PD pathology might be linked with the decline of lymphocyte subsets reflecting the influence of inflammatory and oxidative stress processes (Gruden et al., 2011).

Despite their potential involvement in PD pathogenesis and progression, the role of NK cells in PD has hardly been explored. NK cells are active members of the innate immune system that act as a first-line defence, and also mediate between the innate and adaptive immune systems (Salazar-Mather et al., 1996; Su et al., 2001). Interestingly, a recent study using blood samples from PD patiens indicates that the NK activity increases as the disease advances (Mihara et al., 2008). Moreover, the study also showed that the NK cell content among the total lymphocytes of the PD group was higher than in the control group (Mihara et al., 2008).

7. Prospects for αSyn-based immunotherapy in PD

In addition to its well known importance in the pathogenesis of PD, αSyn is becoming a primary target for preventing or controlling the process of PD. In the late few years, vaccination for treating some neurodegenerative disorders has emerged as a potentially useful approach. Thus far, this avenue has been scarcely explored for PD. Importantly, immunization with αSyn was shown to generate a humoral response in a mouse model of PD (Masliah et al., 2005), producing beneficial albeit modest results on histopathological markers of the disease. On the contrary, using N-αSyn as the immunogen proved to elicit strong antigen-specific effector T cell responses in MPTP-intoxicated mice that caused exacerbated neuroinflammation and neurodegeneration (Benner et al., 2008). This response was further shown to be largely mediated by Th17 cells and causing Treg dysfunction (Reynolds et al., 2010). In addition, the authors demonstrated that Treg cells from mice treated with the neuropeptide VIP, known to promote Treg responses (Delgado et al., 2005; Gonzalez-Rey et al., 2006), can efficiently modulate N-αSyn-generated immunity in MPTP mice and confer neuroprotection (Reynolds et al., 2010), suggesting a possible novel therapeutic avenue for PD.

Given that microglial activation can maintain or even aggravate the disease process, blocking inflammation or shifting the balance between pro-inflammatory and anti-inflammatory states in a controlled manner, offers one of the most promising strategies for developing palliative (and maybe preventive) therapies for PD and related disorders. Epidemiological data have identified the non steroidal anti-inflammatory drug (NSAID) ibuprofen as neuroprotective for PD (Klegeris et al., 2007b). NSAIDs are thought to act on dopamine quinone formation and activation by αSyn of both astrocytes and microglia. On the other hand, Gendelman and colleagues demonstrated that T cells from mice immunized with Copolymer-1 (Cop-1), are able to attenuate microglial responses and lead to neuroprotection in a MPTP mouse model of PD (Benner et al., 2004). This neuroprotective effect was later found to be mediated by the $CD4^+$ type of T cells, suggesting the possible involvement of Treg cells (Laurie et al., 2007). Later work by the same group confirmed this hypothesis by showing that passive transfer to MPTP mice of activated Treg cells, but not effector T cells, efficiently suppressed microglial activation and afforded neuroprotection (Reynolds et al., 2007), suggesting that the immunomodulating abilities of Treg cells could potentially be utilized as a therapeutic approach against PD (Stone et al., 2009).

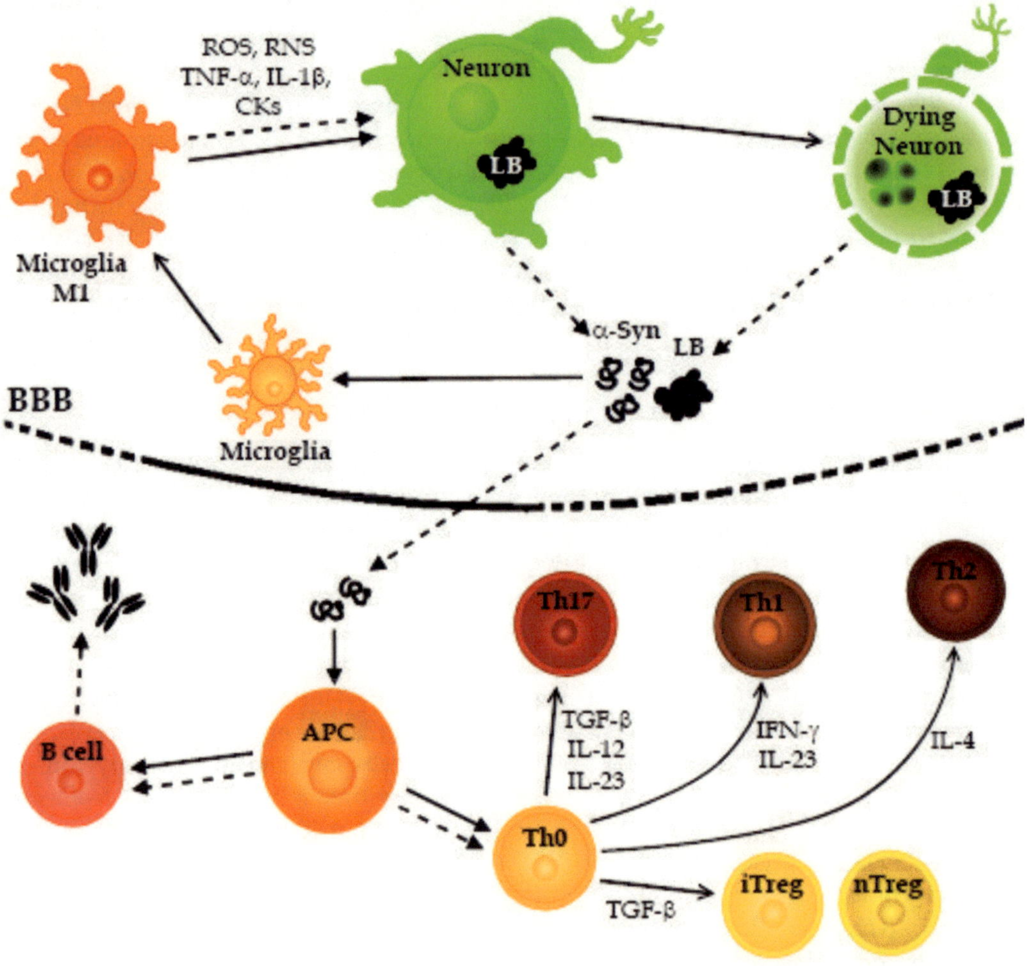

Fig. 1. Links between αSyn and the immune response in PD. Continuous arrows with filled tips: positive effect; continuous arrows with open tips: cell transformation; discontinuous arrows: secretion of cellular factors. APC, Antigen-processing cell; BBB, Blood-brain barrier; CKs, Chemokines; IL, Interleukin; IFN-γ, Interferon γ; LB, Lewy bodies; ROS, Reactive oxygen species; RNS, Reactive nitrogen species; TGF-β, Tumor growth factor β.

8. Conclusion

It is well established that PD onset and progression are characterized by sustained activation of microglia, linked to significant dopaminergic neuron loss in the SN of the brain. Over the last few years, it has become accepted that overexpression and aggregation of αSyn, an amyloid-like protein, is linked to neurotoxicity through various proposed mechanisms, and may be one of the primary causes of the immunological abnormalities observed in PD. Recent studies with cellular and *in vivo* models of the disease indicate that increased levels of extracellular αSyn, both in its aggregated and non-aggregated forms, are found in a PD scenario.

Accumulated evidence has now established that aggregated extracellular αSyn is able to trigger the activation of microglia, inducing a highly detrimental cascade of neuroinflammation and neuronal demise. In addition, recent studies have have demonstrated that non-aggregated αSyn can also have a substantial impact on microglial phenotype and cytokine release profile, especially in the cases of familial PD αSyn mutants. By releasing toxic factors, or by phagocytosing neighbouring cells, activated microglia and astrocytes are believed to form a self-perpetuating neuronal degeneration cycle. On the other hand, recent findings point at a possible role of the adaptive immune system involving αSyn, and the pathological process in PD. Clearly, further studies in this direction are necessary to help understand the complex immunological mechanisms underlying PD and the key, and possibly multiple, links between αSyn and the immune response in relation to in relation to pathogenesis (Figure 1).

In addition to trying to develop effective tools to prevent αSyn aggregation, modulating the innate immune response by intervening microglial activation, promoting a selective aSyn-specific humoral response, and manipulating the balance between effector and immunomodulatory T-cell populations, may be considered as highly promising therapeutic approaches for the treatment of PD and other synucleinopathies.

9. Acknowledgements

We gratefully acknowledge the financial support provided by the Spanish Ministry of Science and Innovation-Carlos III Institute of Health according to the 'Plan Nacional de I+D+I 2008-2011' (PS09-2252 to DP, and CP10/00527 to CR, with cofunding by FEDER), the Andalusian Ministry of Health (PI-2010-0824 to DP), and the PAIDI Program from the Andalusian Government (CTS-677 to DP). ALG holds a FPU predoctoral fellowship from the Spanish Ministry of Education. We are most indebted to Neuroinvest Foundation for its continuing support.

10. References

Aloisi, F. (2001). Immune function of microglia. *Glia*, 36, (2), pp. (165-79).

Alvarez-Erviti, L., et al. (2011). Alpha-synuclein release by neurons activates the inflammatory response in a microglial cell line. *Neurosci Res*, 69, (4), pp. (337-42).

Anderson, J. P., et al. (2006). Phosphorylation of Ser-129 is the dominant pathological modification of alpha-synuclein in familial and sporadic Lewy body disease. *J Biol Chem*, 281, (40), pp. (29739-52).

Appel, S. H., et al. (2010). T cell-microglial dialogue in Parkinson's disease and amyotrophic lateral sclerosis: are we listening? *Trends Immunol*, 31, (1), pp. (7-17).

Auluck, P. K., et al. (2002). Chaperone suppression of alpha-synuclein toxicity in a Drosophila model for Parkinson's disease. *Science*, 295, (5556), pp. (865-8).

Austin, S. A., et al. (2006). Alpha-synuclein expression modulates microglial activation phenotype. *J Neurosci*, 26, (41), pp. (10558-63).

Austin, S. A., et al. (2011). Lack of Alpha-Synuclein modulates microglial phenotype In Vitro. *Neurochem Res*, 36, (6), pp. (994-1004).

Baglioni, S., et al. (2006). Prefibrillar amyloid aggregates could be generic toxins in higher organisms. *J Neurosci*, 26, (31), pp. (8160-7).

Benner, E. J., et al. (2008). Nitrated alpha-Synuclein immunity accelerates degeneration of nigral dopaminergic neurons. *PLoS One*, 3, (1), pp. (e1376).

Benner, E. J., et al. (2004). Therapeutic immunization protects dopaminergic neurons in a mouse model of Parkinson's disease. *Proc Natl Acad Sci U S A*, 101, (25), pp. (9435-40).

Bennett, M. C. (2005). The role of alpha-synuclein in neurodegenerative diseases. *Pharmacol Ther*, 105, (3), pp. (311-31).

Biasini, E., et al. (2004). Proteasome inhibition and aggregation in Parkinson's disease: a comparative study in untransfected and transfected cells. *J Neurochem*, 88, (3), pp. (545-53).

Borghi, R., et al. (2000). Full length alpha-synuclein is present in cerebrospinal fluid from Parkinson's disease and normal subjects. *Neurosci Lett*, 287, (1), pp. (65-7).

Bosco, D. A., et al. (2006). Elevated levels of oxidized cholesterol metabolites in Lewy body disease brains accelerate alpha-synuclein fibrilization. *Nat Chem Biol*, 2, (5), pp. (249-53).

Braak, H., et al. (2003). Staging of brain pathology related to sporadic Parkinson's disease. *Neurobiol Aging*, 24, (2), pp. (197-211).

Braak, H., et al. (2007). Development of alpha-synuclein immunoreactive astrocytes in the forebrain parallels stages of intraneuronal pathology in sporadic Parkinson's disease. *Acta Neuropathol*, 114, (3), pp. (231-41).

Brochard, V., et al. (2009). Infiltration of CD4+ lymphocytes into the brain contributes to neurodegeneration in a mouse model of Parkinson disease. *J Clin Invest*, 119, (1), pp. (182-92).

Bucciantini, M., et al. (2004). Prefibrillar amyloid protein aggregates share common features of cytotoxicity. *J Biol Chem*, 279, (30), pp. (31374-82).

Bucciantini, M., et al. (2002). Inherent toxicity of aggregates implies a common mechanism for protein misfolding diseases. *Nature*, 416, (6880), pp. (507-11).

Cabin, D. E., et al. (2002). Synaptic vesicle depletion correlates with attenuated synaptic responses to prolonged repetitive stimulation in mice lacking alpha-synuclein. *J Neurosci*, 22, (20), pp. (8797-807).

Campbell, B. C., et al. (2001). The solubility of alpha-synuclein in multiple system atrophy differs from that of dementia with Lewy bodies and Parkinson's disease. *J Neurochem*, 76, (1), pp. (87-96).

Castagnet, P. I., et al. (2005). Fatty acid incorporation is decreased in astrocytes cultured from alpha-synuclein gene-ablated mice. *J Neurochem*, 94, (3), pp. (839-49).

Castano, A., et al. (1998). Lipopolysaccharide intranigral injection induces inflammatory reaction and damage in nigrostriatal dopaminergic system. *J Neurochem*, 70, (4), pp. (1584-92).

Colton, C. A., et al. (2006). Expression profiles for macrophage alternative activation genes in AD and in mouse models of AD. *J Neuroinflammation*, 3, pp. (27).

Cookson, M. R. (2009). alpha-Synuclein and neuronal cell death. *Mol Neurodegener*, 4, pp. (9).

Croisier, E.&M. B. Graeber (2006). Glial degeneration and reactive gliosis in alpha-synucleinopathies: the emerging concept of primary gliodegeneration. *Acta Neuropathol*, 112, (5), pp. (517-30).

Croisier, E., et al. (2005). Microglial inflammation in the parkinsonian substantia nigra: relationship to alpha-synuclein deposition. *J Neuroinflammation*, 2, pp. (14).

Chen, H., et al. (2005). Nonsteroidal antiinflammatory drug use and the risk for Parkinson's disease. *Ann Neurol*, 58, (6), pp. (963-7).

Chen, H., et al. (2003). Nonsteroidal anti-inflammatory drugs and the risk of Parkinson disease. *Arch Neurol*, 60, (8), pp. (1059-64).

Chen, S., et al. (1998). Experimental destruction of substantia nigra initiated by Parkinson disease immunoglobulins. *Arch Neurol*, 55, (8), pp. (1075-80).

Chiti, F.&C. M. Dobson (2006). Protein misfolding, functional amyloid, and human disease. *Annu Rev Biochem*, 75, pp. (333-66).

Choi, D. Y., et al. (2010). Aging enhances the neuroinflammatory response and alpha-synuclein nitration in rats. *Neurobiol Aging*, 31, (9), pp. (1649-53).

Chung, C. Y., et al. (2009). Dynamic changes in presynaptic and axonal transport proteins combined with striatal neuroinflammation precede dopaminergic neuronal loss in a rat model of AAV alpha-synucleinopathy. *J Neurosci*, 29, (11), pp. (3365-73).

Danzer, K. M., et al. (2011). Heat-shock protein 70 modulates toxic extracellular alpha-synuclein oligomers and rescues trans-synaptic toxicity. *FASEB J*, 25, (1), pp. (326-36).

Dedmon, M. M., et al. (2005). Heat shock protein 70 inhibits alpha-synuclein fibril formation via preferential binding to prefibrillar species. *J Biol Chem*, 280, (15), pp. (14733-40).

Delgado, M., et al. (2005). Vasoactive intestinal peptide generates CD4+CD25+ regulatory T cells in vivo. *J Leukoc Biol*, 78, (6), pp. (1327-38).

Delgado, M.&D. Ganea (2003). Neuroprotective effect of vasoactive intestinal peptide (VIP) in a mouse model of Parkinson's disease by blocking microglial activation. *FASEB J*, 17, (8), pp. (944-6).

Desplats, P., et al. (2009). Inclusion formation and neuronal cell death through neuron-to-neuron transmission of alpha-synuclein. *Proc Natl Acad Sci U S A*, 106, (31), pp. (13010-5).

El-Agnaf, O. M., et al. (2003). Alpha-synuclein implicated in Parkinson's disease is present in extracellular biological fluids, including human plasma. *FASEB J*, 17, (13), pp. (1945-7).

El-Agnaf, O. M., et al. (2006). Detection of oligomeric forms of alpha-synuclein protein in human plasma as a potential biomarker for Parkinson's disease. *FASEB J*, 20, (3), pp. (419-25).

Fernagut, P. O.&M. F. Chesselet (2004). Alpha-synuclein and transgenic mouse models. *Neurobiol Dis*, 17, (2), pp. (123-30).

Gao, H. M.&J. S. Hong (2008). Why neurodegenerative diseases are progressive: uncontrolled inflammation drives disease progression. *Trends Immunol*, 29, (8), pp. (357-65).

Gao, H. M., et al. (2008). Neuroinflammation and oxidation/nitration of alpha-synuclein linked to dopaminergic neurodegeneration. *J Neurosci*, 28, (30), pp. (7687-98).

Gao, H. M., et al. (2011). Neuroinflammation and alpha-Synuclein dysfunction potentiate each other driving chronic progression of neurodegeneration in a mouse model of Parkinson's disease. *Environ Health Perspect*, pp.

Gasser, T. (2005). Genetics of Parkinson's disease. *Curr Opin Neurol*, 18, (4), pp. (363-9).

Giasson, B. I., et al. (2000). Oxidative damage linked to neurodegeneration by selective alpha-synuclein nitration in synucleinopathy lesions. *Science*, 290, (5493), pp. (985-9).

Giorgi, C., et al. (2008). Ca2+ signaling, mitochondria and cell death. *Curr Mol Med*, 8, (2), pp. (119-30).

Giuliani, F., et al. (2003). Vulnerability of human neurons to T cell-mediated cytotoxicity. *J Immunol*, 171, (1), pp. (368-79).

Glass, C. K., et al. (2010). Mechanisms underlying inflammation in neurodegeneration. *Cell*, 140, (6), pp. (918-34).

Golovko, M. Y., et al. (2009). The role of alpha-synuclein in brain lipid metabolism: a downstream impact on brain inflammatory response. *Mol Cell Biochem*, 326, (1-2), pp. (55-66).

Gonzalez-Rey, E., et al. (2006). Vasoactive intestinal peptide generates human tolerogenic dendritic cells that induce CD4 and CD8 regulatory T cells. *Blood*, 107, (9), pp. (3632-8).

Griffin, W. S., et al. (2006). Interleukin-1 mediates Alzheimer and Lewy body pathologies. *J Neuroinflammation*, 3, pp. (5).

Gruden, M. A., et al. (2011). Immunoprotection against toxic biomarkers is retained during Parkinson's disease progression. *J Neuroimmunol*, pp.

Gu, X. L., et al. (2010). Astrocytic expression of Parkinson's disease-related A53T alpha-synuclein causes neurodegeneration in mice. *Mol Brain*, 3, pp. (12).

Halliday, G. M.&C. H. Stevens (2011). Glia: Initiators and progressors of pathology in Parkinson's disease. *Mov Disord*, 26, (1), pp. (6-17).

Hasegawa, M., et al. (2002). Phosphorylated alpha-synuclein is ubiquitinated in alpha-synucleinopathy lesions. *J Biol Chem*, 277, (50), pp. (49071-6).

He, Y., et al. (2002). Role of Fcgamma receptors in nigral cell injury induced by Parkinson disease immunoglobulin injection into mouse substantia nigra. *Exp Neurol*, 176, (2), pp. (322-7).

Hodara, R., et al. (2004). Functional consequences of alpha-synuclein tyrosine nitration: diminished binding to lipid vesicles and increased fibril formation. *J Biol Chem*, 279, (46), pp. (47746-53).

Huang, C., et al. (2006). Heat shock protein 70 inhibits alpha-synuclein fibril formation via interactions with diverse intermediates. *J Mol Biol*, 364, (3), pp. (323-36).

Jenco, J. M., et al. (1998). Regulation of phospholipase D2: selective inhibition of mammalian phospholipase D isoenzymes by alpha- and beta-synucleins. *Biochemistry*, 37, (14), pp. (4901-9).

Jo, E., et al. (2000). alpha-Synuclein membrane interactions and lipid specificity. *J Biol Chem*, 275, (44), pp. (34328-34).

Kawai, T.&S. Akira (2007). TLR signaling. *Semin Immunol*, 19, (1), pp. (24-32).

Kebir, H., et al. (2007). Human TH17 lymphocytes promote blood-brain barrier disruption and central nervous system inflammation. *Nat Med*, 13, (10), pp. (1173-5).

Kim, S., et al. (2009). Alpha-synuclein induces migration of BV-2 microglial cells by up-regulation of CD44 and MT1-MMP. *J Neurochem*, 109, (5), pp. (1483-96).

Kim, S., et al. (2004a). Alpha-synuclein induces apoptosis by altered expression in human peripheral lymphocyte in Parkinson's disease. *FASEB J*, 18, (13), pp. (1615-7).

Kim, S., et al. (2004b). Alpha-synuclein, Parkinson's disease, and Alzheimer's disease. *Parkinsonism Relat Disord*, 10 Suppl 1, pp. (S9-13).

Kim, Y. S.&T. H. Joh (2006). Microglia, major player in the brain inflammation: their roles in the pathogenesis of Parkinson's disease. *Exp Mol Med*, 38, (4), pp. (333-47).

Klegeris, A., et al. (2007a). Functional ryanodine receptors are expressed by human microglia and THP-1 cells: Their possible involvement in modulation of neurotoxicity. *J Neurosci Res*, 85, (10), pp. (2207-15).

Klegeris, A., et al. (2006). Alpha-synuclein and its disease-causing mutants induce ICAM-1 and IL-6 in human astrocytes and astrocytoma cells. *FASEB J*, 20, (12), pp. (2000-8).

Klegeris, A., et al. (2007b). Therapeutic approaches to inflammation in neurodegenerative disease. *Curr Opin Neurol*, 20, (3), pp. (351-7).

Klegeris, A., et al. (2008). Alpha-synuclein activates stress signaling protein kinases in THP-1 cells and microglia. *Neurobiol Aging*, 29, (5), pp. (739-52).

Klucken, J., et al. (2004). Hsp70 Reduces alpha-Synuclein Aggregation and Toxicity. *J Biol Chem*, 279, (24), pp. (25497-502).

Ko, L., et al. (2000). Sensitization of neuronal cells to oxidative stress with mutated human alpha-synuclein. *J Neurochem*, 75, (6), pp. (2546-54).

Kreutzberg, G. W. (1996). Microglia: a sensor for pathological events in the CNS. *Trends Neurosci*, 19, (8), pp. (312-8).

Kruger, R., et al. (1998). Ala30Pro mutation in the gene encoding alpha-synuclein in Parkinson's disease. *Nat Genet*, 18, (2), pp. (106-8).

Laurie, C., et al. (2007). CD4+ T cells from Copolymer-1 immunized mice protect dopaminergic neurons in the 1-methyl-4-phenyl-1,2,3,6-tetrahydropyridine model of Parkinson's disease. *J Neuroimmunol*, 183, (1-2), pp. (60-8).

Lee, D., et al. (2002). alpha-Synuclein exhibits competitive interaction between calmodulin and synthetic membranes. *J Neurochem*, 82, (5), pp. (1007-17).

Lee, E. J., et al. (2010). Alpha-synuclein activates microglia by inducing the expressions of matrix metalloproteinases and the subsequent activation of protease-activated receptor-1. *J Immunol*, 185, (1), pp. (615-23).

Lee, H. J., et al. (2005). Intravesicular localization and exocytosis of alpha-synuclein and its aggregates. *J Neurosci*, 25, (25), pp. (6016-24).

Lee, J. K., et al. (2009a). Neuroinflammation in Parkinson's disease. *J Neuroimmune Pharmacol*, 4, (4), pp. (419-29).

Lee, J. T., et al. (2008). Ubiquitination of alpha-synuclein by Siah-1 promotes alpha-synuclein aggregation and apoptotic cell death. *Hum Mol Genet*, 17, (6), pp. (906-17).

Lee, P. H., et al. (2006). The plasma alpha-synuclein levels in patients with Parkinson's disease and multiple system atrophy. *J Neural Transm*, 113, (10), pp. (1435-9).

Lee, S. B., et al. (2009b). Identification of the amino acid sequence motif of alpha-synuclein responsible for macrophage activation. *Biochem Biophys Res Commun*, 381, (1), pp. (39-43).

Lee, S. J. (2008). Origins and effects of extracellular alpha-synuclein: implications in Parkinson's disease. *J Mol Neurosci*, 34, (1), pp. (17-22).

Lim, K. L.&J. M. Tan (2007). Role of the ubiquitin proteasome system in Parkinson's disease. *BMC Biochem*, 8 Suppl 1, pp. (S13).

Long-Smith, C. M., et al. (2009). The influence of microglia on the pathogenesis of Parkinson's disease. *Prog Neurobiol*, 89, (3), pp. (277-87).

Mandel, S., et al. (2005). Gene expression profiling of sporadic Parkinson's disease substantia nigra pars compacta reveals impairment of ubiquitin-proteasome subunits, SKP1A, aldehyde dehydrogenase, and chaperone HSC-70. *Ann N Y Acad Sci*, 1053, pp. (356-75).

Martinez, J., et al. (2003). Parkinson's disease-associated alpha-synuclein is a calmodulin substrate. *J Biol Chem*, 278, (19), pp. (17379-87).

Masliah, E., et al. (2005). Effects of alpha-synuclein immunization in a mouse model of Parkinson's disease. *Neuron*, 46, (6), pp. (857-68).

McGeer, P. L., et al. (1988). Reactive microglia are positive for HLA-DR in the substantia nigra of Parkinson's and Alzheimer's disease brains. *Neurology*, 38, (8), pp. (1285-91).

McGeer, P. L.&E. G. McGeer (2008). Glial reactions in Parkinson's disease. *Mov Disord*, 23, (4), pp. (474-83).

Mihara, T., et al. (2008). Natural killer cells of Parkinson's disease patients are set up for activation: a possible role for innate immunity in the pathogenesis of this disease. *Parkinsonism Relat Disord*, 14, (1), pp. (46-51).

Miklossy, J., et al. (2006). Role of ICAM-1 in persisting inflammation in Parkinson disease and MPTP monkeys. *Exp Neurol*, 197, (2), pp. (275-83).

Mori, F., et al. (2002). Demonstration of alpha-synuclein immunoreactivity in neuronal and glial cytoplasm in normal human brain tissue using proteinase K and formic acid pretreatment. *Exp Neurol*, 176, (1), pp. (98-104).

Mount, M. P., et al. (2007). Involvement of interferon-gamma in microglial-mediated loss of dopaminergic neurons. *J Neurosci*, 27, (12), pp. (3328-37).

Orr, C. F., et al. (2005). A possible role for humoral immunity in the pathogenesis of Parkinson's disease. *Brain*, 128, (Pt 11), pp. (2665-74).

Ouchi, Y., et al. (2005). Microglial activation and dopamine terminal loss in early Parkinson's disease. *Ann Neurol*, 57, (2), pp. (168-75).

Papachroni, K. K., et al. (2007). Autoantibodies to alpha-synuclein in inherited Parkinson's disease. *J Neurochem*, 101, (3), pp. (749-56).

Park, D. R., et al. (2003). Fas (CD95) induces proinflammatory cytokine responses by human monocytes and monocyte-derived macrophages. *J Immunol*, 170, (12), pp. (6209-16).

Park, J. Y., et al. (2008). Microglial phagocytosis is enhanced by monomeric alpha-synuclein, not aggregated alpha-synuclein: implications for Parkinson's disease. *Glia*, 56, (11), pp. (1215-23).

Peng, X., et al. (2005). Alpha-synuclein activation of protein phosphatase 2A reduces tyrosine hydroxylase phosphorylation in dopaminergic cells. *J Cell Sci*, 118, (Pt 15), pp. (3523-30).

Perez, R. G.&T. G. Hastings (2004). Could a loss of alpha-synuclein function put dopaminergic neurons at risk? *J Neurochem*, 89, (6), pp. (1318-24).

Polymeropoulos, M. H., et al. (1997). Mutation in the alpha-synuclein gene identified in families with Parkinson's disease. *Science*, 276, (5321), pp. (2045-7).

Ponomarev, E. D., et al. (2007). CNS-derived interleukin-4 is essential for the regulation of autoimmune inflammation and induces a state of alternative activation in microglial cells. *J Neurosci*, 27, (40), pp. (10714-21).

Przedborski, S., et al. (2001). Oxidative post-translational modifications of alpha-synuclein in the 1-methyl-4-phenyl-1,2,3,6-tetrahydropyridine (MPTP) mouse model of Parkinson's disease. *J Neurochem*, 76, (2), pp. (637-40).

Racke, M. K., et al. (2000). The role of costimulation in autoimmune demyelination. *J Neuroimmunol*, 107, (2), pp. (205-15).

Reynolds, A. D., et al. (2007). Neuroprotective activities of CD4+CD25+ regulatory T cells in an animal model of Parkinson's disease. *J Leukoc Biol*, 82, (5), pp. (1083-94).

Reynolds, A. D., et al. (2008a). Nitrated alpha-synuclein-activated microglial profiling for Parkinson's disease. *J Neurochem*, 104, (6), pp. (1504-25).

Reynolds, A. D., et al. (2008b). Nitrated alpha-Synuclein and microglial neuroregulatory activities. *J Neuroimmune Pharmacol*, pp. (54-74)

Reynolds, A. D., et al. (2010). Regulatory T cells attenuate Th17 cell-mediated nigrostriatal dopaminergic neurodegeneration in a model of Parkinson's disease. *J Immunol*, 184, (5), pp. (2261-71).

Reynolds, A. D., et al. (2009a). Nitrated α-synuclein-induced alterations in microglial immunity are regulated by CD4+ T cell subsets. *J Immunol*, 182, (7), pp. (4137-49).

Reynolds, A. D., et al. (2009b). Proteomic studies of nitrated alpha-synuclein microglia regulation by CD4+CD25+ T cells. *J Proteome Res*, 8, (7), pp. (3497-511).

Richter-Landsberg, C., et al. (2000). alpha-synuclein is developmentally expressed in cultured rat brain oligodendrocytes. *J Neurosci Res*, 62, (1), pp. (9-14).

Roodveldt, C., et al. (2009). Chaperone proteostasis in Parkinson's disease: stabilization of the Hsp70/alpha-synuclein complex by Hip. *EMBO J*, 28, (23), pp. (3758-70).

Roodveldt, C., et al. (2008). Immunological features of alpha-synuclein in Parkinson's disease. *J Cell Mol Med*, 12, (5B), pp. (1820-9).

Roodveldt, C., et al. (2010). Glial innate immunity generated by non-aggregated alpha-synuclein in mouse: differences between wild-type and Parkinson's disease-linked mutants. *PLoS One*, 5, (10), pp. (e13481).

Rott, R., et al. (2008). Monoubiquitylation of alpha-synuclein by seven in absentia homolog (SIAH) promotes its aggregation in dopaminergic cells. *J Biol Chem*, 283, (6), pp. (3316-28).

Salazar-Mather, T. P., et al. (1996). NK cell trafficking and cytokine expression in splenic compartments after IFN induction and viral infection. *J Immunol*, 157, (7), pp. (3054-64).

Sanchez-Guajardo, V., et al. (2010). Microglia acquire distinct activation profiles depending on the degree of alpha-synuclein neuropathology in a rAAV based model of Parkinson's disease. *PLoS One*, 5, (1), pp. (e8784).

Sanchez-Pernaute, R., et al. (2004). Selective COX-2 inhibition prevents progressive dopamine neuron degeneration in a rat model of Parkinson's disease. *J Neuroinflammation*, 1, (1), pp. (6).

Schiess, M. C., et al. (2010). CSF from Parkinson disease patients differentially affects cultured microglia and astrocytes. *BMC Neurosci*, 11, pp. (151).

Shin, E. C., et al. (2000). Expression patterns of alpha-synuclein in human hematopoietic cells and in Drosophila at different developmental stages. *Mol Cells*, 10, (1), pp. (65-70).

Shults, C. W., et al. (2005). Neurological and neurodegenerative alterations in a transgenic mouse model expressing human alpha-synuclein under oligodendrocyte promoter: implications for multiple system atrophy. *J Neurosci*, 25, (46), pp. (10689-99).

Souza, J. M., et al. (2000). Dityrosine cross-linking promotes formation of stable alpha - synuclein polymers. Implication of nitrative and oxidative stress in the pathogenesis of neurodegenerative synucleinopathies. *J Biol Chem*, 275, (24), pp. (18344-9).

Spillantini, M. G., et al. (1998). alpha-Synuclein in filamentous inclusions of Lewy bodies from Parkinson's disease and dementia with lewy bodies. *Proc Natl Acad Sci U S A*, 95, (11), pp. (6469-73).

Stefani, M.&C. M. Dobson (2003). Protein aggregation and aggregate toxicity: new insights into protein folding, misfolding diseases and biological evolution. *J Mol Med*, 81, (11), pp. (678-99).

Stone, D. K., et al. (2009). Innate and adaptive immunity for the pathobiology of Parkinson's disease. *Antioxid Redox Signal*, 11, (9), pp. (2151-66).

Su, H. C., et al. (2001). NK cell functions restrain T cell responses during viral infections. *Eur J Immunol*, 31, (10), pp. (3048-55).

Su, X., et al. (2009). Mutant alpha-synuclein overexpression mediates early proinflammatory activity. *Neurotox Res*, 16, (3), pp. (238-54).

Su, X., et al. (2008). Synuclein activates microglia in a model of Parkinson's disease. *Neurobiol Aging*, 29, (11), pp. (1690-701).

Tanji, K., et al. (2002). Upregulation of alpha-synuclein by lipopolysaccharide and interleukin-1 in human macrophages. *Pathol Int*, 52, (9), pp. (572-7).

Tanji, K., et al. (2001). Expression of beta-synuclein in normal human astrocytes. *Neuroreport*, 12, (13), pp. (2845-8).

Terada, S., et al. (2003). Glial involvement in diffuse Lewy body disease. *Acta Neuropathol*, 105, (2), pp. (163-9).

Theodore, S., et al. (2008). Targeted overexpression of human alpha-synuclein triggers microglial activation and an adaptive immune response in a mouse model of Parkinson disease. *J Neuropathol Exp Neurol*, 67, (12), pp. (1149-58).

Thomas, M. P., et al. (2007). Ion channel blockade attenuates aggregated alpha synuclein induction of microglial reactive oxygen species: relevance for the pathogenesis of Parkinson's disease. *J Neurochem*, 100, (2), pp. (503-19).

Tofaris, G. K., et al. (2003). Ubiquitination of alpha-synuclein in Lewy bodies is a pathological event not associated with impairment of proteasome function. *J Biol Chem*, 278, (45), pp. (44405-11).

Tokuda, T., et al. (2006). Decreased alpha-synuclein in cerebrospinal fluid of aged individuals and subjects with Parkinson's disease. *Biochem Biophys Res Commun*, 349, (1), pp. (162-6).

Tokuda, T., et al. (2010). Detection of elevated levels of α-synuclein oligomers in CSF from patients with Parkinson disease. Neurol, 75, (20), pp. (1766-72).

Verreck, F. A., et al. (2004). Human IL-23-producing type 1 macrophages promote but IL-10-producing type 2 macrophages subvert immunity to (myco)bacteria. *Proc Natl Acad Sci U S A*, 101, (13), pp. (4560-5).

Vila, M., et al. (2001). The role of glial cells in Parkinson's disease. *Curr Opin Neurol*, 14, (4), pp. (483-9).

Wakabayashi, K., et al. (2000). NACP/alpha-synuclein-positive filamentous inclusions in astrocytes and oligodendrocytes of Parkinson's disease brains. *Acta Neuropathol*, 99, (1), pp. (14-20).

Wersinger, C.&A. Sidhu (2006). An inflammatory pathomechanism for Parkinson's disease? *Curr Med Chem*, 13, (5), pp. (591-602).

Wu, D. C., et al. (2002). Blockade of microglial activation is neuroprotective in the 1-methyl-4-phenyl-1,2,3,6-tetrahydropyridine mouse model of Parkinson disease. *J Neurosci*, 22, (5), pp. (1763-71).

Wyss-Coray, T.&L. Mucke (2002). Inflammation in neurodegenerative disease--a double-edged sword. *Neuron*, 35, (3), pp. (419-32).

Yamada, T., et al. (1992). Lewy bodies in Parkinson's disease are recognized by antibodies to complement proteins. *Acta Neuropathol*, 84, (1), pp. (100-4).

Yazawa, I., et al. (2005). Mouse model of multiple system atrophy alpha-synuclein expression in oligodendrocytes causes glial and neuronal degeneration. *Neuron*, 45, (6), pp. (847-59).

Yu, S., et al. (2007). Extensive nuclear localization of alpha-synuclein in normal rat brain neurons revealed by a novel monoclonal antibody. *Neuroscience*, 145, (2), pp. (539-55).

Zarranz, J. J., et al. (2004). The new mutation, E46K, of alpha-synuclein causes Parkinson and Lewy body dementia. *Ann Neurol*, 55, (2), pp. (164-73).

Zhang, W., et al. (2007). Microglial PHOX and Mac-1 are essential to the enhanced dopaminergic neurodegeneration elicited by A30P and A53T mutant alpha-synuclein. *Glia*, 55, (11), pp. (1178-88).

Zhang, W., et al. (2005). Aggregated alpha-synuclein activates microglia: a process leading to disease progression in Parkinson's disease. *FASEB J*, 19, (6), pp. (533-42).

Zhou, Y., et al. (2005). Microglial activation induced by neurodegeneration: a proteomic analysis. *Mol Cell Proteomics*, 4, (10), pp. (1471-9).

5

The Knoll-Concept to Decrease the Prevalence of Parkinson's Disease

Ildikó Miklya
Semmelweis University, Department of Pharmacology and Pharmacotherapy
Hungary

1. Introduction

(-)-Deprenyl (D)/Selegiline, introduced under the code name: E-250, in 1964/65 as a new spectrum "psychic energizer" (Knoll et al., 1965), and named (-)-deprenyl from 1970, became famous in 1971/1972 as the first selective inhibitor of B-type monoamine oxidase (MAO-B) (Knoll & Magyar, 1972). D, registered at present in 64 countries, started its world-wide carrier as a therapeutic agent in 1977 as the unique MAO inhibitor free of the cheese-effect (reviewing its early history see Knoll, 1983).

In the early 1960s when Knoll developed D MAO inhibitors were at the center of interest. It was the period when the hypothesis that depression is associated with diminished monoaminergic tone in the brain took root in the scientific community. MAO inhibitors played a key role in the development of this hypothesis. It became clear that MAO inhibitors elated depressed patients because they enhance the biological activity of monoamine transmitters in the central nervous system.

In 1951 isoniazid and its isopropyl-derivative, iproniazid, were successfully introduced for the treatment of tuberculosis and it was an unexpected observation that in contrast to isoniazid, iproniazid produced undesirable central stimulation in some patients. Zeller, who proposed in 1938 the name "monoamine oxidase" for the class of enzymes responsible for the oxidative deamination of monoamines, discovered in 1952 that iproniazid is capable to inhibit MAO activity in the brain and isoniazid is devoid of this property (Zeller & Barsky, 1952). In 1956 Crane analyzed the psychiatric side effects of iproniazid and concluded that it might be beneficial in the treatment of depression (Crane, 1956) and Kline introduced it as a "psychic energizer" (Kline, 1958).

Series of new MAO inhibitors were soon developed. It was, however, observed in 1963 that after eating cheese depressive patients treated with the highly potent MAO inhibitor, tranylcypromine, develop temporary clinical symptoms similar to a paroxysm induced by pheochromocytoma: hypertension, palpitation, neck stiffness, headache, nausea, vomiting. The same was observed also during treatment with nialamid, pargyline, and other MAO inhibitors. Blackwell (1963) realized that the hypertensive crisis is associated with the ingestion of high amounts of tyramine in cheese, the metabolism of which is inhibited by the MAO inhibitors ("cheese-effect"). Similar clinical episodes have also been observed after the ingestion of some other foodstuffs, such as yeast products and chianti wines, pickled herring, chicken liver, which are rich in tyramine, and/or other amine such as β-phenylethylamine (PEA), tryptamine, or L-3,4-dihydroxyphenylalanine (L-DOPA).

Knoll et al. demonstrated in a paper published in 1968 that the new MAO inhibitor, E-250, is free of the cheese-effect, because in contrary to the known MAO inhibitors, it does not potentiate, but inhibits the effect of tyramine (Knoll et al., 1968). The summary of this paper concluded that: "As the so-called cheese reaction, namely clinical symptoms similar to a paroxism induced by pheochromocytoma after cheese consumption is caused by the tyramine potentiating action of the MAO inhibitors, this tyramine inhibiting property of E-250 may be highly valuable for human therapy." Following Knoll's proposal it was shown later that D is free of the cheese effect also in humans (Elsworth et al., 1978; Sandler et al., 1978).

It was Birkmayer in Vienna who first demonstrated that, in contrast to the known MAO inhibitors, D can be combined safely with levodopa in Parkinson's disease (PD). Because of the serious side effect of levodopa in PD, Birkmayer and Hornykiewicz tried earlier to achieve a levodopa-sparing effect by the concurrent administration of levodopa and an MAO inhibitor, but this line of clinical research was soon terminated because the combination elicited serious hypertensive attacks (Birkmayer & Hornykiewicz, 1962). Birkmayer, considering the peculiar pharmacological profile of D dared to combine this MAO inhibitor with levodopa in PD and since the levodopa-sparing effect was achieved without side-effect (Birkmayer et al., 1977), this study initiated, and the Lancet Editorial "Deprenyl in Parkinson's disease" (The Lancet, September 25, 1982) substantially promoted the worldwide use of D in PD. Further studies revealed that D slows the rate of the functional deterioration of the nigrostriatal dopaminergic neurons in patients with early, untreated PD, and thus slows the progress of the disease (Tetrud & Langstone, 1989; Parkinson Study Group, 1989, 1993; Allain et al., 1991; Myttyla et al., 1992; Larsen et al., 1999).

The first two studies to demonstrate the beneficial effect of D in Alzheimer's disease (AD) were published in 1987 (Martini et al., 1987; Tariot et al., 1987) and a stream of clinical studies with small sample sizes, published between 1990 and 1993, confirmed the usefulness of D in the treatment of the disease (for review see Knoll, 2001). Finally, in 1977 a proper controlled trial showed that in patient with moderately severe AD, treatment with D slows the progression of the disease (Sano et al., 1997).

In retrospect it is hard to understand why D was before 2006, thus for 40 years, in striking contrast with the expectation of its developer, nowhere in the world registered with the indication to use it as an antidepressant. Knoll selected E-250 for further development in the hope that it will be used as a new efficient antidepressant. Before publishing the first paper on E-250 he already asked his schoolmate, the psychiatrist Ervin Varga, to test the new compound in depressed patients. The outcome of this preliminary study was cited as personal communication in the first paper (Knoll et al., 1965). Varga presented his results in the same year in a lecture (Varga, 1965) and published with his coworkers two papers on the antidepressant effect of D (Varga & Tringer, 1967; Tringer et al., 1971). Further clinical studies confirmed the antidepressant effect of D (Mann & Gershon, 1980; Youdim, 1980; Tom & Cummings, 1998; Zesiewitz et al., 1999; Miyoshi, 2001) and an analysis of the use of D in major depression was carefully reviewed (Gaszner & Miklya, 2006), nevertheless, only 40 years after Knoll's original proposal in 2006 was a D preparation (Emsam), based on a double-blind placebo-controlled trial performed by Amsterdam (2003), registered in the USA for the treatment of major depression. Emsam is the first transdermally administered antidepressant.

Slowing the age-related deterioration of the catecholaminergic neurons is that still unexploited pharmacological property of D which deserves from practical point of view

favored attention. Although liquid deprenyl citrate preparations (Selepryl, Cyprenil) containing 1 mg D in 1 drop, the proposed daily dose for slowing brain aging, are since years in circulation, a controlled, double-blind clinical trial to lay the firm foundation of the prophylactic antiaging D therapy remained up to the present unperformed.
Since the estimated increase of the number of individuals over 65 will reach by 2050 the 1.1 billion level, thus to decrease the prevalence of age-related neurodegenerative diseases, like Parkinson's and Alzheimer's, is an urgent necessity, the main aim of this review is to sum up the arguments which renders probable the concept that the prophylactic lifelong daily administration of 1 mg D from sexual maturity until death improves the quality of life in senescence and show promise to prevent or delay the onset of PD and AD (Knoll, 2005).

2. The development of deprenyl

Joseph Knoll developed D in the early 1960s. Since 1951 he performed with his two coworkers, Karoly Kelemen and Berta Knoll, behavioral studies with rats, the aim of which was to study the cortical mechanisms which ensure the manipulability of the individual. He essentially developed in those years his working hypothesis that the appearance of the mammalian brain with the ability to acquire drives produced species with manipulability to fit for domestic life, i.e. to life in intimate association with and to the advantage of humans. To study the nature of the acquired drives, a special model was developed, the training of rats in a way that they fix in their cortex an unnatural urge, the so-called glass-cylinder-seeking drive. Those rats that performed best acquired this drive in a stable manner and maintained this unnatural urge for a life time. Knoll summarized the results and described the conclusion of his first 16-year research period with the glass-cylinder-seeking rats in a monograph (Knoll, 1969) and finally presented, after a further 36-year research period, his theory "The Brain and Its Self. A Neurochemical Concept of the Innate and Acquired Drives" in a second monograph (Knoll, 2005). His theory, based on the physiology of the acquired drives, furnishes knowledge about the most important brain mechanisms which created the society: the manipulability of the cortex.
An acquired drive is always built on an inner drive, however, after the acquired drive has been ultimately fixed, its origin, the innate drive, cannot be recognized anymore either in man or a domesticated animal. A glass-cylinder-seeking rat will never acquire this drive under natural conditions. The experimenter manipulated consciously its brain, making use of the innate potential to change a group of cortical neurons via proper training in a way that the rat is fixing an acquired drive. In case of a fully successful training, the glass-cylinder-seeking rat behaves as one who has a fanatical desire for the glass-cylinder. These rats showed the same high-grade adaptability and readiness in overcoming different obstacles during goal-attainment as the ones influenced by innate drives, such as hunger or sexual desire. "Humans possess the most manipulable brain among all living creatures on earth. The brain of a suicide-killer is furtively manipulated. The properly acquired drive develops as a result of long-lasting training. The subject always acts under coercion, under severe mental pressure. Nevertheless, it is the nature of acquired drives that if the manipulation was fully successful the individual ultimately behaves as one possessing a fanatical desire to reach the acquired-drive-motivated goal." (Knoll, 2005, p 139).
It was at the beginning of these behavioral studies that the need for a new type central stimulant, a proper experimental tool for studying the physiology of the acquired drives, emerged. Knoll's aim was to find an amphetamine-like psychic energizer without the side-

effect of the amphetamines that as soon as the dose is surpassing the 1-2 mg/kg level, the drug-induced continuous, irresistible release of catecholamines from their intraneuronal stores in the brain stem neurons arrives to an intensity resulting in aimless hypermotility which blocks purposeful behavior. Since in those times the MAO inhibitors represented a new type of central stimulants, he decided to approach his goal via a structure-activity-relationship study, the starting structure of which was methamphetamine, containing, in order to make the molecule capable to block MAO activity irreversibly, a propargyl-group attached to the nitrogen.

Out of a series of newly synthesized patentable propargyl-group-containing methamphetamine-derivatives Knoll selected finally E-250 for further development. Amphetamines, the synthetic long acting analogues of PEA are like their parent compound releasers of noradrenaline from their intraneuronal stores, thus they increase blood pressure. E-250 behaved anomalously. It did not increase blood pressure; it even inhibited the blood pressure increasing effect of its parent compound (see Knoll et al., 1965, Fig.1). Knoll realized the peculiar practical importance of this behavior and demonstrated that this compound, in contrast to all known MAO inhibitors, does not potentiate, but inhibits the effect of tyramine, thus it is free of the cheese effect (Knoll et al., 1968). This feature of D allowed later to combine it safely with levodopa in PD and initiated its world-wide use as a therapeutic agent (Birkmayer et al., 1977).

3. The period while the selective inhibition of MAO-B in the brain was thought to be fully responsible for the therapeutic effects of deprenyl

In the same year when Knoll demonstrated with two of his coworkers that D is free of the cheese-effect (Knoll et al., 1968), Johnston described a new irreversible MAO inhibitor, MB 9302 (later named clorgyline), which preferentially inhibited the deamination of serotonin (Johnston, 1968). Johnston proposed the existence of two forms of MAO, "type A" and "type B", the former being selectively inhibited by clorgyline and the latter insensitive to it. This nomenclature has become widely accepted and is still in use. The unique substrate specificity of this new MAO inhibitor was soon corroborated (Hall et al., 1969), and clorgyline became the classic experimental tool to inhibit selectively MAO-A.

In MAO research a selective inhibitor of MAO-B was badly needed and Knoll realized that D was the missing link, the highly selective inhibitor of MAO-B. He presented this finding first in 1971 in his lecture at the first international MAO meeting in Cagliari (Sardinia). D was used thereafter as the specific experimental tool to analyze MAO-B. The first paper which described this novel property of D (Knoll & Magyar, 1972) became 10 years later a citation classic (Knoll J., This Week's Citation Classic, January 15, 1982). After the discovery that D is a selective inhibitor of MAO-B this property of the compound remained for years in the center of his interest. He pointed for the first time in his lecture at the second international MAO meeting "Monoamine Oxidase and its Inhibition" organized by the CIBA Foundation in London 1975, to the importance to study carefully the consequence of the relation between PEA and D.

Since PEA, the physiologically important endogenous central nervous system stimulant is a specific substrate for MAO-B, thus D is increasing exceedingly PEA levels in the brain, he mentioned in the summary of this lecture that D in combination with PEA might be efficient in certain types of depression. In the discussion of his lecture (Knoll, 1976, pp 155-160) he referred repeatedly to the importance of this line of further research. A couple of years later, following Knoll's proposal, the antidepressive efficacy of D (5-10 mg daily) plus phenylalanine (250 mg/day), the precursor of PEA, has been evaluated in 155 unipolar depressed patients. Both oral and intravenous administration of the combination showed beneficial effect in 90% of outpatients and 80.5% of inpatients. It was concluded that this combined treatment has a potent antidepressive action based on the accumulation of PEA in the brain (Birkmayer et al., 1984).

In a further study Knoll enlarged his concept that D offers a previously unknown possibility to exploit the natural endowments of PEA and argued as follows (see Knoll, 1978a, p.59):"...a progressive significant decrease in the dopamine content of the nigrostriatum is to be observed at the decline of life....The physiological decrease of the dopamine content of the striatum could easily be prevented by the continuous administration of a small dose of (-)-deprenyl....", moreover: "There is now ample evidence that phenylethylamine is endogenous in the brain and might play a role in affective behavior. Urinary excretion of free phenylethylamine was found to be reduced in depressed patients supporting the hypothesis that phenylethylamine deficit may be one of the biochemical lesions in depression...".

In the same year, in another lecture (Knoll, 1978b) he emphasized the importance to begin the administration of D in the earliest state of parkinsonism. The validity of Knoll's proposal to begin the administration of this drug in the earliest state of PD got splendid verification a decade later in the Deprenyl and Tocopherol Antioxidant Therapy of Parkinsonism (DATATOP) study performed on selected patients with early untreated PD. It was shown that the administration of D delays significantly the onset of disability necessitating levodopa therapy (Tetrud & Langston, 1989; Parkinson Study Group, 1989). Knoll's close reasoning in this time was as follows: "Considering the mechanism of action of (-)-deprenyl it seems to be of high importance to begin the administration of this drug in the earliest state of parkinsonism, in order to preserve as far as possible the physiological control of acetylcholine release in the striatum thereby reducing the amount of the required levodopa to the lowest possible level. Even the known slow degradation of the nigrostriatal dopaminergic neurons, a frequent phenomenon of ageing, might be counteracted by starting long term treatment with low doses of (-)-deprenyl in due time." (Knoll, 1978b, p 195).

Furthermore, it is evident from the discussion quoted from this study that the concept to slow the physiological age-related decline of the dopaminergic machinery in the brain stem via prophylactic low dose D treatment, took slowly its final shape, and we may say in retrospect that Knoll's coming important longevity studies (Knoll, 1988; Knoll et al., 1989, 1994) cast in this paper their shadows before.

We can also follow in these years Knoll's method that whenever he wanted to prove undeniably the relevance of a well defined pharmacological effect of D in its therapeutic efficiency he started a structure-activity-relationship study and fabricated a D-derivative which differed only in its pharmacological spectrum from its parent compound in being devoid of the questionable property. For example, he found that D is a potent inhibitor of the uptake of amines into the nerve endings of catecholaminergic neurons.

Since he wanted to test the significance of the monoamine-uptake inhibitory property of D in its therapeutic effect, he developed selective MAO-B inhibitors, J-508 and U-1424, devoid of this effect (Knoll et al., 1978c). Using N-methyl-N-propargyl-/1-indenyl/-ammonium (J-508) as a reference compound which acts as a highly potent MAO inhibitor, devoid of uptake-inhibitory and releasing effects, the influence of MAO inhibitors on uptake was tested on a battery of isolated organs (cat nictitating membrane, perfused ear artery and strip of pulmonal artery of the rabbit, rat vas deferens).

In contrast to the nonselective and A-selective MAO inhibitors, as well as to the newly introduced selective MAO-B inhibitors (J-508, U-1424), D was unique in inhibiting tyramine-uptake. This means that D is unique in being free of the cheese effect. This was for example the reason why Knoll did not suggest developing J-508 as a therapeutic agent, despite that this compound was found to be a 20-times more potent selective inhibitor of MAO-B than D (Knoll, 1978c, Table 2).

It is remarkable in this context that, about 30 years later, the desmethyl-analogue of J-508 (Rasagiline) was registered as a "new" second generation selective MAO-B inhibitor with the argument that since (-)-methamphetamine is a metabolite of D of which rasagiline is free, this is the advantage of rasagiline over D. Everybody who reads the literature knows that this is a sham-argument in support of a "me too" compound. An exact experimental study (Yasar et al. 1993) proved that D is free of amphetamine-like dependence capacity, they concluded:"…the preclinical findings reviewed generally support the clinical experience that in over 20 years of therapeutic use there has been no established case of human abuse l-deprenyl." (Yasar et al., 1993, p 230). Furthermore, it is absolutely out of the common that there is nowhere the slightest hint in the rapidly increasing rasagiline literature that since this compound is the desmethyl-analogue of J-508, the pharmacology of which was described in detail 30 years ago, the developers carefully compared the pharmacological spectrum of rasagiline and J-508 showing its advantage over its parent compound. Since J-508 is devoid of the catecholaminergic activity enhancer (CAE) effect characteristic to D, we tested in this respect rasagiline in the shuttle box and found that this J-508 analogue bears resemblance to its parent compound and not to D (Miklya, 2008).

Influenced by new experimental data Knoll became suspicious that an unknown stimulatory effect and not MAO-B inhibition might primarily be responsible for the therapeutic benefits of the drug. By changing the propargyl moiety, which binds covalently with the flavin in MAO, to a propyl group, he developed 1-phenyl-2-propylamino-pentane (PPAP), a D-analogue, free of MAO-B inhibitory potency (Knoll et al., 1992a). He described in his monograph (Knoll, 2005) the essence of the PPAP story as follows: "With the development of (-)-1-phenyl-2-propylaminopentane, (-)-PPAP, the (-)-deprenyl analogue free of the MAO-B inhibitory potency, we already furnished direct evidence that the enhanced dopaminergic activity following administration of (-)-deprenyl was unrelated to the inhibition of MAO-B. Because (-)-PPAP, like (-)-deprenyl, inhibited the uptake of tyramine in isolated smooth muscle tests, we first assumed that the drug-induced enhanced dopaminergic activity was due to an uptake inhibitory effect. Further studies revealed that this interpretation was false." The discovery of the CAE effect in the early 1990s clarified the main mechanism through which D is enhancing the activity of the nigrostriatal dopaminergic neurons and terminated the period when the selective inhibition of MAO-B was in the center of interest.

4. Longevity studies. The proof that lifelong administration of deprenyl slows significantly the age-related decline of sexual performance and learning ability and prolongs life

The first paper which furnished experimental evidence for the pressing necessity to start a longevity study is the one entitled "Can the suicide inactivation of MAO by deprenyl explain its pharmacological effects?" (Knoll, 1981a). In this paper the pharmacological spectrum of D was reviewed and experimental and clinical evidence was listed proving that D facilitates via different mechanisms the dopaminergic modulation in the brain. The putative physiological role of extrasynaptosomal MAO, which is of the B-type, in the dopaminergic and "trace aminergic" modulation and its significance in the therapeutic effect of D was analyzed. The working hypothesis was proposed that the age-related increase in MAO-B activity in the human brain is the biochemical lesion in senescence which results in a decline of dopaminergic and "trace aminergic" modulation and triggers many of the phenomena (slight parkinsonian syndrome, anxiety, depressed mood, severely inhibited sexual performance, etc.) known to accompany the aging process. The obvious possibility to prevent or counteract the MAO-B related consequences of aging by long-term treatment with D was discussed. It was shown in this paper first that D is significantly improving the sexual performance of sluggish male rats and clorgyline is devoid of this property. The aphrodisiac effect of D in aged sluggish male rats was further demonstrated in a couple of papers (Knoll, 1981b; Yen et al., 1982; Knoll et al., 1983).

Knoll presented his fully elaborated strategy to improve the quality of life in senescence via the prophylactic life-long administration of D in his lecture delivered at the "Strategy of Drug Research" IUPAC-IUPHAR Symposium in Nordwijkerhout (The Netherlands) in 1981. He summarized his views as follows: "In the aging brain, there is a loss of neurons compensated for by a proliferation of glial cells. We might thus predict that dopaminergic and "trace aminergic" modulation in the brain declines in senescence because of loss of neurons and because of the increased monoamine oxidase (MAO)-B activity present in the glia. The hypothesis was forwarded that the significant increase of the incidence of depression in the elderly, the age-dependent decline in male sexual vigor and the frequent appearance of parkinsonian symptoms in the latter decades of life might be attributed to a decrease of dopamine and "trace amines" in the brain. The possibility to counteract these biochemical lesions of aging by chronic administration of (-)-deprenyl, a selective inhibitor of MAO-B, which facilitates dopaminergic and "trace aminergic" activity in the brain and is a safe drug in man, was analyzed in detail. The restitution and long term maintenance of full scale sexual activity in aged male rats continuously treated with (-)-deprenyl was demonstrated as an experimental model in support of the view that the long term administration of small doses of deprenyl may improve the quality of life in senescence" (Knoll, 1982, p 107).

In one of his following studies "Deprenyl (selegiline): the history of its development and pharmacological action" (Knoll, 1983), he reviewed experimental and clinical data to show the potential benefits of using D in the elderly. He referred for example to a paper which showed that D significantly prolonged the duration of PD, i.e. the lifespan of the D-treated patients was substantially extended (Birkmayer, Knoll et al., 1983). Knoll's hypothesis inspired this clinical analysis and led later to a more extensive analysis of Birkmayer's clinical data which definitely showed increased life expectancy resulting from addition of D to Madopar-treatment in PD (Birkmayer, Knoll et al., 1985).

In 1983 Knoll introduced his concept regarding the peculiar antiaging effect of D to the gerontologists in a lecture presented at the 7th European Symposium on Basic Research in Gerontology (Budapest, Hungary). He presented in this lecture new data to demonstrate that since the dopaminergic system represents the most rapidly aging neuronal network in the human brain, we lose after age 45 about 13% of our dopamine per decade, and D facilitates without side effects in a unique manner dopaminergic activity, which plays a leading role in the age-related decline of learning ability and sexual potency, it is reasonable to try to improve the quality of life in senescence via the prophylactic life-long small-dose administration of D (Knoll, 1985).

Knoll performed on a special, long-living strain of rats (first generation Wistar males x Logan females), with his two coworkers, Dallo and Yen, his first longevity study between 1984 and 1988. The concept and teaching of this study was published in a crucially important paper (Knoll, 1988) and in a brief summary (Knoll et al., 1989).

The study revealed that better performers in the mating test are better learners in the shuttle box and the more active animals live significantly longer than their less active peers. It was established by the aid of D which increased superoxide dismutase activity in the striatum, facilitated the activity of the nigrostriatal dopaminergic neurons with utmost selectivity, and protected these neurons from their age-related decay, that the efficiency of a rat in behavioral test, as well as the duration of its life are striatal dopamine dependent functions.

As a measure of striatal function, sexual activity was tested once a week in a group of male rats (n=132) from 24th month of their life. Because of the age-related decay of this function none of the 2-year-old animals displayed full scale sexual activity. By dividing the group equally the rats were treated with saline and D (0.25 mg/kg sc.), respectively, three times a week. In the saline-treated group (n=66) the last signs of sexual activity vanished to the 33rd week of treatment. D-treatment restored full scale sexual activity in 64 out of 66 rats. The longest living rat in the saline-treated group lived 164 weeks. The average lifespan of the group was 147.05±0.56 weeks. The shortest living animal in the D-treated group lived 171 weeks and the longest living rat died during the 226th week of its life. The average lifespan was 197.98±2.36 weeks, i.e. higher than the estimated maximum age of death in the rat (182 weeks). This was the first instance that by the aid of a well-aimed medication, members of a species lived beyond the known lifespan maximum. Further detailed studies in Knoll's laboratory corroborated the results of the first longevity study. It was demonstrated that rats treated during their post-developmental phase of life with a small dose of D lost their ability to ejaculate later (Knoll et al., 1989; Knoll, 1992; Knoll et al., 1994), showed a slower decline in learning performance with the passing of time (Knoll, 1989; Knoll et al., 1989, 1994), and lived significantly longer than their saline-treated peers (Knoll et al., 1989, 1994).

The original finding that D prolongs life was confirmed in rats (Milgram et al., 1990; Kitani et al., 1993), mice (Yen & Knoll, 1992; Freisleben et al., 1994; Archer et al., 1996), hamsters (Stoll et al., 1997), and dogs (Ruehl et al., 1997). In one strain of mice D-treatment had no beneficial effect on survival (Ingram et al., 1993); and Stoll et al. (1997) found increased lifespan in D-treated female hamsters only. Moreover, in the longevity studies substantial strain differences were found in the efficiency of D. It has to be considered, however, that enhancer substances stimulate the enhancer-sensitive neurons in the brain stem in a peculiar manner. Thus, the same dose of an enhancer drug may exert a peak effect on one strain, a much lower effect on an other strain, and be ineffective on a third strain (see Main Heading 5 for details).

One group found, in striking contrast with all other studies, an increased mortality in male Wistar rats treated with D 0.5 mg/kg for up to 20 months (Gallagher et al., 1998). The toxicological studies performed with D and decades of experiences on thousands of rats make clear that the administration of D 0.5 mg/kg 3 times a week could not be responsible for the observed increased mortality in the rats. It is worth mentioning that even in clinical studies improper combination of levodopa with D led to confusion and misinterpretation as it happened in a study performed by the Parkinson's Disease Research Group of the United Kingdom and published in 1995 (Lees, 1995; for a critical analysis see Knoll, 1998).

5. The catecholaminergic activity enhancer (CAE) effect of deprenyl

The availability of HPLC to measure exactly the catecholamines and serotonin in physiological quantities allowed a new approach. The thorough analysis of the dose-dependent effect of D on the release of catecholamines and serotonin from isolated, discrete, rat brain regions (dopamine from the striatum, substantia nigra and tuberculum olfactorium; noradrenaline from the locus coeruleus; and serotonin from the raphe) pointed to operation of a previously unknown peculiar enhancer regulation in the catecholaminergic neurons in the brain stem.

Rats were treated with 0.01, 0.025, 0.05, 0.1 and 0.25 mg/kg D, respectively, once daily for 21 days. Discrete rat brain regions were isolated 24 hours after the last injection and the biogenic amines released during 20 min from the freshly isolated tissue samples were measured. The amount of dopamine released from the substantia nigra and tuberculum olfactorium clarified that the dopaminergic neurons worked on a significantly higher activity level even in rats treated with the lowest, 0.01 mg/kg dose of D. As this small dose of D leaves the MAO-B activity and the uptake of amines practically unchanged, this study was the first unequivocal demonstration for the operation of a hitherto unknown enhancer mechanism in dopaminergic neurons stimulated by D in very low doses (Knoll & Miklya, 1994). D enhanced also the release of noradrenaline from the locus coeruleus, but did not enhance, even diminished the release of serotonin from the raphe. Thus, D proved to exert a highly specific, previously undetected CAE effect.

Further studies revealed that the parent compounds of D, PEA and methamphetamine, are primarily CAE substances but this property remained undetected because PEA and its long acting derivatives, amphetamine and methamphetamine, induce the continuous release of catecholaminergic transmitters from their neuronal pool which hinders completely the detectability of the CAE effect of these compounds. Since D is the only PEA-derived CAE-substance which is devoid of the catecholamine releasing property, it enabled to discover the enhancer regulation in the catecholaminergic neurons of the brain stem (Knoll et al., 1996a,b).

An additional proof of the operation of the enhancer regulation in the brain stem was the discovery that tryptamine is a natural enhancer substance which acts primarily on the serotonergic neurons (Knoll, 1994, for review see Knoll, 2005, 3.1.1). This experience catalyzed later the structure-activity-relationship study aiming to develop a tryptamine-derived enhancer substance and led finally to the selection of R-(-)-1-(benzofuran-2-yl)-2-propylaminopentane (BPAP), which is in rat experiments about hundred times more potent than D, for further development (Knoll et al., 1999). In contrast to D which is almost ineffective on the serotonergic neurons, BPAP is a highly potent enhancer of the serotonergic neurons.

Fig.1 and 2a,b show the striking difference between the catecholamine-releasing and the CAE effect.

The enhancer substances stimulate the enhancer sensitive neurons in the brain stem in a peculiar manner. Fig.3 shows, as an example, the bi-modal, bell-shaped concentration curve characteristic to the enhancer effect of BPAP, the presently known most potent and selective enhancer substance. The one in the low nanomolar range, with a peak effect at 10^{-13}M concentration, clearly demonstrates the existence of a highly complex, specific form of enhancer regulation in noradrenergic neurons. The second, with a peak effect at 10^{-6}M concentration, shows the operation of a ten million times less sensitive, obviously nonspecific form of the enhancer regulation in these neurons (Knoll et al., 2002).

6. Deprenyl-induced enhancement of scavenger function in the striatum

Knoll brought up for the first time in 1987 his idea that D may facilitate scavenger function in striatal neurons (Knoll, 1987). In a section of this paper, entitled "The putative role of scavenger function changes in the long-term deprenyl treatment induced protection of the nigrostriatal dopaminergic neuron", he referred to their experiences that the physiological consequences of the dopaminergic regulation in the caudate nucleus are detectable by measuring the basal ouabain-stimulated release of acetylcholine (ACh) (Knoll, 1978c).
Dopamine cell bodies dominating in the A9 and A10 of the substantia nigra produce such large amounts of dopamine that the striatum, in which neurons terminate, contains the highest amount of dopamine in the brain. The physiological role of dopamine released in the striatum is the continuous inhibition of the release of ACh from the cholinergic interneurons of the caudate nucleus. According to data shown in this paper (Knoll, 1987, Table 6) the amount of ouabain-induced release of ACh from isolated striatal slices dissected from untreated rats was found to be 366.7±57.3 pmole/g/min and the addition of dopamine (2.6 x 10^{-4} mole/L) increased the amount to 591.0±52.5 pmole/g/min, showing that dopamine stimulated the presynaptic dopamine "autoreceptors". In striatal slices taken from rats pretreated with 6-hydroxydopamine (6-OHDA) the ouabain-induced release of ACh increased to 706.0±60.0 pmole/g/min, similarly to the situation in PD, where loss of the nigrostriatal dopaminergic neurons leads to an uninhibited release of ACh in the

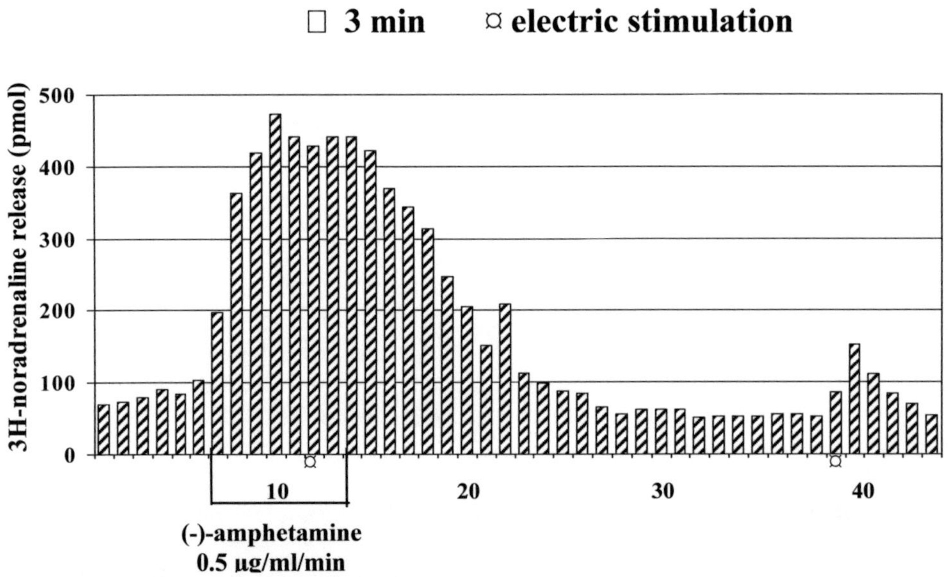

Fig. 1. Demonstration that amphetamine, the synthetic PEA-derivative, is inducing a long lasting spontaneous release of ^{3}[H]-noradrenaline from an isolated rat brain stem and electrical stimulation is ineffective, showing that the detectability of the enhancer effect is hindered.

striatum. The addition of dopamine inhibited to 372.9±93.8 pmole/g/min the ouabain-induced release of ACh, thus acted in the model like levodopa acts in PD.

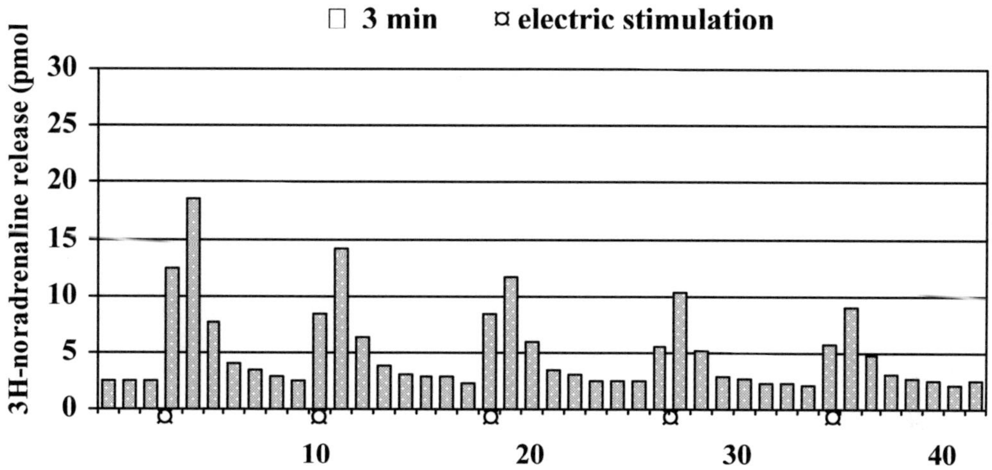

(a)

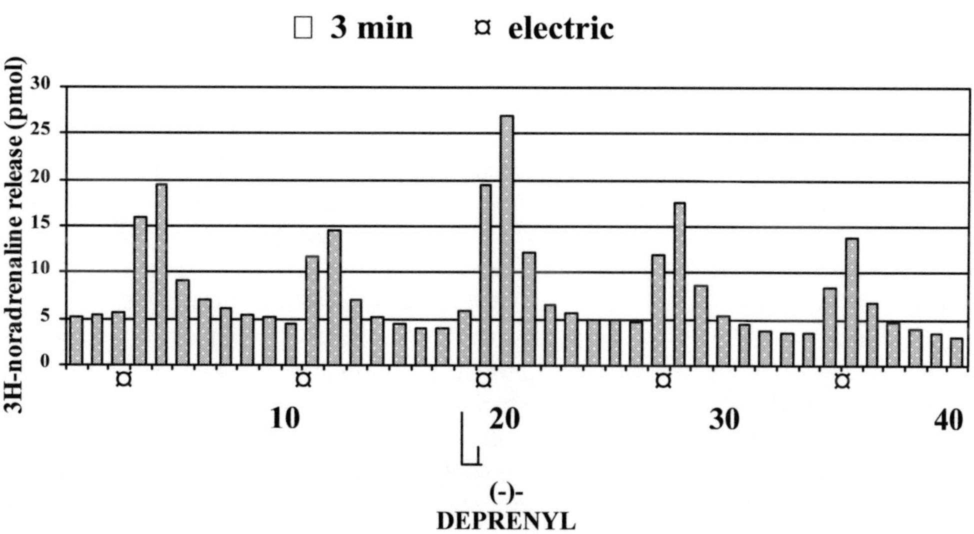

(b)

Fig. 2. a. Release of ^{3}[H]-noradrenaline from an isolated rat brain stem to consecutive electrical stimulations. There is a slow decline in response due to the exhaustion of the isolated organ. b The demonstration that since D is devoid of the spontaneous releasing effect of ^{3}[H]-noradrenaline characteristic to amphetamines, the CAE effect of D, the powerful enhancement of the release of ^{3}[H]-noradrenaline to electrical stimulation, is detectable.

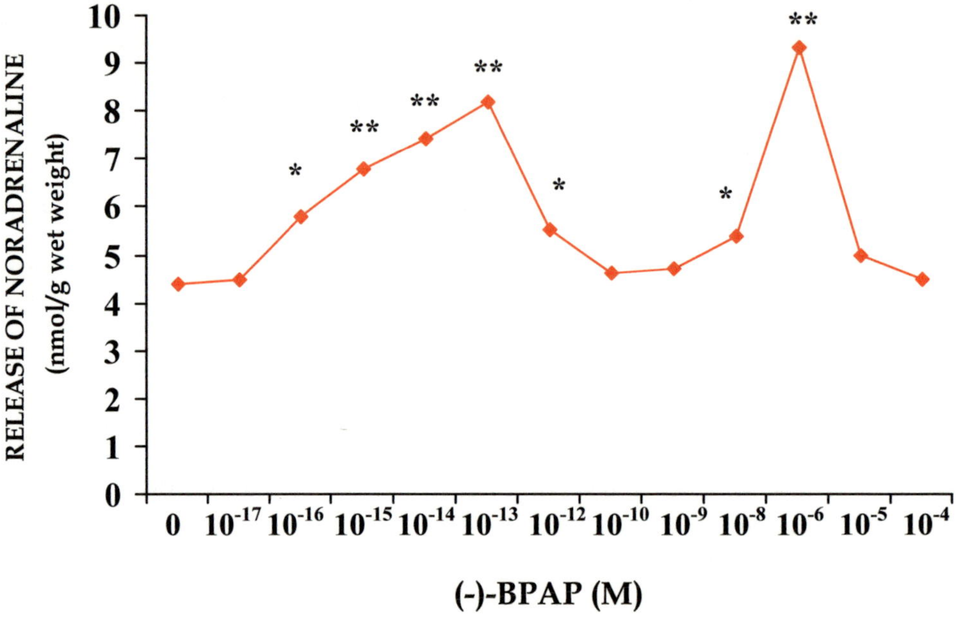

Fig. 3. The concentration effect curve characteristic to the CAE effect of enhancer substances. (The enhancer effect of BPAP on isolated locus coeruleus of rats is shown. For details see Knoll et al., 2002.); $^{*}p<0.01$, $^{**}p<0.001$.

D-treatment protected completely the striatum from the toxic effect of 6-OHDA. The s.c. injection of 0.25 mg/kg D for 3 weeks and the administration of 6-OHDA 24 hours after the last injection of D did not change the ouabain-induced release of ACh. Regarding the mechanism of this protection, Knoll concluded: "…the blockade of B-type MAO, the inhibition of the uptake of 6-OHDA into the neuron and the facilitation of scavenger function, the improvement of the removal of the neurotoxic free radicals may have shares in the highly efficient shielding effect of (-)-deprenyl" (Knoll, 1987, p 57). It was shown later that D increases dopamine transporter (DAT) expression but the new DAT molecules appear not to be functionally active (Lamensdorf et al., 1999).

After this conclusion, it was a reasonable step forward to test the effect of D on the scavenger mechanism in the striatum. And we really find in Knoll's next paper the first data showing that daily administration of D for three weeks is significantly enhancing the activity of superoxide dismutase (SOD) in the striatum of both male and female rats (Knoll, 1988, Table VII). This was an important discovery. The finding was soon confirmed by Carrillo et al. who found that also catalase activity was induced by D (Carrillo et al., 1991).

Knoll showed that D has no direct effect on brain SOD activity in general. Using the cerebellum as a reference tissue, he showed that SOD activity in this area did not change in a statistically significant manner in D-treated male and female rats (Knoll, 1989). Carrillo et al. confirmed also this finding. They showed in rats that activities of both SOD and catalase were significantly increased in striatum and substantia nigra but not in hippocampus, cerebellum and liver (Carrillo et al., 1992a). They also demonstrated that in old male mice D increased SOD and catalase activities in the substantia nigra, striatum and cerebral cortex, but not in hippocampus, cerebellum or liver (Carrillo et al., 1994a). Furthermore, in accordance with the finding in rats, D increased SOD activity in the striatum, but not in the hippocampus of beagle dogs (Carrillo et al., 1994b). Knoll demonstrated that D-induced enhancement of the SOD activity in the striatum of CFY rats was unrelated to the MAO inhibitory effect of the drug. Clorgyline, one of the most potent MAO inhibitors, inhibited rather than enhanced striatal SOD activity in rats (Knoll, 1988, 1990).

As we discussed earlier, the peculiar dose-dependency of the CAE effect of the enhancer substances (see Fig.3) clearly indicates the need of special caution regarding the optimal dosage with respect to each effect of D and other enhancer substances. Regarding the scavenger function of D, Carrillo et al. studied in detail the sex and age-dependency on the optimal dosage of this effect in rats (Carrillo et al., 1992b, 1993). The perplexed problem of the optimal dosage of D for increasing lifespan was analyzed and discussed between 1994 (Carrillo et al., 1994c) and 2006 (Kitani et.al., 2006) in a dozen of papers.

7. Neuroprotective effect of deprenyl

Hundreds of experimental studies prove that D protects against a couple of toxins (MPTP, 6-OHDA, DSP-4, AF64-A) and is a highly potent neuroprotective agent. The first study showing that D reduces PC12 cell apoptosis by inducing new protein synthesis was published by Tatton et al. (1994). Since this effect was exerted in concentrations as low as 10^{-13}M it was clear that the neuroprotective effect of D is unrelated to MAO-B inhibition (Tatton, et al. 1996). The real unanswered question is the mechanism through which D is protecting so many different cells against diverse deleterious effects. Knoll's arguments in support of the assumption that the CAE effect of D might be primarily responsible for most of the beneficial therapeutic effects of the drug (Knoll, 1998) require much thought. As a matter of fact, Tatton's finding was already prima-facie experimental evidence supporting Knoll's concept. D reduced PC12 cell apoptosis in 10^{-13}M concentration, exactly in the range where D exerts its CAE effect. The final proof, however, of the key importance of the enhancer effect in the neuroprotective capacity of the enhancer substances was the development of (-)-BPAP, a more potent enhancer substance than D which has no chemical similarity to the propargylamines. In the first paper which described the pharmacological profile of this new experimental tool, the relation of the neuroprotective property of this compound to its enhancer effect was demonstrated (Knoll et al., 1999). In this study the protective effect of racemic BPAP was measured against β-amyloid induced neurotoxicity on cultured rat hippocampal neurons, showing that enhancer substances might favorable influence AD.

At the 10th day the cultured cells were injured by exposing them for 3 days to a 20 μM concentration of β-amyloid 25-35 fragment. This concentration of β-amyloid decreased the survival of the neurons (control=100%) to 22.4±7.20% (mean±S.D.). BPAP significantly inhibited the β-amyloid induced neurotoxicity in the cultured hippocampal neurons in two distinct ranges of concentration, one with a peak of 10^{-14}M and one with a peak of 10^{-8}M. The peculiar concentration dependency of the effect of BPAP on the hippocampal neurons was surprisingly identical with that on the noradrenergic neurons, showing that the cell device in service of the enhancer regulation might be very similar to each other in the different enhancer-sensitive neurons (see Knoll 2001, Fig 13 and 14).

The interpretation of the finding in the first paper describing the pharmacology of (-)-BPAP (Knoll et al., 1999, p 1731) needs still serious consideration: "As a matter of fact there is a conspicuous similarity between the BPAP induced effect on the cultured rat hippocampal neurons and the one induced by (-)deprenyl in rats treated with the drug for years during their post-developmental phase of life. In the (-)deprenyl experiment we picked out of a population of 1600 rats the animals with the lowest and the highest sexual performance and demonstrated, on the one hand, that the 'high performing' rats lived significantly longer than their 'low performing' peers, and on the other hand, that (-)deprenyl treatment transformed the low performing rats into significantly higher performing ones, which lived then as long as their saline treated high performing peers (Knoll et al., 1994). We assume that high performing, longer living rats possess a more efficient catecholaminergic brain machinery than their low performing peers and the treatment with (-)deprenyl, a CAE substance, acts accordingly. Whatever performance we measure in a random population, we always find a huge variation in efficiency, ranging from very low to very high performing individuals. This is true also regarding the performance of cells in a population of cultured neurons. We may look at the 20% of the cultured hippocampal neurons which survived in the presence of β-amyloid, as 'high performing' cells, those possessing the most efficient BPAP-sensitive activation mechanism. Adding to the cultured neurons BPAP in the optimum concentration (10^{-14}M), the highly potent and selective enhancer of this regulation made each neuron higher performing and the surviving rate increased from 20% to 70%.
BPAP has obviously the same effect on the noradrenergic, dopaminergic, serotoninergic and hippocampal neurons. It may stimulate endogenous substances which enhance the activity of the neurons according to their physiological need. The high potency of BPAP in stimulating this regulation makes search in the brain after much more potent endogenous 'enhancer' substances than PEA and tryptamine, reasonable".
Hundreds of papers were published on the diverse effects of D, among them unexpected ones, like for example antitumor effect (ThyagaRajan & Felten, 2002), peculiar influence on stem cells (Esmaeili et al., 2006), enhancement of the secretion of the neurotrophic factors (Ohta et al., 2002; Shimazu et al., 2003), etc. It is the most important to decide which effect of the drug is primarily responsible for the verified benefits in PD, AD, major depression, and for its antiaging effect. Since the CAE effect of D is still not common knowledge, authors may remain inattentive to their findings which give clear information about this mechanism. An example: Groc et al. (2000) presented evidence of D insensitive apoptosis of nigral neurons during development. They found that apoptotic death of dopamine neurons during development is insensitive to daily treatment of the pregnant mothers and then newborns with D 0.1, 1.0, or 10 mg/kg. This finding informs about the key importance of the enhancer regulation in the effectiveness of D. Since the enhancer regulation in the brain of rats starts working only at the discontinuation of breast feeding (end of the third week of age) (Knoll & Miklya, 1995),it is obvious that apoptotic death of nigral neurons is insensitive to daily treatment of D before that age.
A second example: Ohta et al. (2002) studied the effects of BPAP, the newly developed enhancer substance, on cultured mouse astrocytes, measuring one of their specific functions the secretion of neurotrophins. They found that astrocytes treated for 24 hours with 0.35mM BPAP secreted into the culture medium 120, 2 and 7 times more NGF, BDNF and GDNF, respectively, than the untreated (control) cells. As Fig.3 demonstrates, BPAP exerts a specific enhancer effect in picomolar concentrations and a nonspecific one in micromolar

concentration. Since Ohta et al. investigated the effect of BPAP in high concentration only and because it is well-known that neuroglial cells play an important physiological role in the brain and modulate the function of neurons in a complex manner, but do not participate in the modification of behavioral functions, whereas BPAP is in the low pico/nanomolar concentration range influencing behavior, Knoll performed with coworkers a second study, testing BPAP on cultured mouse astrocytes in a range of 10^{-15}M to $5x10^{-4}$M concentration. This study corroborated the finding of the first one. The synthesis of NGF was significantly enhanced in the high micromolar concentration range with a peak effect at 10^{-4}M concentration, whereas $5x10^{-4}$M was ineffective. BPAP acted similarly on the synthesis of BDNF and GDNF. But the crucial step forward was the proof that, as expected, BPAP was ineffective in the low concentration range. Thus the specific form of enhancer regulation was not detectable in glial cells (Shimazu et al., 2003).

It can be little doubt that to differentiate between the specific and nonspecific enhancer effect of D requires consideration. Nevertheless, it remains for the future to identify the specific macromolecular target(s) that accommodate the endogenous enhancer substances and their synthetic derivatives; to demonstrate the existence of the predicted endogenous enhancer substances that are much more potent than PEA or tryptamine; and to map the enhancer-sensitive neurons and other cells in the brain, even if we know that the neurons of the catecholaminergic and serotonergic systems in the brain are probably the physiologically, biochemically, and pharmacologically best studied constituents of the CNS. For the time being it is unpredictable how many enhancer sensitive-cells exist the activity of which can be influenced by enhancer substances. An example: Denes et al. (2006) demonstrated that like the widely investigated rat PC12 cells, also human brain capillary endothelial cells (HBEC) are enhancer sensitive ones. Both D and BPAP exerted their significant cytoprotective effect on both HBEC and rat PC12 cells with the dose-dependency characteristic to the enhancer substances.

8. The rational of Knoll's concept that prophylactic deprenyl therapy may decrease the prevalence of neurodegenerative diseases, like Parkinson's and Alzheimer's

The dopaminergic system the neurons of which originate in the substantia nigra pars compacta, ventral tegmental area and hypothalamus is influencing many important brain functions playing a key role in the ability of the human brain to acquire new behavior. According to present knowledge the nigrostriatal dopaminergic neurons are the most rapidly aging neurons in the human brain. The dopamine content of the human caudate nucleus decreases steeply, at a rate of 13-15% per decade over age 45. We know that symptoms of PD appear if the dopamine content of the caudate sinks below 30% of the normal level. Aging of the nigrostriatal dopaminergic neurons is essentially similar in rodents and in humans. Direct biochemical evidence for the age-related decline of the dopaminergic function in rat is the loss of striatal D2-receptors in the aging brain.

Dopamine itself might play a main role in the unusually drastic age-related changes of the nigral dopaminergic system. 80% of brain dopamine is localized here. The complex autooxidation of the large amounts of DOPA and dopamine in the striatum continuously generating substantial quantities of toxic free radicals and highly reactive quinones, creates a permanent danger for the nigrostriatal dopaminergic neuron, which has to mobilize its natural defensive measures against these toxic metabolites. Neuromelanin, which is synthesized via the polymerization of oxidative products of dopamine, with the evident aim of finally depositing waste products, is in the substantia nigra the visible sign of successful self defense of the neuron against the free radicals and quinones originating from dopamine metabolism. The sluggish depositing of neuromelanin in the human substantia nigra is in excellent agreement with this view.

Knoll and his coworkers found that small dose D treatment prevented in rats age-related morphological changes in the neurons of the substantia nigra (Knoll et al., 1992b). This experimental study was in harmony with the clinical experience of Rinne et al. (1991) who found that the number of medial nigral neurons was greater and the number of Lewy bodies fewer in those PD patients who had been treated with D in combination with levodopa when compared with patients who had received levodopa alone. Collating the human data with the results of Knoll et al.'s study in rats it is reasonable to assume that D-treatment retards the death of the nigral neurons in the patients.

It is evident that if we focus our attention in our fight against the manifestation of PD via protecting the age-related decay of the dopaminergic machinery in the brain, we must not forget that the prophylactic low dose administration of D is strongly enhancing also the noradrenergic neurons. D and BPAP are highly potent stimulants of the noradrenergic system (Knoll, 2005). Fig.3 shows as an example that BPAP is enhancing the release of ^{3}[H]-noradrenaline from the isolated locus coeruleus in picomolar concentration and D acts similarly (see Fig.2b). Thus, it is of significant importance to follow those experimental and clinical studies which call attention to an inverse relationship between brain noradrenaline level and dopamine loss in PD (Tong et al., 2006). Zarow et al. (2003) showed in a study that in AD and PD neuronal loss in the locus coeruleus is greater than in substantia nigra. Locus coeruleus is a neuromelanin-pigmented neuronal structure (Ararat et al., 1977) and it is known that in PD and AD morphological alterations of the noradrenergic neurons result in a decrease of the neuronal population and this plays a role in depression and dementia in PD (Chan-Palay, 1991). A more recent study described the morphological and morphometric alterations of the locus coeruleus in patients who suffered from PD with normal cognitive function and in patients who suffered from PD associated with dementia, comparing them with normal controls and the morphological alterations of the synapses in cases of PD associated with dementia plead in favor of the importance of the normal circuits of locus coeruleus in cognitive functions (Baloyannis et al., 2006). Furthermore, it was shown that among 20 brain areas dopamine loss in PD was negatively correlated with healthy noradrenaline levels, with regions rich in noradrenaline spared from dopamine loss. The authors concluded that "…therapeutic approaches designed to enhance brain noradrenergic activity … should be considered as possible neuroprotective strategies in PD" (Tong et al., 2006, p. 1727). Thus, the fact that D is a potent enhancer of the noradrenergic neurons is additional important factor which might substantially contribute in slowing the age-related decline of brain functions.

Since on isolated substantia nigra of rats the special CAE effect of D is detectable already at 10^{-14}M concentration and in *in vivo* experiments 0.025 mg/kg D (1/10th of the dose which blocks MAO-B) is sufficient to keep the dopaminergic neurons in the midbrain on a higher activity level, and since decades of clinical experiences showed that the regular daily dose, 10 mg D is very safe, the prophylactic administration of 1 mg D per day lends itself particularly well for life-long treatment.

9. Conclusion

The catecholaminergic machinery, the noradrenergic and dopaminergic neuronal system in the brain plays a key role in the maintenance of vigilance, motivation, alerting and orientation, as well as in learning, sexual activity, drive motivated behavioral performances, cognition, etc. The dopaminergic system is the most rapidly aging neuronal system in the brain. Since the diagnosis of PD is the unequivocal proof that age-related irreversible deterioration of the nigrostriatal dopaminergic neuronal system has already surpassed a critical level in the patient, and the disease is incurable, prevention remains the only chance for the future to fight off PD.

The development of D in 1964/1965 which became famous in 1971/1972 as the first selective inhibitor of MAO-B and started its carrier as a therapeutic agent in 1977 as the unique MAO-B inhibitor which being free of the cheese effect could safely be combined with levodopa in PD and is at present registered in 64 countries and used to treat PD, AD and major depression, is a unique stimulant of catecholaminergic neurons in the brain. D is a derivative of methamphetamine, which is a long acting variant of PEA, the natural brain constituent. Both PEA and methamphetamine are known to act as releasers of catecholamines from their neuronal pool. D is the first PEA/methamphetamine-derivative free of the catecholamine releasing property and this change in the pharmacological spectrum ensured to discover that D is enhancing via a previously undetected mechanism the activity of the catecholaminergic neurons in the brain. This CAE effect of PEA which is exerted in much lower concentration than its catecholamine releasing effect remained undetected because the releasing effect hindered its detectability.

The role of D in the discovery of the enhancer regulation was clarified in a monograph (Knoll, 2005). Data were presented showing that in the course of developmental longevity, from weaning until sexual maturity, a significantly higher level of enhancer regulation is operating in the catecholaminergic neurons. This mechanism is responsible for the exuberant physical strength and mental vigor in the uphill period of life. Sexual hormones terminate this period and bring back the enhancer regulation to the pre-weaning level. This mechanism terminates developmental longevity and constitutes the foundation of the transition from adolescence to adulthood. The postdevelopmental phase of life, the slow continuous aging process, the unfortunate common fate of all mature adults begins and is finally terminated by natural death. Since D as a safe CAE substance works against the slow age-related decline of the catecholaminergic neurons in the brain, prophylactic lifelong administration of 1 mg D per day is proposed to slow the natural aging process.

The longevity studies performed with D furnished unequivocal evidence that life-long prophylactic treatment with D slowed significantly the age-related decline of the sexual performance and learning ability of animals and prolong their life. Furthermore, on the one hand, the retrospective analysis of the survival of patients treated with madopar alone (N=377) and with madopar plus D (N=564) showed that the supplementation of madopar with D significantly prolonged the survival of patients, and on the other hand, the DATATOP study showed that D-treatment slowed down the rate of deterioration of the human striatal dopaminergic system. These experimental and clinical findings guide the way for the long overdue study to select at least 60 year-old healthy males and females, treat half of the population with placebo and half with 1 mg D per day, and follow carefully the changes in their state of health until death. Since the decay of the catecholaminergic machinery with the passing of time plays an obviously important role in brain aging, and there is unequivocal evidence that D slows the aging of the catecholaminergic system, prophylactic D-treatment will not only improve the quality of life in senescence but it seems to be a pharmacologically well-founded expectation that the prevalence of PD and AD might be significantly lower in the D-treated group than in the placebo-treated one. Over 60 the number of the most common age-related neurodegenerative diseases, Parkinson's and Alzheimer's, start to increase because, in a sensitive part of the population the decay of some functionally key important neuronal systems surpass a critical level (like the dopaminergic machinery in case of PD), thus the maintenance of the enhancer regulation on a higher activity level may slow this process. Considering the rapid increase of the population over 65, a collaborative implementation of the proposed clinical trial, which has a fair chance of success, is of greater importance than realized heretofore.

10. References

Allain, H.; Gougnard, J. & Naukirek, H.C. (1991). Selegiline in de novo parkinsonian patients: the French selegiline multicenter trial (FSMT). *Acta Neurologica Scandinavica Suppl* Vol.84, No.136, pp.73-78, ISSN 0065-1427

Amsterdam, J.D. (2003). A double-blind, placebo-controlled trial of the safety and efficacy of selegiline transdermal system without dietary restrictions in patients with major depressive disorder. *Journal of Clinical Psychiatry* Vol.64, No.2, (February 2003), pp. 208-214, ISSN 0160-6689

Ararat, D. & Shinnamon, H. (1977). The locus coeruleus: neurobiology of a central noradrenergic nucleus. *Progress in Neurobiology* Vol.9, pp.147-196

Archer, J.R. & Harrison, D.E. (1996). L-Deprenyl treatment in aged mice slightly increases life spans, and greatly reduces fecundity by aged males. *Journal of Gerontology Series A – Biological Sciences and Medical* Vol.51, No.6 (November 1996) pp. B448-B453, ISSN 1079-5006

Baloyannis, S.J.; Costa, V. & Baloyannis, V.C. (2006). Morphological alterations of the synapses in the locus coeruleus in Parkinson's disease. *Journal of the Neurological Sciences* Vol.248, No.1-2, (October 2006) pp. 35-41,

Birkmayer, W. & Hornykiewicz, O. (1962). Der L-dioxyphenyl-alanin-effekt beim Parkinson syndrom des Menschen. *Archiv für Psychiatrie und Nervenkrankheiten Vereinigt mit Zeitschrift für die Gesamte Neurologie und Psychiatrie* Vol.203, No.5, pp. 560-574, ISSN 0003-9373

Birkmayer, W.; Riederer, P., Ambrozi, L. & Youdim, M.B.H. (1977). Implications of combined treatment with "Madopar" and L-Deprenil in Parkinson's disease. A long term study. *Lancet* Vol.1, No.8009, (February 1977) pp. 439-443, ISSN 0140-6736

Birkmayer, W.; Knoll, J., Riederer, P. & Youdim, M.B.H. (1983). (-)Deprenyl leads to prolongation of l-dopa efficacy in Parkinson's disease. *Modern Problems of Pharmacopsychiatry* Vol.19, pp. 170-176, ISSN 0077-0094

Birkmayer, W.; Riederer, P., Linauer, W. & Knoll, J. (1984). L-Deprenyl plus L-phenylalanine in the treatment of depression. *Journal of Neural Transmission-General Section* Vol.59, No.1, pp. 81-87, ISSN 0300-9564

Birkmayer, W.; Knoll, J., Riederer, P., Youdim, M.B.H., Hars, V. & Marton, V. (1985). Increased life expectancy resulting from addition of L-deprenyl to Madopar treatment in Parkinson's disease: a longterm study. *Journal of Neural Transmission-General Section* Vol.64, No.2, pp. 113-127, ISSN 0300-9564

Blackwell, B. (1963). Hypertensive crisis due to monoamine oxidase inhibitors. *The Lancet* Vol.282, No.7313, pp. 849-851, ISSN 0140-6736

Carrillo, M.C.; Kanai, S., Nokubo, M. & Kitani, K. (1991). (-)-Deprenyl induces activities of both superoxide dismutase and catalase but not of glutathione peroxidase in striatum of young male rats. *Life Sciences* Vol.48, No.6, pp. 517-521, ISSN 0024-3205

Carrillo, M.C.; Kitani, K., Kanai, S. & Ivy, G.O. (1992a). The ability of (-)-deprenyl to increase superoxide dismutase activities in the rat is tissue and brain region selective. *Life Sciences* Vol.50, No.25, pp. 1985-1992, ISSN 0024-3205

Carrillo, M.C.; Kanai, S., Nokubo, M., Ivy, G.O., Sato, Y. & Kitani, K. (1992b). (-)-Deprenyl increases activities of superoxide dismutase and catalase in striatum but not in hippocampus: the sex and age-related differences in optimal dose in the rat. *Experimental Neurology* Vol.116, No.3, pp. 286-294, ISSN 0014-4886

Carrillo, M.C.; Kanai, S., Sato, Y., Nokubo, M., Ivy, G.O. & Kitani, K. (1993). The optimal dosage of (-)deprenyl for increasing superoxidase dismutase activities in several brain regions decreases with age in male Fischer 344 rats. *Life Sciences* Vol.52, No.24, pp. 1925-1934, ISSN 0024-3205

Carrillo, M.C.; Kitani, K., Kanai, S., Sato, Y., Miyasaka, K. & Ivy, G.O. (1994a). (-)-Deprenyl increases activities of superoxide dismutase and catalase in certain brain regions in old male mice. *Life Sciences* Vol.54, No.14, pp. 975-981, ISSN 0024-3205

Carrillo, M.C.; Ivy, G.O., Milgram, N.W., Head, E., Wu, P. & Kitani, K. (1994b). (-)Deprenyl increases activities of superoxide dismutase (SOD) in striatum of dog brain. *Life Sciences* Vol.54, No.20, pp. 1483-1489, ISSN 0024-3205

Carrillo, M.C.; Kitani, K., Kanai, S., Sato, Y., Miyasaka, K. & Ivy, G.O. (1994c). The effect of long term (6 months) treatment with (-)deprenyl on antioxidant enzyme activities in selective brain regions in old female Fischer 344 rats. *Biochemical Pharmacology* Vol.47, No.8, pp. 1333-1338, ISSN 0006-2952

Chan-Palay, V. (1991). Depression and dementia in Parkinson's disease: catecholamine changes in the locus coeruleus - Basis for therapy. *Dementia* Vol.2, No.1, pp. 7-17, ISSN 1013-7424

Crane, G.E. (1956). Psychiatric side effects of iproniazid. *The American Journal of Psychiatry* Vol.112, No.7, pp. 494-501

Esmaeili, F.; Tiraihi, T., Movahedin, M. & Mowla, S.J. (2006). Selegiline induces neuronal phenotype and neurotrophins expression in embryonic stem cells. *Rejuvenation Research* Vol.9, No.4 (Winter, 2006) pp 475-484, ISSN 1549-1684

Freisleben, H.J.; Lehr, F. & Fuchs, J. (1994) Lifespan of immunosuppressed NMRI-mice is increased by deprenyl. *Journal Neural Transmission Supplement* Vol.41, pp. 231-236, ISSN 0303-6965

Gallagher, I.M.; Clow, A. & Glover, V. (1998). Long term administration of (-)deprenyl increases mortality in male Wistar rats. *Journal of Neural Transmission Supplement* No.52, pp. 315-320, ISSN 0303-6995

Gaszner, P. & Miklya, I. (2006). Major depression and the synthetic enhancer substances, (-)-deprenyl and R-(-)-1-(benzofuran-2-yl)-2-propylaminopentane. *Progress in Neuro-Psychopharmacology Biological Psychiatry* Vol.30, No.1, pp. 5-14, ISSN 02778-5846

Groc, L.; Levine, R.A., Foster, J.A., Normile, H.J., Weissmann, D. & Bezin, L. (2000). Evidence of deprenyl-insensitive apoptosis of nigral dopamine neurons during development. *Developmental Brain Research* Vol.120, No.1, pp. 95-98, ISSN 0165-3806

Hall, D.W.R.; Logan, B.W. & Parsons, G.H. (1969). Further studies on the inhibition of monoamine oxydase by MB 9302 (clorgyline)-I. Substrate specificity in various mammalians species. *Biochemical Pharmacology* Vol.18, No.6, pp. 1447-1454, ISSN 0006-2952

Johnston, J.P. (1968). Some observations upon a new inhibitor of monoamine oxidase in human brain. *Biochemical Pharmacology* Vol.17, No.7, pp. 1285-1297, ISSN 0006-2952

Ingram, D.K.; Wiener, H.L., Chachich, M.E., Longo, J.M., Hengemihle, J. & Gupta, M. (1993). Chronic treatment of aged mice with L-deprenyl produced marked MAO-B inhibition but no beneficial effects on survival, motor performance, or nigral lipofuscin accumulation. *Neurobiology of Aging* Vol.14, No.5, pp. 431-440, ISSN 0197-4580

Kitani, K.; Kanai, S., Sato, Y., Ohta, M., Ivy, G.O. & Carrillo, M.C. (1993). Chronic treatment of (-)deprenyl prolongs the life span of male Fischer 344 rats. Further evidence. *Life Sciences* Vol.52, No.3, pp. 281-288, ISSN0024-3205

Kitani, K.; Kanai, S., Miyasaka, K., Carrillo, M.C. & Ivy, G.O. (2006). The necessity of having a proper dose of (-)deprenyl (D) to prolong the life spans of rats explains discrepancies among different studies in the past. *Annals of the New York Academy of Sciences* Vol.1067, No.1, pp. 375-382, ISSN 0077-8923

Kline, N.S. (1958). Clinical experience with iproniazid (marsilid). *Journal of Clinical Experimental Psychophathology Supplement* 1, Vol.19, pp. 72-78

Knoll, J. (1976). Analysis of the pharmacological effects of selective monoamine oxidase inhibitors. In: *Monoamine oxidase and its inhibition.* Ciba Foundation Symposium 39 (new series), G.E.S. Wolstenholme & J. Knight, (Eds), pp. 131-161, ISBN 0444-1525-9, Elsevier, Amsterdam

Knoll, J. (1978a). On the dual nature monoamine oxidase. *Horizons in Biochemistry and Biophysics* Vol.5, pp. 37-64

Knoll, J. (1978b). The possible mechanism of action of (-)deprenyl in Parkinson's disease. *Journal of Neural Transmission – General Section* Vol.43, No.3-4, pp. 177-198

Knoll, J. (1978c). The pharmacology of selective irreversible monoamine oxidase inhibitors. In: *Enzyme-activated irreversible inhibitors,* N. Seiler, M.J. Jung & J. Koch-Weser, (Eds), pp 253-269, ISBN 0-444-80080-8, Elsevier/North Holland

Knoll, J. (1981a). Can the suicide inactivation of MAO by deprenyl explain its pharmacological effects? In: *Molecular Basis of Drug Action,* T. Singer & N. Ondarza, (Eds), pp 185-201, ISBN 0-444-00632-X, Elsevier, Amsterdam

Knoll, J. (1981b). The pharmacology of selective MAO inhibitors. In: *Monoamine Oxidase Inhibitors. The State of the Art,* M.B.H. Youdim & E.S. Paykel, (Eds), pp 45-61, Wiley, New York

Knoll, J. (1982). Selective inhibition of B type monoamine oxidase in the brain: a drug strategy to improve the quality of life in senescence. In: *Strategy in Drug Research,* J.A. Keverling Buisman, (Ed), pp 107-135, ISBN 0-444-42053-3, Elsevier, Amsterdam

Knoll, J. (1983). Deprenyl (selegiline). The history of its development and pharmacological action. *Acta Neurolologica Scandinavica* Vol.68, Suppl 95, pp. 57-80, ISSN 0001-6314

Knoll, J. (1985). The facilitation of dopaminergic activity in the aged brain by (-)deprenyl. A proposal for a strategy to improve the quality of life in senescence. *Mechanisms of Ageing and Development* Vol.30, No.2, pp.109-122, ISSN 0047-6374

Knoll, J. (1987). R-(-)Deprenyl (Selegiline, Movergan R) facilitates the activity of the nigrostriatal dopaminergic neuron. *Journal of Neural Transmission Supplement* 25, pp. 45-66, ISSN 0303-6965

Knoll, J. (1988). The striatal dopamine dependency of lifespan in male rats. Longevity study with (-)deprenyl. *Mechanisms of Ageing and Development* Vol.46, No.1-3, pp. 237-262, ISSN 0047-6374

Knoll, J. (1989). The pharmacology of selegiline /(-)deprenyl/. New aspects. *Acta Neurologica Scandinavica Supplement* 80, No.126, pp. 83-91, ISSN 0065-1427

Knoll, J. (1990). Nigrostriatal dopaminerg activity, deprenyl treatment, and longevity. In: Advances in Neurology.Vol. 53: *Parkinson's disease: anatomy, pathology, and therapy..*: M.M. Streifler, A.D. Korczyn, E. Melamed & M.H.B. Youdim, (Eds), pp 425-429, ISSN 0091-3952, Raven Press, New York

Knoll, J. (1992). Pharmacological basis of the therapeutic effect of (-)deprenyl in age-related neurological diseases. *Medicinal Research Reviews* Vol.12, No.5, pp. 505-524, ISSN 0198-6325

Knoll, J. (1994). Memories of my 45 years in research. *Pharmacology & Toxicology* Vol.75, No.2, pp. 65-72, ISSN 0901-9928

Knoll, J. (1998). (-)Deprenyl (Selegiline), a catecholaminergic activity enhancer (CAE) substance acting in the brain. *Pharmacology & Toxicology* Vol.82, No.2, pp. 57-66, ISSN 0901-9928

Knoll, J. (2001). Antiaging compounds: (-)Deprenyl (Selegiline) and (-)1-(benzofuran-2-yl)-2-propylaminopentane, (-)BPAP, a selective highly potent enhancer of the impulse propagation mediated release of catecholamines and serotonin in the brain. *CNS Drug Reviews* Vol.7, No.3, pp. 317-345, ISSN 1080-563X

Knoll, J. (2005). *The brain and its self. A neurochemical concept of the innate and acquired drives.* ISBN -10 3-540-23969-3, Springer, Berlin, Heidelberg, New York.

Knoll, J. & Magyar, K. (1972). Some puzzling effects of monoamine oxidase inhibitors. *Advances in Biochemical Psychopharmacology* Vol.5, pp. 393-408

Knoll, J. & Miklya, I. (1994). Multiple small dose administration of (-)deprenyl enhances catecholaminergic activity and diminishes serotonergic activity in the brain and these effects are unrelated to MAO-B inhibition. *Archives Internationales de Pharmacodynamie et de Therapie* Vol.328, No.1, pp. 1-15, ISSN 0003-9780

Knoll, J. & Miklya, I. (1995). Enchanced catecholaminergic and serotoninergic activity in rat brain from weaning to sexual maturity: Rationale for prophylactic (-) deprenyl (selegiline) medication. *Life Sciences* Vol.56, No.8, pp. 611-620, ISSN 0024-3205

Knoll, J.; Ecseri, Z., Kelemen, K., Nievel, J. & Knoll, B. (1965). Phenylisopropylmethyl propinylamine (E-250) a new psychic energizer. *Archives Internationales de Pharmacodynamie et de Thérapie* Vol.155, No.1, pp. 154-164, ISSN 0003-9780

Knoll, J.; Vizi, E.S. & Somogyi, G. (1968). Phenylisopropylmethylpropinylamine (E-250), a monoamine oxidase inhibitor antagonizing the effects of tyramine. *Arzneimittelforschung Vol.*18, pp. 109-112

Knoll, J.; Yen, T.T. & Dallo, J. (1983). Long-lasting, true aphrodisiac affect of (-)deprenyl in sexually sluggish old male rats. *Modern Problems of Pharmacopsychiatry* Vol.19, pp. 135-153, ISSN 0077-0094

Knoll, J.; Dallo, J. & Yen, T.T. (1989). Striatal dopamine, sexual activity and lifespan. Longevity of rats treated with (-)deprenyl. *Life Sciences* Vol.45, No.6, pp. 525-531, ISSN 0024-3205

Knoll, J.; Knoll, B., Török, Z., Timar, J. & Yasar, S. (1992a). The pharmacology of 1-phenyl-2-propylamino-pentane (PPAP) a deprenyl-derived new spectrum psycho-stimulant. *Archives Internationales de Pharmacodynamie et de Therapie* Vol.316, pp. 5-29, ISSN 0003-9780

Knoll, J.; Toth, V., Kummert, M. & Sugar, J. (1992b). (-)Deprenyl and (-)parafluorodeprenyl-treatment prevents age-related pigment changes in the substantia nigra. A TV-image analysis of neuromelanin. *Mechanisms of Ageing and Development* Vol.63, No.2, pp. 157-163, ISSN 0047-6374

Knoll, J.; Yen, T.T. & Miklya, I. (1994). Sexually low performing male rats dies earlier than their high performing peers and (-)deprenyl treatment eliminates this difference. *Life Sciences* Vol.54, No.15, pp. 1047-1057, ISSN 0024-3205

Knoll, J., Miklya, I., Knoll, B., Marko, R. & Racz, D. (1996a). Phenylethylamine and tyramine are mixed-acting sympathomimetic amines in the brain. *Life Sciences* Vol.58, No.23, pp. 2101-2114, ISSN 0024-3205

Knoll, J.; Miklya, I., Knoll, B., Marko, R. & Kelemen, K. (1996b). (-)Deprenyl and (-)l-phenyl-2-propilaminopentane, (-)PPAP, act primarly as potent stimulants of actionpotential - transmitter release coupling in the catecholaminergic neurons. *Life Sciences* Vol.58, No.10, pp. 817-827, ISSN 0024-3205

Knoll, J.; Yoneda, F., Knoll, B., Ohde, H. & Miklya, I. (1999). (-)1-(Benzofuran-2-yl)-2-propylaminopentane, /(-)BPAP/, a selective enhancer of the impulse propagation mediated release of catecholamines and serotonin in the brain. *British Journal of Pharmacology* Vol.128, No.8, pp. 1723-1732, ISSN 0007-1188

Knoll, J.; Miklya, I. & Knoll, B. (2002). Stimulation of the catecholaminergic and serotoninergic neurons in the rat brain by R-(-)-1-(benzofuran-2-yl)-2-propylaminopentane, (-)-BPAP. *Life Sciences* Vol.71, No.18, pp. 2137-2144, ISSN 0024-3205

Lancet Editorial. (1982). Deprenyl in Parkinson's Disease. *The Lancet* Vol.2, No.8300, (September 25) pp. 695-696, ISSN 0140-6736

Lamensdorf, I.; Porat, S.; Simantov, R.. & Finberg, J.P. (1999) Effect of low-dose treatment with selegiline on dopamine transporter (DAT) expression and amphetamine-induced dopamine release in vivo. *British Journal of Pharmacology* Vol. 126, No.4, pp.997-1002, ISSN 0007-1188

Larsen, J.P.; Boas, J. & Erdal, J.E. (1999). Does selegiline modify the progression of early Parkinson's disease? Results from a five-year study. The Norwegian-Danish Study Group. *European Journal of Neurology* Vol.6, No.5, pp. 539-547, ISSN 1351-5101

Lees, A.J. (1995). Comparison of therapeutic effects and mortality data of levodopa and levodopa combined with selegiline in patients with early, mild Parkinson's disease *British Medical Journal* Vol.311, No.7020, pp. 1602-1607, ISSN 0959-535X

Mann, J.J. & Gershon, S. (1980). A selective monoamine oxidase-B inhibitor in endogenous depression. *Life Sciences* Vol.26, No.11, pp. 877-882, ISSN 0024-3205

Martini, E.; Pataky, I., Szilagyi, K. & Venter, V. (1987). Brief information on an early phase-II study with (-)deprenyl in demented patients. *Pharmacopsychiatry* Vol.20, No.6, pp. 256-257, ISSN 0176-3679

Miklya, I. (2008). A comparison of the pharmacology of (-)-deprenyl to N-methyl-propargylamine-1-aminoindane (J-508) and rasagiline, the desmethyl-analogue of J-508. *Neuropsychopharmacologia Hungarica* Vol.10, No.1, pp. 15-22

Milgram, M.W.; Racine, R.J., Nellis, P., Mendoca, A. & Ivy, G.O. (1990). Maintenance on L-(-)deprenyl prolongs life in aged male rats. *Life Sciences* Vol.47, No.5, pp. 415-420, ISSN 0024-3205

Miyoshi, K. (2001). Parkinson's disease. *Nippon Rinsho. Japanese Journal of Clinical Medicine* Vol.59, No.8, pp. 1570-1573, ISSN 0047-1852

Myttyla, V.V.; Sotaniemi, K.A., Vourinen, J.A. & Heinonen, E.H. (1992). Selegiline as initial treatment in de novo parkinsonian patiens. *Neurology* Vol.42, pp. 339-343

Ohta, K.; Ohta, M., Mizuta, I., Fujinami, A., Shimazu, S., Sato, N., Yoneda, F., Hayashi, K. & Kuno, S. (2002). The novel catecholaminergic and serotonergic activity enhancer *R*-(-)-1-(benzofuran-2-yl)-2-propylaminopentane up-regulates neurotrophic factor synthesis in mouse astrocytes. *Neuroscience Letters* Vol.328, No.3, pp. 205-208, ISSN 0304-3940

Parkinson Study Group. (1989). Effect of (-)deprenyl on the progression disability in early Parkinson's disease. *New England Journal of Medicine* Vol.321, No.20, pp. 1364-1371, ISSN 0028-4793

Parkinson Study Group. (1993). Effect to tocopherol and (-)deprenyl on the progression of disability in early Parkinson's disease. *New England Journal of Medicine* Vol.328, No.3, pp. 176-183, ISSN 0028-4793

Rinne, J.O.; Röyttä, M., Paljärvi, L., Rummukainen, J. & Rinne, U.K. (1991). Selegiline (deprenyl) treatment and death of nigral neurons in Parkinson's disease. *Neurology* Vol.41, No.6, pp. 859-861, ISSN 0028-3878

Ruehl, W.W.; Entriken, T.L., Muggenberg, B.A., Bruyette, D.S., Griffith, W.G. & Hahn, F.F. (1997). Treatment with L-deprenyl prolongs life in elderly dogs. *Life Sciences* Vol.61, No.11, pp. 1037-1044, ISSN 0024-3205

Sano, M.; Ernesto, C., Thomas, R.G., Klauber, M.R., Schafer, K., Grundman, M., Woodbury, P., Growdon, J., Cotman, C.W., Pfeiffer, E., Schneider, L.S. & Thal, L.J. (1997). A controlled trial of selegiline, alpha-tocopherol, or both as treatment for Alzheimer's disease. *New England Journal of Medicine* Vol.336, No.17, pp. 1216-1222, ISSN 0028-4793

Shimazu, S.; Tanigawa, A., Sato, N., Yoneda, F., Hayashi, K., Knoll, J. (2003). Enhancer substances: Selegiline and *R*-(-)-1-(benzofuran-2-yl)-2-propylaminopentane, [(-)-BPAP] enhance the neurotrophic factor synthesis on cultured mouse astrocytes. *Life Sciences* Vol.72, No.24, pp. 2785-2792, ISSN 0024-3205

Stoll, S.; Hafner, U., Kranzlin, B. & Muller, W.E. (1997). Chronic treatment of Syrian hamsters with low-dose selegiline increases life span in females but not males. *Neurobiology of Aging* Vol.18, Mo.2, pp. 205-211, ISSN 0197-4580

Tariot, P.N.; Cohen, R.M., Sunderland, T., Newhouse, P.A., Yount, D. & Mellow, A.M. (1987). L-(-)Deprenyl in Alzheimer's disease. *Archives of General Psychiatry* Vol.44, No.5, pp. 427-433, ISSN 0003-990X

Tatton, W.G.; Ju, W.Y., Holland, D.P., Tai, C. & Kwan, M. (1994). (-)-Deprenyl reduces PC12 cell apoptosis by inducing new protein synthesis. *Journal of Neurochemistry* Vol.63, No.4, pp. 1572-1575, ISSN 0022-3042

Tatton, W.G.; Wadia, J.S., Ju, W.Y., Chalmers-Redman, R.M. & Tatton, N.A. (1996). (-)-Deprenyl reduces neuronal apoptosis and facilitates neuronal outgrowth by altering protein synthesis without inhibiting monoamine oxidase. *Journal of Neural Transmission Supplement*, Vol.48, pp. 45-59, ISSN 0303-6995

Tetrud, J.W. & Langston, J.W. (1989). The effect of (-)deprenyl (selegiline) on the natural history of Parkinson's disease. *Science* Vol.245, No.4917, pp. 519-522, ISSN 0036-8075

ThyagaRajan, S. & Felten, D.L. (2002). Modulation of neuroendocrine-immune signaling by L-deprenyl and L-desmethyldeprenyl in aging and mammary cancer. *Mechanisms Aging and Development* Vol.123, No.8, (April, 2002), pp.1065-1079, ISSN 0047-6374

Tom, T. & Cummings, J.L. (1998). Depression in Parkinson's disease. Pharmacological characteristics and treatment. *Drugs Aging* Vol.12, No.1, pp. 55-74, ISSN 1170-229X

Tong, J.; Hornykiewicz, O. & Kish, S.J. (2006). Inverse relationship between brain noradrenaline level and dopamine loss in Parkinson Disease. *Archives of Neurology* Vol.63, No.12, pp. 1724-1728, ISSN 0003-9942

Tringer, L., Haits, G. & Varga, E. (1971). The effect of (-)E-250, (-)L-phenyl-isopropylmethyl-propinyl-amine HCl, in depression. In: *V. Conferentia Hungarica pro Therapia et Investigatione in Pharmacologia*, G. Leszkovszky, (Ed), pp 111-114, Publishing House of the Hungarian Academy of Sciences, Budapest,

Varga, E. (1965). Vorläufiger Bericht über die Wirkung des Präparats E-250 (phenyl-isopropyl-methyl-propinylamine-chlorhydrat) In: *III. Conferentia Hungarica pro Therapia et Investigatione in Pharmacologia*, B. Dumbovich, (Ed), pp 197-201, Publishing House of the Hungarian Academy of Sciences, Budapest,

Varga, E. & Tringer, L. (1967). Clinical trial of a new type of promptly acting psychoenergetic agent (phenyl-isopropylmethyl-propinylamine HCl, E-250). *Acta Medica Academiae Scientiarum Hungaricae* Vol.23, No.3, pp. 289-295, ISSN 0001-5989

Yasar, S.; Winger, G., Nickel, B., Schulze, G. & Goldberg, S.R. (1993). Preclinical evaluation of l-deprenyl: Lack of amphetamine-like abuse potential. In: *Inhibitors of Monoamine Oxidase B. Pharmacology and Clinical Use in Neurodegenerative Disorders*, I. Szelenyi, (Ed), pp215-233, ISBN 3-7643-2782-0, Birkhauser Verlag, Basel, Switzerland

Yen, T.T. & Knoll, J. (1992). Extension of lifespan in mice treated with Dinh lang (Policias fruticosum L.) and (-)deprenyl. *Acta Physiologica Hungarica* Vol.79, No.2, pp. 119-124, ISSN 0231-424X

Yen, T.T.; Dallo, J. & Knoll, J. (1982). The aphrodisiac effect of low doses of (-)deprenyl in male rats. *Polish Journal of Pharmacology and Pharmacy* Vol.34, No.5-6, pp. 303-308, ISSN 0301-0244

Youdim, M.B. (1980). Monoamine oxidase inhibitors as anti-depressant drugs and as adjuct to L-dopa therapy of Parkinson's disease. *Journal of Neural Transmission Supplement,* Vol.16, pp. 157-161, ISSN 0303-6995

Zarow, C.; Lynnes, S.A., Mortimer, J.A. & Chui, H.C. (2003). Neuronal loss is greater in the locus coeruleus than nucleus basalis and substantia nigra in Alzheimer and Parkinson disease. *Archives of Neurology* Vol.60, No.3, pp. 337-341, ISSN 0003-9942

Zeller, E.A. & Barsky. J. (1952). In vivo inhibition of liver and brain monoamine oxidase by 1-isonicotinyl-2-isopropylhydrazine. *Proceedings of the Society for Experimental Biology and Medicine* Vol.81, pp. 459-468

Zesiewitz, T.A.; Gold, M,, Chari, G. & Hauser, R.A. (1999). Current issues in depression in Parkinson's disease. *The American Journal of Geriatric Psychiatry* Vol.7, No.2, pp. 110-118

6

Utility of Organotypic Slices in Parkinson's Disease Research

Fabio Cavaliere and Carlos Matute
Neurotek-UPV/EHU, Department of Neuroscience and CIBERNED,
Bizkaia Technology Park, Zamudio
Spain

1. Introduction

Parkinson's disease (PD) is a chronic and progressive neurodegenerative disease of unknown etiology. The pathology involves a degeneration of dopaminergic neurons of the substantia nigra with consequent dopamine (DA) deficiency and neurodegeneration of striatal neurons.

The most effective treatments target compensation for the DA deficit. Among the different strategies applied, the most used is pharmacological substitutive treatment with levodopa (L-DOPA). Nevertheless, all current treatments may be considered palliative and not curative.

Here we review the latest advances in research and preclinical investigation in cell restorative therapy by using slice tissue cultures as a model of PD. This chapter describes in detail the main organotypic models used to study the cellular and molecular mechanisms leading to dopaminergic degeneration. In particular, we move from the simplest organotypic co-cultured model of the substantia nigra-striatum-cortex to the unique slice of nigro-striatal slice used to study endogenous neurogenesis or viral vector-mediated overexpression of α-synuclein in midbrain slices. We discuss the possibility of using such models to induce adult neurogenesis by combining pharmacological treatments or for preclinical studies in cell transplantation.

The strategies in place thus far to restore the dopaminergic system in PD are pharmacological treatments, such as administration of L-DOPA, cell restorative therapy by gene therapy, or cell therapy by stem cell grafting. The main pharmacological treatment for PD symptoms today is the administration of L-DOPA, especially in the first stages of disease. L-DOPA, a DA precursor, acts to counteract the DA deficit in neurons. However, the beneficial effect of the drug lasts only a few years with disease progression and loss of efficacy, followed by onset of secondary effects such as on–off phenomena, dyskinesia, and psychosis. Moreover, recent studies in an animal model (Muller et al., 2004) suggest a toxic effect of prolonged L-DOPA treatment; thus, pharmacological investigation is devoted to studying new compounds or new therapeutic strategies. Inhibitors of an alternative metabolic route of DA such as entacapone and tolcapone are also used in pharmacological treatment (Linazasoro, 2008).

The administration of several neurotrophic factors has been intensively investigated in a rat model as a possible therapeutic strategy for PD (Grandoso et al., 2007). In particular, glial cell line–derived neurotrophic factor (GDNF) has been shown to exert prominent action on dopaminergic neurons by enhancing their survival and stimulating the outgrowth of DA fibers (Kirik et al., 2004). As noted, current pharmacological therapy for PD is considered only palliative and not curative, reflecting the necessity for new strategies and new therapeutic targets.

The principal targets of gene therapy in PD are replacement of tyrosine hydroxylase (TH) striatal neurons and blocking of neurodegeneration of the nigrostriatal pathway. The latter can be accomplished with local expression of neuroprotective neurotrophins such as GDNF. One promising approach to gene therapy for PD is the combined use of craniotomy as a delivery system with viral vectors as a gene expression system. Injection of viral vectors for the expression of neurotrophic factors in primate models allows local production of therapeutic genes. Nevertheless, the single injection into the human or animal brain of either adeno-associated virus (AAV) or herpes simplex virus results in an inflammatory reaction leading to astrogliosis and demyelination (Dewey et al., 1999; McMenamin et al., 1998). Both AAV and retrovirus permanently and randomly integrate into the host genome, but neither AAV nor retrovirus crosses the blood–brain barrier (BBB). Therefore, it is necessary to administer the virus via craniotomy and by intracerebral injection, a very invasive approach. However, the most intense expression of the therapeutic gene is generally limited to the injection site, owing to limited diffusion of the virus within the brain. Current limitations of brain gene therapy approaches can be circumvented with the development of a transvascular delivery as a support for gene therapy. However, this approach would require the formulation of plasmid DNA in a way that allows the exogenous gene to cross the BBB and enter the brain via the transvascular route after an intravenous injection.

Cell therapy for PD is based on neural stem cell transplantation intended to give rise to new dopaminergic neurons. The in vitro features of stem cells include the ability to (1) proliferate in a 3D free-floating system called neurospheres, (2) exhibit self-renewal, (3) generate a large number of progeny through the transient amplification of a population of progenitor cells, and (4) retain their multi-lineage potential over time. These cells must generate new cells in response to injury or disease, create synapses, and integrate into a preexisting neuronal network. Cells that satisfy all of these criteria are defined as stem cells, whereas those cells that satisfy some but not all of the functional criteria listed above and are already committed to one specific lineage are defined as progenitor cells. From a clinical point of view, cell therapy in PD must satisfy the following objectives: (1) the grafted cells must survive and form connections; (2) the patient's brain must integrate and use the grafted neurons; and (3) the grafts must induce measurable clinical improvement (Lindval & Bjiorklund, 2004; Meyer et al., 2010).

Cell regeneration can be obtained also by pharmacological activation of endogenous neurogenesis. Generation of newborn neurons in the adult mammalian brain occurs throughout life in the subventricular zone (SVZ) or in the subgranular zone of the hippocampus. In particular, the SVZ cover an interesting role in new cell regeneration due to the proximity with striatum. Neurogenesis can occur in brain regions which are damaged due to pathological conditions; in this case, the local environment influenced by cellular stress plays a crucial role in modulating the mechanisms of proliferation, migration and differentiation. Adult neurogenesis can be sustained, directly, by activating mechanisms of cell regeneration (e.g. with neurotrophic factors), or by the clearance of local negative environment (e.g. blocking excitotoxicity and apoptosis) (Vergni et al., 2009)

Despite problems, the use of cell therapy for the replacement of dead neurons results an attractive strategy for the treatment of PD. Here we review different in vitro experimental models used to study the cellular mechanisms of PD and highlight the feasibility of such models for each of the use described above (pharmacological treatment, gene therapy or cell transplantation).

2. The advantage of using brain organotypic cultures

The necessity to cultivate slice tissues begins from the needs to find out a valid and reliable model between the monocultures and in vivo models. The organotypic culture resembles the in vivo model better than dissociated cultures. In fact, individual cells are in tight contact with each other, maintain their organotypic architecture, and preserve neuron–glia interactions, tissue-specific transport, and ion diffusion systems. Moreover, the organotypic cultures represent an efficient cellular model to overcome the in vivo impediments of the BBB. The strength of organotypic cultures in neuroscience research has been the opportunity to cultivate for weeks or months CNS tissue, giving open accessibility to complex cellular systems. Organotypic cultures are ideally prepared from P3-P10 animals (rats or mice) even if few attempts have been made to cultivate organotypic slices from adult CNS tissues. Young postnatal animals already possess essential cytoarchitecture, are easily handy -respect to the embryonic tissue- and nerve cells survive explantation more readily –respect to the adult slices. The advantage of use organotypic cultures derives from their versatility in experiments that require long-term survival, such as live recording (Zhang et al., 2007; Lacar et al., 2010) or pharmacology (chronic drug application) as well as electrophysiology.

Many different procedures have been proposed to maintain slice tissues from CNS in culture, but the most successful was the "roller tube" technique. This technique, finally characterized more in detail by Gaehwiler (1988), was developed on the basis of experiences based on multitude of works with explants culture.

In roller tube cultures (Fig. 1A), the tissue is embedded in a plasma clot and attached on a glass coverslip. The coverslip with the embedded slice tissue are located in a tube that undergoes continuous slow rotation in a cell culture incubator. The oxygenation is maintained by continuous exchange of liquid-gas interface generated by the slow rotation. The technique was successively modified several time (e.g. Braschler et al., 1989; Andres et al., 2005) but the roller tube technique always maintain a very thin cultures (from an initial 400μm to about 50μm) with consequential preferential use for experiments that require optimal optical conditions (e.g. electron microscopy or electrophysiology).

At the beginning of 90's Stoppini and colleague (1991) published a new method to cultivate organotypic slices. In this method brain slices were placed on a semiporous membrane and cultivated at the air-liquid interface (fig. 1B). The absence of clot facilitates the studies of synaptic reorganization being a useful tool to study plasticity and sprouting already during the first days of culture. The real advantage of this technique is that cultures are easily prepared and offer great advantages when a 3D structure is desired (from an initial 400μm thickness, slices are cultivated up to 100-150μm). The air-liquid interface has become a key instrument to study the adult neurogenesis. Organotypic cultures match the tri-dimensional space where neural progenitors migrate to reach maturation in vivo. In the paper by Vergni and colleagues (2009) the authors ideally represented the slice culture comprising subventricular zone (SVZ), as the spatial extension to elaborate a mathematical model to describe neuroblast activation and migration following oxygen and glucose deprivation.

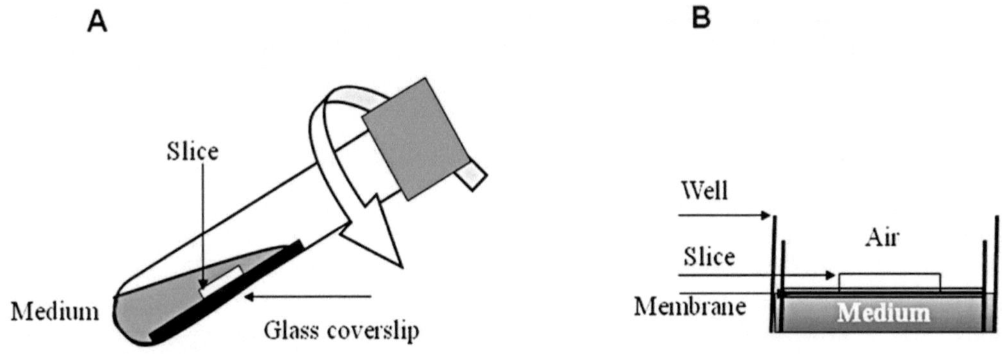

Fig. 1. **Roller tube (A) and semiporous membrane (B) methods used to cultivate organotypic cultures.** In both cases slices are cultivated in air-liquid interface, generated by tube rotation (A) or by the membrane (B) (see text for explanation).

3. Organotypic models for parkinson's disease

The first organotypic models used to study the nigrostriatal pathway were developed as co-cultures of slices from the substantia nigra with cortex and striatum (Ostergaard et al., 1996; Plenz & Kitai, 1998). These organotypic co-cultures, cultivated with using the roller tube method as well as a semiporous membrane, after several days in culture developed dopaminergic fibers connecting the substantia nigra with the striatum. Preservation of function of the newborn fibers was demonstrated by electrophysiology whereas the anatomical connection was shown by immunofluorescence. These organotypic models were used to study the role and the modulation of glutamate in dopaminergic development (Gramsbergen et al., 2002; Ostergaard et al., 1996; Plenz & Kitai, 1998). By confocal laser scanning microscopy, Plenz and Kitai demonstrated that the glutamate system modulated the dopaminergic innervations of the striatum. Activation of glutamate receptors generated sprouting of dopaminergic fibers and increase of innervations in the striatum. First was hypothesized that activation of glutamatergic receptors could induce neurogenesis but no generation of new neurons was observed in the substantia nigra. Increase of striatal neurons innervations was explained as a trophic effect generated by the selective activation of the metabotropic receptors of the mGluR group I, as specific mGluR I antagonists inhibited the dopaminergic innervation in the striatum. Results are sustained also by the mRNA expression of mGluR5 and mGluR5 receptor (Testa et al., 2005; Romano et al., 2005). Because both drugs were added to the medium, no conclusions could be drawn as to the site of drug action. In this case the stereotaxic application of the drug (see below Stahl et al., 2009) may account for a more precise evaluation of the mechanism.
The relevance of the co-culture was addressed later with studies of the effect of donor age on dopaminergic innervations (Gramsbergen et al., 2002). Because the model is composed of three different slices (co-culture), the age of the tissue donor is relevant to slice preservation and dopaminergic innervation. Of interest, it was found that the addition of brain-derived neurotrophic factor (BDNF) had a trophic effect and stimulated an increase in TH immunoreactivity in the striatum as well as protection from apoptotic death. BDNF also induced an increase in cell generation, possibly of progenitor cells, expressing TH immunoreactivity. These observations indicated that BDNF may sustain cell viability and dopaminergic differentiation after grafting of immature DA neurons.

PD in these slices can be modeled by treating organotypic cultures with toxins, selective for DA nigro-striatal degeneration (6-hydroxy DA-6-OHDA, rotenone, MPTP). As in animal model, 6-OHDA in organotypic cultures drives to neuronal death mediated by oxidative stress (Saner et al., 2007) inducing selective degeneration of dopaminergic neurons. However, this toxin doesn't produce extra-nigral pathology or Lewy body-like inclusions (Lane et al., 2007). In order to set up an organotypic culture as a model of PD it is important to take in account how to apply the toxin. Evaluation of neuronal death is different depending on the method of 6-OHDA application (Stahl et al., 2009). If toxin is applied directly in the medium it generates uniform DAergic cell death without accounting for natural variation occurring among slices, whereas local application of the drug at the tissue surface of main dopaminergic nuclei (substantia nigra pars compacta, ventral tegmental area and retrorubral field) of organotypic cultures, cause a precisely localized cell death resembling *in vivo* stereotactic model (Stahl et al., 2009).

Recently, we proposed an innovative organotypic model to study nigrostriatal degeneration and adult cell regeneration (Cavaliere et al., 2010). The presence of the nigrostriatal network with the cortex and subventricular zone (SVZ) in a single slice made possible the study of the mechanisms of nigrostriatal degeneration as well as the mechanisms of adult neurogenesis from the SVZ. This type of slice was made by cutting in a single plane the region between the ventral mesencephalon and the cortex (Fig. 2).

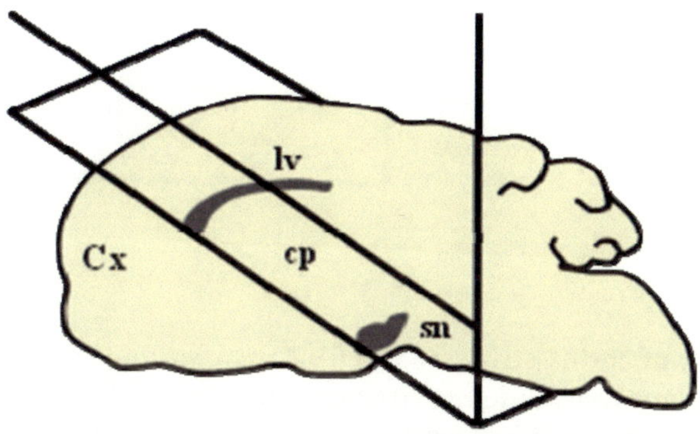

Fig. 2. **Schematic view of organotypic slice preparation preserving the nigrostriatal pathway.** Slices are cut (350μm) at 45° in a single plane to include the substantia nigra (sn), striatum-caudate putamen (cp), subventricular zone of the lateral ventricle (lv), and cerebral cortex (cx).

In this model, nigrostriatal degeneration can be obtained by mechanical transection of nigrostriatal fibers or chemically, for example by treatment with the DA analog 6-OHDA. In both cases, in agreement with the results presented by Gramsbergen and colleagues (2002), the degeneration of the nigrostriatal network induced classic PD features (e.g. α-synuclein inclusions, Halliday and McCann, 2008) and increase in TH expression in the neurogenetic niche of the SVZ. It is still not clear whether the increment of TH in SVZ cells means an increment in protein synthesis or generation of newborn TH^+ cells, but the functional meaning seems to be a response to the damage generated in the striatal area.

PD can also be modeled in organotypic cultures from cortex-striatum and SVZ (Cavaliere et al., 2005; Vergni et al., 2009; Tønnesen et al., 2011; Fig.3) in which dopaminergic inputs from the substantia nigra to the striatum are severed by slicing. This model is extremely useful especially in studying neurogenesis induced after severe nigro-striatal degeneration. Tønnesen and colleagues (2011) used this model to study functional graft of multipotent stem cells in damaged striatum. It is well known that effective synaptic integration into pre-existing neuronal circuitry after stem cell transplantation results difficult to analyze despite integration in the host tissue and robust behavioral rescue (Parish et al., 2008). In this paper the authors overexpressed the gene Wnt5a into TH-GFP derived neurospheres to generate DA neurons. These cells were then transplanted in the cortex-striatum-SVZ organotypic model and patch clamp recording and optogenetic tools were used to study the functional properties and synaptic integration of transplanted DA neurons into host cells. Host brain tissue was modified genetically to respond to optogenetic stimuli. Briefly, optogenetic is the response, in milliseconds time-scale, of cells overexpressing foto-sensitive receptors, like channelrhodopsins (ChR) or halorhodopsin (NpHR). Cells modified in this way can be depolarized (in case of ChR) or hyperpolarized (in case of NpHR) when stimulated with blue or orange light respectively (Miesenböck G. 2009). Optogenetic stimulation of organotypic slices and patch clamp recording of GFP grafted cells revealed synaptic integration and bidirectional connection of grafted cells with cortex and striatum.

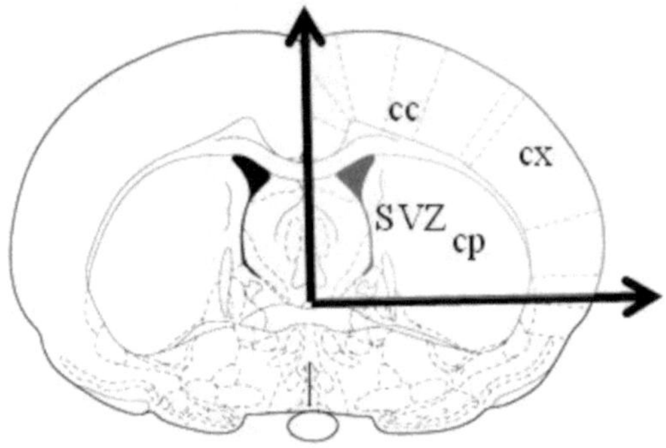

Fig. 3. **Schematic view of cortex-striatum and SVZ organotypic slice**. Slices are cut (350μm) coronally in a single plane to include the striatum-caudate putamen (cp), subventricular zone of the lateral ventricle (SVZ), cerebral cortex (cx) and corpus callosum (cc) and cultivated in air-liquid interface.

Organotypic cultures were used also to study the effect of α-synuclein on midbrain neurons. This model resembles the animal model obtained by viral transduction of human α-synuclein in rodents or non human primates (Kirik et al., 2002, 2003; Eslamboli et al., 2007). Differently from the methods that use drug delivery, this model doesn't address free radical damage and associated mitochondrial dysfunction, moreover the neurotoxin models are essentially non-progressive and do not replicate all aspects of the disease. This model takes advantage of the special property of recombinant vectors generated from adeno-associated viruses (rAAV) to transduce the nigral dopamine neurons with very high efficiency. In the organotypic model, midbrain slices were trasfected with truncated α-synuclein (A53T) fused to EGFP (Zach et al., 2007). Virus exposure resulted in dramatic changes in neurite morphology with α-synuclein locally accumulated in distorted and swollen neuritis. Neuritic swelling was observed especially in long neurites originating from putative projection neurons transduced with truncated more than with the full-length α-synuclein, as already demonstrated in animal model and PD patients.

4. Advances of preclinical cell therapy

Different cell types have been used for experimental and clinical cell therapy, giving in all cases partial PD symptom improvement. Neurospheres from human fetuses have already been used for PD cell therapy (see Brundin et al., 2000, and Lindval & Kokaia, 2006, 2009, for a review). They consist of both multipotent stem cells and more restricted progenitors at different stages of differentiation. Kim and colleagues in 2006 performed a comparative study between neurospheres obtained from different fetal brain tissues, in order to check whether the neural stem and precursor cells have specific regional or temporal characteristics with regard to growth, differentiation, and region-specific gene expression. They found that isolated neurospheres from different CNS compartments expressed distinctive molecular markers of regional identity even if this regional pattern could be reversed by environmental factors.

Transplantation studies in animal models of PD have highlighted the main problems that arise from the stem cell grafts (Table 1). In line with this the preclinical use of organotypic tissue model to study mechanisms and cell regeneration in PD becomes worthy.

In most cases, grafted cells displayed many of the morphological characteristics of DA neurons, with expression of dopaminergic markers and reinnervation of the lesioned striatum. However, cell therapy presents secondary effects. First, the risk of teratoma from embryonic and fetal stem cell transplantation is relatively high. It has to be considered that direct implantation of mouse embryonic stem cells into the rat striatum gives rise to tumor generation in 20% of the cases (Freed et al., 2001). Second, in 15% of the patients transplanted with stem cells of fetal origin, post-operative dyskinesias have been observed in the "off" phase (Bjorklund et al., 2002). In fact, the most important problem with the use of human fetal stem cells, besides the poor availability, is the lack of standardization, which results in a high variability in the degree of symptomatic relief.

CELL	REINNERVATION	SYMPTOMS IMPROVEMENT	LIMITS	REFERENCES
Mouse ESC	Partial	Partial	Risk of teratoma Ethical considerations	Kim et al., 2002
Monkey ESC	Partial	Partial	Risk of teratoma Ethical considerations	Sanchez-Pernaute et al., 2008
Human ESC	Not detected	Partial	Risk of teratoma Ethical considerations	Cho et al., 2008
Rat BMSC	Fibers	Partial	Lack of homogeneous differentiation, no evidence of dopaminergic specialization, low integration into pre-existing neuronal network	Dezawa et al., 2004
EMT	Extensive	Partial	Ethical considerations, Lack of homogeneous differentiation	Winkler et al., 2000

Table 1. Stem cell graft in animal models of PD. ESC, embryonic stem cells; BMSC, bone marrow stem cells; EMT, embryonic mesencephalic tissue.

To overcome the secondary effects of using embryonic and fetal stem cells, several groups have used adult stem cells for transplantation located primarily in the SVZ of the forebrain and in the sub-granular layer of the dentate gyrus of the hippocampal formation (Vergni et al., 2009). However, newly generated cells with a neuronal phenotype can be generated also from adult tissues that are different from the brain. Because of the ease of their isolation and their large potential for differentiation, mesenchymal stem cells are among the first stem cell types to be introduced into clinical studies. Results on differentiation of mesenchymal stem cells derived from such tissues are still controversial; e.g., debate persists about how to isolate a homogeneous population of the cells with specific criteria from the bone marrow, how to expand them ex vivo without affecting their differentiation potential, and how to develop easy methods for quality control of the cellular-based products (Chen et al., 2006; Kassem, 2006).

In addition to the use of the correct cell type (Meyer et al., 2010) and the generation of a standard protocol, other scientific improvements are necessary for the development of a clinically practicable cell therapy in PD. One is the proper selection of patients. It is of primary importance to determine whether a cell graft can be affected by disease progression. Cell regeneration should be done especially in those patients who positively respond to L-DOPA and in those patients for whom the main pathology is a loss of DA neurons, more than debilitating symptoms like dementia or degeneration of the non-dopaminergic system. In this regard, PET analysis before the engraftment is critical to understanding the preoperative degeneration pattern.

5. Conclusion

Cell therapy used to generate new dopaminergic neurons possesses a high potential. Up to now, all of the therapies used to counteract the symptoms of PD are palliative and limited in their therapeutic impact. Furthermore, the lack of standardized protocols and absence of a correct selection protocol for patients in the clinical trials result in a high variability in the degree of symptomatic relief. More efforts to surmount this variability and to achieve success in restorative therapy have to be made in this direction. The selection of a correct model to study the cellular and molecular mechanisms and for preclinical investigations represents a promising strategy to achieve a successful protocol for animal and human cell therapy.

6. Acknowledgment

Supported by MICINN, CIBERNED and Universidad del País Vasco.

7. References

Andres RH., Ducray AD., Pérez-Bouza A., Schlattner U., Huber AW., Krebs SH., Seiler RW., Wallimann T., Widmer HR (2005) Creatine supplementation improves dopaminergic cell survival and protects against MPP+ toxicity in an organotypic tissue culture system. *Cell Transplant*. Vol. 14, pp. 537-550.

Bjorklund, LM., Sanchez-Pernaute, R., Chung, S., Andersson, T., Chen, IY., McNaught, KS., Brownell, AL., Jenkins, BG., Wahlestedt, C., Kim, KS., & Isacson, O. (2002) Embryonic stem cells develop into functional dopaminergic neurons after transplantation in a Parkinson rat model. *Proc Natl Acad Sci USA* Vol. 99, pp. 2344–2349.

Braschler UF., Iannone A., Spenger C., Streit J., Lüscher HR (1989) A modified roller tube technique for organotypic cocultures of embryonic rat spinal cord, sensory ganglia and skeletal muscle. *J Neurosci Methods.* Vol. 29, pp. 121-129.

Brundin, P., Karlsson, J., Emgård, M., Schierle, GS., Hansson, O., Petersén, A., & Castilho, RF. (2000) Improving the survival of grafted dopaminergic neurons: a review over current approaches. *Cell Transplant.* Vol 9, pp. 179-195.

Cavaliere, F., Dinkel, K., & Reymann, K. (2005) Microglia response and P2 receptor participation in oxygen/glucose deprivation-induced cortical damage. *Neuroscience.* Vol. 136, pp. 615-623.

Cavaliere, F., Vicente, ES., & Matute, C. (2010) An organotypic culture model to study nigro-striatal degeneration. *J Neurosci Methods.* Vol. 188, pp. 205-212.

Chen, Y., Teng, FY., & Tang BL (2006) Coaxing bone marrow stromal mesenchymal stem cells towards neuronal differentiation: progress and uncertainties. *Cell Mol Life Sci.* Vol. 63, pp. 1649-1657.

Cho, MS., Lee, YE., Kim, JY., Chung, S., Cho, YH., Kim, DS., Kang, SM., Lee, H., Kim, MH., Kim, JH., Leem, JW., Oh, SK., Choi, YM., Hwang, DY., Chang, JW., & Kim, DW. (2008) Highly efficient and large-scale generation of functional dopamine neurons from human embryonic stem cells. *Proc. Natl. Acad. Sci. U. S. A.* Vol. 105, pp. 3392–3397.

Dewey, RA., Morrissey, G., Cowsill, CM., Stone, D., Bolognani, F., Dodd, NJ., Southgate, TD., Klatzmann, D., Lassmann, H., Castro, MG., & Löwenstein, PR. (1999) Chronic brain inflammation and persistent herpes simplex virus 1 thymidine kinase expression in survivors of syngeneic glioma treated by adenovirus-mediated gene therapy: implications for clinical trials. *Nat Med.* Vol. 5, pp. 1256-1263.

Dezawa, M., Kanno, H., Hoshino, M., Cho, H., Matsumoto, N., Itokazu, Y., Tajima, N., Yamada, H., Sawada, H., Ishikawa, H., Mimura, T., Kitada, M., Suzuki, Y., Ide, C. (2004) Specific induction of neuronal cells from bone marrow stromal cells and application for autologous transplantation. *J. Clin. Invest.* Vol. 113, pp. 1701–1710.

Eslamboli, A., Romero-Ramos, M., Burger, C., Bjorklund, T., Muzyczka, N., Mandel, RJ., Baker, H., Ridley, RM., & Kirik, D. (2007) Long-term consequences of human alpha-synuclein overexpression in the primate ventral midbrain. *Brain.* Vol. 130, pp. 799-815.

Freed, CR., Greene, PE., Breeze, RE., Tsai, WY., DuMouchel, W., Kao, R., Dillon, S., Winfield, H., Culver, S., Trojanowski, JQ., Eidelberg, D., & Fahn, S. (2001) Transplantation of embryonic dopamine neurons for severe Parkinson's disease. *N Engl J Med* Vol. 344, pp. 710–719.

Gähwiler, BH. (1988) Organotypic cultures of neural tissue. *Trends Neurosci.* Vol. 11, pp. 484-489.

Gramsbergen, JB., Sandberg, M., Møller, Dall, A., Kornblit, B., & Zimmer, J. (2002) Glutathione depletion in nigrostriatal slice cultures: GABA loss, dopamine resistance and protection by the tetrahydrobiopterin precursor sepiapterin. *Brain Res.* Vol. 935, pp. 47-58.

Grandoso, L., Ponce, S., Manuel, I., Arrúe, A., Ruiz-Ortega, JA., Ulibarri, I., Orive, G., Hernández, RM., Rodríguez, A., Rodríguez-Puertas, R., Zumárraga, M.,

Linazasoro, G., Pedraz, JL., & Ugedo, L. (2007) Long-term survival of encapsulated GDNF secreting cells implanted within the striatum of parkinsonized rats. *Int J Pharm.* Vol. 343, pp. 69-78.

Halliday, G.M. and McCann, H. (2008) Human-based studies on alpha-synuclein deposition and relationship to Parkinson's disease symptoms. *Exp Neurol.* Vol. 209, pp. 12–21.Kassem, M. (2006) Stem cells: potential therapy for age-related diseases. *Ann N Y Acad Sci.* Vol. 1067, pp. 436-442.

Kim, H., Kim, IS., Lee, IlS., Lee, JP., Snyder, EY., & Park, KI. (2006) Human neurospheres derived from the fetal central nervous system are regionally and temporally specified but are not committed *Exp. Neurol.* Vol. 199, pp. 222-235.

Kim J.H., Auerbach, JM., Rodríguez-Gómez, JA., Velasco, I., Gavin, D., Lumelsky, N., Lee, SH., Nguyen, J., Sánchez-Pernaute, R., Bankiewicz, K., & McKay, R. (2002) Dopamine neurons derived from embryonic stem cells function in an animal model of Parkinson's disease *Nature* Vol. 418, pp. 50–56.

Kirik, D., Annett, LE., Burger, C., Muzyczka, N., Mandel, RJ., & Björklund, A. (2003) Nigrostriatal alpha-synucleinopathy induced by viral vector-mediated overexpression of human alpha-synuclein: a new primate model of Parkinson's disease. *Proc Natl Acad Sci U S A.* Vol. 100, pp. 2884-2889.

Kirik, D., & Björklund, A. (2003) Modeling CNS neurodegeneration by overexpression of disease-causing proteins using viral vectors. *Trends Neurosci.* Vol. 26, pp. 386-392.

Kirik, D., Georgievska, B., & Björklund, A. (2004) Localized striatal delivery of GDNF as a treatment for Parkinson disease. *Nat Neurosci.* Vol. 7, pp. 105-110.

Kirik, D., Rosenblad, C., Burger, C., Lundberg, C., Johansen, TE., Muzyczka, N., Mandel, RJ., & Bjorklund, A. (2002) Parkinson-like neurodegeneration induced by targeted overexpression of alpha-synuclein in the nigrostriatal system. *J Neurosci* Vol. 22, pp. 2780–2791.

Lacar, B., Young, SZ., Platel, JC., & Bordey, A. (2010) Imaging and recording subventricular zone progenitor cells in live tissue of postnatal mice. *Front Neurosci.* Vol. 19; 4. pii: 43.

Lane, E., & Dunnett, S. (2007) Animal models of Parkinson's disease and L-dopa induced dyskinesia: How close are we to the clinic? *Psychopharmacology* doi:10.1007/ s00213−007−0931−8.

Linazasoro G. & On behalf of the Nanotechnologies for Neurodegenerative Diseases Study Group of the Basque Country (NANEDIS). (2008) Potential applications of nanotechnologies to Parkinson's disease therapy *Parkinsonism & Related Disorders* Vol. 14, pp. 383-392.

Lindvall, O., & Björklund, A. (2004) Cell therapy in Parkinson's disease. NeuroRx. Vol. 1, pp. 382-393.

Lindvall O, & Kokaia Z. (2009) Prospects of stem cell therapy for replacing dopamine neurons in Parkinson's disease. *Trends Pharmacol Sci.* Vol. 30, pp. 260-267.

Lindvall O, & Kokaia Z. (2006) Stem cells for the treatment of neurological disorders. *Nature.* Vol. 441, pp. 1094-1096.

McMenamin, MM., Byrnes, AP., Charlton, HM., Coffin, RS., Latchman, DS., & Wood, MJ. (1998) A gamma34.5 mutant of herpes simplex 1 causes severe inflammation in the brain *Neuroscience.* Vol. 83, 1225-1237.

Meyer, AK., Maisel, M., Hermann, A., Stirl, K., & Storch, A. (2010) Restorative approaches in Parkinson's Disease: Which cell type wins the race? *J. Neurol. Sci.* Vol. 289, pp. 93–103.

Miesenböck G. (2009) The optogenetic catechism. *Science.* Vol. 326, pp. 395-359.

Müller, T., Hefter, H., Hueber, R., Jost, WH., Leenders, KL., Odin, P., & Schwarz, J. (2004) Is levodopa toxic? *J Neurol.* Vol. 251 Suppl 6:VI/44-6.

Ostergaard, K., Jones, SA., Hyman, C., & Zimmer, J. (1996) Effects of donor age and brain-derived neurotrophic factor on the survival of dopaminergic neurons and axonal growth in postnatal rat nigrostriatal cocultures. *Exp Neurol.* Vol. 142, pp. 340-350.

Parish CL., Castelo-Branco G., Rawal N., Tonnesen J., Sorensen AT., Salto C et al. (2008) Wnt5a-treated midbrain neural stem cells improve dopamine cell replacement therapy in parkinsonian mice. *J Clin Invest.* Vol. 118, pp. 149-160.

Plenz & Kitai (1998) Regulation of the Nigrostriatal Pathway by Metabotropic Glutamate Receptors during Development. *J. Neuroscience,* Vol. 18, pp. 4133–4144.

Romano C., Van den Pol AN., O'Malley KL (1996) Enhanced early developmental expression of the metabotropic glutamate receptor mGluR5 in rat brain: protein, mRNA splice variants, and regional distribution. *J Comp Neurol* Vol. 367, pp. 403–412.

Sanchez-Pernaute, R., Lee, H., Patterson, M., Reske-Nielsen, C., Yoshizaki, T., Sonntag, KC., Studer, L., & Isacson, O. (2008) Parthenogenetic dopamine neurons from primate embryonic stem cells restore function in experimental Parkinson's disease *Brain* Vol. 131, pp. 2127–2139.

Saner, A., & Thoenen, H. (1971) Model experiments on the molecular mechanism of action of 6-hydroxydopamine. *Mol Pharmacol* Vol. 7, 147–154.

Stahl K., Skare O., Torp R (2009) Organotypic cultures as a model of Parkinson's disease. A twist to an old model *ScientificWorldJournal.* Vol. 9 pp. 811-821.

Stoppini, L., Buchs, PA., & Muller, D. (1991) A simple method for organotypic cultures of nervous tissue. *J. Neurosci Methods.* Vol. 37, pp. 173-182.

Testa CM., Standaert DG., Young AB., Penney Jr JB (1994) Metabotropic glutamate receptor mRNA expression in the basal ganglia of the rat. *J Neurosci* Vol. 14, pp. 3005–3018.

Tønnesen, J., Parish, CL., Sørensen, AT., Andersson, A., Lundberg, C., Deisseroth, K., Arenas, E., Lindvall, O., & Kokaia, M. (2011) Functional Integration of Grafted Neural Stem Cell-Derived Dopaminergic Neurons Monitored by Optogenetics in an In Vitro Parkinson Model. *PLoS ONE* Vol. 6, e17560. doi:10.1371.

Vergni, D., Castiglione, F., Briani, M., Middei, S., Alberdi, E., Reymann, KG., Natalini, R., Volonté, C., Matute, C., & Cavaliere, F. (2009) A model of ischemia-induced neuroblast activation in the adult subventricular zone. *PLoS ONE.* Vol. 4, e5278.

Winkler, C., Kirik, D., Björklund, A., & Dunnett, SB. (2000) Transplantation in the rat model of Parkinson's disease: ectopic versus homotopic graft placement *Prog. Brain Res.* Vol. 127, pp. 233–265.

Zach S., Bueler H., Hengerer B., Gillardon F (2007) Predominant neuritic pathology induced by viral overexpression of alpha-synuclein in cell culture. *Cell Mol Neurobiol.* Vol. 27, pp. 505-515.

Zhang, RL., Le Tourneau, Y., Gregg, SR., Wang, Y., Toh, Y., Robin, AM., Zhang, ZG., & Chopp, M. (2007) Neuroblast division during migration toward the ischemic striatum: a study of dynamic migratory and proliferative characteristics of neuroblasts from the subventricular zone. *J Neurosci*. Vol. 27, pp. 3157-3162.

Part 3

Identified Targets and Growth Factors

7

Therapeutic Potential of Polyphenols in Parkinson's Disease

Rajeswara Babu Mythri[1,*], G. Harish[1,*], N. Raghunath[1] and M.M. Srinivas Bharath[1,**]
National Institute of Mental Health and Neurosciences (NIMHANS), Bangalore, Karnataka India

1. Introduction

Increased human life expectancy has resulted in larger geriatric population throughout the world. Consequently, there is increased prevalence of age-associated neurodegenerative diseases including Parkinson's disease (PD) with serious impact on healthcare. This has intensified the scientific research on the pathology and therapy of the central nervous system (CNS). Although modern approach in biomedical research has made major breakthroughs in understanding the pathological basis of PD, the knowledge about therapy is limited. Consequently, PD does not have a permanent cure.

During recent years, there have been several options for PD therapy including both pharmacological and neurosurgical approaches. These strategies are primarily aimed at improving the motor symptoms without any major side effects ultimately improving the quality of the life of the patient. Drugs such as L-dihydroxyphenyl alanine (levodopa or L-DOPA) replenish the lost dopamine in the brain in early PD and provide symptomatic relief. Apart from L-dopa therapy, other drugs including dopamine receptor agonists, MAO-B inhibitors and anti-cholinergic drugs have been utilized in the pharmacotherapy of PD (Almeida & Hyson, 2008). But, each class of drugs is limited by potential side effects and motor complications with chronic treatment. Further, most PD medications do not effectively tackle tremor, postural instability and cognitive deficits. Moreover, most of these drugs are not completely effective against degeneration of the remaining dopaminergic neurons (Almeida & Hyson, 2008). Due to these serious lacunae, there is a tremendous momentum to develop newer treatments involving disease modifying, restorative, possibly curative drugs with lesser side effects. Most importantly, these drugs should protect the dying neurons thus preventing further neuronal loss. In this direction there have been novel strategies of PD pharmacotherapy applicable either as independent therapies or as a supplement with the existing therapies. These have been tested in experimental models and although many of these molecules show promise, their toxicology, bioavailability and clinical efficacy in human subjects needs to be examined thoroughly before application to PD.

---

* Equal contribution,
** Corresponding author

Neurodegeneration in PD involves multiple pathways such as oxidative stress, mitochondrial damage, protein aggregation, neuroinflammation etc. Modern medicine utilizes a well-defined chemical molecule(s) for pharmacotherapy which might not be effective against different disease pathways. Hence, the challenge is to come up with novel molecules that could simultaneously target multiple disease pathways without significant side-effects, be non-toxic at higher concentrations and have the ability to cross the blood-brain barrier indicating a paradigm shift from monotherapy to multi-therapy based on various targets. Towards this, natural phytochemicals which possess medicinal properties are being exploited (Kumar, 2006) which has increased the interest in the use of herbal products (Tsao, 2010). Consequently, there is increasing support for combination of modern drugs with medicine to evolve better therapies. It is interesting to note that although phytochemicals normally function as toxins and protect the plant source against damage due to pests and harmful organisms, at the lower concentrations consumed by humans, these compounds activate adaptive cellular stress responses *in vivo* ("hormetic mechanisms") thereby providing cytoprotection against exogenous toxins. Such hormetic mechanisms relevant to neuronal survival and improved brain function ultimately elevate the levels of antioxidant enzymes, protein chaperones and neurotrophic factors (Mattson et al., 2007). Polyphenols from various plant sources form a major group of phytochemicals with potential therapeutic and curative properties.

2. Polyphenols: Structure and biological properties

Polyphenols are the most widely distributed natural compounds in the plant kingdom. They are the secondary metabolites which were originally synthesized to protect the plants against microbial attack, pests and ultraviolet radiation. Polyphenols are present in fruits, vegetables, oils etc. and provide plants with brilliant colours and fragrance. Polyphenols might possess many biologically significant functions with implications for human degenerative diseases (Han et al., 2007).

2.1 Chemistry of Polyphenols

Polyphenols in general have a phenolic structure with several hydroxyl groups. Natural polyphenols vary from simple molecules (viz., phenolic acids) to complex polymeric forms (viz., condensed tannins) (Tsao, 2010). Flavonoids are the largest group of polyphenols and have been studied extensively. Currently more than 8000 phenolic structures are known and among them over 4000 flavonoids have been identified (Bravo, 1998, Cheynier, 2005, Harborne & Williams, 2000).They are classified based on the number of phenolic rings and the structural elements that link these rings (Butterfield et al., 2002, Ramassamy, 2006) (Figures 1 and 2) as follows:

a. **Phenolic acids:** These are non-flavonoid polyphenols that constitute less than 1/3 of the phenolic content in our diet and are represented mainly by benzoic acids and cinnamic acid derivatives.

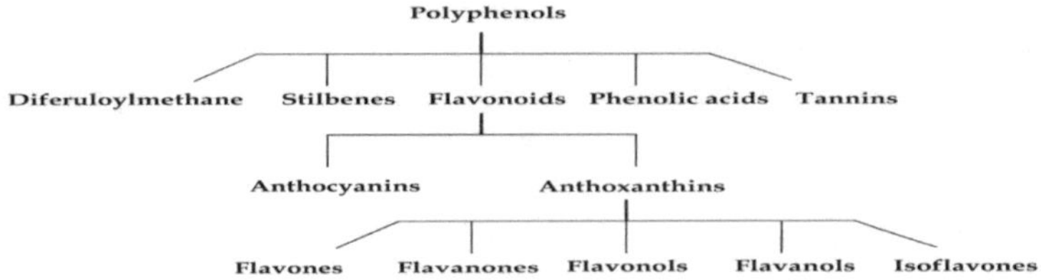

Fig. 1. Classification of polyphenols.

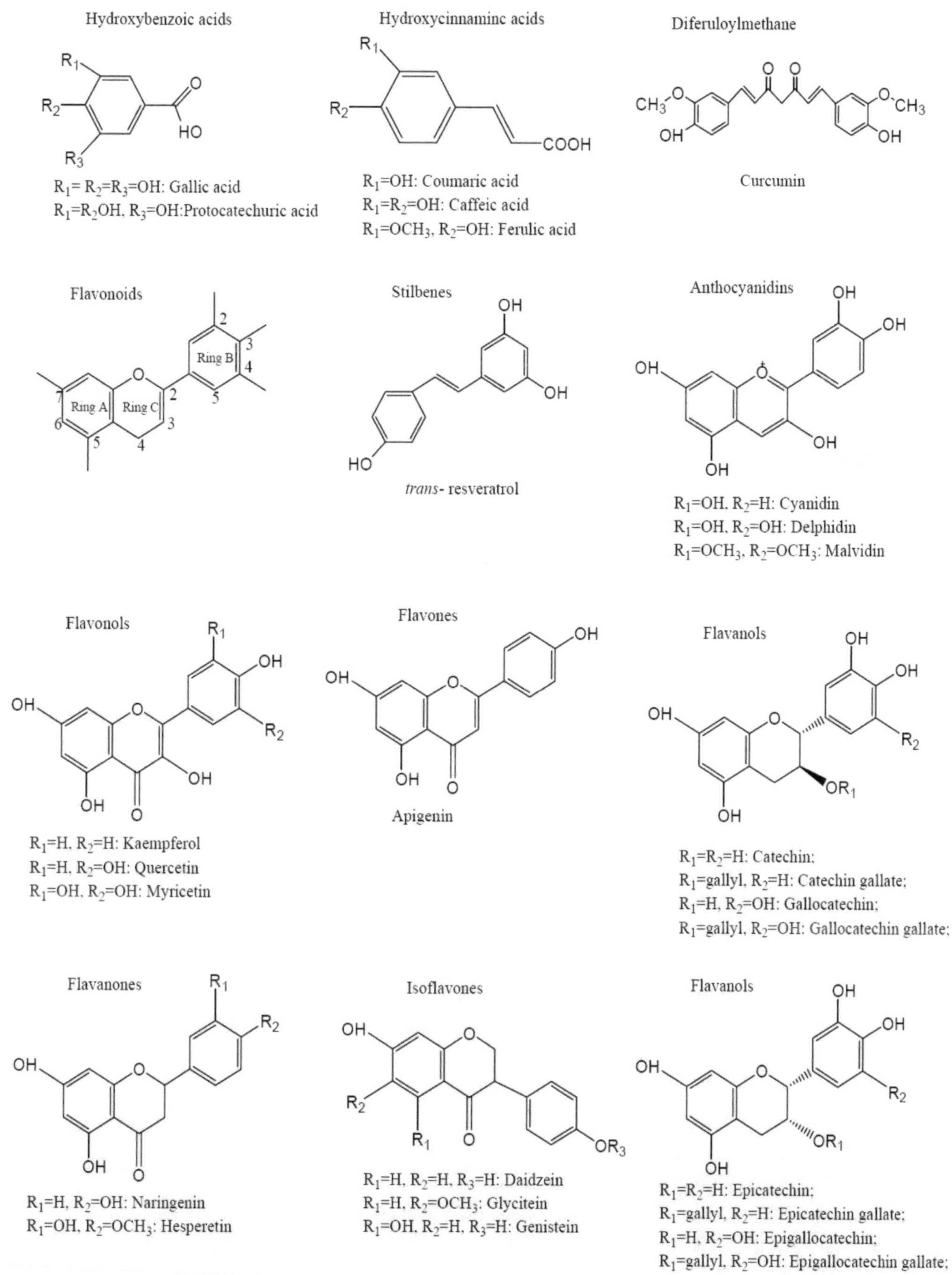

Fig. 2. Chemical structures of common polyphenols.

b. **Flavonoids:** These represent approximately 2/3 of the polyphenolic content in our diet. They have the C6-C3-C6 strucural backbone, of which two are phenolic rings named Ring A and Ring B, and one chromane ring (Tsao 2010). Flavonoids are further classified based on the oxidation state of the chromane ring into Anthocyanins and anthoxanthins. Anthoxanthins are further classified into Flavones, Flavonols, Flavonones, Isoflavones, Flavanols (D'Archivio et al., 2007).
c. **Stilbenes:** Stilbenes are characterized by the presence of 1,2-diphenylethylene nucleus with hydroxyl groups substituted on the aromatic rings (Han et al., 2007). The best known compound among Stilbenes is trans-resveratrol.
d. **Tannins:** Tannins are water soluble polyphenols and are classified into condensed and hydrolysable tannins.
e. **Diferuloylmethanes:** Diferuloylmethanes are characterized by two aromatic rings substituted with hydroxyls, and linked by aliphatic chain containing carbonyl groups. Curcumin is one of the best known polyphenol among diferuloylmethanes.

Most polyphenols are chemically modified by acetylation, hydroxylation, methoxylation. These modifications could significantly influence the physicochemical properties and *in vivo* absorption/degradation of the polyphenols. For e.g., acetylated flavonoids (epicatechin, epigallocatechin) are absorbed without deconjugation and hydrolysis (Rice-Evans & Miller 1996, Scalbert & Williamson 2000). Similarly, polyphenols with most antioxidant potential possess 3- 6 hydroxyl groups. However, hydroxylation in the C3 position significantly inhibits the antioxidant activity and chelation of metals (Huguet et al., 1990, van Acker et al., 1996). Most polyphenols also exist as glycosides with the addition of sugar and acylated sugars at different positions of the polyphenolic structure (one to three moieties per polyphenol) (Tsao, 2010). The attached sugar could be either glucose or rhamnose and each glycosylation influences the physicochemical properties and intestinal absorption of the polyphenol (Rice-Evans & Miller, 1996, Scalbert & Williamson, 2000). Accordingly, if polyphenols are glycosylated with glucose/galactose, they will be absorbed through the small intestine by specific carriers (Scalbert & Williamson, 2000). Those containing rhamnose cannot be absorbed through the small intestine and are degraded by rhamnosidases produced by the colonic microflora. Further, glycosylation of polyphenols might decrease their antioxidant properties (Fukumoto & Mazza, 2000).

2.2 Biological functions of polyphenols

Polyphenols might ameliorate neurodegeneration mainly via (i) intrinsic antioxidant properties and/or by (ii) modulation of cell signalling pathways that control cell survival, death and differentiation (Chen et al., 2000, Molina et al., 2003, Shen et al., 2007, Spencer, 2007).

2.2.1 Antioxidant properties

It has been suggested that consumption of foods or beverages which are rich in polyphenols can increase the antioxidant levels *in vivo* (Frankel et al., 1993). Polyphenols can protect against cellular oxidative stress by directly scavenging free radicals and by chelation of divalent metal ions. The phenolic hydroxyl groups are potent nucleophiles that neutralize free radicals and form aroxyl radicals and this is central to the antioxidant properties of polyphenols. The antioxidant potential is enhanced by the vicinal hydroxyl groups depending on their number and orientation relative to the electron withdrawing groups

such as COOH, CH_2COOH, or $(CH)_2CO_2CH$ (Rice-Evans et al., 1996). The radical scavenging activity of polyphenols is measured by Trolox (a water soluble α-tocopherol analog)-equivalent antioxidant capacity (TEAC) assay and expressed as the millimolar concentration of Trolox (TEAC=1) equivalent to the activity of a 1 mM solution of the given compound (Rice-Evans et al. 1996). Most of the common polyphenols have higher TEAC value compared to the endogenous antioxidant glutathione (GSH), whose TEAC is 1.0.
Since free divalent metal ions such as iron generate free radicals by fenton reaction, chelation of free iron by polyphenols protects neurons from oxidative stress (Li et al., 2010) with implications for PD and Alzheimer's disease (AD) (Sahu & Gray 1997, Sugihara et al., 1999). Flavonoids protect against oxidative damage either by forming complexes with iron or copper or by direct detoxification due to inherent structural characteristics that enhance the antioxidant potential (Bors et al., 1990).

2.2.2 Modulation of cell signalling pathways

Beyond antioxidant activities, polyphenols such as curcumin, resveratrol, quercetin and other flavonoids modulate cellular signalling pathways, that could affect the gene expression and interfere with cell death mechanisms (Williams et al., 2004). Polyphenols exert modulatory effects on neurons by selectively interacting with protein kinase and lipid kinase signalling cascades such as phosphatidylinositol 3-kinase (PI3 kinase or PI3K)/akt, tyrosine kinase, protein kinase C (PKC) and Mitogen activated protein kinase (MAPK) pathways (Agullo et al., 1997, Gamet-Payrastre et al., 1999, Matter et al., 1992, Schroeter et al., 2002, Spencer et al., 2003, Vlahos et al., 1994). Inhibitory or stimulatory actions at these pathways immensely affect the cellular functions by altering the phosphorylation states of target molecules and/or by modulating gene expression (Spencer, 2007). Many Polyphenols bind to ATP binding sites of proteins (Conseil et al., 1998) like PKC (Gamet-Payrastre et al. 1999, Kantengwa & Polla, 1991), protein kinase A (PKA) (Revuelta et al., 1997), calcium plasma membrane ATPase, mitochondrial ATPase and topoisomerase (Boege et al., 1996). For example, the stilbene resveratrol and the citrus flavones, naringenin and hesperetin have been shown to inhibit the activity of a number of protein kinases (Spencer 2007). Flavonoids and their metabolites can selectively interact within MAPK signalling pathways (Kobuchi et al., 1999, Kong et al., 2000).

a. **Extracellular signal-regulated kinase (ERK) pathway:** Some flavonoids are found to have inhibitory effect on the ERK pathway and some others activate this pathway. Flavonoids have close structural homology to specific inhibitors of ERK pathway, such as PD98059 (2'–amino-3'-methoxyflavone), which is a selective non-competitive inhibitor of the mitogen activated kinase, MEK 1 (Alessi et al., 1995). Flavonoids and their metabolites may also act on this pathway in a similar manner. Certain flavonoids such as Quercetin and its O-methylated metabolites are shown to induce neuronal apoptosis by inhibition of ERK pathway (Spencer 2003). The MEK inhibitor PD98059 has been shown to effectively block inducible nitric oxide synthase (iNOS) expression and generation of nitric oxide (NO•) (Bhat et al., 1998), suggesting that flavonoids may also be capable of exerting anti-inflammatory actions via inhibitory actions on MEK1 within the ERK signalling pathway. Studies have indicated that flavanols (Huang et al., 2005, Li et al., 2004), flavones (Chen et al., 2004, Kim et al., 2001, Lee et al., 2003, Shen et al., 2002, Woo et al., 2006), and flavonols (Chen et al., 2005) are all capable of inhibiting the release of NO• by activated microglia via the down-regulation of iNOS gene expression. Epicatechin (EC), and one of its metabolites, 3′-O–methyl-(–)- epicatechin (mEC), have been shown to stimulate phosphorylation of ERK1/2 and the downstream transcription factor cAMP response element binding protein (CREB) at physiological concentrations (Schroeter et al., 2007). Some polyphenols may act on the ERK pathway via acting through steroid-like receptors in neurons to modulate ERK and CREB-mediated gene expression. For example, resveratrol rapidly activates ERK signalling through alpha and beta estrogen receptors (Klinge et al., 2005).

b. **c-Jun-N-terminal kinase (JNK):** There are a number of potential sites where flavonoids may interact in the JNK pathway. EC and mEC have been shown to protect neurons against oxidative damage via a mechanism involving the suppression of JNK, and downstream partners, c-jun and pro-caspase-3 (Schroeter et al., 2001). The flavone, baicalein, significantly inhibits 6-hydroxydopamine (6-OHDA) induced JNK activation and neuronal cell death and quercetin suppresses JNK activity and apoptosis induced by hydrogen peroxide (Ishikawa & Kitamura 2000), 4-hydroxy-2-nonenal (4HNE) (Uchida et al., 1999) and tumour necrosis factor-alpha (TNF-α) (Kobuchi et al. 1999). Flavonoids may inhibit the activation of JNK pathway upstream by decreasing oxidative stress and maintaining calcium homeostasis (Davis 1999). They may also inhibit JNK activation by modulation of the apoptosis signal-regulating kinase 1 (ASK1) phosphorylation state, and its association with 14-3-3 protein, which is essential for suppression of cellular apoptosis (Zhang, L. et al., 1999). Investigations have indicated that flavonoids might have anti-apoptotic property by blocking oxidative stress induced activation of caspase-3 in neurons (Schroeter et al. 2001, Schroeter et al., 2000). Flavonoid o-quinones, formed from the intracellular oxidation of flavonoids also inhibit JNK and other MAPKs via the nucleophilic addition to the cysteine residues of these proteins (Spencer et al., 2004).

c. **PI3 kinase pathway:** Flavonoids can modulate signalling through the serine/threonine kinase, Akt/PKB, one of the main downstream effectors of PI3K in neuronal survival (Coffer et al., 1998). Experimental studies suggest that flavonoids inhibit PI3K via direct interactions with its ATP binding site. Indeed, one of the most selective PI3K inhibitors available, LY294002, was modelled based on the structure of quercetin (Matter et al. 1992).

In the current review, we have discussed the properties and therapeutic potential in PD of three important polyphenols: cucumin, resveratrol and tea polyphenols.

3. Curcumin

Curcumin, the yellow curry spice from the rhizome of turmeric is a polyphenolic compound with several beneficiary properties. Chemically characterized to be diferuloylmethane ($C_{21}H_{20}O_6$) or 1,6-heptadiene-3,5-dione-1,7-bis(4-hydroxy-3-methoxyphenyl), curcumin exists as a group of compounds called curcuminoids.

3.1 Absorption

Although curcumin has several beneficial properties *in vivo*, a major limiting factor is its poor bioavailability. Its poor bioavailability is due to insolubility in aqueous media, poor absorption, rapid metabolism and fast systemic elimination. Following oral administration of curcumin (1.0 g / kg) in mice, 0.13 μg / ml was detected in the plasma after 15 min and peaked at 0.22 μg / ml at 1 hr. Plasma concentration of curcumin however declined to 5 ng /

ml at 6 h. Following intraperitoneal administration of curcumin (0.1 g/kg), only 2.25 μg / ml appeared in the plasma in the first 15 min. Upto 99% of curcumin and 85% of tetrahydrocurcumin was conjugated with glucuronide thus limiting their bioavailability. It has also been suggested that oral administration of curcumin results in very low absorption into the blood. At 1 h time point, the intestine, spleen, liver and kidney had 177.04, 26.06, 26.90, and 7.51 μg/g curcumin respectively, while the brain had as less as 0.41 μg / g. Mass spectrometry analysis suggested that curcumin was first biotransformed to dihydrocurcumin and then tetrahydrocurcumin which were subsequently converted to monoglucuronide conjugates (Pan et al., 1999). In a more recent study, curcumin was administered orally to rats at 500 mg / kg and the peak curcumin concentration of ~36 mg / whole tissue, in the intestine was reached at 1 h time point, while in the blood, liver and kidney, peak concentrations were reached at 6 h (Suresh & Srinivasan 2010). In a pilot human trial on cancer patients, the concentration of curcumin in the liver following oral administration (450 - 3600 mg/ day for 1 week prior to surgery) was measured. The results indicated that only trace levels of curcumin and its metabolites were present in the liver and in circulation and the order of magnitude was too less to exert pharmacological effects (Garcea et al., 2004). As a result of this constraint, research is now directed towards enhancing the bioavailability of curcumin. Animal and human studies suggest that administration of curcumin along with piperine / turmeric oil enhances its bioavailability (Bishnoi et al., 2010, Suresh & Srinivasan 2010). Administration of curcumin along with piperine enables curcumin to stay for longer in the tissues. When administered with piperine, curcumin was detected in the brain at 24, 48 and 96 h and at 48 h the levels of curcumin in the brain exceeded that found in the kidney (5.87 μg vs 1.16 μg) (Suresh & Srinivasan 2010). More recently, curcumin nanoparticles which are entirely water soluble have been suggested to enhance its bioavailability (Ray et al., 2011). Curcumin complexation with phosphatidyl choline (PC) and liposomal curcumin PC complex enhanced its bioavailability in terms of better absorption and improved pharmacokinetics (Gupta & Dixit 2011a, b).

3.2 Antioxidant properties of curcumin

The antioxidant activity of curcumin has been attributed to the various functional groups of curcumin. Jovanovic et al. suggest that the central methylenic group rather than the phenolic group is the H-atom donor, while others attribute its radical scavenging property to the phenolic group (Barclay et al., 2000, Priyadarsini et al., 2003) and the methoxy group further enhances this activity (Priyadarsini et al. 2003). The interactions between curcumin and biological relevant free radicals have been thoroughly investigated. Iwunze and McEwan demonstrated by biophysical techniques that curcumin directly detoxified the reactive nitrogen species peroxynitrite (PN) (Iwunze & McEwan 2004). Our group demonstrated that curcumin can protect neuronal mitochondria against PN induced nitration and nitrosylation of brain mitochondrial proteins (Mythri et al., 2007). It was also shown that curcumin protected against PN induced protein nitration and inhibition of enzyme activity of mitochondrial complex I with implications for PD (Mythri et al. 2007). Recently, we demonstrated that curcumin protects against PN mediated loss of mitochondrial membrane potential and mitochondrial integrity and curcumin derivatives offered improved protection compared to curcumin (Mythri et al. 2011). Mishra et al demonstrated that at low superoxide concentrations, curcumin effectively caused superoxide dismutation without itself undergoing any chemical change, but at higher concentrations of superoxide, curcumin inhibited superoxide activity by reacting with it (Mishra et al., 2004). The enol structure with the intramolecular hydrogen bond of curcumin strongly enhances the free radical scavenging activity (Ohara 2005, Toniolo et al., 2002). *In vivo*, the antioxidant activity of curcumin could be mediated through antioxidant enzymes such as superoxide dismutase (SOD), catalase, and glutathione peroxidase (GPx). Curcumin has been shown to serve as a Michael acceptor, reacting with GSH and thioredoxin (Adams et al., 2005). Curcumin has been found to be at least ten times more active as an antioxidant than even vitamin E (Khopde et al., 2000). The phenolic and the methoxy group on the phenyl ring and the 1,3-diketone system seem to be important structural features of curcumin that can contribute to these effects. The antioxidant activity of curcumin increases when the phenolic group has a methoxy group at the ortho position (Motterlini et al., 2000).

3.3 Intracellular targets

The important molecular targets of curcumin include growth factors, growth factor receptors, transcription factors, transcription factor receptors, cytokines, enzymes and genes which regulate apoptosis. Curcumin activates the NF-E2-related factor 2/ Antioxidant Response Element (Nrf2/ARE) pathway which in turn induces synthesis of phase II antioxidant (Jeyapaul & Jaiswal, 2000, Wild et al., 1999), glutathione-S-transferase (GST) (Chanas et al., 2002, Ye et al., 2007), NADH quinone oxidoreductase 1 (NQO1) (Ye et al., 2007) and hemeoxygenase-1 (HO-1). Curcumin suppresses activation of the pro-survival transcription factor, nuclear factor kappa B (NFκB) by inhibition of IκB kinase (Jobin et al., 1999, Plummer et al., 1999). Suppression of NFκB leads to down regulation of cell cycle regulatory protein cyclin D1, cyclooxygenase 2 (COX2) and matrix metalloproteinase 9 (MMP-9) (Shishodia et al., 2005). Curcumin further, suppresses interleukin 6 (IL-6) mediated signal transducers and activators of transcription (STAT-3) phosphorylation and its subsequent nuclear translocation (Bharti et al., 2003). Curcumin, it has been reported, activates the peroxisome proliferator activated receptor γ (PPAR γ) and hence mediates expression of cyclin D1 and epidermal growth factor receptor (EGFR) (Chen & Xu, 2005). Curcumin down regulates the transcription factor, AP-1, by direct interaction with its DNA binding motif, (Bierhaus et al., 1997, Huang, T. S. et al., 1991) and also inhibits interleukin 1 alpha (IL-1α) and TNF-induced AP-1 activation (Xu, Y. X. et al., 1997). Moreover, curcumin targets the JNK pathway preventing JNK 1/2 and c Jun phosphorylation and caspase 3 activation (Yu et al., 2010). Curcumin probably interferes with the signalling molecules at the same level or proximally upstream of MAPKKK level, hence indirectly affects the JNK pathway (Chen, Y. R. & Tan 1998). Furthermore, curcumin induces anti apoptotic genes such as Bcl-2 and inhibits iNOS resulting in reduction of ROS, abrogates oxidative stress mediated cytochrome c release or caspase 3 activation, significantly increases levels of anti apoptotic proteins Bcl-2 and Bcl-xL and decreases levels of pro-apoptotic proteins Bax and Bad (Chen, J. et al., 2006, Chen, Y. R. & Tan 1998). Curcumin treatment causes a 3-7 fold increase in the modifier subunit of the GSH synthesizing enzyme, gamma-glutamyl cysteine ligase (γ-GCL), in both the neurons and astrocytes (Dale & Russell 1956, Lavoie, S. et al., 2009) and enhances GSH levels (Jagatha et al., 2008) probably by enhancing astrocytic efflux of GSH (Stridh et al., 2010). In addition, curcumin regulates iron metabolism by activation of iron regulatory protein and repression of ferretin, suggesting a role as an iron chelator (Jiao et al., 2006, Jiao et al., 2009).

Curcumin has been used as an antioxidant, antiseptic, anti-inflammatory, antibacterial and antitumor agent and has been used against various disorders such as arthritis, cardiovascular diseases, lung fibrosis, gall stone formation, cardiotoxicity, diabetes, wound healing, AD and many more (Aggarwal 2006, Sharma et al., 2006). Recent studies have also shown curcumin to be protective against cancer (Duvoix et al., 2005), diabetes (Cheng et al., 2009, Peeyush et al., 2009) and for the reduction of blood cholesterol (Alwi et al., 2008, Ejaz et al., 2009, Jang et al., 2008). Curcumin protects against ischemia induced elevation in malondialdehyde (MDA) and lactate dehydrogenase (LDH) release in animal models (Dikshit et al., 1995). Faster restoration of muscle architecture upon curcumin treatment in injury models is probably mediated via NFκB activation (Thaloor et al., 1999).

3.4 Effects of curcumin in models of PD

More recently, curcumin has found its role as a therapeutic agent in models of neurological disorders such as stroke and AD (Lim et al., 2001, Thiyagarajan & Sharma 2004, Yang et al., 2005). Lim et al. have shown that dietary curcumin reduces amyloid pathology, oxidative stress and pro-inflammatory markers in transgenic mice, in addition curcumin reduces the levels of GFAP, a marker of astrocytic proliferation (Lim et al. 2001). Further, curcumin not only prevented formation of abeta aggregates but could also disintegrate preformed aggregates by directly binding to plaques (Yang et al. 2005). Curcumin can cross the blood brain barrier and is found to be least toxic in human subjects at high doses (Lao et al., 2006, Qureshi et al., 1992, Shankar et al., 1980, Shoba et al., 1998). It can detoxify ROS, prevent protein aggregation and induce neurogenesis *in vivo* (Kim, S. J. et al., 2008, Priyadarsini et al. 2003, Xu, Y. et al., 2007).

Since PD is a neurological condition involving oxidative and nitrosative stress pathways, curcumin can serve as a potential therapeutic molecule for PD. Although thiol reducing agents such as GSH have been evaluated for their anti-PD activity, their efficiency is limited due to poor ability to cross the blood brain barrier (Bharath et al., 2002). Curcumin on the other hand can cross the blood brain barrier and can be administered at higher doses without the risk of toxicity. Curcumin treatment protects substantia nigra (SN) neurons, improves striatal dopamine levels and chelates Fe^{2+}, following administration of 6-hydroxy dopamine (6-OHDA) in rats (Zbarsky et al., 2005). Curcumin treatment abrogates dopamine induced striatal neuron cell death (Luo et al., 1999). Curcumin treatment could further increase the density of dopaminergic neurons in the SN (Vajragupta et al., 2003). In all these studies, protection was afforded only by pretreatment with curcumin prior to administration of the toxin. A recent study in our laboratory indicated that chronic dietary consumption of turmeric caused an increase in the tyrosine hydroxylase (TH) positive neurons in the SN (Mythri et al. 2011). This is consistent with earlier reports suggesting that curcumin contributes to neurogenesis (Kim, S. J. et al. 2008, Xu, Y. et al. 2007). Similarly, our laboratory also demonstrated that curcumin derivatives with improved bioavailability offers better defense against 1-methyl-4-phenylpyridinium (MPP^+) in dopaminergic neurons (Mythri et al. 2011).

Curcumin treatment attenuates 3-nitropropionic acid mediated oxidative stress *in vivo* (Kumar, A. et al., 2007). PN is a highly labile reactive nitrogen species which inflicts severe cellular damage by nitrosative protein modifications. However, PN mediated nitrosative stress and mitochondrial dysfunction were attenuated by pretreatment with curcumin *in vitro* (Mythri et al. 2011). Curcumin mediated protection from PN toxicity is probably due to its direct interaction with and inactivation of PN *in vitro* (Iwunze & McEwan 2004, Mythri et al. 2007) or indirectly by enhancing GSH levels *in vivo* ((Jagatha et al. 2008, Mythri et al.

2007). Curcumin down regulates iNOS which is probably mediated by the cJun/AP-1 pathway (Brouet & Ohshima 1995, Chan et al., 1998, Chen, J. et al. 2006). It has been suggested that curcumin binding to the AP-1 binding site on the promoter region of iNOS, results in its inactivation (Brouet & Ohshima 1995). Pan et al. have further reported that curcumin reduces iNOS mRNA levels and blocks induction of NFκB (Pan, M. H. et al., 2000). Rajeswari and colleagues have reported an increase in striatal dopamine and dihydroxy phenyl acetic acid (DOPAC) levels following curcumin injection in 1-methyl-4-phenyl-1,2,3,6-tetrahydropyridine (MPTP)-injected mice (Rajeswari & Sabesan 2008). In addition curcumin restores mitochondrial membrane potential, causes elevation in Cu-Zn SOD and modulates NFκB nuclear translocation (Wang, J. et al., 2009a) by inhibition of IL6 and TNFα (Wang, S. L. et al., 2009b). Curcumin treatment inhibits AP-1 pathway by prevention of c-Jun phosphorylation (Luo et al. 1999) in addition to inhibition of JNK phosphorylation (Sawada et al., 2002, Yu et al. 2010) and caspase 3 activation (Yu et al. 2010). It has been reported that curcumin induces anti apoptotic genes such as Bcl-2 and inhibits iNOS resulting in reduction of ROS, abrogates oxidative stress mediated cytochrome c release or caspase 3 activation, significantly increases levels of anti apoptotic proteins Bcl-2 and Bcl-xL and decreases levels of pro-apoptotic proteins Bax and Bad (Chen, J. et al. 2006, Chen, Y. R. & Tan 1998). Curcumin induced cytoprotection was probably mediated by the Bcl-2 – mitochondria – reactive oxygen species (ROS) – iNOS pathway.

Oxidative damage of lipids results in the formation of aldehydes such as 4HNE and MDA, which can integrate into lipid membranes resulting in disruption of membrane integrity, energy crisis and eventually cell death. Increased levels of 4HNE adducts have been reported in PD brains (Yoritaka et al., 1996). Lipid peroxidation mediated mitochondrial damage and apoptosis were abrogated by curcumin treatment and this was probably by checking cytochrome c release and caspase and PARP activation (Zhu et al., 2004). Curcumin was further able to protect from 4HNE mediated alterations in mitochondrial respiratory function and redox metabolism, cytochrome c release, DNA fragmentation and PARP activation in PC12 cells suggesting a protective function against lipid peroxidation mediated damage (Raza et al., 2008).

Interestingly, not only is curcumin an antioxidant molecule but can also increase the levels of GSH, an endogenous antioxidant molecule, probably by enhancing astrocytic efflux of GSH (Stridh et al. 2010). Results from our laboratory and others have shown that curcumin enhances GSH levels *in vitro* and *in vivo* (Jagatha et al. 2008, Rajeswari 2006), in addition to enhancing the antioxidant enzyme activities of SOD and catalase in the striatum and mid brain of MPTP injected mice (Rajeswari 2006). In addition curcumin treatment results in a 3-7 fold increase in the modifier subunit of the GSH synthesizing enzyme, γ-GCL, in both the neurons and astrocytes (Dickinson et al., 2003, LaVoie, M. J. et al., 2005). Curcumin mediated increase in the transcription of GCL genes is probably via regulation of the binding of transcription factors to the 12-tetradecanoate 13-acetate (TPA)-responsive elements (TRE) and electrophilic response element (EpRE) elements (Dickinson et al. 2003). It further activates the Nrf2/ARE pathway which in turn induces synthesis of phase II antioxidant enzymes such as GCL (Jeyapaul & Jaiswal 2000, Wild et al. 1999), GST (Chanas et al. 2002, Ye et al. 2007), NQO1 (Ye et al. 2007) and HO-1. We have used diester derivatives of curcumin (di-piperoyl, di-valinoyl and di-glutamoyl) with a resultant enhanced protection against GSH depletion mediated oxidative stress and toxin induced cell death in a dopaminergic neuronal cell line (Harish et al., 2010, Mythri et al. 2011). Particularly the di-glutamoyl derivative showed maximum protection due to its deesterification following absorption thus providing glutamate as a precursor for GSH synthesis. Thus one could use such pro drugs with improved uptake and better radical scavenging properties to combat oxidative and nitrosative stress in various neurodegenerative disorders such as PD.

Curcumin further inhibits aggregation of α-synuclein *in vitro* (Pandey et al., 2008, Wang, M. S. et al., 2010) and aggregation of A53T mutant α-synuclein in SH-SY5Y cells in a dose dependent manner. Curcumin, thus enhances α-synuclein solubility rendering them non-toxic (Pandey et al. 2008). It also exhibits neuro-restorative properties as shown by its ability to disintegrate preformed α-synuclein fibrils (Ono & Yamada 2006). Curcumin pre-treatment resulted in a reduction in aggregation of synphilin-1, a component of Lewy neuritis seen during PD, as a function of rotenone induced nitrosative stress, in SH-SY5Y dopaminergic cells suggesting its efficacy in ameliorating nitrosative stress induced damage (Pal et al. 2011).

Curcumin has been suggested to regulate proteins involved in iron metabolism. Increased brain iron content is a major risk factor for PD pathogenesis. It has been reported that the SN of PD brains has increased iron content (Sofic et al., 1988). Not only is iron responsible for the production of ·OH radical, but also promotes dopamine autooxidation in the SN neurons resulting in the release of H_2O_2 (Ben-Shachar et al., 1995). It has been reported that curcumin induces activation of iron regulatory protein and repression of ferretin and a reduction in levels of hepcidin, suggesting a role as an iron chelator (Jiao et al. 2006, Jiao et al. 2009).

Epidemiological studies have suggested that consumption of curcumin by the Asian Indians is probably the reason for the low incidence of AD / PD in India when compared to the Caucasians (Ganguli et al., 2000). A study exploring the effect of race and age on the prevalence of PD reported that there are approximately 40% less melanized nigral neurons in Indian brains when compared to Caucasian brains (Muthane et al., 1998). Furthermore, there was no change in the number of nigral neurons with advancing age in the Asian Indian population (Alladi et al., 2009). Hence the lower prevalence of PD in India despite lower numbers of nigral neurons suggests protective mechanism probably related to the dietary habits. Chronic consumption of spices such as turmeric provide antioxidant defense against various conditions such as diabetes and cancer (Sinha et al., 2003, Srinivasan 2005). We have recently demonstrated that chronic dietary consumption of turmeric ameliorated the MPTP induced neurotoxicity in mice (Mythri et al. 2011). Although curcumin is the most active ingredient of turmeric, it could be more effective in its natural milieu. Also the biological properties of natural extracts would probably be mediated by their various constituents rather than a single compound. Therefore it would be interesting to study the pharmacokinetics and pharmacodynamics of curcumin or the other biologically active components of turmeric in order to completely understand its mechanism of action.

4. Resveratrol

Resveratrol (3,5,4'-trihydroxy-trans-stilbene), a phytoalexin and a stilbenoid derived is a naturally occurring polyphenol with strong antioxidant properties (Baur & Sinclair 2006, Fremont 2000). Resveratrol is a dietary polyphenol found in the skin of grapes, raspberries, mulberries, pistachios and peanuts under normal conditions and synthesized by other medicinal and edible plants under stress conditions (Rocha-Gonzalez et al., 2008, Saiko et al., 2008). It exists as cis- and trans- isomers which are either free or bound to glucose (Mattivi et al., 1995). The trans- form can undergo isomerisation to the cis- form when exposed to ultraviolet irradiation (Lamuela-Raventos et al., 1995). Experimental evidences *in vitro* and *in vivo* have demonstrated the pharmacological potential of resveratrol in human diseases and aging with curative properties against neurodegenerative diseases (Rocha-Gonzalez et al. 2008).

4.1 Absorption of resveratrol

The oral absorption of resveratrol in humans is thought to occur mainly by transepithelial diffusion. However, a major portion of resveratrol administered orally is excreted via feces and urine (Wenzel & Somoza 2005). Following oral ingestion, trans-resveratrol is extensively metabolized in the enterocyte before it enters the blood and target organs. Since trans-resveratrol is photosensitive it is easily oxidized thus presenting unfavorable pharmacokinetics (Frozza et al., 2010). Extensive metabolism in the intestine and liver results in the bioavailability of resveratrol to be <1% and dose escalation and repeated dose administration does not significantly alter the bioavailability. Metabolic studies, both in plasma and in urine, have revealed that resveratrol is modified as glucuronides and sulfates. The sulfated and glucuronidated forms appeared within approximately 15 min of entering the bloodstream, and moderate consumption of red wine results in serum levels of resveratrol that barely reach the micromolar concentrations. In contrast, its metabolites, which may be the active principle, circulate in serum for up to 9 h (Saiko et al. 2008). However, reduced dihydroresveratrol conjugates, in addition to highly polar but unknown products, may account for ~ 50% of resveratrol following oral administration. Apart from the metabolism in the intestine and liver, colonic bacterial metabolism also contributes to resveratrol bioavailability (Walle 2011). Among these, extremely rapid sulfate conjugation by the intestine/liver appears to be the rate-limiting step in resveratrol's bioavailability. Although the systemic bioavailability of resveratrol is very low, accumulation of resveratrol in epithelial cells along the aerodigestive tract and potentially active resveratrol metabolites may still produce *in vivo* effects (North & Verdin 2004). Since low bioavailability of resveratrol is a major obstacle to biomedical applications, efforts are in progress to improve the absorption and slow down its metabolism (Biasutto et al., 2010). Oral and intravenous (i.v.) administration of resveratrol in human volunteers revealed that the absorption following oral administration of 25 mg oral dose was at least 70%, with peak plasma levels of resveratrol and metabolites at 491 ± 90 ng/ml (about 2 μM) and a plasma half-life of 9.2 ± 0.6 h. However, only trace amounts of unchanged resveratrol (<5 ng/ml) could be detected in plasma and most of the oral dose was recovered in urine.

4.2 Effects of resveratrol in models of PD

Similar to curcumin, the effectiveness of resveratrol is due to its ability to simultaneously target multiple pathways and proteins and thus may be effective in restoring homoestasis *in vivo*. The most important property relevant in abrogation of neuronal damage is its antioxidant potential. This has been extensively studied in different models and most of them refer to the systemic effects (Kovacic & Somanathan 2010). Experiments from our laboratory have showed that resveratrol prevented peroxynitrite mediated nitration of mitochondrial proteins and this was significantly higher compared to curcumin (Mythri et al. 2007). Apart from its antioxidant properties, resveratrol displays anti-cancer and anti-inflammatory properties. The anti-cancer properties arise due its ability to inhibit multiple target enzymes including kinases, cyclooxygenases, ribonucleotide reductase and DNA polymerases. Similarly, resveratrol protects the cardiovascular system against ischemic-reperfusion injury, promotes vasorelaxation, protects the endothelium and displays anti-atherosclerotic properties and other functions thereby strongly supporting its role in cardioprotection. Resveratrol displays different properties depending on its concentration and also on the target cell and its physiology (Saiko et al. 2008). Resveratrol and its derivatives have shown promise in AD therapy and other neurodegenerative disorders (Albani et al., 2010) and more specifically on the inhibition of β-amyloid peptide aggregation (Richard et al., 2011).

Interestingly, resveratrol-mediated intracellular effects and protective mechanisms might be via its effects as an agonist of the sirtuins (also called SIRT or silent information regulator two-proteins), which belong to the histone deacetylase family (Pallas et al., 2008, Wang, F. et al., 2007, Zhuang et al., 2003). Sirtuins possess NAD^+ dependent deacetylase activity and mono-ribosyltransferase activity and are found in most organisms (North & Verdin 2004, Yamamoto et al., 2007). SIRT1 is a major modulator of metabolism and displays therapeutic properties (Finkel et al., 2009, Harikumar & Aggarwal 2008, Karuppagounder et al., 2009). It has been hypothesized that by activating SIRT1, resveratrol modulates the activity of numerous proteins, including peroxisome proliferator-activated receptor coactivator-1alpha (PGC-1 alpha), the FOXO family, Akt (protein kinase B) and NFκB (Pallas et al., 2009). The beneficial effects of resveratrol as an anti-aging compound are believed to be mediated via the activation of SIRT1 (Hung et al., 2010).

Resveratrol administration in adult mice protected the SN dopaminergic neurons and striatal dopamine against the neurotoxic effects of MPTP (Anderson et al., 2006, Blanchet et al., 2008). Resveratrol administration also significantly protected mice from MPTP-induced motor coordination impairment, hydroxyl radical overloading, and neuronal loss with implications for PD therapy (Lu et al., 2008). In cell culture, treatment with resveratrol protected against MPP^+ toxicity and oxidative damage by modulating the apoptotic markers (Bournival et al., 2009, Gelinas & Martinoli 2002). It has also been demonstrated that resveratrol effectively blocked the proteolytic cleavage of PKCδ and kinase activity induced by MPP^+. In BV-2 microglial cells activated with lipopolysaccharide (LPS), pretreatment with resveratrol suppressed pro-inflammatory cytokine production and nitric oxide release. It could be surmised that resveratrol protects against the dopaminergic neurodegeneration by modulating the PKCδ dependent proapoptotic signaling pathway and the inflammatory response in activated microglia (Gordon , 2010). Resveratrol significantly reversed the toxic effects of MPTP by increasing the levels of dopamine and its metabolites, GSH and activities of GPx and reducing lipid peroxidation along with enhanced behaviour performance indicating that resveratrol could target multiple pathways with therapeutic potential in PD (Anandhan et al., 2010). Interestingly, transfection with SIRT1 siRNA blocked MPP^+-induced apoptosis in SH-SY5Y cells indicating that the toxicity of MPP^+ was mediated via SIRT1 and possibly through the regulation of another pro-apoptotic protein BCL2/Adinovirus E1B 19kDa Interacting Protein 2 (BNIP2). In a similar study, Alvira and colleagues showed that although resveratrol prevented MPP^+ induced death of cortical neurons in culture, the effect was not mediated via SIRT1 activation, since sirtinol - a SIRT1 inhibitor could not attenuate MPP^+ toxicity (Alvira et al., 2007). Furthermore MPP^+ decreased the expression of SIRT1 indicating that the antiapoptotic effects of resveratrol against MPP^+ are independent of the stimulation of SIRT1 and depend on its antioxidant properties.

Other *in vitro* studies have also demonstrated the effects of Resveratrol against different neurotoxins (Chao et al., 2008, Okawara et al., 2007, Outeiro et al., 2007). The therapeutic role of resveratrol has been demonstrated in 6-OHDA induced *in vivo* model of PD. Ultrastructural analysis showed that resveratrol alleviated 6-OHDA-induced chromatin condensation, mitochondrial dysfunction and vacuolization of SN dopaminergic neurons. Resveratrol also reduced the levels of COX-2 and TNF-α mRNA in the SN suggesting that resveratrol exerts its effects via reduced neuroinflammatory reaction (Jin, F. et al., 2008). Oral treatment with resveratrol and its liposomal form prevented oxidative damage, prevented neuronal damage and restored motor behaviour in a 6-OHDA rat model of PD (Khan et al., 2010, Wang, Y. et al., 2011). The study also showed that resveratrol liposome offered better therapeutic effect than free resveratrol due to increased bioavailability. Oxyresveratrol, a polyhydroxylated stilbene from mulberry showed improved protection against 6-OHDA compared to resveratrol owing to its antioxidant activity, blood-brain barrier permeability and water solubility (Chao et al. 2008). Pinostilbene, a methylated derivative of resveratrol showed improved cellular bioavailability and better defense against 6-OHDA neurotoxicity in neuronal cell culture (Chao et al., 2010b). Lee et al. demonstrated that resveratrol protected SH-SY5Y neuroblastoma cells from apoptosis induced by dopamine (Lee, M. K. et al., 2007).

Experiments in rat primary midbrain neuron-glia cultures demonstrated that resveratrol protected dopaminergic neurons against LPS-induced neurotoxicity in a dose and time-dependent manner via inhibition of microglial activation and suppression of release of proinflammatory factors. The anti-inflammatory effects and therapeutic effects against LPS toxicity was attributed to the inhibition of NADPH oxidase-dependent generation of reactive oxygen species and attenuation of translocation of the cytosolic subunit (p47) of NADPH oxidase to the cell membrane. This mechanism was substantiated when resveratrol was not effective in cultures from NADPH deficient mice. This is also related to an attenuation of MAPK and NFκB signalling pathways in microglia (Zhang, F. et al., 2010). Bureau and colleagues demonstrated that resveratrol reduced apoptotic neuronal cell death induced by neuroinflammation in an LPS cell model and strongly decreased the mRNA expression of two proinflammatory genes, IL-1α and TNF-α (Bureau et al., 2008).

Administration of a botanical extract (Regrapex-R) prepared from whole grape *Vitis vinifera* and *Polygonum cuspidatum*, enriched with polyphenols including resveratrol, to a drosophila transgenic model of PD overexpressing alpha-synuclein caused dose-dependent scavenging effects on ROS, protected mitochondria from oxidative damage and improved locomotor dysfunction and extended lifespan (Long et al., 2009). Resveratrol was able to protect neuronal cells in culture against toxicity arising from two aggregation-prone proteins, the AD-involved amyloid-beta (1-42) peptide (Abeta42) and the familiar PD linked alpha-synuclein (A30P) [alpha-syn(A30P)] (Albani et al., 2009).

5. Tea polyphenols

Tea is one of the most frequently consumed beverage of the world. Out of the 2.5 million metric tons of dried tea manufactured annually, ~20 % is green tea, which is mainly consumed in China and Japan and ~78 % is black tea, which is consumed in Western countries (Chen, L. et al., 1997). Although consumption of tea as an ancient beverage and a lifestyle habit has been recognized, its potential pharmacological actions beneficial to human health have been recently reported (Weinreb et al., 2004). Human epidemiological and animal experiments indicate that consumption of green and black tea might protect the brain against aging and reduce the incidence of dementia, AD and PD, which might be one of the mechanistic factors underlying the significantly lower rates of age-related neurological disorders among Asians compared to European or American populations (Mandel, S. A. et al., 2008). Green tea is non-fermented and contains mainly catechins that accounts for 30-40% of its dry weight. Catechins are polyphenols that have been suggested to contribute to the therapeutic properties of green tea. On the contrary, black and red teas are extensively fermented and oolong tea is semi-fermented which catalyzes the oxidation and polymerization of catechins thereby reducing their content to 3-10 % of dry weight. The catechins from green tea are polyphenols representing flavonoids. The eight major catechins of green tea are (+)-catechin (C), (+)-catechin gallate, (+)-gallocatechin, (+)-gallocatechin gallate, (-)-epicatechin (EC), (-)-epicatechin gallate (ECG), (-)-epigallocatechin (EGC), and (-)-epigallocatechin gallate (EGCG) (+ and - represent *cis* and *trans* isomers respectively). EGCG is the most abundant catechin (Higdon & Frei 2003). Green tea in addition to catechins contain 2-3% of caffeic acid and 1-6% of amino acids (theanine constitutes about 50% amino acid content) (Higdon & Frei 2003).

5.1 Absorption

The *in vivo* metabolism of green tea catechins has been very well documented in humans and laboratory animals (Li, C. et al., 2000, Pietta et al., 1998). In humans, orally administered catechins are absorbed, metabolized and largely excreted within 24 h. Catechins were detected in rat plasma and bile as free or sulphated and glucuronidated conjugates (Harada et al., 1999). The bioavailability of green tea polyphenols *in vivo* depends on the route of administration. After intragastric administration of decaffeinated green tea (DGT) (200 mg/kg) in rats, 13.7 % of EGC and 31.2 % of EC were shown in the plasma, but only 0.1% of EGCG was bioavailable (Chen, L. et al. 1997). Intravenous injection of DGT (25 mg/kg) showed that, the beta-elimination half-lives of EGCG, EGC, and EC were 212, 45, and 41 min respectively (Chen, L. et al. 1997). Recent studies have suggested that the EC metabolites such as epicatechin glucuronide and 3'-O-methylated epicatechin glucuronide formed after oral ingestion in rats were detectable in the brain (Abd El Mohsen et al., 2002). The results from the distribution study suggest that EGCG is mainly excreted through bile, and that EGC and EC are excreted through both the bile and urine (Spencer 2003).

5.2 Antioxidant functions of tea polyphenols

There is growing evidence that catechins exert protective role in neurodegeneration. Several studies have suggested that the potential curative and therapeutic effects of tea polyphenols could be attributed to their free radical scavenging capacity. Catechins are powerful hydrogen donating antioxidants and scavengers of reactive oxygen and nitrogen species *in vitro* (Lee, S. et al., 2000, Matsuoka et al., 1995, Oliver et al., 1990). Tea polyphenols may also regulate antioxidant enzymes like SOD and catalase in mouse striatum (Levites et al., 2001). Progressive iron accumulation in SN pars compacta of PD patients is well established and is considered to be a major contributor to oxidative stress (Gerlach et al., 1994, Riederer et al., 1989). Green tea polyphenols can stoichiometrically bind ferric iron to form an inactive iron polyphenol complex (Grinberg et al., 1997). In rat brain tissue, green tea and black tea extracts were shown to inhibit lipid peroxidation promoted by iron ascorbate in homogenates of brain mitochondrial membranes (Levites et al., 2002b). EGCG inhibited paraquat-induced MDA production in rat liver microsomes by scavenging superoxide radicals and by iron chelating activity (Liou et al., 2001).

5.3 Functions of tea and its constituent polyphenols in PD

Several prospective studies have assessed the association between coffee/tea consumption and PD risk, but the results are inconsistent. Kandinov and colleagues carried out a retrospective study on 278 consecutive PD patients and assessed the data on smoking and coffee or tea consumption and found that disease progression was not affected by cigarette smoking, tea or coffee consumption (Kandinov et al., 2007). In contrast, the same group demonstrated that cigarette smoking, coffee and tea drinking may protect against PD and delay the onset of disease (Kandinov et al., 2009). According to their study in human patients, while consumption of more than 3 cups of tea per day delayed the onset of motor symptoms by 7.7 years, coffee consumption advanced the age of PD onset by 4.8 years. In a related study, Barranco Quintana and colleagues compiled data from human studies carried out by different groups and observed a clear protective effect of tea consumption and this protective effect was more evident in the Chinese populations (Barranco Quintana et al., 2009). They also suggest that the low rate of tea consumption among persons with PD could provide valuable insight into the pathology. A population based study in ethnic Chinese to understand the role of environmental factors and dietary intake demonstrated that while there was a dose-dependent protective effect of PD in coffee and tea drinkers and smokers, a history of exposure to heavy metals increased the risk of PD (Tan, E. K. et al., 2003). Tan et al. observed that while black tea, a caffeine-containing beverage, showed an inverse association with PD risk, green tea drinking was unrelated to PD (Tan, Louis C. et al., 2008). A study among Finnish subjects indicated that coffee drinking is associated with a lower risk of PD and increased tea consumption is associated with a lower risk of PD (Hu et al., 2007). Since most of these studies are based on survey among PD patients, it would be difficult to draw significant conclusions.

However, experiments in cell and animal models have clearly indicated the therapeutic effects of tea extracts and its constituent catechin, EGCG against PD. These curative properties might be due to their ability to act as antioxidants, modulators of intracellular neuronal signalling, metabolism, cell survival/death genes, and mitochondrial function (Mandel, S. A. et al. 2008, Mandel, S. A. et al., 2011). With reference to PD therapy, EGCG has a dual therapeutic effect *in vivo* (Kang et al., *2010)*. Firstly, EGCG is a naturally occurring catechol-O-methyl transferase (COMT) inhibitor which strongly inhibited human liver COMT-mediated O-methylation of L-DOPA in a dose-dependent manner and decreased the accumulation of 3-O-methyldopa in the plasma and striatum *in vivo* following oral administration of L-DOPA + carbidopa. In addition, EGCG also protected against glutamate-induced oxidative cytotoxicity in hippocampal cultures through inactivation of the NFκB-signaling pathway *in vitro* and against kainic acid-induced oxidative damage and neurodegeneration in the hippocampus *in vivo*.

Many studies related to therapeutic effects of tea polyphenols in PD have been carried out in the Parkinsonian model involving the neurotoxin 6-OHDA and have obtained varied results. Rats treated with black tea either prior to or after 6-OHDA provided significant protection in terms of behavioural and motor functions, antioxidant levels, apoptotic markers, dopaminergic neuronal numbers and expression of tyrosine hydroxylase (TH). However, the degree of improvement in motor and neurochemical deficits was more prominent in 6-OHDA rats pre-treated with the extract (Chaturvedi et al., 2006). Green tea polyphenols protected SH-SY5Y neuroblastoma cells against apoptosis induced by 6-OHDA as evidenced by lowered apoptotic markers, restoration of mitochondrial integrity, decreased oxidative damage and intracellular free Ca^{2+} and inhibition of auto-oxidation of 6-OHDA. Further, the cells were protected against 6-OHDA-induced increase in levels of NO and protein nitration, and over-expression of neuronal NOS (nNOS) and iNOS. These results indicate that green tea polyphenols ameliorate 6-OHDA toxicity via attenuation of the ROS-NO pathway (Guo et al., 2005). The same group confirmed these effects against 6-OHDA *in vivo* in mid brain and striatum again emphasizing the involvement of the ROS-NO pathway (Guo et al., 2007). In order to identify the active ingredient against 6-OHDA, five catechins [EGCG, ECG, EGC, EC and (+)-C] representing the most prominent tea polyphenols were compared with regard to their effects on 6-OHDA-induced apoptosis in PC12 cells and the protective effects of the five catechins were in the order ECG > EGCG > EC > (+)-C > EGC and the antiapoptotic activities appear to be structurally related to the 3-gallate group (Jin, C. F. et al., 2001, Nie et al., 2002). In a related study, it was showed that EGCG protected against 6-OHDA via stimulation of PKC and modulation of cell survival/cell cycle genes such as Bax, Bad, Mdm2, Bcl-2, Bcl-w, and Bcl-x(L) and also by potent antioxidant and iron chelating actions thereby preventing nuclear translocation and activation of cell death promoting NFκB (Levites et al., 2002a). Since the stability and bioavailability of EGCG are restricted, Chao et al. generated and tested a pro-drug representing a fully acetylated EGCG (pEGCG) in a PD cell model (Chao et al., 2010a). They found that pEGCG displayed improved protection compared to EGCG against 6-OHDA toxicity in SH-SY5Y neuroblastoma cells probably via activation of Akt pathway and reduced caspase-3 activity. In contrast, when Leaver et al. administered rats with EGCG for 14 days followed by exposure to 6-OHDA, they observed that EGCG produced subtle symptomatic relief in lesioned animals and could not prevent neuronal damage to a significant extent (Leaver et al., 2009).

Tea extracts and EGCG have displayed therapeutic effect in other toxic models of PD. Tea extract and EGCG protected against MPTP mediated dopamine loss and neurotoxicity *in vivo* and this effect could be mediated by inhibition of NOS (Choi et al., 2002, Kim, J. S. et al., 2010, Li, R. et al., 2006). In a related study, it was demonstrated that green tea extract and EGCG protected against MPTP neurotoxicity via antioxidant effects and inhibition of monoamine oxidase-B (MOAB) (Levites et al. 2001). Mechanistically, green tea polyphenols can ameliorate neuronal damage via inhibitory effects on dopamine transporters (DAT), through which they block MPP^+ uptake and protect dopaminergic neurons against MPP^+-induced injury (Pan, T. et al., 2003). Similarly, Hou et al. (2008) demonstrated that EGCG attenuated cell death in PC12 cells induced by the herbicide and PD toxin paraquat (PQ) by maintaining mitochondrial membrane potential, inhibiting caspase-3 activity and down regulating the expression of pro-apoptotic protein second mitochondrial-derived activator of caspase (SMAC) in cytosol. However, in rotenone-treated mesencephalic cultures and organotypic striatal cultures, EGCG protected striatal slices to a limited extent by counteracting NO production by rotenone but was not significantly effective against rotenone toxicity in mesencephalic cultures (Moldzio et al., 2010).

Green tea could also protect against environmental toxin-induced cell injury and neuroinflammation with implications for PD. Tai and Truong (2010) reported that EGCG reduced dichlorodiphenyl-trichloroethane (DDT)-induced cell death in dopaminergic SH-

SY5Y cells suggesting that EGCG might activate a protective mechanism that might alleviate organochlorine pesticide-induced cell injury. Likewise, EGCG also inhibited LPS-activated microglial secretion of NO and TNF-α through the down-regulation of iNOS and TNF-α expression thereby protecting against neuroinflammation and injury in dopaminergic neurons (Li, R. et al. 2004). The antioxidant property of EGCG is also beneficial against protein aggregation in PD. Iron induces toxic aggregation of monomeric alpha synuclein leading to neurodegeneration in dopaminergic neurons. In the MPTP model, iron accumulation is also linked to NO-dependent mechanism. Mandel et al. showed that EGCG prevented the accumulation of iron and alpha-synuclein in SN thereby preventing neuronal damage (Mandel, S. et al., 2004). However, green tea and its constituent polyphenols could not protect PC12 cells against L-glutamate and MPP^+ (Mazzio et al., 2001).

6. Conclusions

Most of the drugs currently used in PD therapy replenish the brain dopamine and provide symptomatic relief during early PD. However, many patients develop motor complications with chronic treatment. Further, these drugs do not slowdown or prevent the progression of the disease since their ability to prevent neuronal damage has not been comprehensively validated in humans. Therefore, novel therapies with possible curative properties are being exploited for adjunctive therapy. It is well documented that neurodegeneration in PD is contributed by several interrelated disease pathways but the molecular mechanisms of their relationships and their chronology have not been completely understood. Therefore, any molecule(s) with therapeutic potential in PD should be simultaneously effective against multiple pathways. In this regard, several *in vitro* and *in vivo* studies using PD models have tested natural antioxidants and molecules for their ability to protect against neurodegeneration with implications for therapy. The most prominent are the polyphenolic antioxidants obtained from plant sources. Most of these compounds display antioxidant, anti-inflammatory and anti-cancer properties, cross the blood-brain barrier and prevent neuronal damage in neurological disorders. Recent studies strongly support the clinical application of these compounds in PD. The current chapter explores the therapeutic potential of polyphenols such as curcumin, resveratrol and tea polyphenols in PD. These three polyphenols share common biological properties including antioxidant function, low toxicity and therapeutic benefits in the brain of different PD models. The available data indeed indicate that these polyphenols could have therapeutic potential in PD. Although several studies have been carried out in the recent years, the biological properties and health benefits of these polyphenols have not been completely understood. However, the most important limiting factor for the therapeutic application of these compounds in PD is their limited bioavailability *in vivo*. Further, the delivery of compounds specifically to mid-brain dopaminergic neurons for maximum therapeutic effect has not been completely standardized. Apart from this, studies are also needed to test the safety and efficacy in humans to translate the experimental results for therapeutic application in PD patients.

7. Acknowledgements

This study was financially supported by the Department of Science and Technology (No. SR/FT/L-152/2005 to MMSB). RBM is supported by an extended senior research fellowship from the Council for Scientific and Industrial Research (CSIR), India. GH is supported by a senior research fellowship from Indian Council for Medical Research (ICMR), India. NR is supported by a junior research fellowship from CSIR, India.

8. References

Abd El Mohsen MM, Kuhnle G, Rechner AR, Schroeter H, Rose S, Jenner P & Rice-Evans CA (2002) Uptake and metabolism of epicatechin and its access to the brain after oral ingestion. *Free Radic Biol Med.* Vol. 33, No. 12, (Dec 15 2002):pp. (1693-1702), 0891-5849 (Print)

Adams BK, Cai J, Armstrong J, Herold M, Lu YJ, Sun A, Snyder JP, Liotta DC, Jones DP & Shoji M (2005) EF24, a novel synthetic curcumin analog, induces apoptosis in cancer cells via a redox-dependent mechanism. *Anticancer Drugs.* Vol. 16, No. 3, (Mar 2005):pp. (263-275), 0959-4973 (Print)

Aggarwal BB, Bhatt, I.D., Ichikawa, H., Ahn, K.S., Sethi, G., Sandur, S.K., Natarajan, C., Seeram, N., Shishodia, S. (2006) Curcumin–biological and medicinal properties. in: *Turmeric: the genus Curcuma,* (ed.), pp (297-368), Taylor and Francis GroupLondon

Agullo G, Gamet-Payrastre L, Manenti S, Viala C, Remesy C, Chap H & Payrastre B (1997) Relationship between flavonoid structure and inhibition of phosphatidylinositol 3-kinase: a comparison with tyrosine kinase and protein kinase C inhibition. *Biochem Pharmacol.* Vol. 53, No. 11, (Jun 1 1997):pp. (1649-1657), 0006-2952 (Print)

Albani D, Polito L, Batelli S, De Mauro S, Fracasso C, Martelli G, Colombo L, Manzoni C, Salmona M, Caccia S, Negro A & Forloni G (2009) The SIRT1 activator resveratrol protects SK-N-BE cells from oxidative stress and against toxicity caused by alpha-synuclein or amyloid-beta (1-42) peptide. *J Neurochem.* Vol. 110, No. 5, (Sep 2009):pp. (1445-1456), 1471-4159 (Electronic)

Albani D, Polito L, Signorini A & Forloni G (2010) Neuroprotective properties of resveratrol in different neurodegenerative disorders. *Biofactors.* Vol. 36, No. 5, (Sep 2010):pp. (370-376), 1872-8081 (Electronic)

Alessi DR, Cuenda A, Cohen P, Dudley DT & Saltiel AR (1995) PD 098059 is a specific inhibitor of the activation of mitogen-activated protein kinase kinase in vitro and in vivo. *J Biol Chem.* Vol. 270, No. 46, (Nov 17 1995):pp. (27489-27494), 0021-9258 (Print)

Alladi PA, Mahadevan A, Yasha TC, Raju TR, Shankar SK & Muthane U (2009) Absence of age-related changes in nigral dopaminergic neurons of Asian Indians: relevance to lower incidence of Parkinson's disease. *Neuroscience.* Vol. 159, No. 1, (Mar 3 2009):pp. (236-245), 0306-4522 (Print)

Almeida QJ, Hyson HC (2008) The evolution of pharmacological treatment for Parkinson's disease. *Recent Pat CNS Drug Discov.* 2008 Jan;Vol 3, No. 1, (Jan 2008): pp. (50-54).

Alvira D, Yeste-Velasco M, Folch J, Verdaguer E, Canudas AM, Pallas M & Camins A (2007) Comparative analysis of the effects of resveratrol in two apoptotic models: inhibition of complex I and potassium deprivation in cerebellar neurons. *Neuroscience.* Vol. 147, No. 3, (Jul 13 2007):pp. (746-756), 0306-4522 (Print)

Alwi I, Santoso T, Suyono S, Sutrisna B, Suyatna FD, Kresno SB & Ernie S (2008) The effect of curcumin on lipid level in patients with acute coronary syndrome. *Acta Med Indones.* Vol. 40, No. 4, (Oct 2008):pp. (201-210), 0125-9326 (Print)

Anandhan A, Tamilselvam K, Vijayraja D, Kumar NA, Rajasankar S & Manivasagam T (2010) *Resveratrol attenuates oxidative stress and improves behaviour in 1-methyl-4-phenyl-1,2,3,6-tetrahydropyridine (MPTP) challenged mice,*

Anderson DW, Bradbury KA & Schneider JS (2006) Neuroprotection in Parkinson models varies with toxin administration protocol. *Eur J Neurosci.* Vol. 24, No. 11, (Dec 2006):pp. (3174-3182), 0953-816X (Print)

Barclay LR, Vinqvist MR, Mukai K, Goto H, Hashimoto Y, Tokunaga A & Uno H (2000) On the antioxidant mechanism of curcumin: classical methods are needed to determine antioxidant mechanism and activity. *Org Lett.* Vol. 2, No. 18, (Sep 7 2000):pp. (2841-2843), 1523-7060 (Print)

Barranco Quintana JL, Allam MF, Del Castillo AS & Navajas RF (2009) Parkinson's disease and tea: a quantitative review. *J Am Coll Nutr.* Vol. 28, No. 1, (Feb 2009):pp. (1-6), 1541-1087 (Electronic)

Baur JA & Sinclair DA (2006) Therapeutic potential of resveratrol: the in vivo evidence. *Nat Rev Drug Discov.* Vol. 5, No. 6, (Jun 2006):pp. (493-506), 1474-1776 (Print)

Ben-Shachar D, Zuk R & Glinka Y (1995) Dopamine neurotoxicity: inhibition of mitochondrial respiration. *J Neurochem.* Vol. 64, No. 2, (Feb 1995):pp. (718-723), 0022-3042 (Print)

Bharath S, Hsu M, Kaur D, Rajagopalan S & Andersen JK (2002) Glutathione, iron and Parkinson's disease. *Biochem Pharmacol.* Vol. 64, No. 5-6, (Sep 2002):pp. (1037-1048), 0006-2952 (Print)

Bharti AC, Donato N & Aggarwal BB (2003) Curcumin (diferuloylmethane) inhibits constitutive and IL-6-inducible STAT3 phosphorylation in human multiple myeloma cells. *J Immunol.* Vol. 171, No. 7, (Oct 1 2003):pp. (3863-3871), 0022-1767 (Print)

Bhat NR, Zhang P, Lee JC & Hogan EL (1998) Extracellular signal-regulated kinase and p38 subgroups of mitogen-activated protein kinases regulate inducible nitric oxide synthase and tumor necrosis factor-alpha gene expression in endotoxin-stimulated primary glial cultures. *J Neurosci.* Vol. 18, No. 5, (Mar 1 1998):pp. (1633-1641), 0270-6474 (Print)

Biasutto L, Marotta E, Garbisa S, Zoratti M & Paradisi C (2010) Determination of Quercetin and Resveratrol in Whole Blood—Implications for Bioavailability Studies. *Molecules.* Vol. 15, No. 9, 2010):pp. (6570-6579), 1420-3049

Bierhaus A, Zhang Y, Quehenberger P, Luther T, Haase M, Muller M, Mackman N, Ziegler R & Nawroth PP (1997) The dietary pigment curcumin reduces endothelial tissue factor gene expression by inhibiting binding of AP-1 to the DNA and activation of NF-kappa B. *Thromb Haemost.* Vol. 77, No. 4, (Apr 1997):pp. (772-782), 0340-6245 (Print)

Bishnoi M, Chopra K, Rongzhu L & Kulkarni SK (2010) Protective Effect of Curcumin and its Combination with Piperine (Bioavailability Enhancer) Against Haloperidol-Associated Neurotoxicity: Cellular and Neurochemical Evidence. *Neurotox Res.* Vol., No. (Nov 13 2010):pp. 1476-3524 (Electronic)

Blanchet J, Longpre F, Bureau G, Morissette M, DiPaolo T, Bronchti G & Martinoli MG (2008) Resveratrol, a red wine polyphenol, protects dopaminergic neurons in MPTP-treated mice. *Prog Neuropsychopharmacol Biol Psychiatry.* Vol. 32, No. 5, (Jul 1 2008):pp. (1243-1250), 0278-5846 (Print)

Boege F, Straub T, Kehr A, Boesenberg C, Christiansen K, Andersen A, Jakob F & Kohrle J (1996) Selected novel flavones inhibit the DNA binding or the DNA religation step of eukaryotic topoisomerase I. *J Biol Chem*. Vol. 271, No. 4, (Jan 26 1996):pp. (2262-2270), 0021-9258 (Print)

Bors W, Heller W, Michel C & Saran M (1990) Flavonoids as antioxidants: determination of radical-scavenging efficiencies. *Methods Enzymol*. Vol. 186, No. 1990):pp. (343-355), 0076-6879 (Print)

Bournival J, Quessy P & Martinoli MG (2009) Protective effects of resveratrol and quercetin against MPP+ -induced oxidative stress act by modulating markers of apoptotic death in dopaminergic neurons. *Cell Mol Neurobiol*. Vol. 29, No. 8, (Dec 2009):pp. (1169-1180), 1573-6830 (Electronic)

Bravo L (1998) Polyphenols: chemistry, dietary sources, metabolism, and nutritional significance. *Nutr Rev*. Vol. 56, No. 11, (Nov 1998):pp. (317-333), 0029-6643 (Print)

Brouet I & Ohshima H (1995) Curcumin, an anti-tumour promoter and anti-inflammatory agent, inhibits induction of nitric oxide synthase in activated macrophages. *Biochem Biophys Res Commun*. Vol. 206, No. 2, (Jan 17 1995):pp. (533-540), 0006-291X (Print)

Bureau G, Longpre F & Martinoli MG (2008) Resveratrol and quercetin, two natural polyphenols, reduce apoptotic neuronal cell death induced by neuroinflammation. *J Neurosci Res*. Vol. 86, No. 2, (Feb 1 2008):pp. (403-410), 1097-4547 (Electronic)

Butterfield D, Castegna A, Pocernich C, Drake J, Scapagnini G & Calabrese V (2002) Nutritional approaches to combat oxidative stress in Alzheimer's disease. *J Nutr Biochem*. Vol. 13, No. 8, (Aug 2002):pp. (444), 1873-4847 (Electronic)

Chan MM, Huang HI, Fenton MR & Fong D (1998) In vivo inhibition of nitric oxide synthase gene expression by curcumin, a cancer preventive natural product with anti-inflammatory properties. *Biochem Pharmacol*. Vol. 55, No. 12, (Jun 15 1998):pp. (1955-1962), 0006-2952 (Print)

Chanas SA, Jiang Q, McMahon M, McWalter GK, McLellan LI, Elcombe CR, Henderson CJ, Wolf CR, Moffat GJ, Itoh K, Yamamoto M & Hayes JD (2002) Loss of the Nrf2 transcription factor causes a marked reduction in constitutive and inducible expression of the glutathione S-transferase Gsta1, Gsta2, Gstm1, Gstm2, Gstm3 and Gstm4 genes in the livers of male and female mice. *Biochem J*. Vol. 365, No. Pt 2, (Jul 15 2002):pp. (405-416), 0264-6021 (Print)

Chao J, Lau WK, Huie MJ, Ho YS, Yu MS, Lai CS, Wang M, Yuen WH, Lam WH, Chan TH & Chang RC (2010a) A pro-drug of the green tea polyphenol (-)-epigallocatechin-3-gallate (EGCG) prevents differentiated SH-SY5Y cells from toxicity induced by 6-hydroxydopamine. *Neurosci Lett*. Vol. 469, No. 3, (Jan 29 2010a):pp. (360-364), 1872-7972 (Electronic)

Chao J, Li H, Cheng KW, Yu MS, Chang RC & Wang M (2010b) Protective effects of pinostilbene, a resveratrol methylated derivative, against 6-hydroxydopamine-induced neurotoxicity in SH-SY5Y cells. *J Nutr Biochem*. Vol. 21, No. 6, (Jun 2010b):pp. (482-489), 1873-4847 (Electronic)

Chao J, Yu MS, Ho YS, Wang M & Chang RC (2008) Dietary oxyresveratrol prevents parkinsonian mimetic 6-hydroxydopamine neurotoxicity. *Free Radic Biol Med*. Vol. 45, No. 7, (Oct 1 2008):pp. (1019-1026), 0891-5849 (Print)

Chaturvedi RK, Shukla S, Seth K, Chauhan S, Sinha C, Shukla Y & Agrawal AK (2006) Neuroprotective and neurorescue effect of black tea extract in 6-hydroxydopamine-lesioned rat model of Parkinson's disease. *Neurobiol Dis*. Vol. 22, No. 2, (May 2006):pp. (421-434), 0969-9961 (Print)

Chen A & Xu J (2005) Activation of PPAR{gamma} by curcumin inhibits Moser cell growth and mediates suppression of gene expression of cyclin D1 and EGFR. *Am J Physiol Gastrointest Liver Physiol*. Vol. 288, No. 3, (Mar 2005):pp. (G447-456), 0193-1857 (Print)

Chen C, Yu R, Owuor ED & Kong AN (2000) Activation of antioxidant-response element (ARE), mitogen-activated protein kinases (MAPKs) and caspases by major green tea polyphenol components during cell survival and death. *Arch Pharm Res*. Vol. 23, No. 6, (Dec 2000):pp. (605-612), 0253-6269 (Print)

Chen CJ, Raung SL, Liao SL & Chen SY (2004) Inhibition of inducible nitric oxide synthase expression by baicalein in endotoxin/cytokine-stimulated microglia. *Biochem Pharmacol*. Vol. 67, No. 5, (Mar 1 2004):pp. (957-965), 0006-2952 (Print)

Chen J, Tang XQ, Zhi JL, Cui Y, Yu HM, Tang EH, Sun SN, Feng JQ & Chen PX (2006) Curcumin protects PC12 cells against 1-methyl-4-phenylpyridinium ion-induced apoptosis by bcl-2-mitochondria-ROS-iNOS pathway. *Apoptosis*. Vol. 11, No. 6, (Jun 2006):pp. (943-953), 1360-8185 (Print)

Chen JC, Ho FM, Pei-Dawn Lee C, Chen CP, Jeng KC, Hsu HB, Lee ST, Wen Tung W & Lin WW (2005) Inhibition of iNOS gene expression by quercetin is mediated by the inhibition of IkappaB kinase, nuclear factor-kappa B and STAT1, and depends on heme oxygenase-1 induction in mouse BV-2 microglia. *Eur J Pharmacol*. Vol. 521, No. 1-3, (Oct 3 2005):pp. (9-20), 0014-2999 (Print)

Chen L, Lee MJ, Li H & Yang CS (1997) Absorption, distribution, elimination of tea polyphenols in rats. *Drug Metab Dispos*. Vol. 25, No. 9, (Sep 1997):pp. (1045-1050), 0090-9556 (Print)

Chen YR & Tan TH (1998) Inhibition of the c-Jun N-terminal kinase (JNK) signaling pathway by curcumin. *Oncogene*. Vol. 17, No. 2, (Jul 16 1998):pp. (173-178), 0950-9232 (Print)

Cheng TC, Lin CS, Hsu CC, Chen LJ, Cheng KC & Cheng JT (2009) Activation of muscarinic M-1 cholinoceptors by curcumin to increase glucose uptake into skeletal muscle isolated from Wistar rats. *Neurosci Lett*. Vol. 465, No. 3, (Nov 20 2009):pp. (238-241), 1872-7972 (Electronic)

Cheynier V (2005) Polyphenols in foods are more complex than often thought. *Am J Clin Nutr*. Vol. 81, No. 1 Suppl, (Jan 2005):pp. (223S-229S), 0002-9165 (Print)

Choi JY, Park CS, Kim DJ, Cho MH, Jin BK, Pie JE & Chung WG (2002) Prevention of nitric oxide-mediated 1-methyl-4-phenyl-1,2,3,6-tetrahydropyridine-induced Parkinson's disease in mice by tea phenolic epigallocatechin 3-gallate. *Neurotoxicology*. Vol. 23, No. 3, (Sep 2002):pp. (367-374), 0161-813X (Print)

Coffer PJ, Jin J & Woodgett JR (1998) Protein kinase B (c-Akt): a multifunctional mediator of phosphatidylinositol 3-kinase activation. *Biochem J*. Vol. 335 (Pt 1), No. (Oct 1 1998):pp. (1-13), 0264-6021 (Print)

Conseil G, Baubichon-Cortay H, Dayan G, Jault JM, Barron D & Di Pietro A (1998) Flavonoids: a class of modulators with bifunctional interactions at vicinal ATP- and steroid-binding sites on mouse P-glycoprotein. *Proc Natl Acad Sci U S A*. Vol. 95, No. 17, (Aug 18 1998):pp. (9831-9836), 0027-8424 (Print)

D'Archivio M, Filesi C, Di Benedetto R, Gargiulo R, Giovannini C & Masella R (2007) Polyphenols, dietary sources and bioavailability. *Ann Ist Super Sanita*. Vol. 43, No. 4, 2007):pp. (348-361), 0021-2571 (Print)

Dale WM & Russell C (1956) A study of the irradiation of catalase by ionizing radiations in the presence of cysteine, cystine and glutathione. *Biochem J*. Vol. 62, No. 1, (Jan 1956):pp. (50-57), 0264-6021 (Print)

Davis RJ (1999) Signal transduction by the c-Jun N-terminal kinase. *Biochem Soc Symp*. Vol. 64, No. 1999):pp. (1-12), 0067-8694 (Print)

Dickinson DA, Iles KE, Zhang H, Blank V & Forman HJ (2003) Curcumin alters EpRE and AP-1 binding complexes and elevates glutamate-cysteine ligase gene expression. *FASEB J*. Vol. 17, No. 3, (Mar 2003):pp. (473-475), 1530-6860 (Electronic)

Dikshit M, Rastogi L, Shukla R & Srimal RC (1995) Prevention of ischaemia-induced biochemical changes by curcumin & quinidine in the cat heart. *Indian J Med Res*. Vol. 101, No. (Jan 1995):pp. (31-35), 0971-5916 (Print)

Duvoix A, Blasius R, Delhalle S, Schnekenburger M, Morceau F, Henry E, Dicato M & Diederich M (2005) Chemopreventive and therapeutic effects of curcumin. *Cancer Lett*. Vol. 223, No. 2, (Jun 8 2005):pp. (181-190), 0304-3835 (Print)

Ejaz A, Wu D, Kwan P & Meydani M (2009) Curcumin inhibits adipogenesis in 3T3-L1 adipocytes and angiogenesis and obesity in C57/BL mice. *J Nutr*. Vol. 139, No. 5, (May 2009):pp. (919-925), 1541-6100 (Electronic)

Finkel T, Deng C-X & Mostoslavsky R (2009) Recent progress in the biology and physiology of sirtuins. *Nature*. Vol. 460, No. 7255, 2009):pp. (587-591), 0028-0836

Frankel EN, Waterhouse AL & Kinsella JE (1993) Inhibition of human LDL oxidation by resveratrol. *Lancet*. Vol. 341, No. 8852, (Apr 24 1993):pp. (1103-1104), 0140-6736 (Print)

Fremont L (2000) Biological effects of resveratrol. *Life Sci*. Vol. 66, No. 8, (Jan 14 2000):pp. (663-673), 0024-3205 (Print)

Frozza RL, Bernardi A, Paese K, Hoppe JB, da Silva T, Battastini AM, Pohlmann AR, Guterres SS & Salbego C (2010) Characterization of trans-resveratrol-loaded lipid-core nanocapsules and tissue distribution studies in rats. *J Biomed Nanotechnol*. Vol. 6, No. 6, (Dec 2010):pp. (694-703), 1550-7033 (Print)

Fukumoto LR & Mazza G (2000) Assessing antioxidant and prooxidant activities of phenolic compounds. *J Agric Food Chem*. Vol. 48, No. 8, (Aug 2000):pp. (3597-3604), 0021-8561 (Print)

Gamet-Payrastre L, Manenti S, Gratacap MP, Tulliez J, Chap H & Payrastre B (1999) Flavonoids and the inhibition of PKC and PI 3-kinase. *Gen Pharmacol*. Vol. 32, No. 3, (Mar 1999):pp. (279-286), 0306-3623 (Print)

Ganguli M, Chandra V, Kamboh MI, Johnston JM, Dodge HH, Thelma BK, Juyal RC, Pandav R, Belle SH & DeKosky ST (2000) Apolipoprotein E polymorphism and Alzheimer disease: The Indo-US Cross-National Dementia Study. *Arch Neurol*. Vol. 57, No. 6, (Jun 2000):pp. (824-830), 0003-9942 (Print)

Garcea G, Jones DJ, Singh R, Dennison AR, Farmer PB, Sharma RA, Steward WP, Gescher AJ & Berry DP (2004) Detection of curcumin and its metabolites in hepatic tissue and portal blood of patients following oral administration. *Br J Cancer*. Vol. 90, No. 5, (Mar 8 2004):pp. (1011-1015), 0007-0920 (Print)

Gelinas S & Martinoli MG (2002) Neuroprotective effect of estradiol and phytoestrogens on MPP+-induced cytotoxicity in neuronal PC12 cells. *J Neurosci Res*. Vol. 70, No. 1, (Oct 1 2002):pp. (90-96), 0360-4012 (Print)

Gerlach M, Ben-Shachar D, Riederer P & Youdim MB (1994) Altered brain metabolism of iron as a cause of neurodegenerative diseases? *J Neurochem*. Vol. 63, No. 3, (Sep 1994):pp. (793-807), 0022-3042 (Print)

Gordon,R. (2010). Resveratrol Protects Dopaminergic Neurons in Parkinson's Disease Models by Modulating the PKC-delta Apoptotic Signaling Pathway & Microglial Activation (24:763.5) Proceedings of FASEB meeting, 0892-6638, conference location, April, 2010

Grinberg LN, Newmark H, Kitrossky N, Rahamim E, Chevion M & Rachmilewitz EA (1997) Protective effects of tea polyphenols against oxidative damage to red blood cells. *Biochem Pharmacol*. Vol. 54, No. 9, (Nov 1 1997):pp. (973-978), 0006-2952 (Print)

Guo S, Bezard E & Zhao B (2005) Protective effect of green tea polyphenols on the SH-SY5Y cells against 6-OHDA induced apoptosis through ROS-NO pathway. *Free Radic Biol Med*. Vol. 39, No. 5, (Sep 1 2005):pp. (682-695), 0891-5849 (Print)

Guo S, Yan J, Yang T, Yang X, Bezard E & Zhao B (2007) Protective effects of green tea polyphenols in the 6-OHDA rat model of Parkinson's disease through inhibition of ROS-NO pathway. *Biol Psychiatry*. Vol. 62, No. 12, (Dec 15 2007):pp. (1353-1362), 1873-2402 (Electronic)

Gupta NK & Dixit VK (2011a) Development and evaluation of vesicular system for curcumin delivery. *Arch Dermatol Res*. Vol. 303, No. 2, (Mar 2011a):pp. (89-101), 1432-069X (Electronic)

Gupta NK & Dixit VK (2011b) Bioavailability enhancement of curcumin by complexation with phosphatidyl choline. *J Pharm Sci*. Vol. 100, No. 5, (May 2011b):pp. (1987-1995), 1520-6017 (Electronic)

Han X, Shen T & Lou H (2007) Dietary Polyphenols and Their Biological Significance. *International Journal of Molecular Sciences*. Vol. 8, No. 9, 2007):pp. (950-988), 1422-0067

Harada M, Kan Y, Naoki H, Fukui Y, Kageyama N, Nakai M, Miki W & Kiso Y (1999) Identification of the major antioxidative metabolites in biological fluids of the rat with ingested (+)-catechin and (-)-epicatechin. *Biosci Biotechnol Biochem*. Vol. 63, No. 6, (Jun 1999):pp. (973-977), 0916-8451 (Print)

Harborne JB & Williams CA (2000) Advances in flavonoid research since 1992. *Phytochemistry*. Vol. 55, No. 6, (Nov 2000):pp. (481-504), 0031-9422 (Print)

Harikumar KB & Aggarwal BB (2008) Resveratrol: a multitargeted agent for age-associated chronic diseases. *Cell Cycle*. Vol. 7, No. 8, (Apr 15 2008):pp. (1020-1035), 1551-4005 (Electronic)

Harish G, Venkateshappa C, Mythri RB, Dubey SK, Mishra K, Singh N, Vali S & Bharath MM (2010) Bioconjugates of curcumin display improved protection against glutathione depletion mediated oxidative stress in a dopaminergic neuronal cell line: Implications for Parkinson's disease. *Bioorg Med Chem*. Vol. 18, No. 7, (Apr 1 2010):pp. (2631-2638), 1464-3391 (Electronic)

Higdon JV & Frei B (2003) Tea catechins and polyphenols: health effects, metabolism, and antioxidant functions. *Crit Rev Food Sci Nutr.* Vol. 43, No. 1, 2003):pp. (89-143), 1040-8398 (Print)

Hou RR, Chen JZ, Chen H, Kang XG, Li MG & Wang BR (2008) Neuroprotective effects of (-)-epigallocatechin-3-gallate (EGCG) on paraquat-induced apoptosis in PC12 cells. *Cell Biol Int.* Vol. 32, No. 1, (Jan 2008):pp. (22-30), 1065-6995 (Print)

Hu G, Bidel S, Jousilahti P, Antikainen R & Tuomilehto J (2007) Coffee and tea consumption and the risk of Parkinson's disease. *Mov Disord.* Vol. 22, No. 15, (Nov 15 2007):pp. (2242-2248), 0885-3185 (Print)

Huang Q, Wu LJ, Tashiro S, Gao HY, Onodera S & Ikejima T (2005) (+)-Catechin, an ingredient of green tea, protects murine microglia from oxidative stress-induced DNA damage and cell cycle arrest. *J Pharmacol Sci.* Vol. 98, No. 1, (May 2005):pp. (16-24), 1347-8613 (Print)

Huang TS, Lee SC & Lin JK (1991) Suppression of c-Jun/AP-1 activation by an inhibitor of tumor promotion in mouse fibroblast cells. *Proc Natl Acad Sci U S A.* Vol. 88, No. 12, (Jun 15 1991):pp. (5292-5296), 0027-8424 (Print)

Huguet AI, Manez S & Alcaraz MJ (1990) Superoxide scavenging properties of flavonoids in a non-enzymic system. *Z Naturforsch C.* Vol. 45, No. 1-2, (Jan-Feb 1990):pp. (19-24), 0939-5075 (Print)

Hung CW, Chen YC, Hsieh WL, Chiou SH & Kao CL (2010) Ageing and neurodegenerative diseases. *Ageing Res Rev.* Vol. 9 Suppl 1, No. (Nov 2010):pp. (S36-46), 1872-9649 (Electronic)

Ishikawa Y & Kitamura M (2000) Anti-apoptotic effect of quercetin: intervention in the JNK- and ERK-mediated apoptotic pathways. *Kidney Int.* Vol. 58, No. 3, (Sep 2000):pp. (1078-1087), 0085-2538 (Print) 0085-2538 (Linking)

Iwunze MO & McEwan D (2004) Peroxynitrite interaction with curcumin solubilized in ethanolic solution. *Cell Mol Biol (Noisy-le-grand).* Vol. 50, No. 6, (Sep 2004):pp. (749-752), 0145-5680 (Print)

Jagatha B, Mythri RB, Vali S & Bharath MM (2008) Curcumin treatment alleviates the effects of glutathione depletion in vitro and in vivo: therapeutic implications for Parkinson's disease explained via in silico studies. *Free Radic Biol Med.* Vol. 44, No. 5, (Mar 1 2008):pp. (907-917), 0891-5849 (Print)

Jang EM, Choi MS, Jung UJ, Kim MJ, Kim HJ, Jeon SM, Shin SK, Seong CN & Lee MK (2008) Beneficial effects of curcumin on hyperlipidemia and insulin resistance in high-fat-fed hamsters. *Metabolism.* Vol. 57, No. 11, (Nov 2008):pp. (1576-1583), 1532-8600 (Electronic)

Jeyapaul J & Jaiswal AK (2000) Nrf2 and c-Jun regulation of antioxidant response element (ARE)-mediated expression and induction of gamma-glutamylcysteine synthetase heavy subunit gene. *Biochem Pharmacol.* Vol. 59, No. 11, (Jun 1 2000):pp. (1433-1439), 0006-2952 (Print)

Jiao Y, Wilkinson Jt, Christine Pietsch E, Buss JL, Wang W, Planalp R, Torti FM & Torti SV (2006) Iron chelation in the biological activity of curcumin. *Free Radic Biol Med.* Vol. 40, No. 7, (Apr 1 2006):pp. (1152-1160), 0891-5849 (Print)

Jiao Y, Wilkinson Jt, Di X, Wang W, Hatcher H, Kock ND, D'Agostino R, Jr., Knovich MA, Torti FM & Torti SV (2009) Curcumin, a cancer chemopreventive and chemotherapeutic agent, is a biologically active iron chelator. *Blood*. Vol. 113, No. 2, (Jan 8 2009):pp. (462-469), 1528-0020 (Electronic)

Jin CF, Shen SR, Sr. & Zhao BL (2001) Different effects of five catechins on 6-hydroxydopamine-induced apoptosis in PC12 cells. *J Agric Food Chem*. Vol. 49, No. 12, (Dec 2001):pp. (6033-6038), 0021-8561 (Print)

Jin F, Wu Q, Lu YF, Gong QH & Shi JS (2008) Neuroprotective effect of resveratrol on 6-OHDA-induced Parkinson's disease in rats. *Eur J Pharmacol*. Vol. 600, No. 1-3, (Dec 14 2008):pp. (78-82), 1879-0712 (Electronic)

Jobin C, Bradham CA, Russo MP, Juma B, Narula AS, Brenner DA & Sartor RB (1999) Curcumin blocks cytokine-mediated NF-kappa B activation and proinflammatory gene expression by inhibiting inhibitory factor I-kappa B kinase activity. *J Immunol*. Vol. 163, No. 6, (Sep 15 1999):pp. (3474-3483), 0022-1767 (Print)

Kandinov B, Giladi N & Korczyn AD (2007) The effect of cigarette smoking, tea, and coffee consumption on the progression of Parkinson's disease. *Parkinsonism Relat Disord*. Vol. 13, No. 4, (May 2007):pp. (243-245), 1353-8020 (Print)

Kandinov B, Giladi N & Korczyn AD (2009) Smoking and tea consumption delay onset of Parkinson's disease. *Parkinsonism Relat Disord*. Vol. 15, No. 1, (Jan 2009):pp. (41-46), 1353-8020 (Print)

Kang KS, Wen Y, Yamabe N, Fukui M, Bishop SC & Zhu BT (2010) Dual beneficial effects of (-)-epigallocatechin-3-gallate on levodopa methylation and hippocampal neurodegeneration: in vitro and in vivo studies. *PLoS One*. Vol. 5, No. 8, 2010):pp. (e11951), 1932-6203 (Electronic)

Kantengwa S & Polla BS (1991) Flavonoids, but not protein kinase C inhibitors, prevent stress protein synthesis during erythrophagocytosis. *Biochem Biophys Res Commun*. Vol. 180, No. 1, (Oct 15 1991):pp. (308-314), 0006-291X (Print)

Karuppagounder SS, Pinto JT, Xu H, Chen HL, Beal MF & Gibson GE (2009) Dietary supplementation with resveratrol reduces plaque pathology in a transgenic model of Alzheimer's disease. *Neurochem Int*. Vol. 54, No. 2, (Feb 2009):pp. (111-118), 0197-0186 (Print)

Khan MM, Ahmad A, Ishrat T, Khan MB, Hoda MN, Khuwaja G, Raza SS, Khan A, Javed H, Vaibhav K & Islam F (2010) Resveratrol attenuates 6-hydroxydopamine-induced oxidative damage and dopamine depletion in rat model of Parkinson's disease. *Brain Res*. Vol. 1328, No. (Apr 30 2010):pp. (139-151), 1872-6240 (Electronic)

Khopde SM, Priyadarsini KI, Guha SN, Satav JG, Venkatesan P & Rao MN (2000) Inhibition of radiation-induced lipid peroxidation by tetrahydrocurcumin: possible mechanisms by pulse radiolysis. *Biosci Biotechnol Biochem*. Vol. 64, No. 3, (Mar 2000):pp. (503-509), 0916-8451 (Print)

Kim H, Kim YS, Kim SY & Suk K (2001) The plant flavonoid wogonin suppresses death of activated C6 rat glial cells by inhibiting nitric oxide production. *Neurosci Lett*. Vol. 309, No. 1, (Aug 17 2001):pp. (67-71), 0304-3940 (Print)

Kim JS, Kim JM, O JJ & Jeon BS (2010) Inhibition of inducible nitric oxide synthase expression and cell death by (-)-epigallocatechin-3-gallate, a green tea catechin, in the 1-methyl-4-phenyl-1,2,3,6-tetrahydropyridine mouse model of Parkinson's disease. *J Clin Neurosci*. Vol. 17, No. 9, (Sep 2010):pp. (1165-1168), 1532-2653 (Electronic)

Kim SJ, Son TG, Park HR, Park M, Kim MS, Kim HS, Chung HY, Mattson MP & Lee J (2008) Curcumin stimulates proliferation of embryonic neural progenitor cells and neurogenesis in the adult hippocampus. *J Biol Chem*. Vol. 283, No. 21, (May 23 2008):pp. (14497-14505), 0021-9258 (Print)

Klinge CM, Blankenship KA, Risinger KE, Bhatnagar S, Noisin EL, Sumanasekera WK, Zhao L, Brey DM & Keynton RS (2005) Resveratrol and estradiol rapidly activate MAPK signaling through estrogen receptors alpha and beta in endothelial cells. *J Biol Chem*. Vol. 280, No. 9, (Mar 4 2005):pp. (7460-7468), 0021-9258 (Print)

Kobuchi H, Roy S, Sen CK, Nguyen HG & Packer L (1999) Quercetin inhibits inducible ICAM-1 expression in human endothelial cells through the JNK pathway. *Am J Physiol*. Vol. 277, No. 3 Pt 1, (Sep 1999):pp. (C403-411), 0002-9513 (Print)

Kong AN, Yu R, Chen C, Mandlekar S & Primiano T (2000) Signal transduction events elicited by natural products: role of MAPK and caspase pathways in homeostatic response and induction of apoptosis. *Arch Pharm Res*. Vol. 23, No. 1, (Feb 2000):pp. (1-16), 0253-6269 (Print)

Kovacic P & Somanathan R (2010) Multifaceted approach to resveratrol bioactivity: Focus on antioxidant action, cell signaling and safety. *Oxid Med Cell Longev*. Vol. 3, No. 2, (Mar-Apr 2010):pp. (86-100), 1942-0994 (Electronic)

Kumar A, Naidu PS, Seghal N & Padi SS (2007) Effect of curcumin on intracerebroventricular colchicine-induced cognitive impairment and oxidative stress in rats. *J Med Food*. Vol. 10, No. 3, (Sep 2007):pp. (486-494), 1096-620X (Print)

Kumar V (2006) Potential medicinal plants for CNS disorders: an overview. *Phytother Res*. Vol. 20, No. 12, (Dec 2006):pp. (1023-1035), 0951-418X (Print)

Lamuela-Raventos RM, Romero-Perez AI, Waterhouse AL & de la Torre-Boronat MC (1995) Direct HPLC Analysis of cis- and trans-Resveratrol and Piceid Isomers in Spanish Red Vitis vinifera Wines. *Journal of Agricultural and Food Chemistry*. Vol. 43, No. 2, 1995):pp. (281-283), 0021-8561

Lao CD, Ruffin MTt, Normolle D, Heath DD, Murray SI, Bailey JM, Boggs ME, Crowell J, Rock CL & Brenner DE (2006) Dose escalation of a curcuminoid formulation. *BMC Complement Altern Med*. Vol. 6, No. 2006):pp. (10), 1472-6882 (Electronic)

LaVoie MJ, Ostaszewski BL, Weihofen A, Schlossmacher MG & Selkoe DJ (2005) Dopamine covalently modifies and functionally inactivates parkin. *Nat Med*. Vol. 11, No. 11, (Nov 2005):pp. (1214-1221), 1078-8956 (Print)

Lavoie S, Chen Y, Dalton TP, Gysin R, Cuenod M, Steullet P & Do KQ (2009) Curcumin, quercetin, and tBHQ modulate glutathione levels in astrocytes and neurons: importance of the glutamate cysteine ligase modifier subunit. *J Neurochem*. Vol. 108, No. 6, (Mar 2009):pp. (1410-1422), 1471-4159 (Electronic)

Leaver KR, Allbutt HN, Creber NJ, Kassiou M & Henderson JM (2009) Oral pre-treatment with epigallocatechin gallate in 6-OHDA lesioned rats produces subtle symptomatic relief but not neuroprotection. *Brain Res Bull*. Vol. 80, No. 6, (Dec 16 2009):pp. (397-402), 1873-2747 (Electronic)

Lee H, Kim YO, Kim H, Kim SY, Noh HS, Kang SS, Cho GJ, Choi WS & Suk K (2003) Flavonoid wogonin from medicinal herb is neuroprotective by inhibiting inflammatory activation of microglia. *FASEB J*. Vol. 17, No. 13, (Oct 2003):pp. (1943-1944), 1530-6860 (Electronic)

Lee MK, Kang SJ, Poncz M, Song KJ & Park KS (2007) Resveratrol protects SH-SY5Y neuroblastoma cells from apoptosis induced by dopamine. *Exp Mol Med*. Vol. 39, No. 3, (Jun 30 2007):pp. (376-384), 1226-3613 (Print)

Lee S, Suh S & Kim S (2000) Protective effects of the green tea polyphenol (-)-epigallocatechin gallate against hippocampal neuronal damage after transient global ischemia in gerbils. *Neurosci Lett*. Vol. 287, No. 3, (Jun 30 2000):pp. (191-194), 0304-3940 (Print)

Levites Y, Amit T, Youdim MB & Mandel S (2002a) Involvement of protein kinase C activation and cell survival/ cell cycle genes in green tea polyphenol (-)-epigallocatechin 3-gallate neuroprotective action. *J Biol Chem*. Vol. 277, No. 34, (Aug 23 2002a):pp. (30574-30580), 0021-9258 (Print)

Levites Y, Weinreb O, Maor G, Youdim MB & Mandel S (2001) Green tea polyphenol (-)-epigallocatechin-3-gallate prevents N-methyl-4-phenyl-1,2,3,6-tetrahydropyridine-induced dopaminergic neurodegeneration. *J Neurochem*. Vol. 78, No. 5, (Sep 2001):pp. (1073-1082), 0022-3042 (Print)

Levites Y, Youdim MB, Maor G & Mandel S (2002b) Attenuation of 6-hydroxydopamine (6-OHDA)-induced nuclear factor-kappaB (NF-kappaB) activation and cell death by tea extracts in neuronal cultures. *Biochem Pharmacol*. Vol. 63, No. 1, (Jan 1 2002b):pp. (21-29), 0006-2952 (Print)

Li C, Lee MJ, Sheng S, Meng X, Prabhu S, Winnik B, Huang B, Chung JY, Yan S, Ho CT & Yang CS (2000) Structural identification of two metabolites of catechins and their kinetics in human urine and blood after tea ingestion. *Chem Res Toxicol*. Vol. 13, No. 3, (Mar 2000):pp. (177-184), 0893-228X (Print)

Li R, Huang YG, Fang D & Le WD (2004) (-)-Epigallocatechin gallate inhibits lipopolysaccharide-induced microglial activation and protects against inflammation-mediated dopaminergic neuronal injury. *J Neurosci Res*. Vol. 78, No. 5, (Dec 1 2004):pp. (723-731), 0360-4012 (Print)

Li R, Peng N, Du F, Li XP & Le WD (2006) Epigallocatechin gallate protects dopaminergic neurons against 1-methyl-4- phenyl-1,2,3,6-tetrahydropyridine-induced neurotoxicity by inhibiting microglial cell activation. *Nan Fang Yi Ke Da Xue Xue Bao*. Vol. 26, No. 4, (Apr 2006):pp. (376-380), 1673-4254 (Print)

Li X, Jankovic J & Le W (2010) Iron chelation and neuroprotection in neurodegenerative diseases. *Journal of Neural Transmission*. Vol., No. 2010):pp. (1-5), 0300-9564

Lim GP, Chu T, Yang F, Beech W, Frautschy SA & Cole GM (2001) The curry spice curcumin reduces oxidative damage and amyloid pathology in an Alzheimer transgenic mouse. *J Neurosci*. Vol. 21, No. 21, (Nov 1 2001):pp. (8370-8377), 1529-2401 (Electronic)

Liou HH, Chen RC, Chen TH, Tsai YF & Tsai MC (2001) Attenuation of paraquat-induced dopaminergic toxicity on the substantia nigra by (-)-deprenyl in vivo. *Toxicol Appl Pharmacol*. Vol. 172, No. 1, (Apr 1 2001):pp. (37-43), 0041-008X (Print)

Long J, Gao H, Sun L, Liu J & Zhao-Wilson X (2009) Grape extract protects mitochondria from oxidative damage and improves locomotor dysfunction and extends lifespan in a Drosophila Parkinson's disease model. *Rejuvenation Res*. Vol. 12, No. 5, (Oct 2009):pp. (321-331), 1557-8577 (Electronic)

Lu F, Zahid M, Wang C, Saeed M, Cavalieri EL & Rogan EG (2008) Resveratrol prevents estrogen-DNA adduct formation and neoplastic transformation in MCF-10F cells. *Cancer Prev Res (Phila)*. Vol. 1, No. 2, (Jul 2008):pp. (135-145), 1940-6215 (Electronic)

Luo Y, Hattori A, Munoz J, Qin ZH & Roth GS (1999) Intrastriatal dopamine injection induces apoptosis through oxidation-involved activation of transcription factors AP-1 and NF-kappaB in rats. *Mol Pharmacol*. Vol. 56, No. 2, (Aug 1999):pp. (254-264), 0026-895X (Print)

Mandel S, Maor G & Youdim MB (2004) Iron and alpha-synuclein in the substantia nigra of MPTP-treated mice: effect of neuroprotective drugs R-apomorphine and green tea polyphenol (-)-epigallocatechin-3-gallate. *J Mol Neurosci*. Vol. 24, No. 3, 2004):pp. (401-416), 0895-8696 (Print)

Mandel SA, Amit T, Kalfon L, Reznichenko L & Youdim MB (2008) Targeting multiple neurodegenerative diseases etiologies with multimodal-acting green tea catechins. *J Nutr*. Vol. 138, No. 8, (Aug 2008):pp. (1578S-1583S), 1541-6100 (Electronic)

Mandel SA, Amit T, Weinreb O & Youdim MB (2011) Understanding the Broad-Spectrum Neuroprotective Action Profile of Green Tea Polyphenols in Aging and Neurodegenerative Diseases. *J Alzheimers Dis*. Vol., No. (Mar 2 2011):pp. 1875-8908 (Electronic)

Matsuoka Y, Hasegawa H, Okuda S, Muraki T, Uruno T & Kubota K (1995) Ameliorative effects of tea catechins on active oxygen-related nerve cell injuries. *J Pharmacol Exp Ther*. Vol. 274, No. 2, (Aug 1995):pp. (602-608), 0022-3565 (Print)

Matter WF, Brown RF & Vlahos CJ (1992) The inhibition of phosphatidylinositol 3-kinase by quercetin and analogs. *Biochem Biophys Res Commun*. Vol. 186, No. 2, (Jul 31 1992):pp. (624-631), 0006-291X (Print)

Mattivi F, Reniero F & Korhammer S (1995) Isolation, Characterization, and Evolution in Red Wine Vinification of Resveratrol Monomers. *Journal of Agricultural and Food Chemistry*. Vol. 43, No. 7, 1995):pp. (1820-1823), 0021-8561

Mattson MP, Son TG & Camandola S (2007) Viewpoint: mechanisms of action and therapeutic potential of neurohormetic phytochemicals. *Dose Response*. Vol. 5, No. 3, 2007):pp. (174-186), 1559-3258 (Electronic)

Mazzio E, Huber J, Darling S, Harris N & Soliman KF (2001) Effect of antioxidants on L-glutamate and N-methyl-4-phenylpyridinium ion induced-neurotoxicity in PC12 cells. *Neurotoxicology*. Vol. 22, No. 2, (Apr 2001):pp. (283-288), 0161-813X (Print)

Mishra B, Priyadarsini KI, Bhide MK, Kadam RM & Mohan H (2004) Reactions of superoxide radicals with curcumin: probable mechanisms by optical spectroscopy and EPR. *Free Radic Res*. Vol. 38, No. 4, (Apr 2004):pp. (355-362), 1071-5762 (Print)

Moldzio R, Radad K, Krewenka C, Kranner B, Duvigneau JC, Wang Y & Rausch WD (2010) Effects of epigallocatechin gallate on rotenone-injured murine brain cultures. *J Neural Transm*. Vol. 117, No. 1, (Jan 2010):pp. (5-12), 1435-1463 (Electronic)

Molina MF, Sanchez-Reus I, Iglesias I & Benedi J (2003) Quercetin, a flavonoid antioxidant, prevents and protects against ethanol-induced oxidative stress in mouse liver. *Biol Pharm Bull*. Vol. 26, No. 10, (Oct 2003):pp. (1398-1402), 0918-6158 (Print)

Motterlini R, Foresti R, Bassi R & Green CJ (2000) Curcumin, an antioxidant and anti-inflammatory agent, induces heme oxygenase-1 and protects endothelial cells against oxidative stress. *Free Radic Biol Med*. Vol. 28, No. 8, (Apr 15 2000):pp. (1303-1312), 0891-5849 (Print)

Muthane U, Yasha TC & Shankar SK (1998) Low numbers and no loss of melanized nigral neurons with increasing age in normal human brains from India. *Ann Neurol.* Vol. 43, No. 3, (Mar 1998):pp. (283-287), 0364-5134 (Print)

Mythri RB, Harish G, Dubey SK, Misra K & Bharath MM (2011) Glutamoyl diester of the dietary polyphenol curcumin offers improved protection against peroxynitrite-mediated nitrosative stress and damage of brain mitochondria in vitro: implications for Parkinson's disease. *Mol Cell Biochem.* Vol. 347, No. 1-2, (Jan 2011):pp. (135-143), 1573-4919 (Electronic)

Mythri RB, Jagatha B, Pradhan N, Andersen J & Bharath MM (2007) Mitochondrial complex I inhibition in Parkinson's disease: how can curcumin protect mitochondria? *Antioxid Redox Signal.* Vol. 9, No. 3, (Mar 2007):pp. (399-408), 1523-0864 (Print)

Nie G, Cao Y & Zhao B (2002) Protective effects of green tea polyphenols and their major component, (-)-epigallocatechin-3-gallate (EGCG), on 6-hydroxydopamine-induced apoptosis in PC12 cells. *Redox Rep.* Vol. 7, No. 3, 2002):pp. (171-177), 1351-0002 (Print)

North BJ & Verdin E (2004) Sirtuins: Sir2-related NAD-dependent protein deacetylases. *Genome Biol.* Vol. 5, No. 5, 2004):pp. (224), 1465-6914 (Electronic)

Ohara K, Mizukami, W., Tokunaga, A., Nagaoka, S., Uno, H., and Mukai (2005) Kinetic Study of the Mechanism of Free-Radical Scavenging Action in Curcumin: Effects of Solvent and pH. *Bull Chem Soc Jpn.* Vol. 78, No. 4, 2005):pp. (615-621), 0009-2673

Okawara M, Katsuki H, Kurimoto E, Shibata H, Kume T & Akaike A (2007) Resveratrol protects dopaminergic neurons in midbrain slice culture from multiple insults. *Biochem Pharmacol.* Vol. 73, No. 4, (Feb 15 2007):pp. (550-560), 0006-2952 (Print)

Oliver CN, Starke-Reed PE, Stadtman ER, Liu GJ, Carney JM & Floyd RA (1990) Oxidative damage to brain proteins, loss of glutamine synthetase activity, and production of free radicals during ischemia/reperfusion-induced injury to gerbil brain. *Proc Natl Acad Sci U S A.* Vol. 87, No. 13, (Jul 1990):pp. (5144-5147), 0027-8424 (Print)

Ono K & Yamada M (2006) Antioxidant compounds have potent anti-fibrillogenic and fibril-destabilizing effects for alpha-synuclein fibrils in vitro. *J Neurochem.* Vol. 97, No. 1, (Apr 2006):pp. (105-115), 0022-3042 (Print)

Outeiro TF, Kontopoulos E, Altmann SM, Kufareva I, Strathearn KE, Amore AM, Volk CB, Maxwell MM, Rochet JC, McLean PJ, Young AB, Abagyan R, Feany MB, Hyman BT & Kazantsev AG (2007) Sirtuin 2 inhibitors rescue alpha-synuclein-mediated toxicity in models of Parkinson's disease. *Science.* Vol. 317, No. 5837, (Jul 27 2007):pp. (516-519), 1095-9203 (Electronic)

Pallas M, Casadesus G, Smith MA, Coto-Montes A, Pelegri C, Vilaplana J & Camins A (2009) Resveratrol and neurodegenerative diseases: activation of SIRT1 as the potential pathway towards neuroprotection. *Curr Neurovasc Res.* Vol. 6, No. 1, (Feb 2009):pp. (70-81), 1875-5739 (Electronic)

Pallas M, Verdaguer E, Tajes M, Gutierrez-Cuesta J & Camins A (2008) Modulation of sirtuins: new targets for antiageing. *Recent Pat CNS Drug Discov.* Vol. 3, No. 1, (Jan 2008):pp. (61-69), 1574-8898 (Print)

Pan MH, Huang TM & Lin JK (1999) Biotransformation of curcumin through reduction and glucuronidation in mice. *Drug Metab Dispos.* Vol. 27, No. 4, (Apr 1999):pp. (486-494), 0090-9556 (Print)

Pan MH, Lin-Shiau SY & Lin JK (2000) Comparative studies on the suppression of nitric oxide synthase by curcumin and its hydrogenated metabolites through down-regulation of IkappaB kinase and NFkappaB activation in macrophages. *Biochem Pharmacol*. Vol. 60, No. 11, (Dec 1 2000):pp. (1665-1676), 0006-2952 (Print)

Pan T, Jankovic J & Le W (2003) Potential therapeutic properties of green tea polyphenols in Parkinson's disease. *Drugs Aging*. Vol. 20, No. 10, 2003):pp. (711-721), 1170-229X (Print)

Pandey N, Strider J, Nolan WC, Yan SX & Galvin JE (2008) Curcumin inhibits aggregation of alpha-synuclein. *Acta Neuropathol*. Vol. 115, No. 4, (Apr 2008):pp. (479-489), 0001-6322 (Print)

Peeyush KT, Gireesh G, Jobin M & Paulose CS (2009) Neuroprotective role of curcumin in the cerebellum of streptozotocin-induced diabetic rats. *Life Sci*. Vol. 85, No. 19-20, (Nov 4 2009):pp. (704-710), 1879-0631 (Electronic)

Pietta PG, Simonetti P, Gardana C, Brusamolino A, Morazzoni P & Bombardelli E (1998) Catechin metabolites after intake of green tea infusions. *Biofactors*. Vol. 8, No. 1-2, 1998):pp. (111-118), 0951-6433 (Print)

Plummer SM, Holloway KA, Manson MM, Munks RJ, Kaptein A, Farrow S & Howells L (1999) Inhibition of cyclo-oxygenase 2 expression in colon cells by the chemopreventive agent curcumin involves inhibition of NF-kappaB activation via the NIK/IKK signalling complex. *Oncogene*. Vol. 18, No. 44, (Oct 28 1999):pp. (6013-6020), 0950-9232 (Print)

Priyadarsini KI, Maity DK, Naik GH, Kumar MS, Unnikrishnan MK, Satav JG & Mohan H (2003) Role of phenolic O-H and methylene hydrogen on the free radical reactions and antioxidant activity of curcumin. *Free Radic Biol Med*. Vol. 35, No. 5, (Sep 1 2003):pp. (475-484), 0891-5849 (Print)

Qureshi S, Shah AH & Ageel AM (1992) Toxicity studies on Alpinia galanga and Curcuma longa. *Planta Med*. Vol. 58, No. 2, (Apr 1992):pp. (124-127), 0032-0943 (Print)

Rajeswari A (2006) Curcumin protects mouse brain from oxidative stress caused by 1-methyl-4-phenyl-1,2,3,6-tetrahydropyridine. *Eur Rev Med Pharmacol Sci*. Vol. 10, No. 4, (Jul-Aug 2006):pp. (157-161), 1128-3602 (Print)

Rajeswari A & Sabesan M (2008) Inhibition of monoamine oxidase-B by the polyphenolic compound, curcumin and its metabolite tetrahydrocurcumin, in a model of Parkinson's disease induced by MPTP neurodegeneration in mice. *Inflammopharmacology*. Vol. 16, No. 2, (Apr 2008):pp. (96-99), 0925-4692 (Print)

Ramassamy C (2006) Emerging role of polyphenolic compounds in the treatment of neurodegenerative diseases: A review of their intracellular targets. Eur J Pharmacol Vol. 545, No. 1, (Sep 2006): pp (51–64)

Ray B, Bisht S, Maitra A & Lahiri DK (2011) Neuroprotective and neurorescue effects of a novel polymeric nanoparticle formulation of curcumin (NanoCurc) in the neuronal cell culture and animal model: implications for Alzheimer's disease. *J Alzheimers Dis*. Vol. 23, No. 1, (Jan 1 2011):pp. (61-77), 1875-8908 (Electronic)

Raza H, John A, Brown EM, Benedict S & Kambal A (2008) Alterations in mitochondrial respiratory functions, redox metabolism and apoptosis by oxidant 4-hydroxynonenal and antioxidants curcumin and melatonin in PC12 cells. *Toxicol Appl Pharmacol*. Vol. 226, No. 2, (Jan 15 2008):pp. (161-168), 0041-008X (Print)

Revuelta MP, Cantabrana B & Hidalgo A (1997) Depolarization-dependent effect of flavonoids in rat uterine smooth muscle contraction elicited by CaCl2. *Gen Pharmacol*. Vol. 29, No. 5, (Nov 1997):pp. (847-857), 0306-3623 (Print)

Rice-Evans CA & Miller NJ (1996) Antioxidant activities of flavonoids as bioactive components of food. *Biochem Soc Trans*. Vol. 24, No. 3, (Aug 1996):pp. (790-795), 0300-5127 (Print)

Rice-Evans CA, Miller NJ & Paganga G (1996) Structure-antioxidant activity relationships of flavonoids and phenolic acids. *Free Radic Biol Med*. Vol. 20, No. 7, 1996):pp. (933-956), 0891-5849 (Print)

Richard T, Pawlus AD, Iglesias ML, Pedrot E, Waffo-Teguo P, Merillon JM & Monti JP (2011) Neuroprotective properties of resveratrol and derivatives. *Ann N Y Acad Sci*. Vol. 1215, No. (Jan 2011):pp. (103-108), 1749-6632 (Electronic)

Riederer P, Sofic E, Rausch WD, Schmidt B, Reynolds GP, Jellinger K & Youdim MB (1989) Transition metals, ferritin, glutathione, and ascorbic acid in parkinsonian brains. *J Neurochem*. Vol. 52, No. 2, (Feb 1989):pp. (515-520), 0022-3042 (Print)

Rocha-Gonzalez HI, Ambriz-Tututi M & Granados-Soto V (2008) Resveratrol: a natural compound with pharmacological potential in neurodegenerative diseases. *CNS Neurosci Ther*. Vol. 14, No. 3, (Fall 2008):pp. (234-247), 1755-5930 (Print)

Sahu SC & Gray GC (1997) Lipid peroxidation and DNA damage induced by morin and naringenin in isolated rat liver nuclei. *Food Chem Toxicol*. Vol. 35, No. 5, (May 1997):pp. (443-447), 0278-6915 (Print)

Saiko P, Szakmary A, Jaeger W & Szekeres T (2008) Resveratrol and its analogs: defense against cancer, coronary disease and neurodegenerative maladies or just a fad? *Mutat Res*. Vol. 658, No. 1-2, (Jan-Feb 2008):pp. (68-94), 0027-5107 (Print)

Sawada H, Ibi M, Kihara T, Honda K, Nakamizo T, Kanki R, Nakanishi M, Sakka N, Akaike A & Shimohama S (2002) Estradiol protects dopaminergic neurons in a MPP+Parkinson's disease model. *Neuropharmacology*. Vol. 42, No. 8, (Jun 2002):pp. (1056-1064), 0028-3908 (Print)

Scalbert A & Williamson G (2000) Dietary intake and bioavailability of polyphenols. *J Nutr*. Vol. 130, No. 8S Suppl, (Aug 2000):pp. (2073S-2085S), 0022-3166 (Print)

Schroeter H, Bahia P, Spencer JP, Sheppard O, Rattray M, Cadenas E, Rice-Evans C & Williams RJ (2007) (-)Epicatechin stimulates ERK-dependent cyclic AMP response element activity and up-regulates GluR2 in cortical neurons. *J Neurochem*. Vol. 101, No. 6, (Jun 2007):pp. (1596-1606), 0022-3042 (Print)

Schroeter H, Boyd C, Spencer JP, Williams RJ, Cadenas E & Rice-Evans C (2002) MAPK signaling in neurodegeneration: influences of flavonoids and of nitric oxide. *Neurobiol Aging*. Vol. 23, No. 5, (Sep-Oct 2002):pp. (861-880), 0197-4580 (Print)

Schroeter H, Spencer JP, Rice-Evans C & Williams RJ (2001) Flavonoids protect neurons from oxidized low-density-lipoprotein-induced apoptosis involving c-Jun N-terminal kinase (JNK), c-Jun and caspase-3. *Biochem J*. Vol. 358, No. Pt 3, (Sep 15 2001):pp. (547-557), 0264-6021 (Print)

Schroeter H, Williams RJ, Matin R, Iversen L & Rice-Evans CA (2000) Phenolic antioxidants attenuate neuronal cell death following uptake of oxidized low-density lipoprotein. *Free Radic Biol Med*. Vol. 29, No. 12, (Dec 15 2000):pp. (1222-1233), 0891-5849 (Print)

Shankar TN, Shantha NV, Ramesh HP, Murthy IA & Murthy VS (1980) Toxicity studies on turmeric (Curcuma longa): acute toxicity studies in rats, guineapigs & monkeys. *Indian J Exp Biol.* Vol. 18, No. 1, (Jan 1980):pp. (73-75), 0019-5189 (Print)

Sharma S, Kulkarni SK, Agrewala JN & Chopra K (2006) Curcumin attenuates thermal hyperalgesia in a diabetic mouse model of neuropathic pain. *Eur J Pharmacol.* Vol. 536, No. 3, (May 1 2006):pp. (256-261), 0014-2999 (Print)

Shen SC, Lee WR, Lin HY, Huang HC, Ko CH, Yang LL & Chen YC (2002) In vitro and in vivo inhibitory activities of rutin, wogonin, and quercetin on lipopolysaccharide-induced nitric oxide and prostaglandin E(2) production. *Eur J Pharmacol.* Vol. 446, No. 1-3, (Jun 20 2002):pp. (187-194), 0014-2999 (Print)

Shen SQ, Zhang Y, Xiang JJ & Xiong CL (2007) Protective effect of curcumin against liver warm ischemia/reperfusion injury in rat model is associated with regulation of heat shock protein and antioxidant enzymes. *World J Gastroenterol.* Vol. 13, No. 13, (Apr 7 2007):pp. (1953-1961), 1007-9327 (Print)

Shishodia S, Sethi G & Aggarwal BB (2005) Curcumin: getting back to the roots. *Ann N Y Acad Sci.* Vol. 1056, No. (Nov 2005):pp. (206-217), 0077-8923 (Print)

Shoba G, Joy D, Joseph T, Majeed M, Rajendran R & Srinivas PS (1998) Influence of piperine on the pharmacokinetics of curcumin in animals and human volunteers. *Planta Med.* Vol. 64, No. 4, (May 1998):pp. (353-356), 0032-0943 (Print)

Sinha R, Anderson DE, McDonald SS & Greenwald P (2003) Cancer risk and diet in India. *J Postgrad Med.* Vol. 49, No. 3, (Jul-Sep 2003):pp. (222-228), 0022-3859 (Print)

Sofic E, Riederer P, Heinsen H, Beckmann H, Reynolds GP, Hebenstreit G & Youdim MB (1988) Increased iron (III) and total iron content in post mortem substantia nigra of parkinsonian brain. *J Neural Transm.* Vol. 74, No. 3, 1988):pp. (199-205), 0300-9564 (Print)

Spencer JP (2003) Metabolism of tea flavonoids in the gastrointestinal tract. *J Nutr.* Vol. 133, No. 10, (Oct 2003):pp. (3255S-3261S), 0022-3166 (Print)

Spencer JP (2007) The interactions of flavonoids within neuronal signalling pathways. *Genes Nutr.* Vol. 2, No. 3, (Dec 2007):pp. (257-273), 1555-8932 (Print)

Spencer JP, Abd-el-Mohsen MM & Rice-Evans C (2004) Cellular uptake and metabolism of flavonoids and their metabolites: implications for their bioactivity. *Arch Biochem Biophys.* Vol. 423, No. 1, (Mar 1 2004):pp. (148-161), 0003-9861 (Print)

Spencer JP, Rice-Evans C & Williams RJ (2003) Modulation of pro-survival Akt/protein kinase B and ERK1/2 signaling cascades by quercetin and its in vivo metabolites underlie their action on neuronal viability. *J Biol Chem.* Vol. 278, No. 37, (Sep 12 2003):pp. (34783-34793), 0021-9258 (Print)

Srinivasan K (2005) Plant foods in the management of diabetes mellitus: spices as beneficial antidiabetic food adjuncts. *Int J Food Sci Nutr.* Vol. 56, No. 6, (Sep 2005):pp. (399-414), 0963-7486 (Print)

Stridh MH, Correa F, Nodin C, Weber SG, Blomstrand F, Nilsson M & Sandberg M (2010) Enhanced glutathione efflux from astrocytes in culture by low extracellular ca(2+) and curcumin. *Neurochem Res.* Vol. 35, No. 8, (Aug 2010):pp. (1231-1238), 1573-6903 (Electronic)

Sugihara N, Arakawa T, Ohnishi M & Furuno K (1999) Anti- and pro-oxidative effects of flavonoids on metal-induced lipid hydroperoxide-dependent lipid peroxidation in cultured hepatocytes loaded with alpha-linolenic acid. *Free Radic Biol Med*. Vol. 27, No. 11-12, (Dec 1999):pp. (1313-1323), 0891-5849 (Print)

Suresh D & Srinivasan K (2010) Tissue distribution & elimination of capsaicin, piperine & curcumin following oral intake in rats. *Indian J Med Res*. Vol. 131, No. (May 2010):pp. (682-691), 0971-5916 (Print)

Tai KK & Truong DD (2010) (-)-Epigallocatechin-3-gallate (EGCG), a green tea polyphenol, reduces dichlorodiphenyl-trichloroethane (DDT)-induced cell death in dopaminergic SHSY-5Y cells. *Neurosci Lett*. Vol. 482, No. 3, (Oct 4 2010):pp. (183-187), 1872-7972 (Electronic)

Tan EK, Tan C, Fook-Chong SMC, Lum SY, Chai A, Chung H, Shen H, Zhao Y, Teoh ML, Yih Y, Pavanni R, Chandran VR & Wong MC (2003) Dose-dependent protective effect of coffee, tea, and smoking in Parkinson's disease: a study in ethnic Chinese. *Journal of the neurological sciences*. Vol. 216, No. 1, 2003):pp. (163-167), 0022-510X

Tan LC, Koh W-P, Yuan J-M, Wang R, Au W-L, Tan JH, Tan E-K & Yu MC (2008) Differential Effects of Black versus Green Tea on Risk of Parkinson's Disease in the Singapore Chinese Health Study. *American Journal of Epidemiology*. Vol. 167, No. 5, (March 1, 2008 2008):pp. (553-560),

Thaloor D, Miller KJ, Gephart J, Mitchell PO & Pavlath GK (1999) Systemic administration of the NF-kappaB inhibitor curcumin stimulates muscle regeneration after traumatic injury. *Am J Physiol*. Vol. 277, No. 2 Pt 1, (Aug 1999):pp. (C320-329), 0002-9513 (Print)

Thiyagarajan M & Sharma SS (2004) Neuroprotective effect of curcumin in middle cerebral artery occlusion induced focal cerebral ischemia in rats. *Life Sci*. Vol. 74, No. 8, (Jan 9 2004):pp. (969-985), 0024-3205 (Print)

Toniolo R, Di Narda F, Susmel S, Martelli M, Martelli L & Bontempelli G (2002) Quenching of superoxide ions by curcumin. A mechanistic study in acetonitrile. *Ann Chim*. Vol. 92, No. 3, (Mar 2002):pp. (281-288), 0003-4592 (Print)

Tsao R (2010) Chemistry and Biochemistry of Dietary Polyphenols. *Nutrients*. Vol. 2, No. 12, 2010):pp. (1231-1246), 2072-6643

Uchida K, Shiraishi M, Naito Y, Torii Y, Nakamura Y & Osawa T (1999) Activation of stress signaling pathways by the end product of lipid peroxidation. 4-hydroxy-2-nonenal is a potential inducer of intracellular peroxide production. *J Biol Chem*. Vol. 274, No. 4, (Jan 22 1999):pp. (2234-2242), 0021-9258 (Print)

Vajragupta O, Boonchoong P, Watanabe H, Tohda M, Kummasud N & Sumanont Y (2003) Manganese complexes of curcumin and its derivatives: evaluation for the radical scavenging ability and neuroprotective activity. *Free Radic Biol Med*. Vol. 35, No. 12, (Dec 15 2003):pp. (1632-1644), 0891-5849 (Print)

van Acker SA, de Groot MJ, van den Berg DJ, Tromp MN, Donne-Op den Kelder G, van der Vijgh WJ & Bast A (1996) A quantum chemical explanation of the antioxidant activity of flavonoids. *Chem Res Toxicol*. Vol. 9, No. 8, (Dec 1996):pp. (1305-1312), 0893-228X (Print)

Vlahos CJ, Matter WF, Hui KY & Brown RF (1994) A specific inhibitor of phosphatidylinositol 3-kinase, 2-(4-morpholinyl)-8-phenyl-4H-1-benzopyran-4-one (LY294002). *J Biol Chem*. Vol. 269, No. 7, (Feb 18 1994):pp. (5241-5248), 0021-9258 (Print)

Walle T (2011) Bioavailability of resveratrol. *Ann N Y Acad Sci*. Vol. 1215, No. (Jan 2011):pp. (9-15), 1749-6632 (Electronic)

Wang F, Nguyen M, Qin FX & Tong Q (2007) SIRT2 deacetylates FOXO3a in response to oxidative stress and caloric restriction. *Aging Cell*. Vol. 6, No. 4, (Aug 2007):pp. (505-514), 1474-9718 (Print)

Wang J, Du XX, Jiang H & Xie JX (2009a) Curcumin attenuates 6-hydroxydopamine-induced cytotoxicity by anti-oxidation and nuclear factor-kappa B modulation in MES23.5 cells. *Biochem Pharmacol*. Vol. 78, No. 2, (Jul 15 2009a):pp. (178-183), 1873-2968 (Electronic)

Wang MS, Boddapati S, Emadi S & Sierks MR (2010) Curcumin reduces alpha-synuclein induced cytotoxicity in Parkinson's disease cell model. *BMC Neurosci*. Vol. 11, No. 2010):pp. (57), 1471-2202 (Electronic)

Wang SL, Li Y, Wen Y, Chen YF, Na LX, Li ST & Sun CH (2009b) Curcumin, a potential inhibitor of up-regulation of TNF-alpha and IL-6 induced by palmitate in 3T3-L1 adipocytes through NF-kappaB and JNK pathway. *Biomed Environ Sci*. Vol. 22, No. 1, (Feb 2009b):pp. (32-39), 0895-3988 (Print)

Wang Y, Xu H, Fu Q, Ma R & Xiang J (2011) Protective effect of resveratrol derived from Polygonum cuspidatum and its liposomal form on nigral cells in Parkinsonian rats. *J Neurol Sci*. Vol., No. (Mar 2 2011):pp. 1878-5883 (Electronic)

Weinreb O, Mandel S, Amit T & Youdim MB (2004) Neurological mechanisms of green tea polyphenols in Alzheimer's and Parkinson's diseases. *J Nutr Biochem*. Vol. 15, No. 9, (Sep 2004):pp. (506-516), 0955-2863 (Print)

Wenzel E & Somoza V (2005) Metabolism and bioavailability of trans-resveratrol. *Mol Nutr Food Res*. Vol. 49, No. 5, (May 2005):pp. (472-481), 1613-4125 (Print)

Wild AC, Moinova HR & Mulcahy RT (1999) Regulation of gamma-glutamylcysteine synthetase subunit gene expression by the transcription factor Nrf2. *J Biol Chem*. Vol. 274, No. 47, (Nov 19 1999):pp. (33627-33636), 0021-9258 (Print)

Williams RJ, Spencer JP & Rice-Evans C (2004) Flavonoids: antioxidants or signalling molecules? *Free Radic Biol Med*. Vol. 36, No. 7, (Apr 1 2004):pp. (838-849), 0891-5849 (Print)

Woo KJ, Lim JH, Suh SI, Kwon YK, Shin SW, Kim SC, Choi YH, Park JW & Kwon TK (2006) Differential inhibitory effects of baicalein and baicalin on LPS-induced cyclooxygenase-2 expression through inhibition of C/EBPbeta DNA-binding activity. *Immunobiology*. Vol. 211, No. 5, 2006):pp. (359-368), 0171-2985 (Print)

Xu Y, Ku B, Cui L, Li X, Barish PA, Foster TC & Ogle WO (2007) Curcumin reverses impaired hippocampal neurogenesis and increases serotonin receptor 1A mRNA and brain-derived neurotrophic factor expression in chronically stressed rats. *Brain Res*. Vol. 1162, No. (Aug 8 2007):pp. (9-18), 0006-8993 (Print)

Xu YX, Pindolia KR, Janakiraman N, Chapman RA & Gautam SC (1997) Curcumin inhibits IL1 alpha and TNF-alpha induction of AP-1 and NF-kB DNA-binding activity in bone marrow stromal cells. *Hematopathol Mol Hematol*. Vol. 11, No. 1, 1997):pp. (49-62), 1082-8893 (Print)

Yamamoto H, Schoonjans K & Auwerx J (2007) Sirtuin Functions in Health and Disease. *Mol Endocrinol*. Vol. 21, No. 8, (August 1, 2007 2007):pp. (1745-1755),

Yang F, Lim GP, Begum AN, Ubeda OJ, Simmons MR, Ambegaokar SS, Chen PP, Kayed R, Glabe CG, Frautschy SA & Cole GM (2005) Curcumin inhibits formation of amyloid beta oligomers and fibrils, binds plaques, and reduces amyloid in vivo. *J Biol Chem*. Vol. 280, No. 7, (Feb 18 2005):pp. (5892-5901), 0021-9258 (Print)

Ye SF, Hou ZQ, Zhong LM & Zhang QQ (2007) Effect of curcumin on the induction of glutathione S-transferases and NADP(H):quinone oxidoreductase and its possible mechanism of action. *Yao Xue Xue Bao*. Vol. 42, No. 4, (Apr 2007):pp. (376-380), 0513-4870 (Print)

Yoritaka A, Hattori N, Uchida K, Tanaka M, Stadtman ER & Mizuno Y (1996) Immunohistochemical detection of 4-hydroxynonenal protein adducts in Parkinson disease. *Proc Natl Acad Sci U S A*. Vol. 93, No. 7, (Apr 2 1996):pp. (2696-2701), 0027-8424 (Print)

Yu S, Zheng W, Xin N, Chi ZH, Wang NQ, Nie YX, Feng WY & Wang ZY (2010) Curcumin prevents dopaminergic neuronal death through inhibition of the c-Jun N-terminal kinase pathway. *Rejuvenation Res*. Vol. 13, No. 1, (Feb 2010):pp. (55-64), 1557-8577 (Electronic)

Zbarsky V, Datla KP, Parkar S, Rai DK, Aruoma OI & Dexter DT (2005) Neuroprotective properties of the natural phenolic antioxidants curcumin and naringenin but not quercetin and fisetin in a 6-OHDA model of Parkinson's disease. *Free Radic Res*. Vol. 39, No. 10, (Oct 2005):pp. (1119-1125), 1071-5762 (Print)

Zhang F, Shi JS, Zhou H, Wilson B, Hong JS & Gao HM (2010) Resveratrol protects dopamine neurons against lipopolysaccharide-induced neurotoxicity through its anti-inflammatory actions. *Mol Pharmacol*. Vol. 78, No. 3, (Sep 1 2010):pp. (466-477), 1521-0111 (Electronic)

Zhang L, Chen J & Fu H (1999) Suppression of apoptosis signal-regulating kinase 1-induced cell death by 14-3-3 proteins. *Proc Natl Acad Sci U S A*. Vol. 96, No. 15, (Jul 20 1999):pp. (8511-8515), 0027-8424 (Print)

Zhu YG, Chen XC, Chen ZZ, Zeng YQ, Shi GB, Su YH & Peng X (2004) Curcumin protects mitochondria from oxidative damage and attenuates apoptosis in cortical neurons. *Acta Pharmacol Sin*. Vol. 25, No. 12, (Dec 2004):pp. (1606-1612), 1671-4083 (Print)

Zhuang H, Kim YS, Koehler RC & Dore S (2003) Potential mechanism by which resveratrol, a red wine constituent, protects neurons. *Ann N Y Acad Sci*. Vol. 993, No. (May 2003):pp. (276-286; discussion 287-278), 0077-8923 (Print)

8

Inhibition of Tau Phosphorylation as a Potential Strategy in Treatment of Parkinson's Disease

Wang Wenya
School of Pharmaceutical Sciences, Southern Medical University
China

1. Introduction

At present, Parkinson's disease (PD) has become the third most common neuropathy following cerebrovascular diseases and epilepsy, and is the second most common neurodegenerative disease after Alzheimer's disease (AD). There is growing evidence that neuronal apoptosis plays a key role in the mechanism in PD, AD and other neurodegenerative diseases [Mattson, 2000; Yuan & Yankner, 2000]. Therefore, regulating neuronal apoptosis signaling pathway will provide a theoretical basis to reveal the mechanism of neuronal apoptosis; and on the basis of research, development of anti-neuronal apoptosis drugs to selectively interfere with critical target of apoptosis signaling pathway would be an important means in prevention of neurodegenerative diseases effectively.

Although subject to intensive research, the etiology of PD is still enigmatic, which in turn has hindered the development of effective treatment. Today, PD treatment is basically symptomatic, and no neuroprotective therapies are available. The current therapy for PD mainly aims at replacing the lost neurotransmitters. The signs and symptoms of PD can be alleviated with drugs that enhance dopamine function, among which, levodopa is considered the most effective one. The most severe shortcoming of levodopa treatment is that it fails to alter the progression of PD. Patients with advanced PD may develop a variety of motor complications associated with levodopa therapy, such as switching phenomena and dyskinesia [Rylander et al., 2010]. More disappointing is the therapeutic effect of levodopa weakens after about two years (Marsden & Parkes, 1977). Therefore, there is still an urgent need of finding more beneficial treatment strategy for the disease. Here, we proposed a neuroprotective drugs to effectively control the course of PD: it can inhibit substantia nigra dopaminergic neurons from "primary" progressive loss, so as to achieve the purpose of effective treatment of Parkinson's Disease.

2. Inhibition of tau phosphorylation as a potential strategy in treating PD

Dopamine neurons have a strong ability of physiological compensation before the disease is clinically evident. Generally, the disease become clinically evident (decompensated state) when the dopamine neuron loss is sufficiently severe (greater than 75% of nigrostriatal dopamine neurons) [Lloyd, 1977]. It is well known that programmed cell death (apoptosis) plays a key role in the neurodegenerative processes in PD [Büeler, 2010; Nagatsu & Sawada,

2007]. Several intraneuronal pathways are implicated in N-methyl-4-phenyl-1, 2, 3, 6-tetrahydropyridine (MPTP) -induced neuronal apoptosis [Chung et al., 2010; Ethell & Fei, 2009; Karunakaran et al., 2008; Saporito et al., 2010]. These include c-Jun N-terminal kinases (JNK) signaling, p53 activation, cell cycle re-activation, Glycogen synthase kinase-3 (GSK-3)/Tau signaling pathway, signaling through bcl-2 family proteins and so on. The neurotoxin MPTP is converted in the brain into 1-methyl-4-phenylpyridinium iodide [MPP (+)] by the enzyme monoamine oxidase B (MAO-B). MPP (+) is a selective inhibitor of mitochondrial complex I and is widely used in rodent and cell models to elicit neurochemical alterations associated with PD. We had found 10μmol/L MPP (+) activated JNK, phosphorylated c-Jun and induced neuronal apoptosis. It decreased the number of tyrosine hydroxylase (TH) immunopositive cells and reduced cytoplasmic volume. SP600125 [Bennet et al., 2001], the specific inhibitor of JNK protected dopaminergic neurons and increased the number of TH immunopositive cells via inhibiting c-Jun phosphorylation. These results indicated that SP600125 inhibited the activation of JNK and therefore protected dopaminergic mesencephalic neurons from apoptosis induced by MPP(+), which suggested that JNK might be a new target of influencing neuronal apoptosis [Wang et al., 2004]. Therefore, we had first proposed a new strategy for PD treatment, which is using a specific inhibitor of JNK. Of course, there are a great number of "targets" to interfere with nigral dopaminergic neuronal apoptosis, such as GSK-3β, also named as Tau protein kinase I (TPK I).

2.1 The tau protein

Tau is a low molecular weight component of cytoskeletal structures. It is one of several types of microtubule-associated proteins (MAPs) which regulate the assembly and stability of microtubule networks. Although microtubule networks exist in all kinds of animal and plant cells, the mRNAs encoding tau proteins are expressed predominantly in neurons, where these tau proteins are localized mostly to axons [Higuchi et al., 2002]. They are abundant in neurons in the central nervous system and are less common elsewhere. This unique feature suggests that Tau may have neuron-specific functions. In a healthy person, tau protein interacts with a compound called tubulin to strengthen the neural tubes in the axons of neurons. The neural tubes essentially act like train tracks for signals to pass along the axon. Disruption in the level of tau protein can lead to instability in the neural tubes, which makes it difficult for neurons to pass signals along [Kowall & Kosik, 1987]. When tau proteins are defective, and no longer stabilize microtubules properly, they can result in dementias, such as Alzheimer's disease [Sergeant et al., 2008].

2.2 Normal functions of tau phosphorylation

Protein phosphorylation is widely used to regulate cellular processes, because it can affect binding between two proteins. Phosphorylation is a process that adds a phosphate group to a protein, particularly on the amino acid serine, threonine or tyrosine. For the Tau protein, its association with microtubules is inhibited if certain residues in its microtubule binding domain are phosphorylated [Gendron & Petrucelli, 2009]. The phosphorylation of tau plays a physiological role in regulating the affinity of tau for microtubules. Though less well studied, phosphorylation also regulates the binding of tau to signaling molecules and could thus influence tau-mediated signaling [Reynolds et al., 2008]. The kinases that phosphorylate tau can be divided into two major groups, according to motif specificity: proline-directed protein kinases (PDPK) and non-proline-directed protein kinases (non-

PDPK). The PDPK include cyclin-dependent kinase 5 (cdk5), mitogen-activated protein kinase (MAPK), and several stress-activated protein kinases. GSK3-β is often described as a PDPK but the proline is not always required for phosphorylation by GSK3-β.The phosphorylation of tau by these kinases inhibits the ability of tau to promote microtubule assembly and facilitates the polymerization of tau into paired helical filaments (PHFs) [Evans et al., 2000]. Among the non-PDPK are cyclic AMP-dependent protein kinase (PKA), calcium- and calmodulin-dependent protein kinase II (CaMKII), and microtubule affinity regulating kinase (MARK). Unbound tau may then be hyperphosphorylated by other kinases. In fact, the phosphorylation of tau by MARK may be a prerequisite for the action of downstream kinases, including GSK-3β and Cdk5 [Nishimura et al., 2004].

Recently, Tau has received great attention because mounting evidence has indicated that hyperphosphorylation of Tau is the origin of Alzheimer's disease (AD). In an AD brain, too many residues in the Tau protein are phosphorylated [Buerger et al., 2006; Schönknecht et al., 2003]

2.3 Phosphorylation of tau in PD

Hyperphosphorylation and accumulation of Tau in neurons and glial cells result in PHFs and is one of the main pathologic hallmarks in many neurodegenerative disorders such as AD and other Tauopathies [Sato et al., 2006]. Phospho-Tau (Ser396) has been found in synaptic-enriched fractions in AD frontal cortex at entorhinal/transentorhinal, limbic and neocortical stages [Muntané et al., 2008]. GSK-3β- immunoprecipitated sarcosyl-insoluble fractions from AD patients can phosphorylate recombinant Tau [Ferrer et al., 2005]. Densitometric studies show between 20% and 40% phospho-Tau (Ser396) in synaptic-enriched fractions of the frontal cortex in PD [Muntané et al., 2008]. Moreover, Tau- immunoreactive Lewy bodies (LBs) are detected in the medulla of 80% of individuals with sporadic PD or dementia with LBs, where Tau is often localized at the periphery of LBs [Ishizawa et al., 2003]. We also found MPP (+)/MPTP induced abnormal phosphorylation of Tau at Ser396 in nigra in PD models. To investigate whether Tau is phosphorylated in MPTP-treated dopaminergic neurons, we examined the histochemical localization of Tau (Ser396) phosphorylation level in SNc following treatment with MPTP. TH immunofluorescence was used to detect DA neurons. Three months old adult male C_{57} black mice were given MPTP at a dose of 30mg/kg ip. once daily for 7 days. SNc slices were prepared 6 h after the third MPTP injection, and double-labeled with antibodies against TH and phospho-Tau (Ser396). We found that in MPTP-treated mice, nearly all TH positive cells exhibited the increased levels in phopspho-Tau, whereas no loss of TH positive cells was observed. Furthermore, many TH negative cells were stained with phopspho-Tau, but the levels were unchanged between MPTP-treated and untreated mice [Wang et al., 2007]. Cell counting results showed that in MPTP-treated group the percentage of phopspho-Tau stained neurons in TH positive cells was increased to 98%, while the control was just 37%. These results suggest that after MPTP treatment, Tau is selectively phosphorylated in dopaminergic neurons. Similarly, Qureshi HY found that exposure of human neuroblastoma M17 cells to MPTP enhances intracellular alpha-synuclein protein level, stimulates Tau protein phosphorylation at Ser262 and induces apoptosis [Qureshi & Paudel, 2010].

2.4 Preventing tau phosphorylation rescued neurons

A cdk5 inhibitory peptide (CIP) selectively inhibited p25/Cdk5 activity and suppressed the aberrant Tau phosphorylation and reduced apoptosis in cortical neurons [Zheng et al.,

2005]. In SH-SY5Y-cotransfected cells expressing α-Syn and human dopamine transporter (hDAT), both LiCl and TDZD-8 blocked GSK-3β activation in a dose-dependent manner, with concomitant decreases in hyperphosphorylation of Tau and cell death [Duka & Sidhu, 2006; Duka et al., 2009]. A GSK-3beta specific inhibitor, L803-mt, attenuated Tau phosphorylation and rescued DA neurons from cell death in mesencephalic cultures [Chung et al., 2010]. We had reported that AR-A014418, a specific inhibitor of GSK-3β, reduced the levels of phospho-Tau (Ser396), protected nigral neurons from apoptosis, and restored the depletion of dopamine evoked by MPTP in C_{57}BL/6N mice [Wang et al.,2007].

2.5 Two anticancer drugs dephosphorylated tau and rescued dopaminergic neurons

2.5.1 Chromomycin A3 protected cultured dopaminergic neurons from apoptosis induced by MPP(+)

Chromomycin A3 (Fig.1.) is a glycosidic antibiotic produced at the fermentation of a strainof *Streptomyces griseus*. It is also called toyomycin or aburamycin. It is not only an antibacterial antibiotic, but also an antitumor antibiotic that inhibits RNA synthesis, especially in solid tumors. Chromomycin belongs to the DNA-interactive Drugs. The compound blocks macromolecule synthesis by a specific, reversible interaction with DNA in the presence of bivalent metal ions. Binding to DNA minor groove mediates an efficient competitive inhibition of DNA gyrase and significantly affects topoisomerase II activity [Hou et al., 2008].

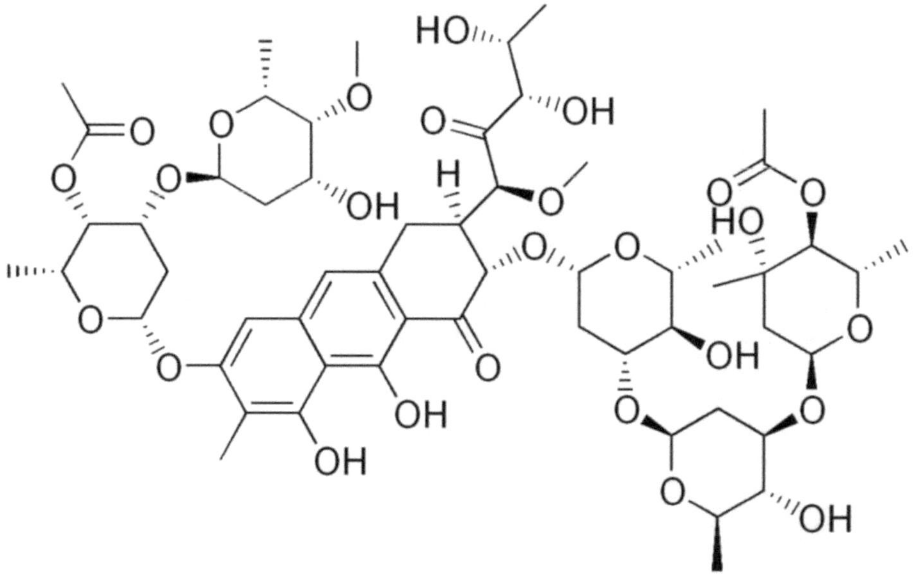

Fig. 1. Chemical structure of Chromomycin A3 [from sigmaaldrich]

Chromomycin A3 has also been shown to be a potent inhibitor of neuronal apoptosis induced by glutathione depletion-induced oxidative stress and DNA-damaging agent Camptothecin [Chatterjee et al., 2001]. Mechanistic studies suggest that chromomycin A3 antagonizes enhanced DNA binding of the transcription factors Sp1 and Sp3 to their cognate "G-C" box, induced by oxidative stress or DNA damage [Chatterjee et al., 2001]. Furthermore, by inhibiting transcription, chromomycin A3 can inhibit protein biosynthesis.

Miller identified chromomycin A3 that inhibited NF-kappaB signaling in a NF-kappaB mediated beta-lactamase reporter gene assay. It induced caspase 3/7 activity and had an inhibitory effect on cervical cancer cell growth [Miller et al., 2010]. We know that oxidative stress and elevation of intracellular calcium levels are particularly important inducers of NF-kappaB activation. Activation of NF-kappaB can interrupt apoptotic biochemical cascades at relatively early steps, before mitochondrial dysfunction and oxyradical production. The available data identify NF-kappaB as an important regulator of evolutionarily conserved biochemical and molecular cascades designed to prevent cell death and promote neuronal plasticity [Mattson et al., 2000]. Together, these results suggest that chromomycin A3 may be effective agents for the treatment of neurological diseases associated with aberrant activation of apoptosis and highlight the potential use of sequence-selective DNA-binding drugs as neurological therapeutics. Last year, we reported that chromomycin A3 inhibited Tau phosphorylation at Ser396 and therefore protected dopaminergic mesencephalic neurons from apoptosis induced by MPP (+) [Wang et al., 2010].

2.5.2 Mithramycin prevented MPP(+)-induced cultured neuronal apoptosis

Chromomycin A3 and mithramycin (also known as MIT and plicamycin) are two DNA binding anticancer antibiotics, acting via inhibition of replication and transcription during macromolecular biosynthesis. The clinical use of chromomycin A3 is limited because of its immuno suppressive properties and greater cytotoxic effects. But mithramycin is one of the older chemotherapy drugs, which has been in use for decades. Mithramycin (Fig.2.) selectively binds to G-C-rich DNA in the presence of Mg (2+) or Zn (2+), inhibiting RNA and DNA polymerase action [Majee & Chakrabarti, 1999]. It also inhibits c-myc expression and induces myeloid differentiation of HL-60 promyelocytic leukemia cells [Dutcher, 1997]. This drug is prescribed primarily in the treatment of malignant tumors of the testis. It is also prescribed in the treatment of hypercalcemia and hypercalciuria associated with cancer [Rosol & Capen, 1987]. It is given by intravenous route only. It was discontinued as of 2000 by the manufacturer based on decreased demand.

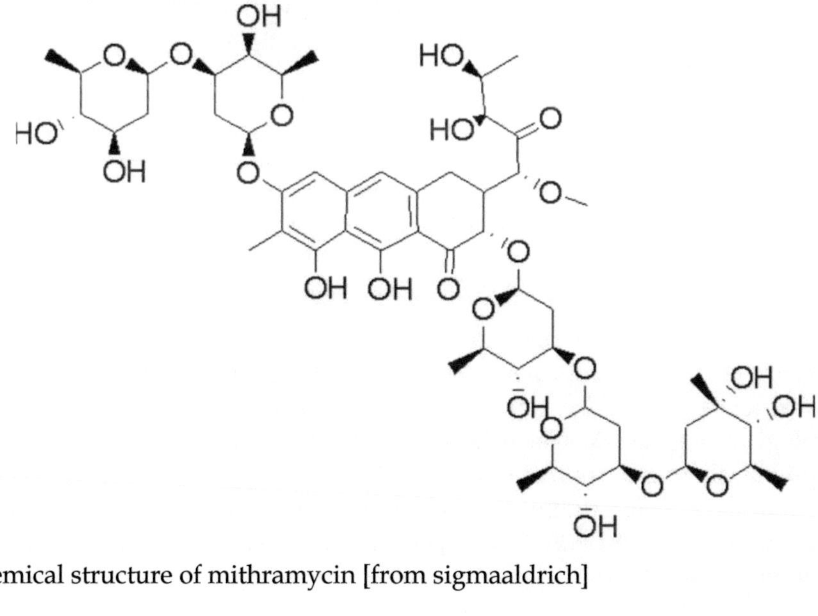

Fig. 2. Chemical structure of mithramycin [from sigmaaldrich]

Renewed interest in mithramycin resulted in about 50 mithramycin related publications in the first half of 2010 alone. Most publications mentioned anti-cancer abilities of the compound, but other medical conditions were also referred, such as: Huntington's disease (HD) neurodegeneration [BirZeit P.A, on line]. Recent research shows that it is helpful in treating motor symptoms and prolonging life in a mouse model of HD [Ferrante et al., 2004].

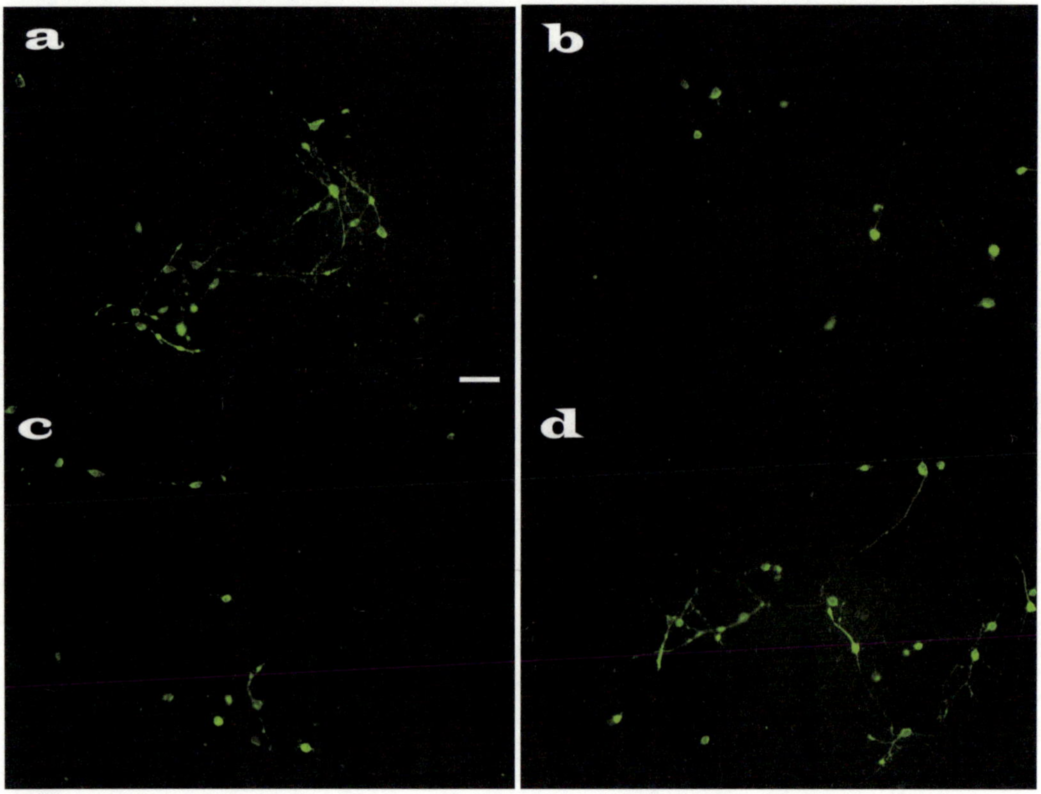

Fig. 3. Mithramycin inhibited MPP (+)-induced apoptosis in cultured dopaminergic neurons. Dopaminergic mesencephalic neurons were obtained from 14-day-old fetal rats. At DIV5, 10 µM MPP(+) was used to induce neuronal apoptosis for 48h. Specific TH-antibody was used to detect dopaminergic neurons. (a) control, Fluorescent micrograph by fluorescence microscope showing TH positive cells visualized with FITS (green); (b) 10µM MPP(+) decreased TH positive cells and reduced cytoplasmic volume; (c) 0.2µM mithramycin, and (d) 0.5µM mithramycin rescued TH positive cells. Scale bar = 50µm.

Pharmacological treatment of a transgenic mouse model of HD (R6/2) with mithramycin extended survival by 29.1%, greater than any single agent reported to date. Increased survival was accompanied by improved motor performance and markedly delayed neuropathological sequelae. Voisin screened candidate therapeutic compounds that were identified previously in cell culture/animal studies in a *C. elegans* HD model and found that two FDA approved drugs, lithium chloride and mithramycin, independently and in combination suppressed HD neurotoxicity [Voisine et al., 2007]. Because it is Food and Drug Administration-approved, researchers thought mithramycin is a promising drug for the treatment of HD. Since mithramycin has enhanced neuronal survival and neuroprotection, it may protect dopaminergic neurons. We also use cultured dopaminergic mesencephalic neurons with MPP (+) as PD cell model.

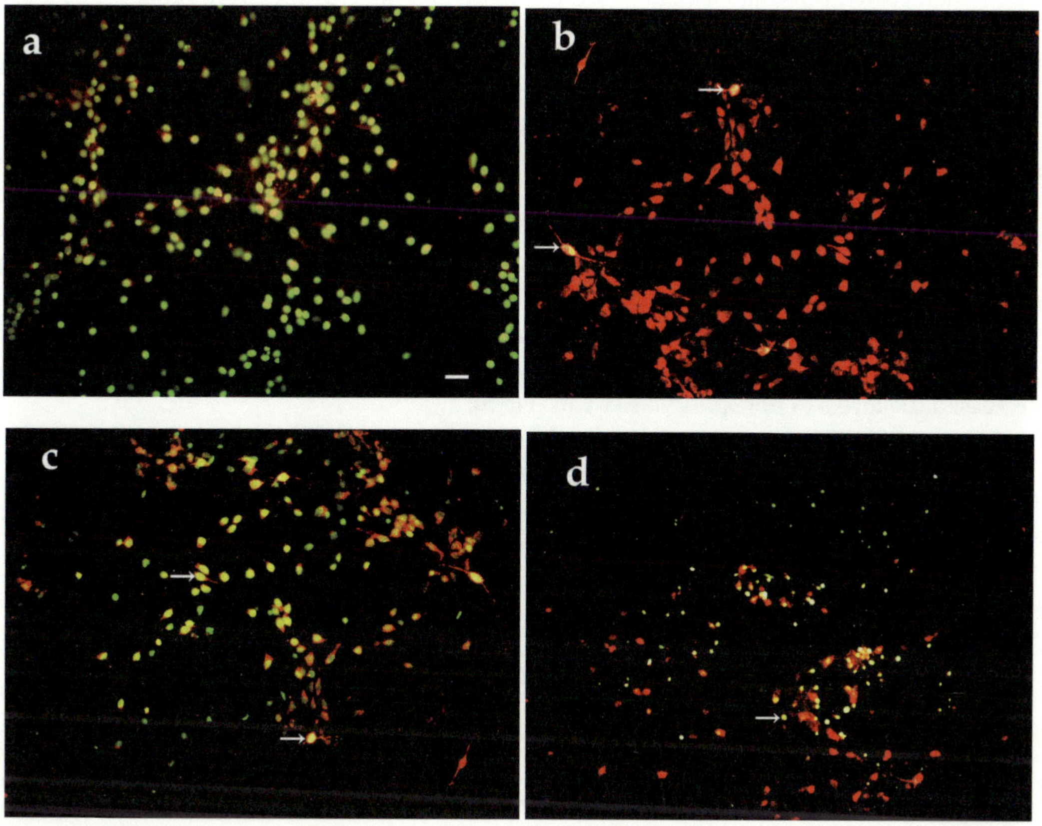

Fig. 4. TUNEL figures of inhibitory effect of mithramycin on dopaminergic neuronal apoptosis induced by MPP (+). Dopaminergic mesencephalic neurons were obtained from 14-day-old fetal rats. At DIV5, 10 μM MPP(+) was used to induce neuronal apoptosis for 48h. Specific TH-antibody was used to detect dopaminergic neurons. (a) Positive control. Strong TUNEL labeling showed apoptotic bodies in all kinds of cells; (b) control, vehicle-treated Neurons;(c) 10 μM MPP (+) induced neurons apoptosis (green) and decreased TH immunopositive cells (red). White arrow showed apoptotic dopaminergic neurons (yellow). (d) Fewer TUNEL-positive cells were shown with 1.0 μM mithramycin treatment. Scale bar = 50μm.

The embryos were removed at embryonic day 14 from pregnant Sprague-Dawley rats that had been anesthetized, then decerebrated. Ventral mesencephalon were dissected and collected. Cell suspensions prepared by mechanical trituration precoated overnight with 1 mg/ml polyethylenimine in borate buffer, pH 8.3. The cells were then maintained for maturation and differentiation in DMEM/F12 culture medium. Cultures were treated at DIV1 and every three days 250 μL of culture medium were replaced by medium supplemented with treatments. At DIV5, 250 μL of 500 μL medium were replaced by fresh medium supplemented or not with mithramycin at 200, 500, 1000 nM and 10 μM of MPP (+) were added. After 48 h, cells were fixed for 15 min with a 4% formaldehyde solution, washed three times with 500 μL PBS then submitted to TH immunostaining to allow analysis of DA neurons. Undoubtedly, MPP (+) induced apoptosis in cultured dopaminergic mesencephalic neurons. It decreased the number of TH positive cells and reduced cytoplasmic volume. 200, 500 and 1000 nM mithramycin rescued TH immunopositive cells from cytotoxic MPP (+) (Fig.3.). To detect DNA fragmentation, we used TUNEL. TUNEL is one of the main methods for detecting apoptotic programmed cell death. We found 1.0 μM mithramycin reduced MPP (+)-caused TUNEL-positive cells (Fig.4.)

Mithramycin not only increased the number of TH immunopositive cells, but also showed protective action in a dose-dependent manner (Table 1). Interesting, mithramycin also decreased the levels of phosphorylated Tau (Fig.5).

Mithramycin (μmol/L)	Neuronal Survival (% control)
0	32.8 ± 2.7
0.2	42.8 ± 5.2 *
0.5	57.1 ± 6.3 **
1.0	65.9 ± 7.3 **
2.0	76.3 ± 8.7 **
5.0	87.3 ± 8.4 **

* $P<0.05$, ** $P<0.01$, compared with control. Control neurons were maintained in DMEM/F12 medium. Neuronal survival was calculated as percentage neuronal survival = (TH positive cells with different concentrations of mithramycin and 10 μM MPP (+) for 48 h / TH positive cells in control medium) x100. Mean±S.E. (n = 3 independent experiments).

Table 1. Protective effect of mithramycin on dopaminergic neuronal apoptosis induced by MPP (+) in a concentration-denpendent manner.

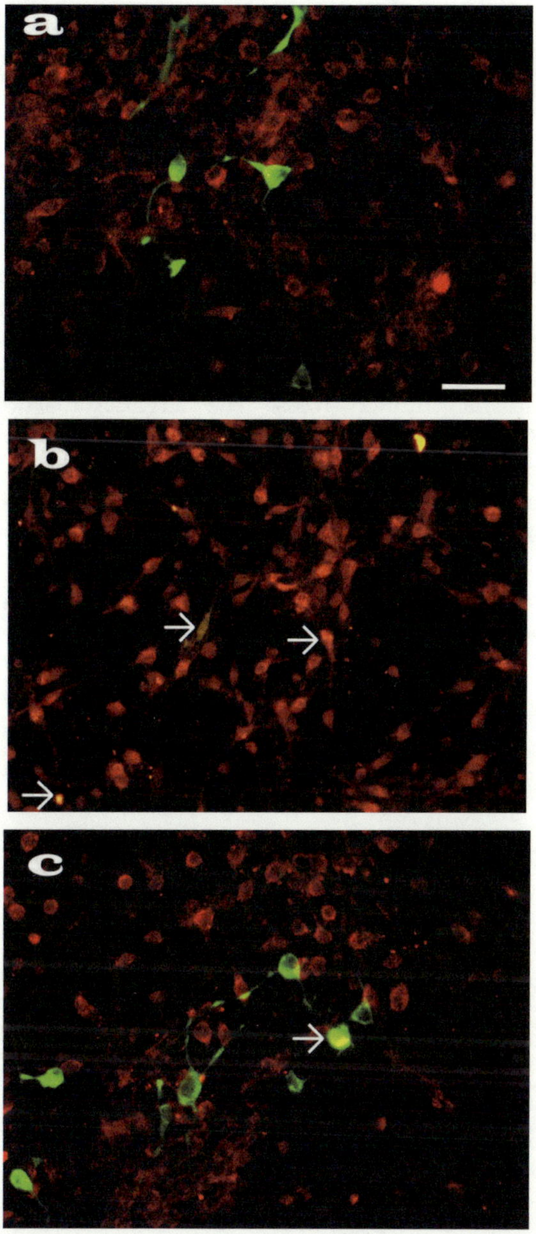

Fig. 5. Mithramycin attenuated Tau (Ser396) phosphorylation induced by MPP (+) in cultured dopaminergic neurons. Detection of p-Tau (Ser396) expression in cultured fetal dopaminergic mesencephalic neurons by immunohistochemistry was at 12 h after MPP (+) treatment. Specific TH-antibody was used to detect dopaminergic neurons. (a) Control, vehicle-treated cultures stained for TH (green) and phospho-Tau (Ser396) (red). (b) A culture treated with 10 μM MPP(+) for 12 h. Note more Tau (Ser396) were phosphorylated, resulting in neurons staining with salmon pink (white arrows). (c) Photomicrograph of a culture treated with 1.0 μM mithramycin. Note MPP (+) increased Tau (ser396) phosphorylation in TH positive neurons which can be prevented by mithramycin. Scale bar=50μm.

Because mithramycin is Food and Drug Administration-approved, it may be a promising drug for the treatment of PD.

3. Conclusions

Among kinases involved in Tau modifications, two are the most relevant: Tau protein kinase I (TPK I) also named GSK-3β and Tau kinase II (TPK II), which is a complex of two subunits: cdk5 and p35 [Alejandra et al., 1999]. In addition to hyperphosphorylation of Tau, p-GSK-3β has the capacity to phosphorylate several transcription factors (such as Jun, Myc, HSF-1, and cAMP response element-binding protein within the nucleus) and the multifunctional protein-catenin, as well as the nerve growth factor receptor [Muntané et al., 2008]. This means different roads meat in Tau (Fig.6). As one of the numerous substrates of GSK-3β/cdk5/p35, Tau has limited roles. The adverse reactions of inhibiting Tau phosphorylation must be less than those of inhibiting GSK-3β activity. Since tau plays an important role in the pathogenesis of Parkinson's disease [Lei et al., 2010], blockade of tau by specific inhibitors may prevent or effectively slow the progression of PD and other neurodegenerative diseases. It is exciting possibility a drug will soon be developed, as there is a patent for the use of aminoindazole derivatives for the inhibition of tau phosphorylation (United States Patent 7629374). This made it possible, which is inhibiting Tau phosphorylation as a potential strategy in treating PD. On the other side, mithramycin and chromomycin A3 are both in clinical use to treat malignant neoplasms. Ultilising approved drugs in "off label" indications can speed up the delivery of new therapies.

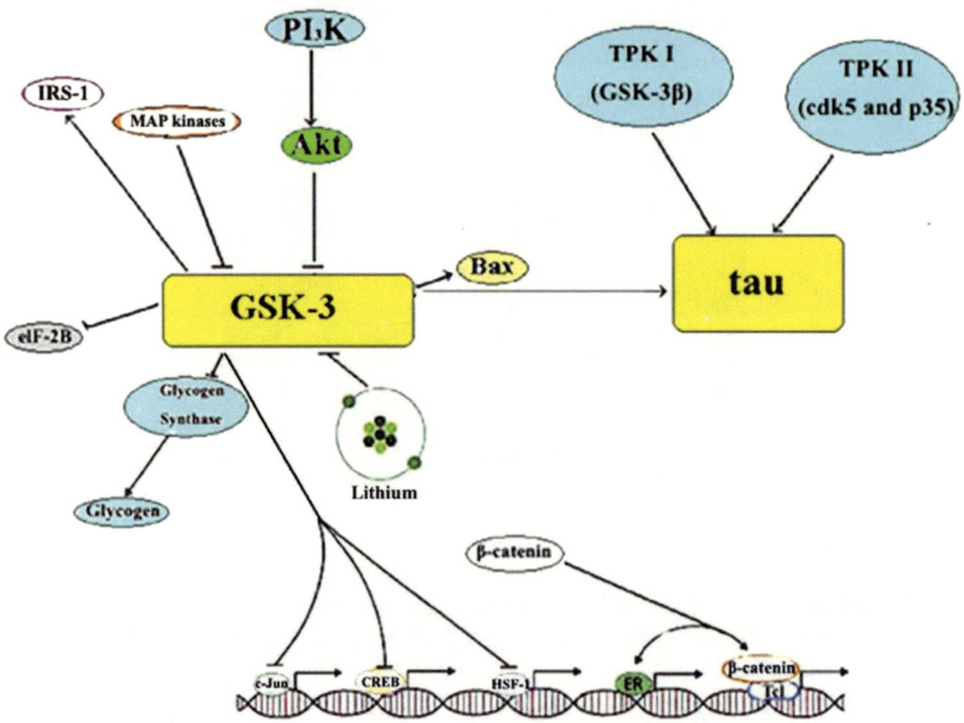

Fig. 6. The Simple diagram of GSK-3β/Tau signal pathways.

4. Acknowledgment

This work was supported by the National Natural Science Foundation of China (Grants No.30400124 and No.81030024); the Natural Science Foundation of Guangdong Province (Grants No.9351008901000003); the funds for good middle-aged/young technology talents of Southern Medical University (Grants No. C1010098).

5. References

Alejandra Alvarez, Rodrigo Toro, Alfredo ceres & Ricardo B. Maccioni. (1999). Inhibition of Tau phosphorylating protein kinase cdk5 prevents L-amyloid-induced neuronal death. *FEBS Letters*, Vol.459, pp.421-426, ISSN 0014-5793

Bennet BL, Sasaki DT, Murray BW, O'Leary EC, Sakata S T, Xu W. Leisten JC, Motiwala A, Pierce S, Satoh Y, Bhagwat SS, Manning AM & Anderson DW. (Nov 2001) SP600125, an anthrapyrazolone inhibitor of Jun N-terminal kinase. *Proc Natl Acad Sci USA*, Vol.98, No.20, pp.13681-13686, ISSN 0027-8424

Büeler H. (Nov 2010). Mitochondrial dynamics, cell death and the pathogenesis of Parkinson's disease. *Apoptosis*, Vol.15, No.11, pp.1336-1353, ISSN 1360-8185

Buerger K, Ewers M, Pirttilä T, Zinkowski R, Alafuzoff I, Teipel SJ, DeBernardis J, Kerkman D, McCulloch C, Soininen H & Hampel H.(Sep 2006). CSF phosphorylated tau protein correlates with neocortical neurofibrillary pathology in Alzheimer's disease. *Brain*, Vol.129, No.Pt 11, pp.3035-3041, ISSN 0006-8950

Chatterjee S, Zaman K, Ryu H, Conforto A & Ratan RR.(Mar 2001) Sequence-selective DNA binding drugs mithramycin A and chromomycin A3 are potent inhibitors of neuronal apoptosis induced by oxidative stress and DNA damage in cortical neurons. *Ann Neurol*, Vol.49, No.3, pp.345-354, ISSN 0364-5134

Chung ES, Bok E, Sohn S, Lee YD, Baik HH & Jin BK. (Jun 2010). GT1b-induced neurotoxicity is mediated by the Akt/GSK-3/Tau signaling pathway but not caspase-3 in mesencephalic dopaminergic neurons. *BMC Neurosci*, Vol.11, pp.74, ISSN 1471-2202. Available from:
http://www.biomedcentral.com/1471-2202/11/74

Duka T, Duka V, Joyce JN & Sidhu A. (Apr 2009). Alpha-Synuclein contributes to GSK-3beta-catalyzed Tau phosphorylation in Parkinson's disease models. *FASEB J*, Vol.23, No.9, (Sep 2009), pp.2820-30, ISSN 1742-464X

Duka T & Sidhu A. (2006). The neurotoxin, MPP(+), induces hyperphosphorylation of Tau, in the presence of alpha-Synuclein, in SH-SY5Y neuroblastoma cells. *Neurotox Res*, Vol.10, No.1, pp.1-10, ISSN 1029-8428

Dutcher JP, Coletti D, Paietta E & Wiernik PH. (May 1997). A pilot study of alpha-interferon and plicamycin for accelerated phase of chronic myeloid leukemia. *Leuk Res*, Vol.21, No.5, pp.375–380, Available from
http://linkinghub.elsevier.com/retrieve/pii/S0145212696001087.

Ethell DW & Fei Q. (Mar 2009). Parkinson-linked genes and toxins that affect neuronal cell death through the Bcl-2 family. *Antioxid Redox Signal*, Vol.11, No.3, pp.529-540, ISSN 1523-0864

Evans DB, Rank KB, Bhattacharya K, Thomsen DR, Gurney ME & Sharma SK.(2000). Tau phosphorylation at serine 396 and serine 404 by human recombinant tau protein kinase II inhibits tau's ability to promote microtubule assembly. *J Biol Chem*, Vol.275, pp.24977–24983, ISSN 0021-9258. doi: 10.1074/jbc.M000808200.

Ferrer I, Gomez-Isla T, Puig B, Freixes M, Ribé E, Dalfó E & Avila J. (2005). Current advances on different kinases involved in Tau phosphorylation, and implications in Alzheimer's disease and Tauopathies. *Curr Alzheimer Res*, Vol.2, No.1, pp.3-18, ISSN 1567-2050

Ferrante RJ, Ryu H, Kubilus JK, D'Mello S, Sugars KL, Lee J, Lu P, Smith K, Browne S, Beal MF, Kristal BS, Stavrovskaya IG, Hewett S, Rubinsztein DC, Langley B & Ratan RR. (Nov 2004). Chemotherapy for the Brain: The Antitumor Antibiotic Mithramycin Prolongs Survival in a Mouse Model of Huntington's Disease. *J Neurosci*, Vol.24, No.46, pp.10335-10342, ISSN 0270-6474

Gendron TF & Petrucelli L. (Mar 2009). The role of tau in neurodegeneration. *Mol Neurodegener*. Vol.4, pp.13, Available from:
http://www.Molecularneuro- degeneration.com/content/4/1/13

Higuchi M, Lee VM & Trojanowski JQ.(2002). Tau and axonopathy in neurodegenerative disorders (Review). *Neuromol Med*, Vol.2, No.2, pp.131-150, ISSN 1535-1084

Hou MH, Lu WJ, Lin HY & Yuann JM. (Apr 2008). Studies of sequence-specific DNA binding, DNA cleavage, and topoisomerase I inhibition by the dimeric chromomycin A3 complexed with Fe(II). *Biochemistry*, Vol.47, No.20, pp.5493-5502, ISSN 0006-2960.

Ishizawa T, Mattila P, Davies P, Wang D & Dickson DW. (2003). Colocalization of Tau and alpha-synuclein epitopes in Lewy bodies. *J Neuropathol Exp Neurol*, Vol.62, No.4, (Apr 2003), pp.389-397, ISSN 0022-3069

Karunakaran S, Saeed U, Mishra M, Valli RK, Joshi SD, Meka DP, Seth P & Ravindranath V. (Nov 2008). Selective activation of p38 MAPK in dopaminergic neurons of substantia nigra leads to nuclear translocation of p53 in MPTP-treated mice. *J Neurosci*, Vol.28, No47, pp.12500-12509, ISSN 0270-6474

Kowall NW & Kosik KS.(Nov 1987). Axonal disruption and aberrant localization of tau protein characterize the neuropil pathology of Alzheimer's disease. *Ann Neurol*, Vol.22, No.5, pp.639-643, ISSN 0364-5134

Lei P, Ayton S, Finkelstein DI, Adlard PA, Masters CL & Bush AI. (Aug 2010). Tau protein: relevance to Parkinson's disease. *Int J Biochem Cell Biol*, Vol.42, No.11, pp.1775-1778, ISSN 1357-2725

Lloyd KG. (1977). CNS compensation to dopamine neuron loss in Parkinson's disease. *Adv Exp Med Biol*, Vol.90, pp.255-266, ISSN 0065-2598

Majee S & Chakrabarti A. (1999). Membrane interaction of an antitumor antibiotic, mithramycin, with anionic phospholipid vesicles. *Biochemical Pharmacology, Vol.*57, No.9, pp.981–987, ISSN . doi:10.1016/S0006-2952(98)00374-8. PMID 10796068.

Marsden CD & Parkes JD. (Feb 1977). Success and problems of long-term levodopa therapy in Parkinson's disease. *Lancet*, Vol.1, No.8007, pp.345-349, ISSN 0140-6736

Mattson MP. (Nov 2000). Apoptosis in neurodegenerative disorders (Review). *Nat Rev Mol Cell Bio*, Vol.1, No.2, pp.120–129, ISSN 1471-0072

Miller SC, Huang R, Sakamuru S, Shukla SJ, Attene-Ramos MS, Shinn P, Van Leer D, Leister W, Austin CP & Xia M.(Jan 2010) Identification of known drugs that act as inhibitors of NF-kappaB signaling and their mechanism of action. *Biochem Pharmacol*, Vol.79, No.9, (May 2010), pp.1272-1280, ISSN 0006-2952

Muntané G, Dalfó E, Martinez A & Ferrer I. (Feb 2008). Phosphorylation of Tau and alpha-synuclein in synaptic-enriched fractions of the frontal cortex in Alzheimer's disease, and in PD and related alpha-synucleinopathies. *Neuroscience*, Vol.152, No.4, (Apr 2008), pp.913-923, ISSN 0306-4522

Nagatsu T & Sawada M. (2007). Biochemistry of postmortem brains in Parkinson's disease: historical overview and future prospects (Review). *J Neural Transm-Supp*, Vol.2007, No.72, pp.113-120, ISSN 0303-6995

Nishimura I, Yang Y & Lu B.(2004). PAR-1 kinase plays an initiator role in a temporally ordered phosphorylation process that confers tau toxicity in Drosophila. *Cell*, Vol.116, pp.671–682, ISSN 0092-8674. doi: 10.1016/S0092-8674(04)00170-9.

Qureshi HY & Paudel HK. (Dec 2010). Parkinsonian neurotoxin MPTP and alpha- synuclein mutations promote Tau protein phosphorylation at Ser262 and destabilize microtubule cytoskeleton in vitro. *J Biol Chem*, Vol.286, No.7, (Feb 2011), pp.5055-5068, ISSN 0021-9258

Reynolds CH, Garwood CJ, Wray S, Price C, Kellie S, Perera T, Zvelebil M, Yang A, Sheppard PW, Varndell IM, Hanger DP & Anderton BH.(May 2008). Phosphorylation regulates tau interactions with Src homology 3 domains of phosphatidylinositol 3-kinase, phospholipase Cgamma1, Grb2, and Src family kinases. *J Biol Chem*, Vol.283, No.26, pp.18177-18186, ISSN 0021-9258

Rosol TJ & Capen CC. (Oct 1987). The effect of low calcium diet, mithramycin, and dichlorodimethylene bisphosphonate on humoral hypercalcemia of malignancy in nude mice transplanted with the canine adenocarcinoma tumor line (CAC-8). *J Bone Miner Res*, Vol.2, No.5, pp.395-405, ISSN 0884-043

Rylander D, Parent M, O'Sullivan SS, Dovero S, Lees AJ, Bezard E, Descarries L & Cenci MA. (2010). Maladaptive plasticity of serotonin axon terminals in levodopa-induced dyskinesia. *Ann Neurol*, Vol.68, No.5, (Nov 2010), pp. 619-628, ISSN 0364-5134

Saporito MS, Thomas BA & Scott RW. (Sep 2000). MPTP activates c-Jun NH (2)-terminal kinase (JNK) and its upstream regulatory kinase MKK4 in nigrostriatal neurons in vivo. *J Neurochem*, Vol.75, No.3, pp.1200-1208, ISSN 0022-3042

Sato S, Cerny RL, Buescher JL & Ikezu T. (2006). Tau-tubulin kinase 1 (TTBK1), a neuron-specific Tau kinase candidate, is involved in Tau phosphorylation and aggregation. *J Neurochem*, Vol.98, No.5, (Sep 2006), pp.1573-1584, ISSN 0022-3042

Schönknecht P, Pantel J, Hunt A, Volkmann M, Buerger K, Hampel H & Schröder J. (Mar 2003). Levels of total tau and tau protein phosphorylated at threonine 181 in patients with incipient and manifest Alzheimer's disease. *Neurosci Lett*, Vol.339, No.2, pp.172-174, ISSN 0304-3940

Sergeant N, Bretteville A, Hamdane M, Caillet-Boudin ML, Grognet P, Bombois S, Blum D, Delacourte A, Pasquier F, Vanmechelen E, Schraen-Maschke S & Buée L.(Apr 2008). Biochemistry of Tau in Alzheimer's disease and related neurological disorders. *Expert Rev Proteomics*, Vol.5, No.2, pp.207-224, ISSN 1478-9450

Voisine C, Varma H, Walker N, Bates EA, Stockwell BR, et al (2007) Identification of Potential Therapeutic Drugs for Huntington's Disease using Caenorhabditis elegans. In: *PLoS ONE*, 06,06,2007, Available from:
http://www.plosone.org/ article/info%3Adoi%2F10.1371%2Fjournal.pone.0000- 504

Wang WY, Li MT, Rao JJ & Zhu NM. (2010). The protective action of chromomycin on dopaminergic neurons. *Chinese Pharmacological Bulletin*, Vol.26, No.4, pp.522-526, ISSN 1001-1978

Wang W, Shi L, Xie Y, Ma C, Li W, Su X, Huang S, Chen R, Zhu Z, Mao Z, Han Y& Li M. (Feb 2004). SP600125, a new JNK inhibitor, protects dopaminergic neurons in the MPTP model of PD. *Neurosci Res*, Vol.48, No.2, pp.195-202, ISSN 0168-0102

Wang W, Yang Y, Ying C, Li W, Ruan H, Zhu X, You Y, Han Y, Chen R, Wang Y & Li M. (Apr 2007). Inhibition of GSK-3beta protects dopaminergic neurons from MPTP toxicity. *Neuropharmacology*, Vol.52, No.8, (Jun 2007), pp. 1678-1684, ISSN 0028-3908

Yuan J & Yankner BA.(Oct 2000). Apoptosis in the nervous system (Review). *Nature*, Vol.407, No.6805, pp.802–809, ISSN 0028-0836

Zheng YL, Kesavapany S, Gravell M, Hamilton RS, Schubert M, Amin N, Albers W, Grant P & Pant HC. (2005). A Cdk5 inhibitory peptide reduces Tau hyperphosphorylation and apoptosis in neurons. *EMBO l*, Vol.24, pp.209-220, ISSN 0261-4189

The Protective Effects of Pre-Treatment with Glutamate Metabotropic Receptor Agonists on the Development of Parkinsonian Movements

Munir Qazzaz[1], Rateb M. Husein[1],
Munther Metani[1] and Abdul-Salam Abdul-Ghani[2]
[1]*Birzeit University, Faculty of Science, Biology and Biochemistry Department, West-Bank,*
[2]*Al-Quds University, Faculty of Medicine, Physiology and Pharmacology Department, East Jerusalem, West-Bank,*
Palestine

1. Introduction

The subcortical nuclei of the basal ganglia are of great importance in initiation of normal body motor activities. Degeneration of nigrostriatal dopaminergic neurons in the substantia nigra pars compacta has been shown to be the main cause of Parkinson's disease (PD) (Phillips & Brown, 1999; Phillips et al., 2006; and Truong et al., 2006).

Degeneration of dopaminergic neurons within the nigrostriatal pathway following treatment with the neurotoxin 6-hydroxy dopamine (6-OHDA) has been accepted widely as a good model of PD (Wichmann et al., 2002; Willis & Kennedy, 2004; Vernon et al., 2005; Troung et al., 2006; Chaturvedi et al., 2006; Phillips et al., 2006).

Excitatory amino acids play an important role, not only in epilepsy (Coutinhio-Netto et al., 1981; Bradford 1995; Abdul-Ghani et al 1997) but also in some neurodegenerative diseases (Wilkinski & Acosta 1995). Excitation of sub-thalamic nucleus neurons in vitro was achieved by activation of group I metabotropic glutamate receptors by (S,R)-dihydroxy-phenylglycine (DHPG), and was blocked by the receptor antagonist (+)-alpha-methyl-4-carboxyphenylglycine (MCPG). No effects were obtained with the selective agonists of group II and group III metabotropic receptors such as L-2-amino-4-phosphonobutyrate (LAP4) and (2S,2'R,3'R)-2-(2',3'-dicarboxycyclopropyl) glycine (DCG-IV) (Abbott et al., 1997). Intra-sub-thalamic injection of (1S,3S)-1-aminocyclopentane-1,3-dicarboxylic acid (1S,3R)-ACPD produced marked contra-lateral rotation, similar to that seen after intra-striatal injection of (1S,3S)-ACPD, suggesting that metabotropic glutamate receptors as a possible target for the treatment of Parkinson's disease (Sacaan et al., 1991: 1992; Kaatz & Albin, 1995). Further more Group-III mGlu receptors stimulation by LAP4 was found to improve akinesia in a rat model of Parkinson's disease (Cuomo et al., 2009). Recently attention has focused on seeking alternative non-dopaminergic strategies in the treatment of basal ganglia disorders, and is now shifting to glutamatergic pathways.

In the current experiments we have tested the effect of pre-treatment with a glutamate metabotropic receptor agonist Sub-type III, LAP4 and a glutamate metabotropic receptor antagonist, MPPG, injected into the median forebrain bundle or to the striatum, on rats made Parkinsonian by intra-cerebral microinjection of 6-OHDA, as described by Willis and Kennedy (2004).

2. Materials and methods

2.1 Drugs and chemicals

All chemicals and drugs were of analytical grade and were purchased from Sigma Chemicals Co., USA.

2.2 Animals and surgery

Sprague-Dawley rats weighing 180 to 250g were used in all experiments. Rats were kept under environmentally controlled conditions (ambient temperature 22 - 23°C; Humidity 40-50% on a 12 hour light dark cycle with food and water available to ad libitum. Experiments were performed following the guidelines of animal care of the national institute of health, and experiments were approved by the ethical committee in our faculty of medicine. The animals were anaesthetized by intra-peritoneal injection of sodium pentobarbital, 60mg/kg. They were kept under light anaesthesia characterized by a negative response to pain and a positive corneal reflex and the level of anaesthesia was periodically verified via the hind limb compression reflex. Rats were placed on a stereotaxic apparatus; the scalp was then incised to expose the parietal bone. After drilling through the bone, a stainless steel cannula was implanted into the median forebrain bundle, using the following coordinates from the bregma: AP= -1.8 mm, L= ± 1.8 mm and V = - 6.1 mm, as described by Willis and Armstrong (1999) (The size of the lesion was not confirmed) for the injection of 6-OHDA (16 µg in 2 µL BPS), and pre-treatment with LAP4 or MPPG. In other experiments a second cannula was implanted in the striatum, coordinates: AP= 1.3 mm, L= ± 2.4 mm and V = - 7.8 mm, for the injection of LAP4 (40ng / 2µl BP) or MPPG (40ng / 2µL BPS). The volume of 2 µL buffer phosphate solution or the same volume of the drugs solution, were slowly micro-injected in a speed of 2 µL per 2 min. to avoid brain damage.
Animals were rendered Parkinsonian by the intra-cerebral microinjection of 6-hydroxy-dopamine (6-OHDA; 16 µg in 2 µL BPS) into the above coordinates at a flow rate of 1 µL/min. LAP4, a selective agonist, or MPPG, a selective antagonist of glutamate metabotropic receptors sub-type III, were unilaterally microinjected into the median forebrain bundle or to the striatum at the same rate of flow, for 15 min before treatment with 6-OHDA.

2.3 Measurement of motor activities

Rats were left to move freely over a 20 meters long and 15 meters wide floor with a 20 × 20 centimetre squared grid. Locomotion (spontaneous movement) was measured daily by counting the number of squares crossed and calculating the speed of movement in centimetres per second. The number of rearing and rotation episodes were measured daily by counting the events over 10 minutes. Averages were then calculated per minute. Body weight was measured weekly as an index of eating behaviour and as the percentage change per month was calculated.

2.4 Statistics

Values were expressed as mean ± standard error of the mean (SEM) for the number of experiments indicated in parentheses. Results were compared, where appropriate, using a

One Way ANOVA with Dunnets post hoc test against 6-OHDA treated animals. Differences were considered statistically significant if $P < 0.05$. Statistical analyses were performed using Graph Pad Prism v 3.03.

3. Results

3.1 Induction of Parkinsonism by 6-OHDA

After microinjection of rats with 6-OHDA into the median forebrain bundle, there was a reduction in locomotion speed from 15.15 ± 0.61 (13) to 8.22 ± 1.03 (36) cm/sec. ($P \leq 0.005$) after one week, and progressively reduced to 3.78 ± 0.54 (36) after 4 weeks. Rotation movements were elevated significantly to 2.64 ± 0.29 (36) times per min. after one week and to 3.58 ± 0.26 (24) after 4 weeks. Rearing was increased to 2.25 ± 0.33 (36) and to 4.75 ± 0.41 (24) times per min. after one week and 4 weeks respectively. The normal increase in body weight was reduced from 38% to 2%. (Fig. 1 and Table 1). 6-OHDA progressively reduced spontaneous movements which became minimal after 4 to 5 weeks (Fig. 2).

		Rotation (No/min)	Rearing (No/min)	% change Body Weight
Sham Control (2μL BPS)		0.31 ± 0.24 (13)	0.15 ± 0.10 (13)	↑38%
6-OHDA (16μg/2μL)	1st Week	2.64 ± 0.29 (36) $^{+}$	2.25 ± 0.33 (36)$^{++}$	
	4th Week	3.58 ± 0.26 (24)$^{++}$	4.75 ± 0.41 (24)$^{++}$	↑2%
LAP4 (40ng/2μL) + **6-OHDA** (16μg/2μL)	1st Week	1.47 ± 0.26 (47)* ↓35%	0.39 ± 0.11 (48)*** ↓83%	
	4th Week	1.41 ± 0.17 (44)*** ↓61%	0.35 ± 0.12 (45)*** ↓93%	↑37%
MPPG (40ng/2μL) + **6-OHDA** (16μg/2μL)	1st Week	1.84 ± 0.33 (31)	1.90 ± 0.35 (31)	
	4th Week	1.57 ± 0.19 (49)** ↓56%	3.90 ± 0.43 (38)	↑22%

Table 1. Effect of pre-treatment with LAP4 and MPPG on motor disorders induced by 6-OH-Dopamine

LAP4 or MPPG (40 ng/2μL) were injected intra-cerebrally into the same site in the median forebrain bundle (Coordinates (AP= -1.8; L=1.8; V= -6.1) 15 min. before injection of 6-OHDA (16 μg / 2μL BPS). Sham control was injected for the same period with the same volume of BPS. Percentage change in body weight and other motor disorders were recorded during the first and the fourth weeks of treatment.

Values are Mean ± SEM and the number of experiments is indicated between brackets.

$^{+}$ $P \leq 0.001$; $^{++}$ $P \leq 0.0005$ Compared to Sham control animals

* $P \leq 0.05$; ** $P \leq 0.002$; *** $P \leq 0.0005$ Compared to 6-OHDA treated animals

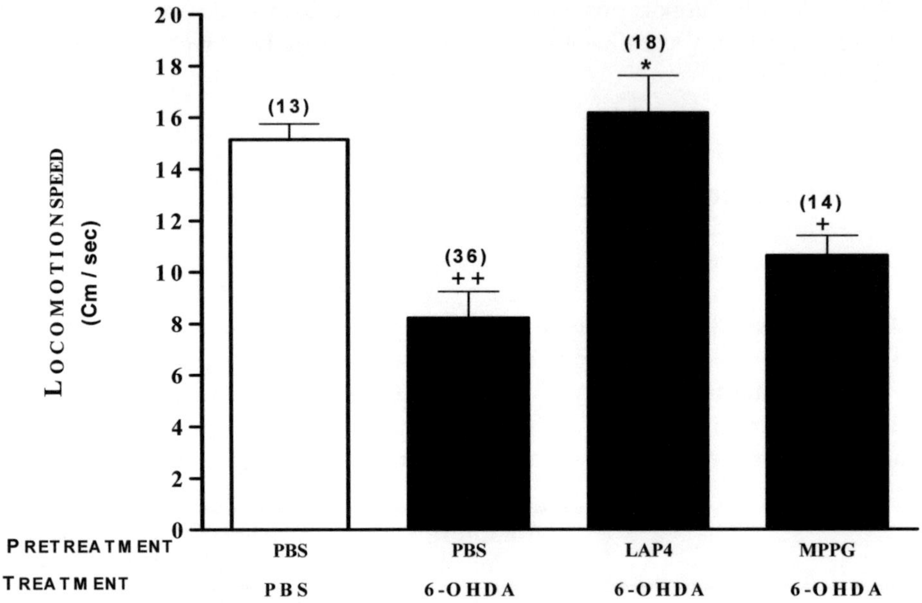

Fig. 1. Effect of pre-treatment with LAP4 and MPPG on Locomotion Disorders induced by injection of 6-OH-Dopamine

LAP4 or MPPG (40 ng / 2µL BPS) were injected intra-cerebrally into the same site in the median forebrain bundle coordinates (Coordinates: AP=-1.8; L=1.8; V=-6.1) 15 min. before injection of 6-OHDA (16 µg / 2µl BPS). Sham control animals were injected for the same period with the same volume of BPS. Locomotion measurements were recorded after one week of treatment.

Values are mean ± SEM for the number of experiments indicated in brackets.

* $P \leq 0.005$	Compared to 6-OHDA treated animals
$^{+}P \leq 0.01$	Compared to sham control animals
$^{++}P \leq 0.005$	Compared to sham control animals

3.2 Pre-treatment with LAP4

Pre-treatment with LAP4 before injection of 6-OHDA increased locomotion by 97 % after one week, from 8.22 ± 1.03 (36) to 16.17 ± 1.46 (18) ($P \leq 0.005$), and by 146% after 4 weeks, from 3.78 ± 0.54 (36) to 9.29 ± 1.28 (14) ($P \leq 0.01$) (Figs 1 and Table 2). Rotation was reduced significantly by 57% from 3.58 ± 0.26 (24) to 1.55 ± 0.26 (18) ($P \leq 0.0005$) after 4 weeks. Rearing was reduced by 85% from 2.25 ± 0.33 (36) to 0.33 ± 0.21(12) after one week, and with the same percentage after 4 weeks, from 4.75 ± 0.41 (24) to 0.73 ± 0.07 (15) ($P \leq 0.0005$). LAP4 prevented the effect of 6-OHDA on body weight, percentage change in body weight was increase from 2% to 38 % (Table 1). The protective effect of LAP4 was consistent for one to 5 weeks after injection of 6-OH Dopamine. (Fig.2)

LAP4 or MPPG (40 ng/2µL) were injected intra-cerebrally into the median forebrain bundle coordinates (AP= -1.8; L=1.8; V= -6.1) 15 min. before injection of 6-OHDA (16 µg / 2µL BPS) into the same site. Sham control values of locomotion 15.15 ± 1.61 (13) cm/sec at 0 time and after 5 weeks 14.38 ± 1.25 (13) cm/sec. Values are Mean ± SEM.

* $P \leq 0.05$; ** $P \leq 0.01$; *** $P \leq 0.005$ compared to animals treated with 6-OHDA alone.

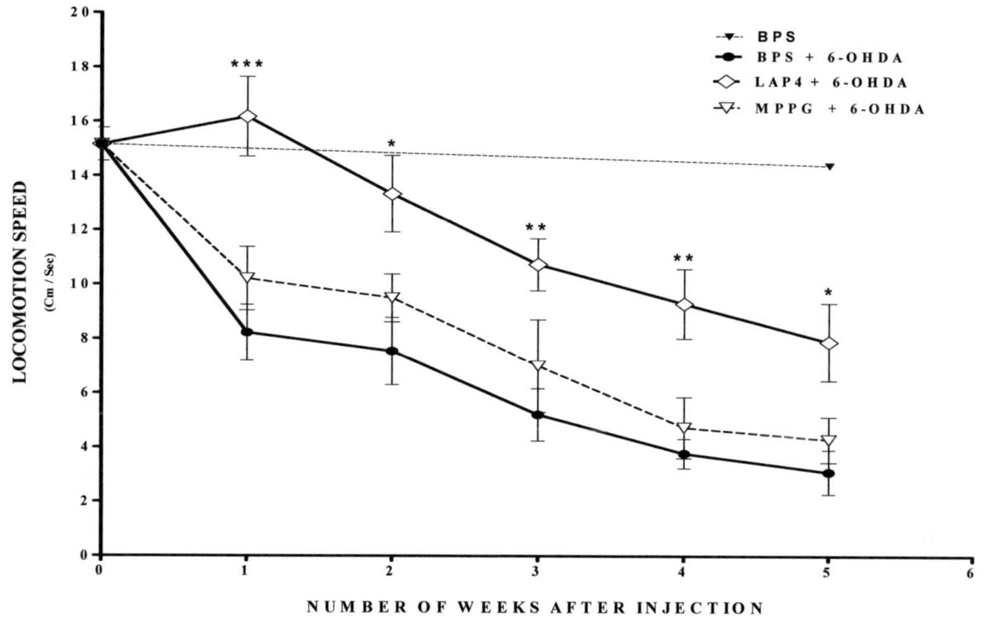

Fig. 2. Effect of pre-treatment with LAP4 and MPPG in Locomotion Disorders induced by 6-OHDA

3.3 Pre-treatment with MPPG

Injection of the glutamate metabotropic antagonist, MPPG, into the striatum instead of LAP4 15 min. before injection of 6-OHDA had no significant effect on motor disorders induced by 6-OHDA (Fig. 1 and Tables 1). However, the effect of 6-OHDA on body weight was largely reversed, from 2% to 22%, and rearing was reduced by 56% after one month of treatment (Table 1).

3.4 Comparison between Injection of LAP4 into the Median Forebrain Bundle (MFB) and Striatum

When LAP4 was intra-cerebrally micro-injected into MFB or Striatum 15 min. prior to the injection of 6-OHDA, it produced significant increase in locomotion one week after the injection (97% increase and 82% increase respectively). The increase was even more after one month (146% and 138% respectively).

There was a small decrease in rotational movement after one week of injection (9% decrease when LAP4 was injected into MFB and 36% decrease when LAP4 was injected into Striatum). The decrease was even higher one month later (57% and 63% respectively).

Similar results were obtained when rearing movement was calculated. A significant decrease was produced one week after LAP4 injection into MFB or striatum (85% and 81% respectively). The decrease persists after one month (85% and 87% respectively).

These results showed no significant difference in the protective effect of LAP4 on motor disorders produced by the injection of 6-OHDA according to its site of injection.

LAP4 or MPPG (40 ng/2μL) were injected intra-cerebrally into the median forebrain bundle (NSB) coordinates (AP= -1.8; L=1.8; V= -6.1) or into the striatum coordinates (AP= 1.3;

L=±2.4; V= -7.8) 15 min. before injection of 6-OHDA (16 µg / 2µL BPS) into the median forebrain bundle. Sham control was injected for the same period with the same volume of BPS. Percentage change in body weight and other motor disorders were recorded during the first and the fourth weeks of treatment.

		Without LAP4		**With LAP4**	
		Sham Control	**6-OHDA**	**MFB** V= - 6.1	**Striatum** V= - 7.8
Locomotion (cm/sec.)	1st Week	15.15 ± 0.61 (13)	8.22 ± 1.03 (36)	**16.17 ± 1.46 (18)** ↑97%**	**14.96 ± 0.99 (26)** ↑82%**
	4th Week		3.78 ± 0.54 (36)	**9.29 ± 1.28 (14)* ↑146%**	**9.00 ± 1.13 (18)** ↑138%**
Rotation (times/min.)	1st Week	0.31 ± 0.24 (13)	2.64 ± 0.29 (36)	**2.39 ± 0.46 (18)**	**1.69 ± 0.33 (36)**
	4th Week		3.58 ± 0.26 (24)	**1.55 ± 0.26 (18)*** ↓57%**	**1.31± 0.23 (26) **** ↓63%**
Rearing (times/min.)	1st Week	0.15 ± 1.0 (13)	2.25 ± 0.33 (36)	**0.33 ± 0.21 (12)** ↓85%**	**0.42 ± 0.13 (36)*** ↓81%**
	4th Week		4.75 ± 0.41 (24)	**0.73 ± 0.07 (15)**** ↓85%**	**0.63 ± 0.22 (35)**** ↓87%**

Table 2. Differences between the intra-cerebral injection of LAP4 into the Median Forebrain Bundle (MFB) or the striatum

Percentage change in LAP4 pre-treated animals are compared to animals treated with 6-OHDA without pre-treatment with LAP4.
Values are Mean ± SEM and the number of experiments is indicated between brackets.
* $P \leq 0.01$; ** $P \leq 0.005$; *** $P \leq 0.001$; **** $P \leq 0.0005$ compared to 6-OHDA treated animals

4. Discussion

Our results show that nigrostriatal micro-injection of 6-OHDA reduced significantly spontaneous locomotion in rats by 46% after one week and 75% after 4 weeks, and reduced the normal gain in body weight by 95%, which indicates a reduction in feeding. Rearing and rotation movements increased by 15 and 9-fold respectively after one week, and by 32 and 12-fold respectively after four weeks. Other workers have made rats Parkinsonian by micro-injection of 6-OHDA into the striatum (Kirik et al., 1989; Chaturvedi et al., 2006), the nigrostriatal bundle (Willis & Kennedy, 2004) or the substantia nigra pars compacta (Vernon et al., 2005). Lopez et al. (2007) found that LAP4 infusion into the globus pallidus reduced abnormal activities associated with Parkinsonism, as did our infusion into the nigrostrial bundle.

LAP4, a selective agonist of group III metabotropic receptors, had a protective effect against the development of motor disorders induced by 6-OHDA when it was micro-injected into the median forebrain bundle. It increased locomotion significantly and reduced motor disorders induced by 6-OHDA by an average of 39% during the first month. It also prevented the effect of 6-OHDA on body weight. In addition LAP4 has reduced significantly motor disorders like rotations and rearing by 61% and 93% respectively. The neuroprotective effect of LAP4 was reported in vitro against rotenone which causes Parkinsonian features in rats (Jiang et al., 2006) and in vivo against 6-OHDA toxicity (Lafon-Cazal et al., 1999; Bruno et al., 2000; Vernon et al., 2005; 2007). The potent and systemically active group II mGlu2/3 receptor agonist (-)-2-oxa-4-aminocyclo[3.1.0]hexane-4,6-dicarboxylic acid (LY379268), was found to provided some protection against nigral and striatal infusion of 6-OHDA (Murray et al., 2002).

We found that in-vivo intra-nigrostriatal injection of glutamate metabotropic antagonist (MPPG) before injection of 6-OHDA had no significant effect on locomotion, rotation movement or rearing, but had a significant effect on body weight changes. Therefore, whereas the development of locomotion disorders induced by injection of 6-OHDA was reduced by pre-treatment with LAP4, a glutamate presynaptic agonist, it was not affected by the selective antagonist, MPPG. Glutamate metabotropic antagonists are known to increase calcium ion uptake in presynaptic membranes (Abdul-Ghani et al., 1997) and increase glutamate release from presynaptic membranes. This could explain the lack of effect of the antagonist on locomotion which we have observed. Similar protective activity was achieved when LAP4 was injected at the same volume and concentration to the striatum coordinates: (AP= 1.3 mm, L= ± 2.4 mm and V = - 7.8). Significant histological and functional protection of the nigrostriatal tract against 6-OHDA toxicity by LAP4 was reported by Vernon et al 2005.

Excessive release of glutamate by neurons feeding into the striatum and substantia nigra could stimulate NO production and iron release, causing an increase in free radicals and oxidative damage to neurons (Snyder & Bredt, 1992; Youdim et al., 1993; Gerlach et al., 1994; Hugon et al., 1996). Perhaps, therefore, agents which inhibit glutamate release in the substantia nigra and striatum may be expected to protect neurons in patients with Parkinson's disease. Vernon et al. (2006) have shown that acute or sub-chronic intra-nigral injection of LAP4 provides significant protection of the nigrostriatal system against 6-OHDA toxicity, and this effect was blocked when LAP4 was co-administered with the selective group III metabotropic glutamate receptor antagonist (R,S)-alpha-methylserine-O-phosphate (MSOP), confirming a receptor-mediated mechanism of action. Whether the neuroprotective effect is due to reduction in glutamate release or due to possible glial cell-related mechanism which may involve increased glutamate uptake by astrocytes (Yao et al., 2005), or production of neurotrophic factors which limit nigrostriatal damage as reported by (Bruno et al., 1997, 1998; Ciccarelli et al., 1999; Matarredona et al., 2001).

It is known that LAP4 is a glutamate presynaptic agonist, with selective activity against group III receptors, and that it inhibits Ca^{++} uptake into presynaptic membranes and inhibits the release of glutamate and aspartate (Vazquez et al., 1995; Abdul-Ghani et al., 1997; Han et al., 2004 and Vernon et al., 2005), likely by negatively modulating voltage-dependent Ca^{++} channels and Ca^{++}-dependent neurotransmitter release (Conn & Pin 1997). These actions explain its anti-epileptogenic and anti-seizure activity, as reported by Abdul-Ghani et al., (1997), and its anti-Parkinsonian activity shown in the present paper. As long ago as 1996, Nicoletti et al suggested that pharmacological agents which reduce glutamate transmission in the basal ganglia might have a neuroprotective effect in patients with Parkinson's disease. The results we report here show that LAP4 is one such agent whose potential in controlling Parkinsonian features warrants further exploration.

5. Conclusion

Our results show that the glutamate metabotropic agonist LAP4 opposes the development of Parkinsonian features induced in rats by infusing 6-OHDA into the corpus striatum. Such agents may offer a non-dopaminergic method of treating Parkinson's disease.

6. Acknowledgement

This work was supported by a grant from the Academy for Educational Development (AED).

7. References

Abbott A, Wigmore M. A. and Lacey M. G. (1997). Excitation of rat sub-thalamic nucleus neurons in vitro by activation of a group I metabotropic glutamate receptor. *Brain Research* 766 (1-2) 162-167.

Abdul-Ghani, A-S., Attwell, P. J. E. Kent, N. S., Bradford, H. F., Croucher, M. J. and Jane, D. E. (1997a). Anti-epileptogenic and anti-convulsant activity of L-2-amino- 4-phosphonobutyrate, a presynaptic glutamate receptor agonist. *Brain Research,* 755, 202-212.

Bradford, H. F. (1995). Glutamate, GABA and Epilepsy. *Progress in Neurobiology.* 47, 477-511.

Bruno V., Sureda F.X., Storto M., Casabona G., Caruso A., Knopfel T., Kuhn R., Nicoletti F. (1998). The neuroprotective activity of group-II metabotropic glutamate receptors requires new protein synthesis and involves a glial neuronal signaling. *J. Neuroscience,* 17, 1891-1897.

Bruno V., Battaglia G., Casabona G., Copani A., Caciagli F., Nicoletti F. (1998). Neuroprotection by glial metabotropic glutamate receptors is mediated by transforming growth factor-β. *J. Neuroscience,* 18, 9594-9600.

Bruno V; Battaglia G; Ksiazek I; Van der Puten H; Catania MV; Giuffrida R; Lukic S; Leonhardt T; Inderbitzin W; Gasparini F; Kuhn R; Hampson D.R; Nicoletti F; Flor P.J (2000). Selective activation of mGlu4 metabotropic glutamate receptors is protective against excitotoxic neuronal death. *J. Neurosci* 20 :6413 – 6420.

Chaturvedi R.K; Shukla S; Seth K; Chauhan S; Sinha C; Shukla Y; Agrawal A.K. (2006) Neuroprotective and neurorescue effect of black tea extract in 6-OH dopamine-lesioned rat model of Parkinsons' disease. *Neurobiology of Disease.* 22; 421-434

Ciccarelli R., Di Iorio P., Bruno V., Battaglia G., D'Alimonte I., D'Onofrio M., Nicolotti F., Caciagli F., (1999). Activation of A1 adenosine or mGlu3 metabotropic glutamate receptors enhances the release of nerve growth factor and S-100β protein from cultured astrocytes. *Glia,* 27, 275-281.

Conn P.J., Pin J. (1997). Pharmacology and functions of metabotropic glutamate receptors. *Annu. Rev. Pharmacol. Toxicol. 37,* 205 -237.

Coutinho-Netto, J., Abdul-Ghani, A-S., Collins, J. F. and Bradford H. F (1981). Is glutamate a trigger factor in epileptic hyperactivity? *Epilepsia,* 22, 289-296.

Cuomo D., Martella G., Barabino E., Plantania P., Vita D., Madeo G., Selvam C., Goudet C., Oueslati N., Pin J.P., Acher F., Pisani A., Beurrier C., Melon C., Goff L.K., Gubellini P. (2009). Metabotropic glutamate receptor subtype 4 selectively modulates both glutamate and GABA transmission in striatum: implications for Parkinson's disease treatment. J. *Neurochemistry* 109; 1096-1105.

Gerlach M., Ben-Shacher, D., Riederer P. and Youdim, M. B. H. (1994). Alerted brain metabolism of iron as a cause of neurodegenerative diseases. *J. Neurochemistry,* 63, (3) 793-807.

Han J.S; Bird G.C; Neugebauer V (2004) Enhanced group III mGluR-mediated inhibition of pain-related synaptic plasticity in the amygdale. *Neuropharmacology* 46: 918-926.

Hugon J., Vallat J. M. and Dumas M. (1996). Role of glutamate and excitotoxicity in neurological diseases. *Rev. Neurol. (Paris)* 152 (4) 239-248.

Jane D.E; Pettaway K; Sunter D.C; Thomas N.K; Watkins J.C.(1995) New phenylglycine derivatives with potent and selective antagonist activity at presynaptic glutamate receptor in neonatal rat spinal cord. *Neuropharmacology* 34 : 851-656.

Jiang Q; Yan Z; Feng J. (2006) Activation of group III metabotropic glutamate receptors attenuates rotenone toxicity on dopaminergic neurons through a microtubule-dependent mechanism. *J. Neurosci.* 26 : 4318-4328.

Kaatz K. W. and Albin R. L. (1995). Intra-striatal and intra-subthalamic stimulation of metabotropic glutamate receptors. *Neuroscience* 66 (1) 55-65.

Kirik D; Rosenblad C; Bjorklund A (1998). Characterization of behavioral and neurodegenerative changes following partial lesions of the nigrostriatal dopamine system, induced by intra-striatal 6-hydroxydopamine in the rat. *Exp. Neurol.* 152 : 259-277

Lafon-Cazal M; Fagni L; Guiraud M.J; Mary S; Lerner-Natoli M; Pin J.P (1999) mGluR7-like metabotropic glutamate receptors inhibit NMDA-mediated excitotoxicity in cultured mouse cerebellar granule neurons. *Eur. J. Neurosci.* 11 :663-672.

Lopez S; Turle-Lorenzo N; Acher F; De Leonibus E; Mele A; Amalric M. (2007) Targeting group III metabotropic glutamate receptors produces complex behavioral effects in rodent models of Parkinsons disease. *J. Neuroscience* 27 (25): 6701 – 6711.

Matarredona E.R., Santiago M., Venero J.L., Cano J., Machado A. (2001)Group II metabotropic glutamate receptor activation protects striatal dopaminergic nerve terminals against MPPI-induced neurotoxicity along with brain-derived neurotrophic factor induction. *J. Neurochem,* 76, 351-360.

Murray T.K.; Messenger M.J; Ward M.A; Woodhouse S; Osbourne D.J; Duty S; ONiell M.J. (2002) Evaluation of the mGlu2/3 agonist LY379268 in rodent models of Parkinsons disease. *Pharmacol. Biochem. Behav.* 73 : 455-466.

Nicoletti F; Bruno V; Copani A; Casabona G; Knopfel T (1996) Metabotropic glutamate receptors: a new target for the therapy of neurodegenerative disorders? *Trends Neurosci.* 19 : 267-271.

Phillips JM, and Brown V.J (1999) Reaction time performance following unilateral striatal dopamine depletion and lesions of the subthalamic nucleus in the rat. *Eur. J. Neuroscience* 11: 1003-1010

Phillips J. M; Lam HA; Ackerson L.C; Maidment N.T (2006) Blockad of mGluR5 glutamate receptors in the sub-thalamic nucleus ameliorates motor asymmetry in an animal model of Parkinsons disease. *Eur. J. Neuroscience* 23, 151-160.

Sacaan A.I; Monn J.A; and Schoepp D.D (1991) Interstriatal injection of a selective metabotropic excitatory amino acid receptor agonist induces contralateral turning in the rat. *J. Pharmacol. Exp. Ther.* 259: 1366-1370.

Sacaan A. I; and Schoepp, D. D. (1992) Activation of hippocampal metabotropic excitatory amino acid receptors leads to seizures and neuronal damage. *Neurosci. Lett.* 139: 77-82

Snyder, S. H. and Bredt, D. S. (1992) . Biological roles of Nitric Oxide. *Scientific American* 68-77.

Troung L; Allbutt H; Kassiou M; Henderson J.M. (2006) Developing a pre-clinical model for parkinsons disease: A study of behaviour in rats with graded 6-OHDA lesions. *Behavioural Brain Res.* 169: 1-9.

Vazquez E; Budd D.C; Herrero I; Nicholls D.G; Sanchez-Prieto J. (1995) Co-existence and interaction between facilitatory and inhibitory metabotropic glutamate receptors and the inhibitory adenosine A receptor in cerebrocortical nerve terminals. *Neuropharmacol.* 34: 919-927.

Vernon A.C; Palmer S; Datla K.P; Zbarsky V; Croucher M.J; Dexter D.T. (2005) Neuroprotective effects of metabotropic glutamate receptor ligands in a 6-hydroxydopamine rodent model of Parkinsons disease. *Eur. J. Neurosciences* 22: 1799-1806.

Vernon A.C; Zbarsky V; Datla K.B; Dexter D.T ; Croucher M.J. (2007) Selective activation of group III metabotropic glutamate receptors by L-(+)-2-amino-4-phosphonobutyric acid protects the nigrostriatal system against 6-hydroxydopamine toxicity in vivo. *J. Pharmacol. Exper. Therap.* 320 (1) 397-409.

Wichman T; Marino M.J; Conn P.J. (2002) Dopamine modulates the function of group II and group III metabotropic glutamate receptors in the substansia nigra pars reticulate. *J. Pharmacol. Exp. Ther.* 302 : 433-441.

Wilkinski S. I. and Acosta G. B. (1995). Role of excitatory amino acids in neuropathology. *Medicina (B. Aires)* 55 (4) 355-365.

Willis G.L and Armstrong S.M (1999). A therapeutic role for melatonin antagonism in experimental models of Parkinsons disease. *Physiological Behavior,* 66: 785-795.

Willis G. L and Kennedy G. A (2004) The implementation of acute versus chronic animal models for treatment discovery in Parkinson's disease. *Reviews in the Neurosciences,* 15, 75-87

Yao H.H., Ding J.H., Zhou F., Wang F., Hu L.F., Sun T., Hu G. (2005). Enhancement of glutamate uptake mediated the neuroprotection exerted by activating group II or III metabotropic glutamate receptors on astrocytes. *J. Neurochem.* 92, 948-961.

Youdim M. B. H. Ben-Shacher, D. and Riederer, P. (1993). Iron-Melanin interaction and Parkinson's disease. *News in Physiological Sciences,* 8, 45-49.

10

GDNF and PD: Less Common Points of View

Ana Saavedra[1,2,3] and Graça Baltazar[4]
[1]*Departament de Biologia Cel·lular, Immunologia i Neurociències, Facultat de Medicina, Universitat de Barcelona, Barcelona,*
[2]*Institut d'Investigacions Biomèdiques August Pi i Sunyer (IDIBAPS), Barcelona,*
[3]*Centro de Investigación Biomédica en Red sobre Enfermedades Neurodegenerativas (CIBERNED),*
[4]*CICS-Centro de Investigação em Ciências da Saúde, Universidade da Beira Interior, Covilhã,*
[1,2,3]*Spain*
[4]*Portugal*

1. Introduction

Glial cell line-derived neurotrophic factor (GDNF) was identified in 1993 (Lin et al., 1993), and since then it has been considered a strong survival factor for dopaminergic neurons of the nigrostriatal pathway that degenerate in Parkinson's disease (PD). This has led to the proposal of GDNF as a potential therapy to slow down, halt or reverse neurodegeneration in PD. Thus, the link GDNF-PD is quite instantaneous, and difficult to keep away from. In this chapter we want to explore less common perspectives in this relationship, and we propose to look at this association from unconventional/emerging points of view, one might say, beyond the typical top10. We will discuss some aspects of PD pathophysiology and alternative therapeutic approaches in PD from a GDNF point of view.

Epidemiological studies show a greater prevalence of PD in men than in women, and there are also gender differences in the progression of the symptoms and responses to L-DOPA treatment (Miller & Cronin-Golomb, 2010). Although the reasons for these gender differences in PD remain to be elucidated, there is growing evidence that estrogen may play a role in this phenomenon. We will present evidences that GDNF may account for the neuroprotection of dopaminergic neurons promoted by estrogen and thereby help to explain the lower incidence of PD in women.

Neuroinflammation is recognized as a major factor in PD pathogenesis, and increasing evidence suggest that microglia is the main source of inflammation contributing to dopaminergic degeneration (Tansey & Goldberg, 2009). Astrocytes, on the other hand, can act as physiological regulators preventing excessive microglial responses (Lynch, 2009). We propose that GDNF can be a key player in astrocytes modulation of microglia activation in the *substantia nigra*. Therefore, a GDNF therapy to PD may not only act directly on dopaminergic neurons themselves, but also indirectly through the modulation of glial crosstalk and neuroinflammation.

Several attempts have been made to increase GDNF at lesion sites aiming at neuroprotection/neuroregeneration. However, the delivery of GDNF to the central nervous system (CNS) is challenging because GDNF is unable to cross the blood–brain barrier. One possibility to overcome this limitation is to conjugate or fuse GDNF with viral proteins, antibodies for transferrin or insulin receptors, or with a fragment of the tetanus toxin, which enable it to cross the blood–brain barrier. Another option is to use molecules that induce GDNF expression or enhance its signaling, and we will emphasize natural compounds. These molecules may prove to be an alternative therapeutic option for PD as herbal extracts are increasingly being reported to be neuroprotective in animal models of PD. Unconventional ways to increase GDNF levels in the brain include dietary manipulations, physical exercise, cognitive stimulation or acupuncture, and these may represent novel drug-free and non-invasive approaches for disease prevention and treatment, an issue that will also be addressed.

Neurodegenerative diseases are puzzling and there is still a long way before we can have answers to all our questions and concerns. In this chapter we hope to disclose new links between GDNF and the pathophysiology of PD, and bring together data that enable a new view on the protective actions of several compounds and lifestyles capable of modulating GDNF levels, which may have therapeutic implications. We believe that this chapter may help in some way to draw attention to new directions of research, and to explore the GDNF-PD route with new eyes.

2. Gender differences in PD

Epidemiological studies have suggested gender differences in PD risk, symptom severity, and treatment outcome (Miller & Cronin-Golomb, 2010). A higher prevalence of PD in men (Baldereschi et al., 2000; Kurtzke & Goldberg, 1988; Marder et al., 1996; Mayeux et al., 1992; Wooten et al., 2004), with a two-fold greater relative risk of PD in men than women (Gillies & McArthur, 2010b), were also reported. In what concerns symptom severity, males present worse rigidity, more frequent symptoms such as writing difficulties, fumblingness, speech and gait problems, whereas women exhibit more levodopa-induced dyskinesia (Miller & Cronin-Golomb, 2010). In addition, sex differences in response to anti-parkinsonism medications have also been reported (Brann et al., 2007). There is greater levodopa bioavailability in women, with higher plasma concentration, so the mean levodopa dosage is lower for women than for men (reviewed by Shulman, 2007). Furthermore, the treatment with levodopa promotes more significant improvements of motor function in women than in men (reviewed by Brann et al., 2007).

While the reason for the sex differences in PD remains to be elucidated, there is growing evidence that estrogen may play a neuroprotective role. This hypothesis is also supported by data showing that shorter exposures to estrogen during life, including fertile life length shorter than 36 years, and cumulative length of pregnancies longer than 30 months, are associated with younger age at onset of PD. In contrast, the use of postmenopausal estrogen replacement therapy seems to reduce the risk of developing the disease (Currie et al., 2004). Also supportive of the protective role of estrogen are data showing that situations corresponding to low endogenous estrogen levels, such onset of menses and menopause or withdrawal of hormone replacement therapy, result in a worsening of parkinsonian symptoms (Gillies & McArthur, 2010b). In contrast, the results obtained in gonadectomized adult male rats and mice exposed to testosterone and dihydrotestosterone indicate that androgens repress the expression of a midbrain dopaminergic phenotype (M.L. Johnson et al., 2010).

In addition to the pro-dopaminergic action of estrogen, an increasing amount of evidence suggests an inherent sex dimorphism in the nigrostriatal pathway. *In vivo* real-time imaging techniques in healthy humans showed greater amphetamine-stimulated striatal dopamine release in men than in women (Munro et al., 2006), and significantly higher striatal 18F-fluorodopa uptake in women (Laakso et al., 2002). Moreover, it has been shown that the activation of estrogen receptors induces differentiation of human neural stem cells, giving rise to dopaminergic neurons (Diaz et al., 2009), a process that may facilitate the replacement of neurons in the course of the disease progression. In addition, the healthy male nigrostriatal dopaminergic pathway expresses higher levels of genes implicated in PD pathogenesis such as α-synuclein and PTEN-induced putative kinase 1 (PINK-1) (Cantuti-Castelvetri et al., 2007).

2.1 Estrogen-mediated neuroprotection in PD models

17β-estradiol, the estrogen stereoisomer with female hormone activity and with high affinity to estrogen receptors, has been shown, both *in vitro* and *in vivo*, at least in female rodents, to protect dopaminergic neurons from different toxic insults such as 6-hydroxydopamine (6-OHDA) (Murray et al., 2003), 1-methyl-4-phenyl-1,2,3,6-tetrahydropyridine (MPTP) or methamphetamine (Bourque et al., 2009). In MPTP mouse models of PD, 17β-estradiol prevents the depletion of striatal dopamine, the reduction of dopamine transporter (DAT) binding and expression, and the decrease of tyrosine hydroxylase (TH)-immunoreactive cells (Callier et al., 2001; D'Astous et al., 2004; Dluzen et al., 1996; Jourdain et al., 2005; Ramirez et al., 2003). Moreover, male mice have been reported to be more sensitive to the toxicity induced by MPTP or methamphetamine than female mice (Bourque et al., 2009). In addition, 17β-estradiol was also shown to be protective against superoxide-, H_2O_2- or glutamate-induced neurotoxicity in primary neuronal mesencephalic cultures (Sawada et al., 1998).

Most studies on the neuroprotective effects of 17β-estradiol have been developed in female rodents, and the results on the protective effects of estrogen in male rodents are still controverse (Bourque et al., 2009; Murray et al., 2003). Both the dose of the hormone and the time of administration in relation to the lesion induction seem to be determinant to the results achieved. Although there are reports showing that 17β-estradiol therapy reduces dopaminergic lesion in females but not in males (Bourque et al., 2009; B. Liu & Dluzen, 2007), recent results from our group show that 17β-estradiol, administered to male rats at a dose regimen that mimics the female physiological levels of the steroid protects dopaminergic cells from a mild lesion induced by intrastriatal administration of 6-OHDA (De Campos et al., 2010). The discrepancies between the results obtained in different studies may also be influenced by differences in the lesion model/volume, or the use of intact or gonadectomized animals, thus altering the contribution of androgens.

2.2 Estrogen receptors involved in the neuroprotection of dopaminergic neurons

The expression of estrogen receptors (ERs) in the *substantia nigra* and striatum, as assessed by *in situ* hybridization, autoradiography, immunohistochemistry or Western blot analysis, has been reported as sparse or absent (Gillies & McArthur, 2010a). ERβ has been reported to be absent from the male mouse *substantia nigra,* and ERα expression was shown not to colocalize with TH (Gillies & McArthur, 2010a). Moreover, in rodents the striatum seems to lack ERβ, whereas ERα is present at low levels, although possibly at higher levels in female compared with male mice (Rodriguez-Navarro et al., 2008). Nevertheless, the modulation of dopamine D2 receptors and DAT by 17β-estradiol has been suggested to involve ERβ, whereas studies using selective ER ligands favor a role for ERα over ERβ in mediating estrogenic neuroprotection (Morissette et al., 2008). Taken together, the results may also suggest that the effect of 17β-estradiol on the nigrostriatal pathway could involve alternative targets (Dluzen, 2005).

It is now well documented that estrogen produces its effects by classic (also called genomic) and non-classic (or non-genomic) actions. The classic pathway involves the activation of intracellular receptors and the regulation of gene transcription. The non-classical pathway is generally associated with more rapid effects (from seconds to minutes) and is initiated by the interaction of 17β-estradiol with receptors in the plasma membrane (Bourque et al., 2009). In the brain, the actions of 17β-estradiol mediated through membrane-associated receptors involve the activation of two different signaling pathways, the mitogen-activated protein kinase (MAPK) and the phosphatidylinositol-3 kinase (PI3-K)/Akt pathway (Morissette et al., 2008).

2.3 Contribution of GDNF to estrogen-mediated neuroprotection

The interactions between 17β-estradiol and neurotrophic factors, namely the ability of the former to regulate the expression of neurotrophic factors such as brain-derived neurotrophic factor (BDNF), insulin-like growth factor-I (IGF-I), artemin, their receptors or signaling pathways, are well documented (Dittrich et al., 1999; Garcia-Segura et al., 2007; Ivanova et al., 2001; J. Kang et al., 2010; Pan et al., 2010; Pietranera et al., 2010; J. Zhou et al., 2005). The expression of GDNF is also modulated by estrogens. As mentioned above, 17β-estradiol, through membrane-associated receptors, can activate the PI3-K/Akt pathway and regulate transcription factors such as NF-kB and cAMP response element binding protein (CREB) (Bourque et al., 2009), which are known to be involved in the control of GDNF expression (Saavedra et al., 2008). 17β-estradiol induces the expression of GDNF in spinal cord astrocyte cultures, and this increase in GDNF rescues spinal motoneurons from AMPA-induced toxicity (Platania et al., 2005). In hypothalamic cultures, 17β-estradiol up-regulates the expression of GDNF in neurons but not in astrocytes (Ivanova et al., 2002). These observations suggest a region-dependent effect on the cell type responsible for GDNF production in response to 17β-estradiol, which may be related to the presence/absence of estrogen receptors in different cell types depending on their location.

The induction of GDNF expression by 17β-estradiol in hypothalamic cell cultures is not prevented by the nuclear receptor antagonist ICI 182,780, indicating that it is mediated by non-classical estrogen signaling. In contrast, it is inhibited by cAMP/PKA and calcium signaling antagonists, suggesting that intracellular calcium and cAMP/PKA signaling are required for GDNF increase in neuronal cells in response to 17β-estradiol. GDNF regulation by 17β-estradiol was also investigated in neonatal astroglial and embryonic mesencephalic neuronal cultures (Kipp et al., 2006). In this case, the up-regulation of GDNF transcription occurs in astrocytes but not in neurons, and the effect is not prevented by ICI 182,780, but is abrogated by interrupting the intracellular calcium signaling or the MAPK signal transduction system (Kipp et al., 2006). In addition, unpublished results from our group show that 17β-estradiol up-regulates GDNF levels in neuron-glia ventral midbrain postnatal cultures, and potentiates the reported L-DOPA- or H_2O_2-induced GDNF up-regulation in the same model (Saavedra et al., 2005, 2006). Estradiol-induced increase of GDNF levels is not blocked by ICI 182,780, and can be induced by estradiol-BSA, a membrane impermeable form, thus supporting the idea that 17β-estradiol is acting through a non-classical pathway (Fig. 1). Although GDNF up-regulation occurs in astrocytes, it is dependent on the presence of neurons indicating that neurons play a crucial role in the signaling process. GDNF neutralization and siRNA-mediated GDNF knockdown experiments clearly demonstrate the participation of this GDNF up-regulation in the neuroprotection provided by 17β-estradiol in 6-OHDA-challenged cultures (De Campos et al., 2010).

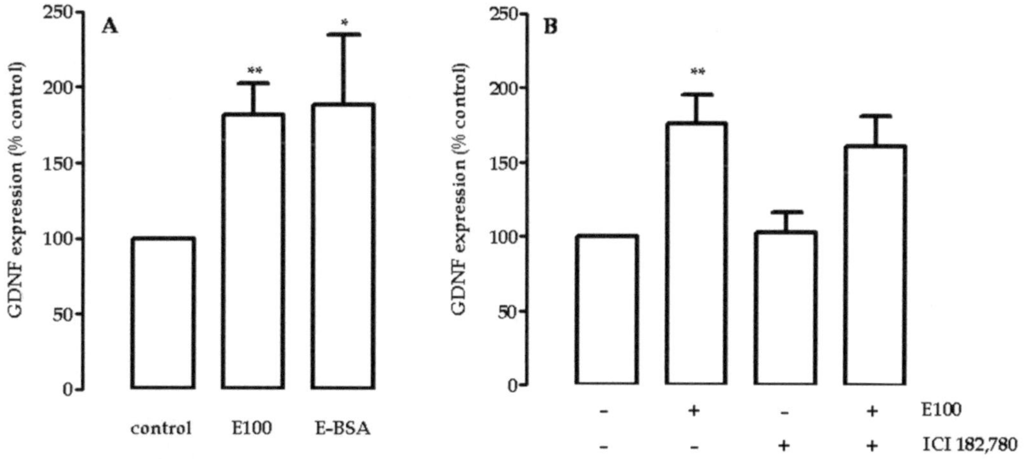

Fig. 1. Contribution of membrane and intracellular estrogen receptors to 17β-estradiol-induced GDNF expression in *substantia nigra* cultures. Cells were incubated for 48 h with 100 nM 17β-estradiol (E100) or with 10 nM membrane-impermeable conjugate estradiol-BSA (E-BSA) **(A)**, or with 100 nM 17β-estradiol in the absence (-) or presence (+) of 10 mM ICI 182,780, a specific blocker of intracellular estrogen receptors **(B)**. Cell extracts were prepared for Western blot analysis of GDNF levels. Data shown are the mean ± S.E.M. of up to nine independent experiments performed in triplicate. Statistical analysis was performed using one-way ANOVA followed by Dunnett's (A) or Bonferroni's test (B). $^{*}P < 0.05$ and $^{**}P < 0.01$ as compared to control.

2.4 Does GDNF contribute to the antioxidant actions of estrogen?

Oxidative stress is considered an important contributor to the neurodegeneration associated with PD, and several markers of oxidative damage are increased in the *substantia nigra pars compacta* of PD patients (Jenner, 2003; Przedborski & Ischiropoulos, 2005). The antioxidant properties of estradiol have long been recognized (Mooradian, 1993), and have been related with the hydroxyl group in the C3 position on the A ring of the steroid structure (Behl et al., 1997). The ability of estrogen to potently restrain free radical production provides an additional mechanism for estrogen-mediated neuroprotection in PD. Accordingly, estradiol suppresses oxidative stress and protects neuronal cells from death induced by oxidant agents (Behl et al., 1997; Mooradian, 1993; Sawada et al., 1998). Interestingly, the ability of GDNF to protect dopaminergic neurons has also been related with antioxidant properties involving the up-regulation of the antioxidant enzymes glutathione peroxidase, superoxide dismutase and catalase (Chao & Lee, 1999; Cheng et al., 2004). Since one of the mechanisms responsible for the neuroprotective effects of estradiol is a reduction in oxidative stress, and the protective effects of GDNF involve a decrease in oxidative stress (M.P. Smith & Cass, 2007), it is tempting to speculate that GDNF may contribute to 17β-estradiol-induced reduction of oxidative stress. Indeed, in a recent work from our group we demonstrate that pre-treatment with 17β-estradiol, which increases GDNF expression, completely prevents the increase of 4-hydroxynonenal levels induced by 6-OHDA in the *substantia nigra* (De Campos et al., 2010).

2.5 Anti-apoptotic role of estrogen

Oxidative stress can cause neuronal apoptosis (Ratan et al., 1994; Tan et al., 1998) and has been considered as one of the major causes of dopaminergic degeneration (Mochizuki et al., 1996; Przedborski & Ischiropoulos, 2005). The neuroprotection mediated by estrogen involves the modulation of apoptosis-related genes (Garcia-Segura et al., 1998; Singer et al., 1998; Vegeto et al., 1999). Sawada and colleagues (2000) studied the anti-apoptotic mechanism induced by estradiol on nigral dopaminergic neurons. They show that estradiol suppresses gene transcription through the AP-1 element, inhibits the transcription of pro-apoptotic genes, and up-regulates the anti-apoptotic Bcl-2, with the consequent reduction of caspase activation. Interestingly, GDNF is able to support the viability of postnatal nigral dopaminergic neurons and embryonic human mesencephalic neurons by inhibiting apoptotic cell death naturally occurring *in vitro* (Burke et al., 1998; Clarkson et al., 1997). Moreover, GDNF also attenuates 6-OHDA- (Ding et al., 2004), bleomycin sulfate- and L-buthionine-[S,R]-sulfoximine-induced apoptosis in cultured dopaminergic neurons (Sawada et al., 2000b). Recent results from our group show a reduction in the number of annexin V-positive dopaminergic neurons in the *substantia nigra* of animals treated with 17β-estradiol before 6-OHDA injection compared with animals injected with 6-OHDA alone (De Campos et al., 2010). Since 17β-estradiol treatment increases GDNF levels in these animals, one may hypothesize that GDNF up-regulation contributes to the anti-apoptotic effect of 17β-estradiol treatment upon a 6-OHDA challenge.

2.6 Anti-inflammatory role of estrogen and dopaminergic neuroprotection

Estrogens control glial activation and the expression of inflammatory mediators implicated in neuroinflammation and neurodegeneration, such as cytokines and chemokines (reviewed by Morale et al., 2006). 17β-estradiol down-regulates glial activation promoted by MPTP in the *substantia nigra* and striatum (Tripanichkul et al., 2006), and it is also able to prevent the increase in the levels of inflammatory mediators, such as the inducible form of nitric oxide synthase (NOS) in response to lipopolysaccharide (LPS), a component of the cell wall of gram-negative bacteria (Vegeto et al., 2001). Activation of ERs in microglial cells blocks nitric oxide (NO) production (Vegeto et al., 2001) and prevents toxicity in mesencephalic neuronal cultures exposed to conditioned medium from LPS-activated microglia (Block & Hong, 2005). In mesencephalic cultures, 17β-estradiol inhibits microglial activation and promotes neuroprotective effects through the activation of both ERα and ERβ (X. Liu et al., 2005). Therefore, estrogens were suggested to promote the switch of microglia from a neurotoxic to a neuroprotective state (Morale et al., 2006). GDNF may also contribute to the anti-inflammatory activity of estrogen. Indeed, we have shown the effectiveness of GDNF in maintaining microglia in a resting state (Rocha et al., 2010). Moreover, Xing and collegues (2010), using midbrain slice cultures, demonstrated that GDNF can inhibit both LPS-induced microglia activation and dopaminergic cell death (see more details in the next section).

3. The vigilant glia

Microglia are the surveillance cells in the CNS, exquisitely sensitive to brain injury and disease, altering their morphology and phenotype to adopt an activated state in response to pathophysiological brain insults. In the adult healthy brain, the majority of microglia is in a "resting" state, monitoring for pathogens and changes in the surrounding microenvironment. Neurons express cell-surface ligands that interact with receptors on the surface of microglia to induce these highly specialized cells to adopt a resting phenotype. For example, CD200 expressed by neurons binds to its receptor CD200R on the microglial cell surface. The regulatory role of CD200-CD200R signaling has been compared to a "break" on innate immunity (X.J. Wang et al., 2007). Moderately activated microglia plays a homeostatic role in the CNS by scavenging neurotoxins, removing dying cells and cellular debris, and promoting collateral sprouting through the release of trophic factors (Block et al., 2007). The designation "activated microglia" comprises highly plastic cells with numerous functionally distinct phenotypes that are not readily apparent from either their morphology or from a limited number of cell-surface antigens that they are known to express (Perry et al., 2010).

3.1 Protective microglia

In the nigrostriatal system, activated microglia and macrophages promote axonal growth and sprouting of dopaminergic neurons after a mechanical lesion to the striatum (Batchelor et al., 1999). After striatal injury, sprouting dopaminergic fibers grow towards and surround macrophages expressing GDNF and BDNF mRNA (Batchelor et al., 1999). The dopaminergic sprouting after striatal injury was shown to involve the production of GDNF by macrophages at the wound site, since preventing GDNF expression with antisense oligonucleotides resulted in a marked decrease in the intensity of the periwound sprouting as revealed by immunohistochemistry and activity of DAT (Batchelor et al., 2000). Moreover, dopaminergic sprouting was related to a gradient of GDNF (Batchelor et al., 2002). These data clearly show that activated microglia and macrophages induce dopaminergic sprouting through synthesis of neurotrophic factors. Interleukin-1 (IL-1) is also involved in dopaminergic sprouting since IL-1 receptor knockout mice do not show neuronal sprouting after a 6-OHDA lesion (Parish et al., 2002). IL-1, produced by reactive microglia and macrophages, induces astrogliosis. Therefore, activated microglia and macrophages appear to stimulate dopaminergic sprouting both directly, by the secretion of neurotrophic factors, and indirectly by the secretion of IL-1 and the stimulation of reactive astrocytosis (Ho & Blum, 1998; Parish et al., 2002). Furthermore, a protective role of microglia in the dopaminergic system was also suggested by results showing that striatal injection of 6-OHDA increases the number of neuron/glial 2 (NG2) cells coexpressing the microglia marker Iba1 and GDNF, both in the striatum and *substantia nigra*. Morevover, 64% of the surviving TH-positive cells are localized in the vicinity of NG2/Iba1/GDNF-positive cells (Kitamura et al., 2010). In addition to the production of GDNF by activated microglia and macrophages upon a mechanical injury to the striatum (Batchelor et al., 1999; Liberatore et al., 1997), it was also described to occur in the injured spinal cord (Satake et al., 2000; Widenfalk et al., 2001), and in cultured macrophages (Hashimoto et al., 2005). Ischemia also induces microglia in cerebral cortex to express GDNF (Wei et al., 2000a). Besides, blockade of ischemia-induced microglia activation leads to a decrease in GDNF production and, in parallel, to a decrease in the expression of the neuronal plasticity proteins synaptophysin and GAP-43, which may indicate a contribution of microglia to brain plasticity (Madinier et al., 2009). Similarly, increased expression of BDNF by microglial cells may contribute to the axonal regeneration after mesencephalic trigeminal nerve injury (Ichikawa et al., 2011). A neuroprotective role of microglia against excitotoxic stimuli was also suggested by results showing that stimulation of microglia with glutamate receptor agonists induces the expression of GDNF, BDNF and nerve growth factor (NGF) (J. Liang et al., 2010).

3.2 PD and neuroinflammation: a toxic version of microglia

Neuroinflammation is a pathological hallmark in patients and experimental models of PD. Both present the classical features of inflammation, with evidence of an uncontrolled process. Moreover, microglia may become activated early in the disease process and remain primed, responding strongly to subsequent stimuli, and thereby enhancing inflammation-induced oxidative stress and cytokine-dependent toxicity in vulnerable neuronal populations (Halliday & Stevens, 2011). In PD, for unknown reasons microglia become persistently overactivated, leading to the overproduction of cytokines (e.g. tumour necrosis factor (TNF)-α, IL-1β and IL-6), and other pro-inflammatory mediators, as well as the release of reactive oxygen species (ROS) (Y.S. Kim & Joh, 2006). A high number of activated microglia has been found in the *substantia nigra pars compacta* of post-mortem PD patients, in the vicinity of the degenerating dopaminergic neurons (Tansey & Goldberg, 2009). Additionally, elevated concentrations of IL-2, IL-6 and TNF-α in the serum, and of IL-6 and IL-1β in the cerebrospinal fluid have been reported in PD patients (E.C. Hirsch & Hunot, 2009). These observations, together with positron emission tomography (PET) imaging studies, support a role for neuroinflammation in PD that appears early and persists throughout the disease course (Tansey & Goldberg, 2009). However, microglial activation in PD is not limited to the *substantia nigra*, and is also found in the putamen, hippocampus, transenthorinal cortex, cingulate cortex and temporal cortex (Block et al., 2007). The selective loss of dopaminergic neurons from the *substantia nigra* might be due to their glutathione deficiency, high content of dopamine, elevated iron concentrations and increased number of microglia in the *substantia nigra* compared with other regions. Therefore, dopaminergic neurons in the *substantia nigra* might be particularly vulnerable to inflammatory insults owing to their precarious redox equilibrium and the large neighboring population of microglia (Block et al., 2007). Indeed, a great body of evidence supports the role of microglia in the degeneration of dopaminergic neurons. In the MPTP mouse model, inhibition of microglial activation with minocycline decreases dopaminergic death (Y. He et al., 2001; D.C. Wu et al., 2002), and neuronal death is greatly diminished in mutant mice deficient in NOS (Dehmer et al., 2000; Liberatore et al., 1999), or deficient in NADPH-oxidase, the enzyme that catalyzes the production of superoxide (D.C. Wu et al., 2003). Moreover, a model of PD was created by infusing LPS in the *substantia nigra*, which activates microglial cells and selectively kills dopaminergic neurons (Block & Hong, 2005). In cell culture models, dopaminergic cell death induced by 1-methyl-4-phenylpyridinium (MPP^+) is greatly reduced in neuron-enriched cultures as compared to neuron-glia cultures, and the addition of microglia to neuron-enriched cultures restablishes MPP^+-induced dopaminergic death (Block & Hong, 2005). The detrimental role of microglia in PD has lead to an attempt of using anti-inflammatory therapies in the treatment of PD (E.C. Hirsch & Hunot, 2009).

3.3 Role of GDNF in controlling microglia activation

Consistent with the role of microglia in the pathogenesis and progression of PD, it has been demonstrated that an attenuation of dopaminergic neurodegeneration may be achieved by regulating microglial activation. There is a good deal of evidence suggesting that astrocytes are capable of reducing the potentially damaging effects of microglia. One of the mechanisms may be through the regulation of microglial expression of the antioxidant enzyme heme oxygenase-1 (HO-1) (Min et al., 2006). Astrocytes are also able to reduce LPS-induced NOS expression and NO production by microglia (Lynch, 2009). Besides, coculture with astrocytes or exposure to astrocyte conditioned media has been shown to reduce microglial phagocytic activity, and the production of IL-12 induced by LPS or interferon (IFN)-γ (Lynch, 2009). Astrocyte-derived transforming growth factor (TGF)-β and IL-10 are known to suppress microglial activation (Y.S. Kim & Joh, 2006). Recent work from our group has shown that soluble mediators released by cultured ventral midbrain astrocytes are able to prevent microglial activation induced by the pro-inflammatory agent Zymosan A (Rocha et al., 2010). We have found that low molecular weight (< 10 kDa) astrocyte-derived soluble mediators, including metallothionein-I/II, a small astrocytic protein with protective roles in the CNS, are able to suppress microglial activation induced by 0.5 μg/mL Zymosan A (Fig. 2). However, when a higher concentration of Zymosan A was used (5 μg/mL), these low molecular weight mediators were insufficient to prevent microglial activation. Under these conditions, we found that among three neurotrophic factors expressed by midbrain astrocytes (GDNF, cerebral dopamine neurotrophic factor (CDNF) and BDNF), only GDNF was able to modulate microglial activation induced by 5 μg/mL Zymosan A. This result was confirmed using several approaches, namely GDNF neutralization experiments, GDNF silencing in astrocyte cultures, and exogenous addition of GDNF to non-conditioned astrocyte culture media. Our results also show that the action of GDNF in microglial cells depends on GDNF family receptor (GFR)α1 (Rocha et al., 2010), a component of the receptor complex that can comprise also the transmembrane Ret tyrosine kinase or the neural cell adhesion molecule (NCAM) (Ibanez, 2010). Thus, the binding of astrocyte-derived GDNF to microglial GFRα1 receptors activates intracellular signaling cascade(s) responsible for inhibiting microglial activation. Our results are in accordance with the finding that exogenous GDNF inhibits LPS-induced increase of NO production and in the number of OX-6-positive cells in the *substantia nigra* in a cortex-striatum-midbrain organotypic culture (Xing et al., 2010), and also with the increased microglial activation observed in the *substantia nigra*, but not in the striatum, of GDNF heterozygous mice (Boger et al., 2010). It was also shown that the anticonvulsant and mood stabilizer valproate, and other histone deacetylase inhibitors, which increase the expression of GDNF and BDNF in astrocytes (P.S. Chen et al., 2006), are capable of reducing microglial activation (Peng et al., 2005; X. Wu et al., 2008).

This regulation of microglial activation by GDNF is of particular interest since GDNF is a potent neurotrophic factor for dopaminergic neurons in the nigrostriatal pathway (Duarte et al., 2007). Previous studies from our group have shown that upon neuronal injury, astrocytic expression of GDNF is increased as a neuroprotective strategy (Saavedra et al., 2006). Astrocytic GDNF up-regulation was found to involve the release of soluble mediators, namely IL-1β, that signal ventral midbrain astrocytes to increase GDNF expression (Saavedra et al., 2007). Furthermore, we have found that injured nigral neurons trigger GDNF up-regulation in striatal cells (Fig. 3), a mechanism that can be relevant to the neuroprotection of dopaminergic terminals in the striatum. Altogether, these data raise the hypothesis that the neuroprotective effect of GDNF in the nigrostriatal system can result not only from a direct effect on dopaminergic neurons, but also from an indirect action through the modulation of glial crosstalk and the neuroinflammatory cascade occurring in PD.

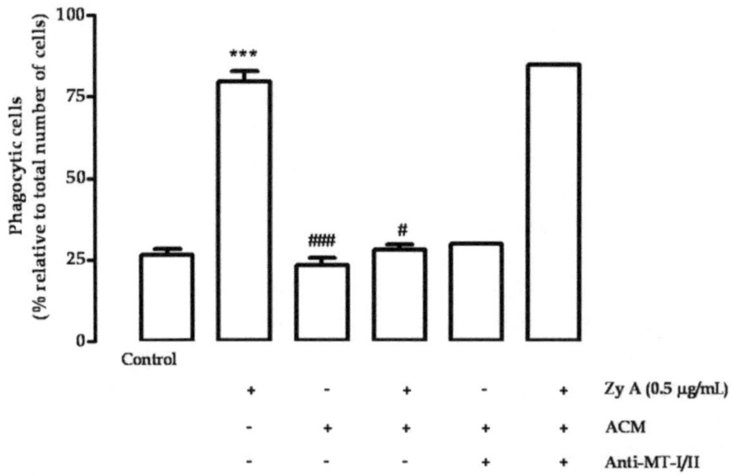

Fig. 2. Quantification of the number of phagocytic cells in *substantia nigra* microglia control cultures and in cultures incubated for 24 h with a low molecular weight fraction (< 10 kDa) of ventral midbrain astrocyte conditioned media (ACM), prior to exposure to 0.5 mg/mL Zymosan A (ZyA) for an additional period of 24 h. The effects of blocking the action of metalothionein (MT)-I/II present in ACM using a specific antibody (anti-MT-I/II; 1:1000; Dako), prior to exposure to 0.5 mg/mL ZyA, are presented. Data shown are the mean ± S.E.M. of up to four independent experiments performed in triplicate. Statistical analysis was performed using one-way ANOVA followed by Bonferroni's test. *** $P < 0.001$ as compared to control; # $P < 0.05$ and ### $P < 0.001$ as compared to ZyA.

Interestingly, inflammatory stimuli are among the candidate signals involved in the intercellular talk that induces glial GDNF expression after injury. Indeed, elevated GDNF expression is observed in response to LPS and to the pro-inflammatory cytokines IL-1β, IL-6, TNF-α and TNF-β in C6 cells (Appel et al., 1997; Verity et al., 1998), and in U-87MG glioblastoma cells (Verity et al., 1999). In cultured astrocytes both exogenous TNF-α, via TNF receptors, and endogenously produced TNF-α induce GDNF expression suggesting that an autocrine loop contributes to the production of neurotrophic factors in response to inflammation (Kuno et al., 2006). In contrast, TNF-α, TNF-β, IL-1β and LPS repress GDNF release in SK-N-AS neuroblastoma cells (Verity et al., 1999). Therefore, it has been proposed that GDNF synthesis and release in response to inflammatory molecules may be differentially regulated in cells of glial and neuronal phenotype (Verity et al., 1999). LPS also increases GDNF secretion (McNaught & Jenner, 2000) as well as GDNF mRNA expression in rodent primary astrocyte cultures (Kuno et al., 2006; Remy et al., 2003). *In vivo*, a high-dose of LPS, rather than a low dose, improves locomotor function after spinal cord injury in rats consistent with GDNF expression in microglia/macrophages (Hashimoto et al., 2005). This

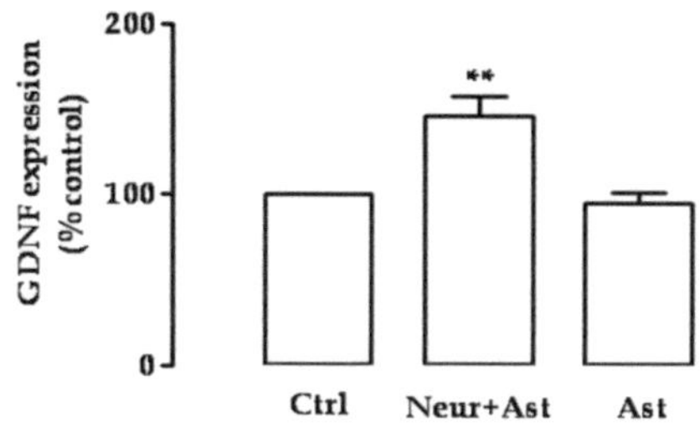

Fig. 3. GDNF expression in striatal cultures exposed to conditioned media from H_2O_2-challenged nigral mixed cultures (Neur+Ast) or ventral midbrain astrocyte cultures (Ast). Ventral midbrain astrocytes or nigral neuron-glial cells were exposed to 50 mM H_2O_2 or vehicle (control - Ctrl) for 1 h. The conditioned media were transferred to striatal cultures for 24 h and cell extracts were prepared for Western blot analysis of GDNF levels. Data shown are the mean ± S.E.M. of up to seven independent experiments performed in triplicate. Statistical analysis was performed using one-way ANOVA followed by Dunnett's test. $^{**}P < 0.01$ as compared to control.

suggests that repair of CNS injuries can occur through GDNF produced by activated microglia/macrophages. Summarizing, growing evidence indicates that microglial activation promotes GDNF expression, and more recent data indicate that GDNF in turn inhibits microglia reactivity which may indicate that GDNF is involved in a process that self-limits microglial neurotoxicity, thus avoiding neuronal injury. These observations lead us to propose that this process to control microglia activation via GDNF fails in PD, and highlight the importance of better understanding the mechanisms implicated in the control of microglia activation by GDNF, and whether changes in these processes occur during the progression of PD.

4. Treating PD with neurotrophic factors: the GDNF candidate

Neurotrophic factors have emerged as key factors in the survival and phenotypic differentiation of neuronal cells during development, in the maintenance of mature neurons in the adult, as well as in their protection/repair upon injury (Benn & Woolf, 2004). It was proposed that changes in the levels of neurotrophic factors, due to alterations in the synthesis, release or activity associated with aging or genetic factors, might be involved in the neuronal loss observed in neurodegenerative diseases as PD (Mattson & Magnus, 2006; Siegel & Chauhan, 2000). The last years have registered increasing interest in the application of neurotrophic factors to the therapeutic field, and PD is a neurodegenerative disease whose treatment with trophic factors has been the focus of extensive research. The potential of GDNF, the prototypical neurotrophic factor for dopaminergic neurons, as a neuroprotective and neurorestorative agent to slow down or halt PD progression, has been vastly debated in the last years (e.g. Aron & Klein, 2011; Evans & Barker, 2008; Hong et al., 2008; Peterson & Nutt, 2008; Ramaswamy et al., 2009; Vastag, 2010).

It has been proposed that those neurons more vulnerable in PD *substantia nigra* (ventral tier *versus* dorsal tier) display an increased expression of proteins that may contribute to vulnerability, together with a deficient expression of neuroprotective molecules. Interestingly, GDNF is among the neurotrophic factors whose differential pattern of expression between the ventral and the dorsal tiers of the *substantia nigra* might account for their distinct vulnerability in PD (Double et al., 2010). GDNF mRNA levels are significantly higher in the ventral striatum, the target region of the ventral tegmental area (VTA) and rostromedial *substantia nigra* cells, than in the dorsal striatum, the target region of dopaminergic neurons from the caudoventral *substantia nigra* (Barroso-Chinea et al., 2005). This correlates with VTA and rostromedial *substantia nigra* cells being more resistant to 6-OHDA toxicity than dopaminergic neurons from the caudoventral *substantia nigra* as occurs in PD (Barroso-Chinea et al., 2005), and supports the idea that the heterogeneous expression of GDNF is a factor involved in the differential vulnerability of midbrain dopaminergic neurons in PD.

Post-mortem studies investigating GDNF distribution in the human parkinsonian brain have yielded conflicting results (Saavedra et al., 2008), and clinical trials performed in advanced PD patients have generated quite disappointing outcomes (see below, 4.1 Clinical trials using GDNF), but many studies in animal models show that GDNF delivery can have trophic effects and restore motor function (Soderstrom et al., 2006). Additionally, GDNF is essential for the maintenance of adult nigrostriatal dopaminergic neurons and other central and peripheral nuclei affected in PD (Pascual et al., 2008). Therefore, the idea of using GDNF as a neuroprotective/neurorestorative therapy for PD is still being pursuited.

Mesencephalic astrocyte-derived neurotrophic factor (MANF), identified as selectively trophic for dopaminergic neurons *in vitro* (Petrova et al., 2003), and CDNF, which exhibits trophic and neurorestorative effects as potent as GDNF both *in vitro* and *in vivo* (Lindholm et al., 2007), might also be relevant targets for the development of alternative or complementary therapeutic approaches for PD.

4.1 Clinical trials using GDNF

Several clinical trials have been performed using the direct intracerebral infusion of GDNF. Despite the extensive literature supporting the neuroprotective role of GDNF on the nigrostriatal pathway most of the clinical trials performed in advanced PD patients have generated rather disappointing results (Aron & Klein, 2011).

The first clinical trial consisted in a randomized controlled trial using recombinant GDNF (r-metHuGDNF, Liatermin®, Amgen) and placebo delivered monthly as bolus via an intraventricular (ICV) catheter to patients with idiopathic PD (Nutt et al., 2003). No clinical benefits were registered at doses sufficient to induce side effects, and the post-mortem analysis of one patient revelead no evidence of rescue of dopaminergic fibers in the striatum or cells in the *substantia nigra* suggesting that insufficient GDNF reached its targets after ICV injection (Nutt et al., 2003). The following clinical trials addressed this issue by using continuous intraputaminal GDNF infusion. In an open-label clinical trial performed on five PD patients, Gill et al. (2003) reported excellent tolerance, few side effects, a significant decrease in total Unified Parkinson's Disease Rating Score (UPDRS) in the 'off' state, elimination of severe akinetic episodes, significant reduction of dyskinesias and improvements in quality of life. 18F-dopa PET scanning showed a significant increase in the uptake around the infusion site and in the *substantia nigra*. A report on one patient autopsied 43 months later showed evident increased TH-positive nerve fibers in the infused putamen indicating that GDNF stimulated axonal sprouting (Love et al., 2005). An independent open-label clinical trial using a different delivery protocol performed unilaterally on ten PD patients also reported positive results at six months and minimal side effects (Slevin et al., 2005). These promising results lead to the design of a randomized placebo-controlled trial involving 34 PD patients. Nevertheless, no significant clinical differences were detected at six months between patients receiving GDNF or placebo (Lang et al., 2006), and the open-label extension of the study was interrupted because three patients developed neutralizing antibodies, which could potentially cross-react with endogenous GDNF (Tatarewicz et al., 2007). Moreover, a parallel toxicologic study showed that infusion of GDNF into the putamen induced cerebellar damage in some monkeys (Hovland et al., 2007).

The overall discouraging results from these clinical trials may be related to poor diffusion of GDNF, the development of anti-GDNF antibodies, or other unindentified effects, while the different outcomes have been proposed to rely on differences in GDNF doses or catheter properties, patient cohort selection, or the choice of unsuitable endpoints, with suboptimal brain delivery of GDNF considered the major limiting factor (Aron & Klein, 2011; Sherer et al., 2006).

A phase I trial involving the delivery of neurturin, another member of the GDNF family, to the striatum of PD patients via adeno-associated virus (AAV) vector showed tolerability, safety, and also potential efficacy (Marks et al., 2008), and a phase II trial was carried out. In this clinical trial there was no significant difference in the UPDRS motor score at 12 months between patients treated with AAV2-neurturin compared with control individuals, and some patients developed tumours (Marks et al., 2010). Currently, a new trial involving the delivery of a four-fold higher dose of AAV2-neurturin to both the putamen and *substantia nigra* is ongoing (Vastag, 2010).

4.2 The ups and downs of GDNF

Although GDNF overexpression is neuroprotective, uncontrolled GDNF levels could lead to unexpected side effects. High doses of exogenously delivered GDNF induce dyskinesias and weight loss in monkeys (Z. Zhang et al., 1997). Additionally, compensatory down-regulation of TH in response to GDNF overexpression in the nigrostriatal system has been reported, both in intact (Georgievska et al., 2004; Rosenblad et al., 2003) and lesioned (Georgievska et al., 2002) rats. An important issue with possible functional consequences that was not addressed in these studies is whether prolonged GDNF infusion alters GDNF receptors Ret, GFRα1 and/or NCAM levels. There is evidence that BDNF infusion into the hippocampus for 6 days (Frank et al., 1996), or prolonged BDNF treatment of primary cortical (Knusel et al., 1997) or hippocampal (Haapasalo et al., 2002) cultures can down-regulate TrkB receptor levels. However, more recent studies in cultured hippocampal slices argue against the possibility that sustained periods of increased BDNF levels will initiate compensatory responses at the receptor level, and suggest that chronic up-regulation of BDNF is accompanied by increased activation of the neurotrophin receptor at spine synapses (Lauterborn et al., 2009). Thus, it is relevant to assess the effect of sustained high levels of GDNF in the nigrostriatal system on GDNF receptor levels as a possible compensatory down-regulation can limit GDNF-mediated neuroprotection. A potential approach to prevent the negative consequences of chronic GDNF infusion in the brain might be to use a regulated viral vector system (Manfredsson et al., 2009). Once optimized, such a system will offer the possibility to fine-tune the therapeutic dose to each PD patient, and to quickly stop GDNF overexpression in case toxicity emerges by adjusting the administration of the controlling agent (Manfredsson et al., 2009).

Several efforts are being made to solve the problems associated with the delivery, targeting, safety, and distribution of trophic factors to the CNS, which need to be overcome before GDNF therapy for PD becomes a reality (Sherer et al., 2006). The delivery of GDNF to the

CNS is challenging because GDNF is unable to cross the blood-brain barrier (Kastin et al., 2003; Kirik et al., 2004). A possibility to overcome this limitation is to conjugate or fuse GDNF with other molecules that enable it to cross the blood-brain barrier. Fusion with viral proteins (Dietz et al., 2006), conjugation with antibodies for transferrin (Albeck et al., 1997; Xia et al., 2008; Q.H. Zhou et al., 2010) or insulin (Boado & Pardridge, 2009; Boado et al., 2007) receptors, or with a fragment of the tetanus toxin (Larsen et al., 2006) provides an efficient way of delivering GDNF to the CNS. Recently, GDNF delivery to the CNS using bone marrow stem cell-derived macrophages, which are able to pass the blood-brain barrier, was proven to ameliorate MPTP-induced degeneration of TH-positive neurons and terminals, stimulate axon regeneration, and reverse hypoactivity in the open field test (Biju et al., 2010).

4.3 Inducing endogenous GDNF expression/signaling

Molecules that induce the endogenous expression of trophic factors or enhance their signaling are receiving increasing attention as alternative therapeutic options for PD. Therefore, in addition to a therapeutic tool itself, GDNF constitutes also a target for the development of new therapeutics. Interestingly, it was suggested that XIB4035, a non-peptidyl small molecule that acts as a GFRα1 agonist and mimics the neurotrophic effects of GDNF in Neuro-2A cells, might have beneficial effects for the treatment of PD (Tokugawa et al., 2003). Leucine-isoleucine (Leu-Ile), a hydrophobic dipeptide that partially resembles the site on FK506 that binds to immunophilin (Schreiber, 1991), significantly increases GDNF and BDNF levels in the conditioned medium from cultured hippocampal neurons, and protects both dopaminergic and non-dopaminergic neurons from natural cell death in low density cultures (Nitta et al., 2004). Interestingly, the effect is lost when cultures are prepared from mice lacking the *GDNF* or *BDNF* gene (Nitta et al., 2004). Moreover, Leu-Ile increases GDNF and BDNF striatal content in mice, inhibits 6-OHDA-induced dopaminergic denervation, and reduces rotational behavior after methamphetamine challenge (Nitta et al., 2004). The ability of Leu-Ile to cross the blood-brain barrier, and to promote GDNF expression without exhibiting immunosuppressive properties, makes it a novel tool for the treatment of PD or other neurodegenerative diseases. More recently, incubation with PYM50028 (Cogane™; common name smilagenin), a novel non-peptide neurotrophic factor inducer, was shown to protect cultured dopaminergic neurons from the toxic effect of MPP^+, an effect almost completely lost in the presence of anti-GDNF and/or anti-GFRα1 antibody. Moreover, GDNF mRNA expression was markedly increased by smilagenin treatment (Y. Zhang et al., 2008). Oral administration of smilagenin to MPTP-lesioned mice resulted in a significant elevation of striatal GDNF levels and attenuated the loss of dopaminergic neurons from the *substantia nigra* (Visanji et al., 2008). Interestingly, smilagenin is now undergoing phase I clinical testing (Aron & Klein, 2011). Finding molecules like XIB4035, Leu-Ile or smilagenin, capable of stimulating GDNF expression/signaling may prove beneficial to the treatment of PD, and would overcome most of the problems associated with the delivery of GDNF protein into the brain, with GDNF expression induced by viral vectors, or with the use of encapsulated GDNF producing cells (Bespalov & Saarma, 2007).

5. Complementary and alternative ways of getting GDNF?

PD patients commonly use complementary and alternative therapies, including altered diet, dietary supplements, herbal supplements, caffeine, nicotine, exercise, physical and massage therapy, melatonin, bright-light therapy and acupuncture (Lokk & Nilsson, 2010; Pecci et al., 2010; Zesiewicz & Evatt, 2009). What is the impact of these complementary and alternative therapies on GDNF levels?

5.1 Is there a GDNF diet?

Compelling evidence from epidemiological and animal studies highlights the importance of dietary factors in counteracting dopaminergic degeneration occurring in PD, so that healthy dietary choices might be relevant to reduce the risk of PD (Di Giovanni, 2009; Gao et al., 2007). Therefore, dietary intervention on PD has emerged as a new way to halt disease progression, or even prevent it.

Some studies show that caloric restriction and intermittent fasting diets are neuroprotective and improve functionality in animal models of stroke, Parkinson's, Huntington's (Mattson, 2005) and Alzheimer's (Halagappa et al., 2007) disease. Moreover, data from epidemiological studies suggest that individuals with low-calorie, low-fat diets may have reduced risk of PD (C.C. Johnson et al., 1999; Logroscino et al., 1996), while the potential association between obesity (Abbott et al., 2003; Hu et al., 2006; Ikeda et al., 2007), or cholesterol intake (Miyake et al., 2010) and the risk of PD have been shown. Accordingly, MPTP treatment produces greater striatal dopamine depletion in high-fat-fed than in control mice (J.Y. Choi et al., 2005). Likewise, rats under high-fat diet for 5 weeks before 6-OHDA infusion into the medial forebrain bundle exhibit greater dopamine depletion in the *substantia nigra* and striatum, and increased oxidative stress than control rats (Morris et al., 2010). Confirming the protective effect of caloric restriction, susceptibility to a neurotoxic insult to dopaminergic neurons is exacerbated in obese mice (Sriram et al., 2002). Conversely, dietary restriction protects adult mice against MPTP-induced dysfunction and degeneration of nigrostriatal dopaminergic neurons, and deficits in motor function decrease markedly in these animals (Duan & Mattson, 1999). Dietary restriction mimicked using a non-metabolizable analogue of glucose (2-deoxy-D-glucose) reduces damage to dopaminergic neurons in the *substantia nigra*, and improves the behavioral outcome following MPTP treatment (Duan & Mattson, 1999). Moreover, treatment with 2-deoxy-D-glucose protects cultured dopaminergic cells against oxidative and metabolic insults (Duan & Mattson, 1999). Surprisingly, caloric restriction was not neuroprotective against 6-OHDA toxicity in rats (Armentero et al., 2008). This lack of effect was likely due to the short duration of dietary restriction, and to a more pronounced neurotoxic insult compared with that registered in previous studies (Duan & Mattson, 1999; Maswood et al., 2004).

Caloric restriction and reduced meal frequency/intermittent fasting are dietary manipulations thought to prolong the health span of the nervous system by acting upon important metabolic and cellular signalling pathways to stimulate the production of protein chaperones, antioxidant enzymes, and neurotrophic factors that help cells to deal with stress and resist disease (Martin et al., 2006). The effect of dietary restriction on GDNF levels was not addressed by Duan & Mattson (1999), but an increase in GDNF levels in the nigrostriatal system may play a role in the positive effect of dietary restriction on MPTP-damaged dopaminergic neurons and motor impairment reported by these authors. In fact, more recent observations indicate that a low-calorie diet reduces the loss of dopaminergic neurons from the *substantia nigra*, the severity of neurochemical deficits, and motor dysfunction in a non-human primate model of PD (Maswood et al., 2004). Furthermore, monkeys maintained for 6 months on a 30% caloric restriction diet exhibit significantly higher levels of GDNF in the caudate nucleus compared with control monkeys, suggesting that the protective effect of reduced calorie diet may result from up-regulation of GDNF expression and consequent activation of neuroprotective signal transduction pathways in dopaminergic neurons (Maswood et al., 2004).

Since caloric restriction increases the amount of endogenous GDNF in the brain of monkeys, it may be possible to ameliorate PD, at least partially, through dietary manipulations. It is also worthy to mention that, for instance, hippocampal BDNF levels are reduced in rats subjected to a saturated-fat diet (H.R. Park et al., 2010; D.C. Wu et al., 2003) which leads us to hypothesize that a similar reduction of GDNF levels might also occur under a high-fat diet. Consistent with the observation that caloric restriction attenuates MPTP-induced depletion of dopamine, the distance moved and speed of movement increased more than two-fold in caloric restricted monkeys compared with those on control diet (Maswood et al., 2004). From an evolutionary point of view, and based on experimental data, it was speculated that the neuroprotective effects of caloric restriction could be due to the induction of growth factors by increased motor activity (Finch, 2004). In fact, activation of the same cellular and molecular pathways that occur in response to mild dietary restriction and intermittent fasting-induced stress can occur in response to physical exercise and cognitive stimulation (Mattson et al., 2004).

Taken together, these evidences support the relevance that dietary intervention might assume as a non-invasive and drug-free strategy for PD management, and suggest that an amelioration of GDNF levels may be involved in the protective effects of a healthy diet and caloric restriction on the nigrostriatal pathway.

5.2 Exercising for GDNF expression?

Substantial evidence suggests a positive role of exercise in slowing the progression of PD (Crizzle & Newhouse, 2006; Falvo et al., 2008; Goodwin et al., 2008), and beneficial effects of exercise on motor and non-motor PD symptoms have been described (Gage & Storey, 2004; Lehman et al., 2005; Logroscino et al., 2006). In addition, epidemiological studies show a negative correlation between the regular practice of exercise and the prevalence of PD (H. Chen et al., 2005; Sasco et al., 1992; Tsai et al., 2002; Q. Xu et al., 2010). Interestingly, it has been recently reported that forced exercise is more beneficial for people with PD than voluntary exercise (Ridgel et al., 2009). Thus, exercise might constitute a non-pharmacological neuroprotective therapy for PD contributing to slow the progressive degeneration of dopaminergic neurons. However, there is a lack of consensus on the optimal delivery and extent of exercise (dosing, type, etc) appropriate at each stage of the disease (Dibble et al., 2009; Goodwin et al., 2008). The mechanisms implicated in the beneficial effect of exercise in PD patients are now being uncovered (M.A. Hirsch & Farley, 2009). In particular, several trophic factors might be involved in the beneficial effects of exercise (e.g. Cotman et al., 2007; Gomez-Pinilla et al., 1998; Widenfalk et al., 1999; Yasuhara et al., 2007).

The data from animal models parallel the observations in PD patients as increased physical activity is neuroprotective/neurorestorative in models of nigrostriatal injury. However, despite the findings supporting the view that exercise protects against the behavioral effects of 6-OHDA and MPTP, data on the protection of dopaminergic neurons from 6-OHDA- or MPTP-induced toxicity are mixed (Zigmond et al., 2009). It has been reported that running for 3 months prior to acute MPTP administration completly protects from TH cell loss

(Gerecke et al., 2010). On the other hand, exercise for 2 weeks after intrastriatal injection of 6-OHDA results in partial recovery of TH labeling and axonal fiber projection to the striatum (Yoon et al., 2007). Treadmill exercise starting the day after intrastriatal 6-OHDA infusion induces significant preservation of TH-positive fibers in the striatum and TH-positive neurons in the *substantia nigra pars compacta* as compared to the non-exercised group (Tajiri et al., 2010). An increase in TH labeling in the *substantia nigra pars compacta* of MPTP-treated mice receiving treadmill exercise was also recently reported (B.A. Smith et al., 2011). In contrast, other authors find no reduction in the loss of dopaminergic neurons in exercised animals (Fisher et al., 2004; O'Dell et al., 2007). Improvements in motor performance in animals undergoing exercise may not necessarily be accompanied by changes in total striatal dopamine levels after exercise (O'Dell et al., 2007; Petzinger et al., 2007). Compensatory changes in stimulus-evoked release and a decrease in dopamine decay might play a relevant role (Petzinger et al., 2007). Some studies show that exercise leads to DAT down-regulation in MPTP-treated mice (Fisher et al., 2004; Petzinger et al., 2007), suggesting that increased synaptic availability of dopamine may underlie behavioral improvements in response to exercise. In contrast, an increase in DAT protein expression has been recently reported in MPTP-treated mice receiving treadmill exercise (B.A. Smith et al., 2011). These discrepancies might be related to differences in the lesion regimen/extension and exercise paradigm.

Physical exercise increases the expression of GDNF in the nigrostriatal system, and this correlates with the protection of dopaminergic neurons against MPTP toxicity (Faherty et al., 2005), and amelioration of motor impairment due to a 6-OHDA lesion (Cohen et al., 2003; Tajiri et al., 2010). Exercise in the running-wheel markedly accelerates spontaneous recovery after a 6-OHDA lesion as animals exercised on the running-wheel prior or after a unilateral striatal 6-OHDA injection show a faster motor recovery compared to non-exercised animals (O'Dell et al., 2007). Recently, daily treadmill exercise similar to clinical settings (30 min/day, 5 days/week for 4 weeks) was shown to up-regulate both GDNF and BDNF in the lesioned and intact sides of the striatum (Tajiri et al., 2010). In a chronic MPTP mouse model with moderate neurodegeneration treadmill exercise during 18 weeks drastically increased GDNF levels in the striatum but not in the *substantia nigra*, and the opposite was observed for BDNF (Lau et al., 2011). The improvement of motor function observed in many studies of forced limb use, treadmill running or running-wheel exercise in both 6-OHDA (Mabandla et al., 2004; Tillerson et al., 2001; 2003; Yoon et al., 2007) and MPTP (Fisher et al., 2004; Tillerson et al., 2003) models of PD raised the hypothesis that up-regulation of GDNF might mediate, or at least contribute to, the protection of the nigrostriatal pathway observed in those reports (A.D. Smith & Zigmond, 2003). How does exercise increase GDNF expression? Since GDNF production is activity-dependent, dopamine is known to stimulate GDNF expression (Saavedra et al., 2008), and exercise increases dopamine in the striatum (Sutoo & Akiyama, 2003), one may envisage that increased dopamine levels during activity of the striatal circuitry may mediate increased GDNF expression in the nigrostriatal system upon physical exercise.

5.3 A stimulating GDNF lifestyle?

Environmental enrichment is characterized by housing conditions that facilitate sensory, motor and cognitive stimuli, accompanied by voluntary physical activity and social interactions. An enriched environment is neuroprotective in animal models of PD. Mice reared in an enriched environment are more resistant to MPTP compared with mice raised in a standard environment (Bezard et al., 2003; Faherty et al., 2005). Moreover, environmental enrichement also improves motor function after unilateral 6-OHDA injection in rats (Jadavji et al., 2006; Steiner et al., 2006). More recently, continuous exposure to environmental enrichement during 3 weeks before and after 6-OHDA injection was reported to prevent dopaminergic neuronal death, protect the nigrostriatal pathway, and reduce motor impairment (Anastasia et al., 2009). The molecular mechanisms involved in the neuroprotective effect of environmental enrichement observed in several rodent models of brain disorders are not clear, but the synthesis and release of neurotrophic factors may play a crucial role (Nithianantharajah & Hannan, 2006). In fact, environmental enrichment increases GDNF mRNA in the *substantia nigra* and striatum, and totally protects against MPTP-induced parkinsonism (Faherty et al., 2005). Bezard et al. (2003) and Turner & Lewis (2003) showed that enriched environment also increases the expression of BDNF in the striatum but, unfortunately, the effect on GDNF levels was not addressed in these studies. In a previous work, an enriched environment was shown to induce the expression of GDNF and to increase the phosphorylation of the transcription factor CREB, while reducing the spontaneous apoptosis in the rat hippocampus by 45%, and protecting against kainate-induced seizures and excitotoxic injury (Young et al., 1999).

What is the relevance of the results obtained in animal models of PD to humans suffering the disease? Most individuals are exposed to a high degree of environmental complexity and novelty. However, the level of cognitive, social and physical stimulation can vary significantly from one person to another, so that correlative and epidemiological data shows that lifestyle, including occupation, leisure activities and physical exercise, has a direct effect on the risk of cognitive decline (Baroncelli et al., 2010). In fact, there is an association between higher educational accomplishment and reduced risk of PD-related dementia (Glatt et al., 1996). Since PD patients suffer from impaired cognitive functions (Jokinen et al., 2009 and references therein), and GDNF contributes to synaptic transmission (Saavedra et al., 2008). Thus, getting engaged in higher levels of mental and physical activity through education, occupation and recreation might constitute a non-invasive and drug-free approach to increase GDNF levels, which, in turn, might both protect the nigrostriatal pathway and reduce the cognitive impairment affecting PD patients.

5.4 Green GDNF?

Consistent with the considerable effort in identifying naturally occurring neuroprotective substances, growing evidence indicates that many oriental herbs and extracts attenuate the degeneration of dopaminergic neurons, and ameliorate the parkinsonism induced by MPTP and 6-OHDA (for a review see L.W. Chen et al., 2007). The number of reports supporting the neuroprotective action of several herbs and herbal extracts on PD models continues to rise, and here we briefly overview the most recent studies.

In vitro, protection against 6-OHDA toxicity was demonstrated using Cyperi rhizoma, the rhizome of *Cyperus rotundus* L. (Lee et al., 2010), while *Chrysanthemum morifolium* Ramat (I.S. Kim et al., 2009) and Yi-Gan San (Doo et al., 2010b) protect cells from MPP^+ toxicity. *In vivo,* Yi-Gan San (Doo et al., 2010b), *Withania somnifera* root extract/Ashwagandha/Indian ginseng (Rajasankar et al., 2009a,b), panaxatriol saponins, the main constituents extracted from *Panax notoginseng* (Luo et al., 2011), pycnogenol, an extract of *Pinus maritime* bark (Khan et al., 2010), *Gynostemma pentaphyllum* (H.S. Choi et al., 2010), and epigallocatechin-3-gallate, a green tea catechin (J.S. Kim et al., 2010), were shown to be neuroprotective in the MPTP model of PD.

Several mechanisms have been proposed to contribute to the neuroprotective effect of herbs and herbal extracts. These include their function as antioxidants to alleviate oxidative stress, inhibitors of monoamine oxidase B to decrease neurotoxicity, scavengers of free radicals, chelators of harmful metals, modulators of cell survival genes and apoptotic signals (L.W. Chen et al., 2007). As a result, herbs and herbal extracts are receiving increasing attention as therapeutic agents for the treatment of PD. The efficacy and safety of their use in adjunct or monotherapy in PD management is under consideration (Chung et al., 2006). Unfortunately, the effect on GDNF expression has not yet been addressed for many of them. It would be very interesting to investigate if these and other herbal extracts are able to increase GDNF expression, as well as whether their protective effects in PD models are mediated, or not, by the up-regulation of GDNF expression. The available data on GDNF induction by herbs or herbal compounds is reviewed below.

Rehmannia glutinosa, a traditional Chinese medicine herb frequently used in the therapy of dementia, induces GDNF gene expression in C6 cells and in primary cortical astrocytes (H. Yu et al., 2006). The stimulation of GDNF gene expression by *Rehmannia glutinosa* in C6 cells can be independently up-regulated through PKC and ERK1/2 pathways (H. Yu et al., 2006). Recently, the protective effect of catalpol, an active component extracted and purified from *Rehmannia glutinosa* was investigated in a chronic MPTP mouse model and in MPP^+-treated mesencephalic neurons. The oral administration of catalpol for 8 weeks dose-dependently improves locomotor ability, significantly elevates striatal dopamine levels and the number of TH-positive neurons in the *substantia nigra pars compacta,* and the striatal DAT density. Interestingly, catalpol treatment also increases GDNF striatal levels, and both the number of dopaminergic neurons and DAT density are positively correlated with GDNF levels (G. Xu et al., 2010). Moreover, catalpol protects cultured mesencephalic neurons against MPP^+ toxicity and up-regulates GDNF mRNA levels in neurons intoxicated with MPP^+, but not in control cultures. Importantly, the protective effect of catalpol against dopaminergic degeneration is abolished by the presence of the GDNF receptor tyrosine kinase Ret inhibitor 4-amino-5-(4-methyphenyl)-7-(t-butyl)-pyrazolo-[3,4-d]pyrimidine (G. Xu et al., 2010). Catalpol has antioxidant (Bi et al., 2008; Tian et al., 2007) and anti-apoptotic (Bi et al., 2009) effects, properties also displayed by GDNF (Saavedra et al., 2008), which suggest that GDNF up-regulation could be an essential step in catalpol-induced neuroprotection, but this is currently unknown.

Smilagenin is a compound extracted from *Rhizoma anemarrhenae* and *Radix asparagi,* medicinal herbs frequently used in the traditional Chinese medicine. A recent work shows that smilagenin, added prior to MPP^+, protects cultured mesencephalic dopaminergic neurons against MPP^+-induced toxicity. GDNF mRNA levels, but not those of GFRα1 or Ret, are markedly elevated in the presence of smilagenin. Moreover, the neuroprotective effect is partially lost in the presence of GDNF and/or GFRα1 antibodies (Y. Zhang et al., 2008). Oral administration of smilagenin to MPTP-lesioned mice elevates striatal GDNF levels and attenuates the loss of dopaminergic neurons (Visanji et al., 2008). Since smilagenin can be taken orally, readily crosses the blood-brain barrier, stimulates GDNF expression, and has neuroprotective effects in the MPTP mouse model of PD, hopefully it is a good candidate for the treatment of PD.

Rhus verniciflua Stokes, commonly known as lacquer tree, has been used for centuries in Korea as a food supplement and a traditional herbal medicine. Recently, the detoxified extract of *Rhus verniciflua* was shown to induce GDNF mRNA and protein expression, both in dopaminergic-like SH-SY5Y cells, and in the rat brain after oral administration (Sapkota et al., 2010). Moreover, GDNF immunoreactivity is markedly enhanced in the *substantia nigra* of rats treated with *Rhus verniciflua* extract. Interestingly, the neuroprotective effects of *Rhus verniciflua* against rotenone-induced toxicity in SH-SY5Y cells include the prevention of GDNF and BDNF down-regulation in rotenone-treated cells (Sapkota et al., 2011).

Ibogaine is a psychoactive compound extracted from *Tabernanthe iboga*, and used for decades in African folklore medicine and rituals. Many studies indicate that ibogaine reduces craving and withdrawal symptoms of several drugs of abuse (Ron & Janak, 2005). This anti-addiction drug increases GDNF levels in SH-SY5Y cells, and up-regulates the GDNF pathway as assessed by the phosphorylation of the GDNF receptor Ret and the downstream kinase ERK1 (D.Y. He et al., 2005). A MEK inhibitor impede ibogaine-induced GDNF up-regulation (D.Y. He & Ron, 2006). In addition, after systemic administration to rodents, ibogaine increases GDNF expression in the VTA (D.Y. He et al., 2005). Since GDNF has been implicated as a negative regulator of drug and alcohol addiction (Ron & Janak, 2005), the effect of ibogaine on GDNF expression likely contributes to its positive impact on the treatment of addiction. Despite its properties, ibogaine is not approved as an addiction treatment because it induces hallucinations, which will impede its use in PD therapeutics too.

Given the neuroprotective effect of some herbal extracts on animal and cellular models of PD, and the ability to induce GDNF expression reported for some of them, it may prove useful to screen traditional therapies for their effect on GDNF levels in the nigrostriatal system, as they might reveal to be valuable GDNF inducers and alternative therapeutic approaches to PD.

5.5 'GDNF-Acupuncture'?

Acupuncture is among the complementary and/or alternative therapies most widely used by PD patients (Lokk & Nilsson, 2010; Pecci et al., 2010). Interestingly, increasing evidence supports a beneficial effect of acupuncture on MPTP (Y.G. Choi et al., 2011; Doo et al., 2010a; Jeon et al., 2008; J.M. Kang et al., 2007), 6-OHDA (Y.K. Kim et al., 2005; H.J. Park et al., 2003; Y.P. Yu et al., 2010) and medial forebrain bundle transection (Jia et al., 2009, 2010; X.B. Liang et al., 2003) PD models, and also in PD patients (Chang et al., 2008; Zhuang & Wang, 2000). Acupuncture can enhance the therapeutic effects of western medicine and reduce the need of medication (Ren, 2008). Relevant in the context of the present sinopsis is the fact that acupuncture therapy increases various neuroprotective agents (Joh et al., 2010), namely GDNF. In medial forebrain bundle-transected rats, high frequency electroacupunture stimulation up-regulates GDNF mRNA levels in both sides of the globus pallidus, suggesting that the retrograde nourishment of GDNF to dopaminergic neurons may contribute to the behavioral improvement observed in these rats (X.B. Liang et al., 2003). Another study shows that the number of GDNF-positive cells and the content of Ret receptor increased significantly in 6-OHDA-injected rats subjected to electroacupuncture (Y.C. Wang et al., 2010). At this point it is also worthy to mention that acupuncture attenuates microglial activation and inflammatory events in MPTP-treated mice (J.M. Kang et al., 2007). Since acupuncture increases GDNF expression, and GDNF is an important inhibitor of microglia activation (see section 3.3 Role of GDNF in controlling microglia activation), it is tempting to speculate that acupuncture might reduce microglia activity through GDNF up-regulation. Interestingly, electroacupuncture increases GDNF signaling in other disease models. Electroacupuncture activates the endogenous GDNF signaling system by increasing the mRNA and protein levels of GDNF and its receptor GFRα1 in dorsal root ganglions of neuropathic pain rats (Dong et al., 2005). In contrast, electroacupuncture-induced analgesia in a rat model of neuropathic pain is significantly attenuated by the down-regulation of GFRα1 expression with antisense oligodeoxynucleotides (Dong et al., 2006). Electroacupuncture also up-regulates GDNF expression in a model of transient focal cerebral ischemia, thereby extending the duration of the endogenous GDNF up-regulation, which may be one of the pathways involved in the protective effect of electroacupuncture against ischemic injury (Wei et al., 2000b). Since the stimulatory effects of electroacupuncture on GDNF/GFRα1 levels have been demonstrated in different models, it would be relevant to address whether they underlie the beneficial effects of electroacupuncture in PD animals models.

6. Conclusion

Male gender, together with the sex dimorphism in the nigrostriatal system, can contribute to the gender differences in PD. The estrogen 17β-estradiol plays a determinant protective role through its antioxidant, anti-inflammatory, and anti-apoptotic actions. Moreover, 17β-estradiol is capable of inducing the expression of neurotrophic factors, namely GDNF, which can have a determinant contribution to the aforementioned protective effects of 17β-estradiol. Although the protective effect of 17β-estradiol in females is consensual, the role of this hormone in males is still not broadly accepted.

Microglia plays a protective role by removing apoptotic neurons and by promoting neuronal survival through the release of neurotrophic factors. However, microglia activation can also play a particularly deleterious role in the nigrostriatal system, contributing to further enhance neuronal injury in PD. Substantial evidence suggests that microglial activation is capable of inducing GDNF expression, and more recent data indicate that GDNF in turn inhibits microglia activation. This may indicate that GDNF is involved in a process that self-limits microglial neurotoxicity thus preventing neuronal injury. The extensive neuroinflammation observed in PD brain indicates that this mechanism of control is no longer effective in the diseased brain. Although the results obtained so far with anti-inflammatory drugs were not conclusive, it would be important to determine what causes the disruption or alteration of this feedback mechanism in the course of PD.

The possibility of manipulating endogenous GDNF expression can have clinical implications for the management of PD, and prove to be useful as an alternative or a complement to pharmacological or more invasive approaches. Growing evidence shows the possibility of reducing the risk for age-related neurodegenerative disorders through dietary and behavioral changes inducing neuronal survival and plasticity. Thus, dietary manipulations, physical exercise and cognitive stimulation, which are known to induce GDNF up-regulation, represent novel drug-free and non-invasive approaches that may help preventing the onset of degeneration or, in combination with pharmacological treatments, reduce the severity of the motor symptoms through the modulation of GDNF levels. Moreover, the use of alternative therapies like herbal supplements and acupuncture might also prove to be neuroprotecive via GDNF up-regulation in the nigrostriatal system. Thus, these approaches to increase endogenous GDNF levels deserve further investigation. Likewise, the impact on GDNF levels of other complementary and alternative therapies used by PD patients should also be addressed in the future. Moreover, given its involvement in synaptic plasticity and synaptogenesis, GDNF also plays a role in learning and memory. One may therefore speculate that increasing the endogenous GDNF expression would also contribute to fight the cognitive decline observed in PD patients. Additionally, it would be interesting to examine the effect of caloric restriction, physical exercise, enriched environment, herbal extracts or acupuncture, which increase GDNF expression in the nigrostriatal system and are neuroprotective in PD models, on the levels of MANF and CDNF, two other dopaminotrophic factors.

7. Acknowledgment

We would like to thank Esther Perez-Navarro for her comments and suggestions.

8. References

Abbott R. D., Ross G. W., White L. R., Sanderson W. T., Burchfiel C. M., Kashon M., Sharp D. S., Masaki K. H., Curb J. D. & Petrovitch H. (2003) Environmental, life-style, and physical precursors of clinical Parkinson's disease: recent findings from the Honolulu-Asia Aging Study. *Journal of Neurology*, Vol. 250 Suppl 3, pp. III30-III39, ISSN 0340-5354

Albeck D. S., Hoffer B. J., Quissell D., Sanders L. A., Zerbe G. & Granholm A. C. (1997) A non-invasive transport system for GDNF across the blood-brain barrier. *Neuroreport*, Vol. 8, No. 9-10, pp. 2293-2298, ISSN 959-4965

Anastasia A., Torre L., de Erausquin G. A. & Masco D. H. (2009) Enriched environment protects the nigrostriatal dopaminergic system and induces astroglial reaction in the 6-OHDA rat model of Parkinson's disease. *Journal of Neurochemistry*, Vol. 109, No. 3, pp. 755-765, ISSN 0022-3042

Appel E., Kolman O., Kazimirsky G., Blumberg P. M. & Brodie C. (1997) Regulation of GDNF expression in cultured astrocytes by inflammatory stimuli. *Neuroreport*, Vol. 8, No. 15, pp. 3309-3312, ISSN 0959-4965

Armentero M. T., Levandis G., Bramanti P., Nappi G. & Blandini F. (2008) Dietary restriction does not prevent nigrostriatal degeneration in the 6-hydroxydopamine model of Parkinson's disease. *Experimental Neurology*, Vol. 212, No. 2, pp. 548-551, ISSN 0014-4886

Aron L. & Klein R. (2011) Repairing the parkinsonian brain with neurotrophic factors. *Trends in Neuroscience*, Vol. 34, No. 2, pp. 88-100, ISSN 0166-2236

Baldereschi M., Di Carlo A., Rocca W. A., Vanni P., Maggi S., Perissinotto E., Grigoletto F., Amaducci L. & Inzitari D. (2000) Parkinson's disease and parkinsonism in a longitudinal study: two-fold higher incidence in men. ILSA Working Group. Italian Longitudinal Study on Aging. *Neurology*, Vol. 55, No. 9, pp. 1358-1363, ISSN 0028-3878

Baroncelli L., Braschi C., Spolidoro M., Begenisic T., Sale A. & Maffei L. (2010) Nurturing brain plasticity: impact of environmental enrichment. *Cell Death & Differentiation*, Vol. 17, No. 7, pp. 1092-1103, ISSN 1350-9047

Barroso-Chinea P., Cruz-Muros I., Aymerich M. S., Rodriguez-Diaz M., Afonso-Oramas D., Lanciego J. L. & Gonzalez-Hernandez T. (2005) Striatal expression of GDNF and differential vulnerability of midbrain dopaminergic cells. *European Journal of Neuroscience,* Vol. 21, No. 7, pp. 1815-1827, ISSN 0953-816X

Batchelor P. E., Liberatore G. T., Porritt M. J., Donnan G. A. & Howells D. W. (2000) Inhibition of brain-derived neurotrophic factor and glial cell line-derived neurotrophic factor expression reduces dopaminergic sprouting in the injured striatum. *European Journal of Neuroscience,* Vol. 12, No. 10, pp. 3462-3468, ISSN 0953-816X

Batchelor P. E., Liberatore G. T., Wong J. Y., Porritt M. J., Frerichs F., Donnan G. A. & Howells D. W. (1999) Activated macrophages and microglia induce dopaminergic sprouting in the injured striatum and express brain-derived neurotrophic factor and glial cell line-derived neurotrophic factor. *Journal of Neuroscience,* Vol. 19, No. 5, pp. 1708-1716, ISSN 0270-6474

Batchelor P. E., Porritt M. J., Martinello P., Parish C. L., Liberatore G. T., Donnan G. A. & Howells D. W. (2002) Macrophages and microglia produce local trophic gradients that stimulate axonal sprouting toward but not beyond the wound edge. *Molecular and Cellular Neurosciences,* Vol. 21, No. 3, pp. 436-453, ISSN 1044-7431

Behl C., Skutella T., Lezoualc'h F., Post A., Widmann M., Newton C. J. & Holsboer F. (1997) Neuroprotection against oxidative stress by estrogens: structure-activity relationship. *Molecular Pharmacology,* Vol. 51, No. 4, pp. 535-541, ISSN 0026-895X

Benn S. C. & Woolf C. J. (2004) Adult neuron survival strategies - slamming on the brakes. *Nature Reviews Neuroscience,* Vol. 5, No. 9, pp. 686-700, ISSN 1471-003X

Bespalov M. M. & Saarma M. (2007) GDNF family receptor complexes are emerging drug targets. *Trends Pharmacology Sciences,* Vol. 28, No. 2, pp. 68-74, ISSN 0165-6147

Bezard E., Dovero S., Belin D., Duconger S., Jackson-Lewis V., Przedborski S., Piazza P. V., Gross C. E. & Jaber M. (2003) Enriched environment confers resistance to 1-methyl-4-phenyl-1,2,3,6-tetrahydropyridine and cocaine: involvement of dopamine transporter and trophic factors. *Journal of Neuroscience,* Vol. 23, No. 35, pp. 10999-11007, ISSN 1529-2401

Bi J., Jiang B., Liu J. H., Lei C., Zhang X. L. & An L. J. (2008) Protective effects of catalpol against H_2O_2-induced oxidative stress in astrocytes primary cultures. *Neuroscience Letters,* Vol. 442, No. 3, pp. 224-227, ISSN 0304-3940

Bi J., Jiang B., Hao S., Zhang A., Dong Y., Jiang T. & An L. (2009) Catalpol attenuates nitric oxide increase via ERK signaling pathways induced by rotenone in mesencephalic neurons. *Neurochemistry International,* Vol. 54, No. 3-4, pp. 264-270, ISSN 0197-0186

Biju K., Zhou Q., Li G., Imam S. Z., Roberts J. L., Morgan W. W., Clark R. A. & Li S. (2010) Macrophage-mediated GDNF delivery protects against dopaminergic neurodegeneration: a therapeutic strategy for Parkinson's disease. *Molecular Therapy,* Vol. 18, No. 8, pp. 1536-1544, ISSN 1525-0016

Block M. L. & Hong J. S. (2005) Microglia and inflammation-mediated neurodegeneration: multiple triggers with a common mechanism. *Progress in Neurobiology,* Vol. 76, No. 2, pp. 77-98, ISSN 0301-0082

Block M. L., Zecca L. & Hong J. S. (2007) Microglia-mediated neurotoxicity: uncovering the molecular mechanisms. *Nature Reviews. Neuroscience,* Vol. 8, No. 1, pp. 57-69, ISSN 1471-003X

Boado R. J. & Pardridge W. M. (2009) Comparison of blood-brain barrier transport of glial-derived neurotrophic factor (GDNF) and an IgG-GDNF fusion protein in the rhesus monkey. *Drug Metababolism Disposition*, Vol. 37, No. 12, pp. 2299-2304, ISSN 0090-9556

Boado R. J., Zhang Y., Zhang Y., Wang Y. & Pardridge W. M. (2007) GDNF fusion protein for targeted-drug delivery across the human blood-brain barrier. *Biotechnology & Bioengineering*, Vol. 100, No. 2, pp. 387-396, ISSN 1097-0290

Boger H. A., Granholm A. C., McGinty J. F. & Middaugh L. D. (2010) A dual-hit animal model for age-related parkinsonism. *Progress in Neurobiology*, Vol. 90, No. 2, pp. 217-229, ISSN 1873-5118

Bourque M., Dluzen D. E. & Di Paolo T. (2009) Neuroprotective actions of sex steroids in Parkinson's disease. *Frontiers in Neuroendocrinology*, Vol. 30, No. 2, pp. 142-157, ISSN 1095-6808

Brann D. W., Dhandapani K., Wakade C., Mahesh V. B. & Khan M. M. (2007) Neurotrophic and neuroprotective actions of estrogen: basic mechanisms and clinical implications. *Steroids*, Vol. 72, No. 5, pp. 381-405, ISSN 0039-128X

Burke R. E., Antonelli M. & Sulzer D. (1998) Glial cell line-derived neurotrophic growth factor inhibits apoptotic death of postnatal substantia nigra dopamine neurons in primary culture. *Journal of Neurochemistry*, Vol. 71, No. 2, pp. 517-525, ISSN 0022-3042

Callier S., Morissette M., Grandbois M., Pelaprat D. & Di Paolo T. (2001) Neuroprotective properties of 17beta-estradiol, progesterone, and raloxifene in MPTP C57Bl/6 mice. *Synapse*, Vol. 41, No. 2, pp. 131-138, ISSN 0887-4476

Cantuti-Castelvetri I., Keller-McGandy C., Bouzou B., Asteris G., Clark T. W., Frosch M. P. & Standaert D. G. (2007) Effects of gender on nigral gene expression and parkinson disease. *Neurobiology of Disease*, Vol. 26, No. 3, pp. 606-614, ISSN 0969-9961

Chang X. H., Zhang L. Z. & Li Y. J. (2008) [Observation on therapeutic effect of acupuncture combined with medicine on Parkinson disease]. *Zhongguo ZhenJiu*, Vol. 28, No. 9, pp. 645-647, ISSN 0255-2930

Chao C. C. & Lee E. H. (1999) Neuroprotective mechanism of glial cell line-derived neurotrophic factor on dopamine neurons: role of antioxidation. *Neuropharmacology*, Vol. 38, No. 6, pp. 913-916, ISSN 028-3908

Chen H., Zhang S. M., Schwarzschild M. A., Hernan M. A. & Ascherio A. (2005) Physical activity and the risk of Parkinson disease. *Neurology*, Vol. 64, No. 4, pp. 664-669, ISSN 1526-632X

Chen L. W., Wang Y. Q., Wei L. C., Shi M. & Chan Y. S. (2007) Chinese herbs and herbal extracts for neuroprotection of dopaminergic neurons and potential therapeutic treatment of Parkinson's disease. *CNS & Neurological Disorders - Drug Targets*, Vol. 6, No. 4, pp. 273-281, ISSN 1871-5273

Chen P. S., Peng G. S., Li G., Yang S., Wu X., Wang C. C., Wilson B., Lu R. B., Gean P. W., Chuang D. M. & Hong J. S. (2006) Valproate protects dopaminergic neurons in midbrain neuron/glia cultures by stimulating the release of neurotrophic factors from astrocytes. *Molecular Psychiatry*, Vol. 11, No. 12, pp. 1116-1125, ISSN 1359-4184

Cheng H., Fu Y.-S. & Guo J.-W. (2004) Ability of GDNF to diminish free radical production leads to protection against kainate-induced excitotoxicity in hippocampus. *Hippocampus*, Vol. 14, No. 1, pp. 77-86, ISSN 1050-9631

Choi H. S., Park M. S., Kim S. H., Hwang B. Y., Lee C. K., & Lee, M. K. (2010) Neuroprotective effects of herbal ethanol extracts from Gynostemma pentaphyllum in the 6-hydroxydopamine-lesioned rat model of Parkinson's disease. *Molecules,* Vol. 15, No. 4 pp. 2814-2824, ISSN 1420-3049

Choi J. Y., Jang E. H., Park C. S. & Kang J. H. (2005) Enhanced susceptibility to 1-methyl-4-phenyl-1,2,3,6-tetrahydropyridine neurotoxicity in high-fat diet-induced obesity. *Free Radical Biology & Medicine,* Vol. 38, No. 6, pp. 806-816, ISSN 0891-5849

Choi Y. G., Yeo S., Hong Y. M. & Lim S. (2011) Neuroprotective changes of striatal degeneration-related gene expression by acupuncture in an MPTP mouse model of parkinsonism: microarray analysis. *Cellular & Molecular Neurobiology,* Vol. 31, No. 3, pp. 377-391, ISSN 1420-3049

Chung V., Liu L., Bian Z., Zhao Z., Leuk F. W., Kum W. F., Gao J. & Li M. (2006) Efficacy and safety of herbal medicines for idiopathic Parkinson's disease: a systematic review. *Movement Disorders,* Vol. 21, No. 10, pp. 1709-1715, ISSN 0885-3185

Clarkson E. D., Zawada W. M. & Freed C. R. (1997) GDNF improves survival and reduces apoptosis in human embryonic dopaminergic neurons in vitro. *Cell & Tissue Research,* Vol. 289, No. 2, pp. 207-210, ISSN 0302-766X

Cohen A. D., Tillerson J. L., Smith A. D., Schallert T. & Zigmond M. J. (2003) Neuroprotective effects of prior limb use in 6-hydroxydopamine-treated rats: possible role of GDNF. *Journal of Neurochemistry,* Vol. 85, No. 2, pp. 299-305, ISSN 0022-3042

Cotman C. W., Berchtold N. C. & Christie L. A. (2007) Exercise builds brain health: key roles of growth factor cascades and inflammation. *Trends in Neuroscience,* Vol. 30, No. 9, pp. 464-472, ISSN 0166-2236

Crizzle A. M. & Newhouse I. J. (2006) Is physical exercise beneficial for persons with Parkinson's disease? *Clinical Journal of Sport Medicine,* Vol. 16, No. 5, pp. 422-425, ISSN 1050-642X

Currie L. J., Harrison M. B., Trugman J. M., Bennett J. P. & Wooten G. F. (2004) Postmenopausal estrogen use affects risk for Parkinson disease. *Archives of Neurology,* Vol. 61, No. 6, pp. 886-888, ISSN 0003-9942

D'Astous M., Morissette M. & Di Paolo T. (2004) Effect of estrogen receptor agonists treatment in MPTP mice: evidence of neuroprotection by an ER alpha agonist. *Neuropharmacology,* Vol. 47, No. 8, pp. 1180-1188, ISSN 0028-3908

De Campos F., Cristovão A. C. & Baltazar G. (2010). Does GDNF contribute to estrogen-mediated neuroprotection?, *FENS Abstr., vol. 5, 050.28,* FENS Fórum 2010, Amsterdam, The Nederlands. July *2010.*

Dehmer T., Lindenau J., Haid S., Dichgans J. & Schulz J. B. (2000) Deficiency of inducible nitric oxide synthase protects against MPTP toxicity in vivo. *Journal of Neurochemistry,* Vol. 74, No. 5, pp. 2213-2216, ISSN 0022-3042

Di Giovanni G. (2009) A diet for dopaminergic neurons? *Journal of Neural Transmission. Supplementa,* Vol. 73, pp. 317-331, ISSN 0303-6995

Diaz N. F., Diaz-Martinez N. E., Camacho-Arroyo I. & Velasco I. (2009) Estradiol promotes proliferation of dopaminergic precursors resulting in a higher proportion of dopamine neurons derived from mouse embryonic stem cells. *International Journal of Developmental Neuroscience,* Vol. 27, No. 5, pp. 493-500, ISSN 1873-474X

Dibble L. E., Addison O. & Papa E. (2009) The effects of exercise on balance in persons with Parkinson's disease: a systematic review across the disability spectrum. *Journal of Neurologic Physical Therapy,* Vol. 33, No. 1, pp. 14-26, ISSN 1557-0576

Dietz G. P., Valbuena P. C., Dietz B., Meuer K., Mueller P., Weishaupt J. H. & Bahr M. (2006) Application of a blood-brain-barrier-penetrating form of GDNF in a mouse model for Parkinson's disease. *Brain Research*, Vol. 1082, No. 1, pp. 61-66, ISSN 0006-8993

Ding Y. M., Jaumotte J. D., Signore A. P. & Zigmond M. J. (2004) Effects of 6-hydroxydopamine on primary cultures of substantia nigra: specific damage to dopamine neurons and the impact of glial cell line-derived neurotrophic factor. *Journal of Neurochemistry*, Vol. 89, No. 3, pp. 776-787, ISSN 0022-3042

Dittrich F., Feng Y., Metzdorf R. & Gahr M. (1999) Estrogen-inducible, sex-specific expression of brain-derived neurotrophic factor mRNA in a forebrain song control nucleus of the juvenile zebra finch. *Proceedings of the National Academy of Sciences of the United States of America*, Vol. 96, No. 14, pp. 8241-8246, ISSN 0027-8424

Dluzen D. E. (2005) Unconventional effects of estrogen uncovered. *Trends in Pharmacological Sciences*. Vol. 26, No. 10, pp. 485-487, ISSN 0165-6147

Dluzen D. E., McDermott J. L. & Liu B. (1996) Estrogen alters MPTP-induced neurotoxicity in female mice: effects on striatal dopamine concentrations and release. *Journal of Neurochemistry*, Vol. 66, No. 2, pp. 658-666, ISSN 0022-3042

Dong Z. Q., Ma F., Xie H., Wang Y. Q. & Wu G. C. (2005) Changes of expression of glial cell line-derived neurotrophic factor and its receptor in dorsal root ganglions and spinal dorsal horn during electroacupuncture treatment in neuropathic pain rats. *Neuroscience Letters*, Vol. 376, No. 2, pp. 143-148, ISSN 0304-3940

Dong Z. Q., Ma F., Xie H., Wang Y. Q. & Wu G. C. (2006) Down-regulation of GFRalpha-1 expression by antisense oligodeoxynucleotide attenuates electroacupuncture analgesia on heat hyperalgesia in a rat model of neuropathic pain. *Brain Research Bulletin*, Vol. 69, No. 1, pp. 30-36, ISSN 0361-9230

Doo A. R., Kim S. T., Kim S. N., Moon W., Yin C. S., Chae Y., Park H. K., Lee H. & Park H. J. (2010a) Neuroprotective effects of bee venom pharmaceutical acupuncture in acute 1-methyl-4-phenyl-1,2,3,6-tetrahydropyridine-induced mouse model of Parkinson's disease. *Neurological Research*, Vol. 32 Suppl 1, No. pp. 88-91, ISSN 0161-6412

Doo A. R., Kim S. N., Park J. Y., Cho K. H., Hong J., Eun-Kyung K., Moon S. K., Jung W. S., Lee H., Jung J. H. & Park H. J. (2010b) Neuroprotective effects of an herbal medicine, Yi-Gan San on MPP+/MPTP-induced cytotoxicity in vitro and in vivo. *Journal of Ethnopharmacology*, Vol. 131, No. 2, pp. 433-442, ISSN 0378-8741

Double K. L., Reyes S., Werry E. L. & Halliday G. M. (2010) Selective cell death in neurodegeneration: why are some neurons spared in vulnerable regions? *Progress in Neurobiology*, Vol. 92, No. 3, pp. 316-329, ISSN 0301-0082

Duan W. & Mattson M. P. (1999) Dietary restriction and 2-deoxyglucose administration improve behavioral outcome and reduce degeneration of dopaminergic neurons in models of Parkinson's disease. *Journal of Neuroscience Research*, Vol. 57, No. 2, pp. 195-206, ISSN 0360-4012

Duarte E. P., Saavedra A. & Baltazar G. (2007) GDNF: a key player in neuron-glia crosstalk and survival of nigrostriatal dopaminergic neurons, In: *Interaction between neurons and glia in aging and disease*, Malva J. O., Rego A. C., Cunha R. & Oliveira C. R., pp. 173-192, Springer-Verlag, ISBN 9780387708300, Berlin

Evans J. R. & Barker R. A. (2008) Neurotrophic factors as a therapeutic target for Parkinson's disease. *Expert Opinion on Therapeutic Targets*, Vol. 12, No. 4, pp. 437-447, ISSN 1472-8222

Faherty C. J., Raviie S. K., Herasimtschuk A. & Smeyne R. J. (2005) Environmental enrichment in adulthood eliminates neuronal death in experimental parkinsonism. *Brain Research Molecular Brain Research,* Vol. 134, No. 1, pp. 170-179, ISSN 0169-328X

Falvo M. J., Schilling B. K. & Earhart G. M. (2008) Parkinson's disease and resistive exercise: rationale, review, and recommendations. *Movement Disorders,* Vol. 23, No. 1, pp. 1-11, ISSN 0885-3185

Finch C. E. (2004) The neurotoxicology of hard foraging and fat-melts. *Proceedings of the National Academy of Sciences of the United States of America,* Vol. 101, No. 52, pp. 17887-17888, ISSN 0027-8424

Fisher B. E., Petzinger G. M., Nixon K., Hogg E., Bremmer S., Meshul C. K. & Jakowec M. W. (2004) Exercise-induced behavioral recovery and neuroplasticity in the 1-methyl-4-phenyl-1,2,3,6-tetrahydropyridine-lesioned mouse basal ganglia. *Journal of Neuroscience Research,* Vol. 77, No. 3, pp. 378-390, ISSN 0360-4012

Frank L., Ventimiglia R., Anderson K., Lindsay R. M. & Rudge J. S. (1996) BDNF down-regulates neurotrophin responsiveness, TrkB protein and TrkB mRNA levels in cultured rat hippocampal neurons. *European Journal of Neuroscience,* Vol. 8, No. 6, pp. 1220-1230, ISSN 0953-816X

Gage H. & Storey L. (2004) Rehabilitation for Parkinson's disease: a systematic review of available evidence. Clinical rehabilitation., Vol. 18, No. 5, pp. 463-482, ISSN 0269-2155

Gao X., Chen H., Fung T. T., Logroscino G., Schwarzschild M. A., Hu F. B. & Ascherio A. (2007) Prospective study of dietary pattern and risk of Parkinson disease. *The American Journal of Clinical Nutrition,* Vol. 86, No. 5, pp. 1486-1494, ISSN 0002-9165

Garcia-Segura L. M., Cardona-Gomez P., Naftolin F. & Chowen J. A. (1998) Estradiol upregulates Bcl-2 expression in adult brain neurons. *Neuroreport,* Vol. 9, No. 4, pp. 593-597, ISSN 0959-4965

Garcia-Segura L. M., Diz-Chaves Y., Perez-Martin M. & Darnaudery M. (2007) Estradiol, insulin-like growth factor-I and brain aging. *Psychoneuroendocrinology,* Vol. 32 Suppl 1, pp. S57-61, ISSN 0306-4530

Georgievska B., Kirik D. & Bjorklund A. (2002) Aberrant sprouting and downregulation of tyrosine hydroxylase in lesioned nigrostriatal dopamine neurons induced by long-lasting overexpression of glial cell line derived neurotrophic factor in the striatum by lentiviral gene transfer. *Experimental Neurology,* Vol. 177, No. 2, pp. 461-474, ISSN 0014-4886

Georgievska B., Kirik D. & Bjorklund A. (2004) Overexpression of glial cell line-derived neurotrophic factor using a lentiviral vector induces time- and dose-dependent downregulation of tyrosine hydroxylase in the intact nigrostriatal dopamine system. *Journal of Neuroscience,* Vol. 24, No. 29, pp. 6437-6445, ISSN 0270-6474

Gerecke K. M., Jiao Y., Pani A., Pagala V. & Smeyne R. J. (2010) Exercise protects against MPTP-induced neurotoxicity in mice. *Brain Research,* Vol. 1341, pp. 72-83, ISSN 0006-8993

Gill S. S., Patel N. K., Hotton G. R., O'Sullivan K., McCarter R., Bunnage M., Brooks D. J., Svendsen C. N. & Heywood P. (2003) Direct brain infusion of glial cell line-derived neurotrophic factor in Parkinson disease. *Nature Medicine,* Vol. 9, No. 5, pp. 589-595, ISSN 1078-8956

Gillies G. E. & McArthur S. (2010a) Independent influences of sex steroids of systemic and central origin in a rat model of Parkinson's disease: A contribution to sex-specific neuroprotection by estrogens. *Hormones and Behavior*, Vol. 57, No. 1, pp. 23-34, ISSN 1095-6867

Gillies G. E. & McArthur S. (2010b) Estrogen actions in the brain and the basis for differential action in men and women: a case for sex-specific medicines. *Pharmacological Reviews*, Vol. 62, No. 2, pp. 155-198, ISSN 1521-0081

Glatt S. L., Hubble J. P., Lyons K., Paolo A., Troster A. I., Hassanein R. E. & Koller W. C. (1996) Risk factors for dementia in Parkinson's disease: effect of education. *Neuroepidemiology*, Vol. 15, No. 1, pp. 20-25, ISSN 0251-5350

Gomez-Pinilla F., So V. & Kesslak J. P. (1998) Spatial learning and physical activity contribute to the induction of fibroblast growth factor: neural substrates for increased cognition associated with exercise. *Neuroscience*, Vol. 85, No. 1, pp. 53-61, ISSN 0306-4522

Goodwin V. A., Richards S. H., Taylor R. S., Taylor A. H. & Campbell J. L. (2008) The effectiveness of exercise interventions for people with Parkinson's disease: a systematic review and meta-analysis. *Movement Disorders*, Vol. 23, No. 5, pp. 631-640, ISSN 0885-3185

Haapasalo A., Sipola I., Larsson K., Akerman K. E., Stoilov P., Stamm S., Wong G. & Castren E. (2002) Regulation of TRKB surface expression by brain-derived neurotrophic factor and truncated TRKB isoforms. *Journal of Biological Chemistry*, Vol. 277, No. 45, pp. 43160-43167, ISSN 0021-9258

Halagappa V. K., Guo Z., Pearson M., Matsuoka Y., Cutler R. G., Laferla F. M. & Mattson M. P. (2007) Intermittent fasting and caloric restriction ameliorate age-related behavioral deficits in the triple-transgenic mouse model of Alzheimer's disease. *Neurobiology of Disease*, Vol. 26, No. 1, pp. 212-220, ISSN 0969-9961

Halliday G. M. & Stevens C. H. (2011) Glia: Initiators and progressors of pathology in Parkinson's disease. *Movement Disorders*, Vol. 26, No. 1, pp. 6-17, ISSN 1531-8257

Hashimoto M., Nitta A., Fukumitsu H., Nomoto H., Shen L. & Furukawa S. (2005) Inflammation-induced GDNF improves locomotor function after spinal cord injury. *Neuroreport*, Vol. 16, No. 2, pp. 99-102, ISSN 0959-4965

He D. Y. & Ron D. (2006) Autoregulation of glial cell line-derived neurotrophic factor expression: implications for the long-lasting actions of the anti-addiction drug, Ibogaine. *The FASEB Journal*, Vol. 20, No. 13, pp. 2420-2422, ISSN 1530-6860

He D. Y., McGough N. N., Ravindranathan A., Jeanblanc J., Logrip M. L., Phamluong K., Janak P. H. & Ron D. (2005) Glial cell line-derived neurotrophic factor mediates the desirable actions of the anti-addiction drug ibogaine against alcohol consumption. *Journal of Neuroscience*, Vol. 25, No. 3, pp. 619-628, ISSN 1529-2401

He Y., Appel S. & Le W. (2001) Minocycline inhibits microglial activation and protects nigral cells after 6-hydroxydopamine injection into mouse striatum. *Brain Research*, Vol. 909, No. 1-2, pp. 187-193, ISSN 0006-8993

Hirsch E. C. & Hunot S. (2009) Neuroinflammation in Parkinson's disease: a target for neuroprotection? *Lancet Neurology*, Vol. 8, No. 4, pp. 382-397, ISSN 1474-4422

Hirsch M. A. & Farley B. G. (2009) Exercise and neuroplasticity in persons living with Parkinson's disease. *European Journal of Physical and Rehabilitation Medicine*, Vol. 45, No. 2, pp. 215-229, ISSN 1973-9087

Ho A. & Blum M. (1998) Induction of interleukin-1 associated with compensatory dopaminergic sprouting in the denervated striatum of young mice: model of aging and neurodegenerative disease. *Journal of Neuroscience*, Vol. 18, No. 15, pp. 5614-5629, ISSN 0270-6474

Hong M., Mukhida K. & Mendez I. (2008) GDNF therapy for Parkinson's disease. *Expert Review of Neurotherapeutics*, Vol. 8, No. 7, pp. 1125-1139, ISSN 1744-8360

Hovland D. N., Jr., Boyd R. B., Butt M. T., Engelhardt J. A., Moxness M. S., Ma M. H., Emery M. G., Ernst N. B., Reed R. P., Zeller J. R., Gash D. M., Masterman D. M., Potter B. M., Cosenza M. E. & Lightfoot R. M. (2007) Six-month continuous intraputamenal infusion toxicity study of recombinant methionyl human glial cell line-derived neurotrophic factor (r-metHuGDNF in rhesus monkeys. *Toxicologic Pathology*, Vol. 35, No. 7, pp. 1013-1029, ISSN 0192-6233

Hu G., Jousilahti P., Nissinen A., Antikainen R., Kivipelto M. & Tuomilehto J. (2006) Body mass index and the risk of Parkinson disease. *Neurology*, Vol. 67, No. 11, pp. 1955-1959, ISSN 0028-3878

Ibanez C. F. (2010) Beyond the cell surface: new mechanisms of receptor function. *Biochemical and Biophysical Research Communications*, Vol. 396, No. 1, pp. 24-27, ISSN 1090-2104

Ichikawa H., Sato T., Kano M., Suzuki T., Matsuo S., Kanetaka H. & Shimizu Y. (2011) Masseteric nerve injury increases expression of Brain-Derived Neurotrophic Factor in microglia within the rat mesencephalic trigeminal tract nucleus. *Cellular and Molecular Neurobiology*, Vol. 31, No. 4, pp. 551-559, ISSN 1573-6830

Ikeda K., Kashihara H., Tamura M., Kano O., Iwamoto K. & Iwasaki Y. (2007) Body mass index and the risk of Parkinson disease. *Neurology*, Vol. 68, No. 24, pp. 2156-2157, ISSN 0028-3878

Ivanova T., Karolczak M. & Beyer C. (2002) Estradiol stimulates GDNF expression in developing hypothalamic neurons. *Endocrinology*, Vol. 143, No. 8, pp. 3175-3178, ISSN 0013-7227

Ivanova T., Kuppers E., Engele J. & Beyer C. (2001) Estrogen stimulates brain-derived neurotrophic factor expression in embryonic mouse midbrain neurons through a membrane-mediated and calcium-dependent mechanism. *Journal of Neuroscience Research*, Vol. 66, No. 2, pp. 221-230, ISSN 0360-4012

Jadavji N. M., Kolb B. & Metz G. A. (2006) Enriched environment improves motor function in intact and unilateral dopamine-depleted rats. *Neuroscience*, Vol. 140, No. 4, pp. 1127-1138, ISSN 0306-4522

Jenner P. (2003) Oxidative stress in Parkinson's disease. *Annals of Neurology*, Vol. 53 Suppl 3, pp. 26-36, ISSN 0364-5134

Jeon S., Kim Y. J., Kim S. T., Moon W., Chae Y., Kang M., Chung M. Y., Lee H., Hong M. S., Chung J. H., Joh T. H., Lee H. & Park H. J. (2008) Proteomic analysis of the neuroprotective mechanisms of acupuncture treatment in a Parkinson's disease mouse model. *Proteomics*, Vol. 8, No. 22, pp. 4822-4832, ISSN 1615-9853

Jia J., Li B., Sun Z. L., Yu F., Wang X. & Wang X. M. (2010) Electro-acupuncture stimulation acts on the basal ganglia output pathway to ameliorate motor impairment in Parkinsonian model rats. *Behavioral Neuroscience*, Vol. 124, No. 2, pp. 305-310, ISSN 0735-7044

Jia J., Sun Z., Li B., Pan Y., Wang H., Wang X., Yu F., Liu L., Zhang L. & Wang X. (2009) Electro-acupuncture stimulation improves motor disorders in Parkinsonian rats. *Behavioural Brain Research,* Vol. 205, No. 1, pp. 214-218, ISSN 0166-4328

Joh T. H., Park H. J., Kim S. N. & Lee H. (2010) Recent development of acupuncture on Parkinson's disease. *Neurological Research,* Vol. 32 Suppl 1, pp. 5-9, ISSN 0161-6412

Johnson C. C., Gorell J. M., Rybicki B. A., Sanders K. & Peterson E. L. (1999) Adult nutrient intake as a risk factor for Parkinson's disease. *International Journal of Epidemiology,* Vol. 28, No. 6, pp. 1102-1109, ISSN 0300-5771

Johnson M. L., Day A. E., Ho C. C., Walker Q. D., Francis R. & Kuhn C. M. (2010) Androgen decreases dopamine neurone survival in rat midbrain. *Journal of Neuroendocrinology,* Vol. 22, No. 4, pp. 238-247, ISSN 1365-2826

Jokinen P., Bruck A., Aalto S., Forsback S., Parkkola R. & Rinne J. O. (2009) Impaired cognitive performance in Parkinson's disease is related to caudate dopaminergic hypofunction and hippocampal atrophy. *Parkinsonism & Related Disorders,* Vol. 15, No. 2, pp. 88-93, ISSN 1353-8020

Jourdain S., Morissette M., Morin N. & Di Paolo T. (2005) Oestrogens prevent loss of dopamine transporter (DAT) and vesicular monoamine transporter (VMAT2) in substantia nigra of 1-methyl-4-phenyl-1,2,3,6-tetrahydropyridine mice. *Journal of Neuroendocrinology,* Vol. 17, No. 8, pp. 509-517, ISSN 0953-8194

Kang J., Qian P. X., Pandey V., Perry J. K., Miller L. D., Liu E. T., Zhu T., Liu D. X. & Lobie P. E. (2010) Artemin is estrogen regulated and mediates antiestrogen resistance in mammary carcinoma. *Oncogene,* Vol. 29, No. 22, pp. 3228-3240, ISSN 1476-5594

Kang J. M., Park H. J., Choi Y. G., Choe I. H., Park J. H., Kim Y. S. & Lim S. (2007) Acupuncture inhibits microglial activation and inflammatory events in the MPTP-induced mouse model. *Brain Research,* Vol. 1131, No. 1, pp. 211-219, ISSN 0006-8993

Kastin A. J., Akerstrom V. & Pan W. (2003) Glial cell line-derived neurotrophic factor does not enter normal mouse brain. *Neuroscience Letters,* Vol. 340, No. 3, pp. 239-241, ISSN 0304-3940

Khan M. M., Hoda M. N., Ishrat T., Ahmad A., Khan M. B., Khuwaja G., Raza S. S., Safhi M. M. & Islam F. (2010) Amelioration of 1-methyl-4-phenyl-1,2,3,6-tetrahydropyridine-induced behavioural dysfunction and oxidative stress by Pycnogenol in mouse model of Parkinson's disease. *Behavioural Pharmacology,* Vol. 21, No. 5-6, pp. 563-571, ISSN 0955-8810

Kim I. S., Koppula S., Park P. J., Kim E. H., Kim C. G., Choi W. S., Lee K. H. & Choi D. K. (2009) Chrysanthemum morifolium Ramat (CM) extract protects human neuroblastoma SH-SY5Y cells against MPP+-induced cytotoxicity. *Journal of Ethnopharmacology,* Vol. 126, No. 3, pp. 447-454, ISSN 0378-8741

Kim J. S., Kim J. M., Jj O. & Jeon B. S. (2010) Inhibition of inducible nitric oxide synthase expression and cell death by (-)-epigallocatechin-3-gallate, a green tea catechin, in the 1-methyl-4-phenyl-1,2,3,6-tetrahydropyridine mouse model of Parkinson's disease. *Journal of Clinical Neuroscience,* Vol. 17, No. 9, pp. 1165-1168, ISSN 0967-5868

Kim Y. K., Lim H. H., Song Y. K., Lee H. H., Lim S., Han S. M. & Kim C. J. (2005) Effect of acupuncture on 6-hydroxydopamine-induced nigrostratal dopaminergic neuronal cell death in rats. *Neuroscience Letters,* Vol. 384, No. 1-2, pp. 133-138, ISSN 0304-3940

Kim Y. S. & Joh T. H. (2006) Microglia, major player in the brain inflammation: their roles in the pathogenesis of Parkinson's disease. *Experimental & Molecular Medicine*, Vol. 38, No. 4, pp. 333-347, ISSN 1226-3613

Kipp M., Karakaya S., Pawlak J., Araujo-Wright G., Arnold S. & Beyer C. (2006) Estrogen and the development and protection of nigrostriatal dopaminergic neurons: concerted action of a multitude of signals, protective molecules, and growth factors. *Frontiers in Neuroendocrinology*, Vol. 27, No. 4, pp. 376-390, ISSN 0091-3022

Kirik D., Georgievska B. & Bjorklund A. (2004) Localized striatal delivery of GDNF as a treatment for Parkinson disease. *Nature Neuroscience*, Vol. 7, No. 2, pp. 105-110, ISSN 1097-6256

Kitamura Y., Inden M., Minamino H., Abe M., Takata K. & Taniguchi T. (2010) The 6-hydroxydopamine-induced nigrostriatal neurodegeneration produces microglia-like NG2 glial cells in the rat substantia nigra. *Glia*, Vol. 58, No. 14, pp. 1686-1700, ISSN 1098-1136

Knusel B., Gao H., Okazaki T., Yoshida T., Mori N., Hefti F. & Kaplan D. R. (1997) Ligand-induced down-regulation of Trk messenger RNA, protein and tyrosine phosphorylation in rat cortical neurons. *Neuroscience*, Vol. 78, No. 3, pp. 851-862, ISSN 0306-4522

Kuno R., Yoshida Y., Nitta A., Nabeshima T., Wang J., Sonobe Y., Kawanokuchi J., Takeuchi H., Mizuno T. & Suzumura A. (2006) The role of TNF-alpha and its receptors in the production of NGF and GDNF by astrocytes. *Brain Research*, Vol. 1116, No. 1, pp. 12-18, ISSN 0006-8993

Kurtzke J. F. & Goldberg I. D. (1988) Parkinsonism death rates by race, sex, and geography. *Neurology*, Vol. 38, No. 10, pp. 1558-1561, ISSN 0028-3878

Laakso A., Vilkman H., Bergman J., Haaparanta M., Solin O., Syvalahti E., Salokangas R. K. & Hietala J. (2002) Sex differences in striatal presynaptic dopamine synthesis capacity in healthy subjects. *Biological Psychiatry*, Vol. 52, No. 7, pp. 759-763, ISSN 0006-3223

Lang A. E., Gill S., Patel N. K., Lozano A., Nutt J. G., Penn R., Brooks D. J., Hotton G., Moro E., Heywood P., Brodsky M. A., Burchiel K., Kelly P., Dalvi A., Scott B., Stacy M., Turner D., Wooten V. G., Elias W. J., Laws E. R., Dhawan V., Stoessl A. J., Matcham J., Coffey R. J. & Traub M. (2006) Randomized controlled trial of intraputamenal glial cell line-derived neurotrophic factor infusion in Parkinson disease. *Annals of Neurology*, Vol. 59, No. 3, pp. 459-466, ISSN 0364-5134

Larsen K. E., Benn S. C., Ay I., Chian R. J., Celia S. A., Remington M. P., Bejarano M., Liu M., Ross J., Carmillo P., Sah D., Phillips K. A., Sulzer D., Pepinsky R. B., Fishman P. S., Brown R. H., Jr. & Francis J. W. (2006) A glial cell line-derived neurotrophic factor (GDNF):tetanus toxin fragment C protein conjugate improves delivery of GDNF to spinal cord motor neurons in mice. *Brain Research*, Vol. 1120, No. 1, pp. 1-12, ISSN 0006-8993

Lau Y. S., Patki G., Das-Panja K., Le W. D. & Ahmad, S.O. (2011) Neuroprotective effects and mechanisms of exercise in a chronic mouse model of Parkinson's disease with moderate neurodegeneration. *European Journal of Neuroscience*, Vol. 33, No. 7, pp. 1264-1274, ISSN 0953-816X

Lauterborn J. C., Pineda E., Chen L. Y., Ramirez E. A., Lynch G. & Gall C. M. (2009) Ampakines cause sustained increases in brain-derived neurotrophic factor signaling at excitatory synapses without changes in AMPA receptor subunit expression. *Neuroscience*, Vol. 159, No. 1, pp. 283-295, ISSN 0306-4522

Lee C. H., Hwang D. S., Kim H. G., Oh H., Park H., Cho J. H., Lee J. M., Jang J. B., Lee K. S. & Oh M. S. (2010) Protective effect of Cyperi rhizoma against 6-hydroxydopamine-induced neuronal damage. *Journal of Medicinal Food*, Vol. 13, No. 3, pp. 564-571, ISSN 1096-620X

Lehman D. A., Toole T., Lofald D. & Hirsch M. A. (2005) Training with verbal instructional cues results in near-term improvement of gait in people with Parkinson disease. *Journal of Neurologic Physical Therapy*, Vol. 29, No. 1, pp. 2-8, ISSN 1557-0576

Liang J., Takeuchi H., Jin S., Noda M., Li H., Doi Y., Kawanokuchi J., Sonobe Y., Mizuno T. & Suzumura A. (2010) Glutamate induces neurotrophic factor production from microglia via protein kinase C pathway. *Brain Research*, Vol. 1322, pp. 8-23, ISSN 1872-6240

Liang X. B., Luo Y., Liu X. Y., Lu J., Li F. Q., Wang Q., Wang X. M. & Han J. S. (2003) Electro-acupuncture improves behavior and upregulates GDNF mRNA in MFB transected rats. *Neuroreport*, Vol. 14, No. 8, pp. 1177-1181, ISSN 0959-4965

Liberatore G. T., Wong J. Y., Porritt M. J., Donnan G. A. & Howells D. W. (1997) Expression of glial cell line-derived neurotrophic factor (GDNF) mRNA following mechanical injury to mouse striatum. *Neuroreport*, Vol. 8, No. 14, pp. 3097-3101, ISSN 0959-4965

Liberatore G. T., Jackson-Lewis V., Vukosavic S., Mandir A. S., Vila M., McAuliffe W. G., Dawson V. L., Dawson T. M. & Przedborski S. (1999) Inducible nitric oxide synthase stimulates dopaminergic neurodegeneration in the MPTP model of Parkinson disease. *Nature Medicine*, Vol. 5, No. 12, pp. 1403-1409, ISSN 1078-8956

Lin, L. F., Doherty, D. H., Lile, J. D., Bektesh, S. & Collins, F. (1993) GDNF: a glial cell line-derived neurotrophic factor for midbrain dopaminergic neurons. *Science*, Vol. 260, No. 5111, pp. 1130-1132, ISSN 0036-8075

Lindholm P., Voutilainen M. H., Lauren J., Peranen J., Leppanen V. M., Andressoo J. O., Lindahl M., Janhunen S., Kalkkinen N., Timmusk T., Tuominen R. K. & Saarma M. (2007) Novel neurotrophic factor CDNF protects and rescues midbrain dopamine neurons in vivo. *Nature*, Vol. 448, No. 7149, pp. 73-77, ISSN1476-4687

Liu B. & Dluzen D. E. (2007) Oestrogen and nigrostriatal dopaminergic neurodegeneration: animal models and clinical reports of Parkinson's disease. *Clinical and Experimental Pharmacology & Physiology*, Vol. 34, No. 7, pp. 555-565, ISSN 0305-1870

Liu X., Fan X.-L., Zhao Y., Luo G.-R., Li X.-P., Li R. & Le W.-D. (2005) Estrogen provides neuroprotection against activated microglia-induced dopaminergic neuronal injury through both estrogen receptor-alpha and estrogen receptor-beta in microglia. *Journal of Neuroscience Research*, Vol. 81, No. 5, pp. 653-665, ISSN 0360-4012

Logroscino G., Sesso H. D., Paffenbarger R. S., Jr. & Lee I. M. (2006) Physical activity and risk of Parkinson's disease: a prospective cohort study. *Journal of Neurology, Neurosurgery, and Psychiatry*, Vol. 77, No. 12, pp. 1318-1322, ISSN 1468-330X

Logroscino G., Marder K., Cote L., Tang M. X., Shea S. & Mayeux R. (1996) Dietary lipids and antioxidants in Parkinson's disease: a population-based, case-control study. *Annals of Neurology*, Vol. 39, No. 1, pp. 89-94, ISSN 0364-5134

Lokk J. & Nilsson M. (2010) Frequency, type and factors associated with the use of complementary and alternative medicine in patients with Parkinson's disease at a neurological outpatient clinic. *Parkinsonism & Related Disorders*, Vol. 16, No. 8, pp. 540-544, ISSN 1353-8020

Love S., Plaha P., Patel N. K., Hotton G. R., Brooks D. J. & Gill S. S. (2005) Glial cell line-derived neurotrophic factor induces neuronal sprouting in human brain. *Nature Medicine*, Vol. 11, No. 7, pp. 703-704, ISSN 1078-8956

Luo F. C., Wang S. D., Qi L., Song J. Y., Lv T. & Bai J. (2011) Protective effect of panaxatriol saponins extracted from Panax notoginseng against MPTP-induced neurotoxicity in vivo. *Journal of Ethnopharmacology*, Vol. 133, No. 2, pp. 448-453, ISSN 0378-8741

Lynch M. A. (2009) The multifaceted profile of activated microglia. *Molecular Neurobiology*, Vol. 40, No. 2, pp. 139-156, ISSN 0893-7648

Mabandla M., Kellaway L., St Clair G. A. & Russell V. A. (2004) Voluntary running provides neuroprotection in rats after 6-hydroxydopamine injection into the medial forebrain bundle. *Metabolic Brain Disease*, Vol. 19, No. 1-2, pp. 43-50, ISSN 0885-7490

Madinier A., Bertrand N., Mossiat C., Prigent-Tessier A., Beley A., Marie C. & Garnier P. (2009) Microglial involvement in neuroplastic changes following focal brain ischemia in rats. *PLoS One*, Vol. 4, No. 12, pp. e8101, ISSN 1932-6203

Manfredsson F. P., Okun M. S. & Mandel R. J. (2009) Gene therapy for neurological disorders: challenges and future prospects for the use of growth factors for the treatment of Parkinson's disease. *Current Gene Therapy*, Vol. 9, No. 5, pp. 375-388, ISSN 1566-5232

Marder K., Tang M. X., Mejia H., Alfaro B., Cote L., Louis E., Groves J. & Mayeux R. (1996) Risk of Parkinson's disease among first-degree relatives: A community-based study. *Neurology*, Vol. 47, No. 1, pp. 155-160, ISSN 0028-3878

Marks W. J., Jr., Ostrem J. L., Verhagen L., Starr P. A., Larson P. S., Bakay R. A., Taylor R., Cahn-Weiner D. A., Stoessl A. J., Olanow C. W. & Bartus R. T. (2008) Safety and tolerability of intraputaminal delivery of CERE-120 (adeno-associated virus serotype 2-neurturin) to patients with idiopathic Parkinson's disease: an open-label, phase I trial. *Lancet Neurology*, Vol. 7, No. 5, pp. 400-408, ISSN 1474-4422

Marks W. J., Jr., Bartus R. T., Siffert J., Davis C. S., Lozano A., Boulis N., Vitek J., Stacy M., Turner D., Verhagen L., Bakay R., Watts R., Guthrie B., Jankovic J., Simpson R., Tagliati M., Alterman R., Stern M., Baltuch G., Starr P. A., Larson P. S., Ostrem J. L., Nutt J., Kieburtz K., Kordower J. H. & Olanow C. W. (2010) Gene delivery of AAV2-neurturin for Parkinson's disease: a double-blind, randomised, controlled trial. *Lancet Neurology*, Vol. 9, No. 12, pp. 1164-1172, ISSN 1474-4422

Martin B., Mattson M. P. & Maudsley S. (2006) Caloric restriction and intermittent fasting: two potential diets for successful brain aging. *Ageing Research Reviews*, Vol. 5, No. 3, pp. 332-353, ISSN 1568-1637

Maswood N., Young J., Tilmont E., Zhang Z., Gash D. M., Gerhardt G. A., Grondin R., Roth G. S., Mattison J., Lane M. A., Carson R. E., Cohen R. M., Mouton P. R., Quigley C., Mattson M. P. & Ingram D. K. (2004) Caloric restriction increases neurotrophic factor levels and attenuates neurochemical and behavioral deficits in a primate model of Parkinson's disease. *Proceedings of the National Academy of Sciences of the United States of America*, Vol. 101, No. 52, pp. 18171-18176, ISSN 0027-8424

Mattson M. P. (2005) Energy intake, meal frequency, and health: a neurobiological perspective. *Annual Review of Nutrition*, Vol. 25, No. pp. 237-260, ISSN 0199-9885

Mattson M. P. & Magnus T. (2006) Ageing and neuronal vulnerability. *Nature Reviews Neuroscience*, Vol. 7, No. 4, pp. 278-294, ISSN 1471-003X

Mattson M. P., Duan W., Wan R. & Guo Z. (2004) Prophylactic activation of neuroprotective stress response pathways by dietary and behavioral manipulations. *NeuroRx*, Vol. 1, No. 1, pp. 111-116, ISSN 1545-5343

Mayeux R., Denaro J., Hemenegildo N., Marder K., Tang M. X., Cote L. J. & Stern Y. (1992) A population-based investigation of Parkinson's disease with and without dementia. Relationship to age and gender. *Archives of Neurology*, Vol. 49, No. 5, pp. 492-497, ISSN 0003-9942

McNaught K. S. & Jenner P. (2000) Dysfunction of rat forebrain astrocytes in culture alters cytokine and neurotrophic factor release. *Neuroscience Letters*, Vol. 285, No. 1, pp. 61-65, ISSN 0304-3940

Miller I. N. & Cronin-Golomb A. (2010) Gender differences in Parkinson's disease: clinical characteristics and cognition. *Movement Disorders*, Vol. 25, No. 16, pp. 2695-2703, ISSN 1531-8257

Min K. J., Yang M. S., Kim S. U., Jou I. & Joe E. H. (2006) Astrocytes induce hemeoxygenase-1 expression in microglia: a feasible mechanism for preventing excessive brain inflammation. *Journal of Neuroscience*, Vol. 26, No. 6, pp. 1880-1887, ISSN 1529-2401

Miyake Y., Sasaki S., Tanaka K., Fukushima W., Kiyohara C., Tsuboi Y., Yamada T., Oeda T., Miki T., Kawamura N., Sakae N., Fukuyama H., Hirota Y. & Nagai M. (2010) Dietary fat intake and risk of Parkinson's disease: a case-control study in Japan. *Journal of the Neurological Sciences*, Vol. 288, No. 1-2, pp. 117-122, ISSN 0022-510X

Mochizuki H., Goto K., Mori H. & Mizuno Y. (1996) Histochemical detection of apoptosis in Parkinson's disease. *Journal of the Neurological Sciences*, Vol. 137, No. 2, pp. 120-123, ISSN 0022-510X

Mooradian A. D. (1993) Antioxidant properties of steroids. *Journal of Steroid Biochemistry and Molecular Biology*, Vol. 45, No. 6, pp. 509-511, ISSN 0960-0760

Morale M. C., Serra P. A., L'Episcopo F., Tirolo C., Caniglia S., Testa N., Gennuso F., Giaquinta G., Rocchitta G., Desole M. S., Miele E. & Marchetti B. (2006) Estrogen, neuroinflammation and neuroprotection in Parkinson's disease: glia dictates resistance versus vulnerability to neurodegeneration. *Neuroscience*, Vol. 138, No. 3, pp. 869-878, ISSN 0306-4522

Morissette M., Le Saux M., D'Astous M., Jourdain S., Al Sweidi S., Morin N., Estrada-Camarena E., Mendez P., Garcia-Segura L. M. & Di Paolo T. (2008) Contribution of estrogen receptors alpha and beta to the effects of estradiol in the brain. *Journal of Steroid Biochemistry and Molecular Biology*, Vol. 108, No. 3-5, pp. 327-338, ISSN 0960-0760

Morris J. K., Bomhoff G. L., Stanford J. A. & Geiger P. C. (2010) Neurodegeneration in an animal model of Parkinson's disease is exacerbated by a high-fat diet. *American Journal of Physiology-Regulatory, Integrative and Comparative Physiology*, Vol. 299, No. 4, pp. R1082-R1090, ISSN 0363-6119

Munro C. A., McCaul M. E., Wong D. F., Oswald L. M., Zhou Y., Brasic J., Kuwabara H., Kumar A., Alexander M., Ye W. & Wand G. S. (2006) Sex differences in striatal dopamine release in healthy adults. *Biological Psychiatry*, Vol. 59, No. 10, pp. 966-974, ISSN 0006-3223

Murray H. E., Pillai A. V., McArthur S. R., Razvi N., Datla K. P., Dexter D. T. & Gillies G. E. (2003) Dose- and sex-dependent effects of the neurotoxin 6-hydroxydopamine on the nigrostriatal dopaminergic pathway of adult rats: differential actions of estrogen in males and females. *Neuroscience*, Vol. 116, No. 1, pp. 213-222, ISSN 0306-4522

Nithianantharajah J. & Hannan A. J. (2006) Enriched environments, experience-dependent plasticity and disorders of the nervous system. *Nature Reviews Neuroscience*, Vol. 7, No. 9, pp. 697-709, ISSN 1471-003X

Nitta A., Nishioka H., Fukumitsu H., Furukawa Y., Sugiura H., Shen L. & Furukawa S. (2004) Hydrophobic dipeptide Leu-Ile protects against neuronal death by inducing brain-derived neurotrophic factor and glial cell line-derived neurotrophic factor synthesis. *Journal of Neuroscience Research*, Vol. 78, No. 2, pp. 250-258, ISSN 0360-4012

Nutt J. G., Burchiel K. J., Comella C. L., Jankovic J., Lang A. E., Laws E. R., Jr., Lozano A. M., Penn R. D., Simpson R. K., Jr., Stacy M. & Wooten G. F. (2003) Randomized, double-blind trial of glial cell line-derived neurotrophic factor (GDNF) in PD. *Neurology*, Vol. 60, No. 1, pp. 69-73, ISSN 0028-3878

O'Dell S. J., Gross N. B., Fricks A. N., Casiano B. D., Nguyen T. B. & Marshall J. F. (2007) Running wheel exercise enhances recovery from nigrostriatal dopamine injury without inducing neuroprotection. *Neuroscience*, Vol. 144, No. 3, pp. 1141-1151, ISSN 0306-4522

Pan M., Li Z., Yeung V. & Xu R. J. (2010) Dietary supplementation of soy germ phytoestrogens or estradiol improves spatial memory performance and increases gene expression of BDNF, TrkB receptor and synaptic factors in ovariectomized rats. *Nutrition & Metabolism (Lond)*, Vol. 7, pp. 75, ISSN 1743-7075

Parish C. L., Finkelstein D. I., Tripanichkul W., Satoskar A. R., Drago J. & Horne M. K. (2002) The role of interleukin-1, interleukin-6, and glia in inducing growth of neuronal terminal arbors in mice. *Journal of Neuroscience*, Vol. 22, No. 18, pp. 8034-8041, ISSN 1529-2401

Park H. J., Lim S., Joo W. S., Yin C. S., Lee H. S., Lee H. J., Seo J. C., Leem K., Son Y. S., Kim Y. J., Kim C. J., Kim Y. S. & Chung J. H. (2003) Acupuncture prevents 6-hydroxydopamine-induced neuronal death in the nigrostriatal dopaminergic system in the rat Parkinson's disease model. *Experimental Neurology*, Vol. 180, No. 1, pp. 93-98, ISSN 0014-4886

Park H. R., Park M., Choi J., Park K. Y., Chung H. Y. & Lee J. (2010) A high-fat diet impairs neurogenesis: involvement of lipid peroxidation and brain-derived neurotrophic factor. *Neuroscience Letters*, Vol. 482, No. 3, pp. 235-239, ISSN 0304-3940

Pascual A., Hidalgo-Figueroa M., Piruat J. I., Pintado C. O., Gomez-Diaz R. & Lopez-Barneo J. (2008) Absolute requirement of GDNF for adult catecholaminergic neuron survival. *Nature Neuroscience*, Vol. 11, No. 7, pp. 755-761, ISSN 1097-6256

Pecci C., Rivas M. J., Moretti C. M., Raina G., Ramirez C. Z., Diaz S., Uribe R. C. & Micheli F. E. (2010) Use of complementary and alternative therapies in outpatients with Parkinson's disease in Argentina. *Movement Disorders*, Vol. 25, No. 13, pp. 2094-2098, ISSN 0885-3185

Peng G. S., Li G., Tzeng N. S., Chen P. S., Chuang D. M., Hsu Y. D., Yang S. & Hong J. S. (2005) Valproate pretreatment protects dopaminergic neurons from LPS-induced neurotoxicity in rat primary midbrain cultures: role of microglia. *Brain Research-Molecular Brain Research*, Vol. 134, No. 1, pp. 162-169, ISSN 0169-328X

Peterson A. L. & Nutt J. G. (2008) Treatment of Parkinson's disease with trophic factors. *Neurotherapeutics*, Vol. 5, No. 2, pp. 270-280, ISSN 1878-7479

Petrova P., Raibekas A., Pevsner J., Vigo N., Anafi M., Moore M. K., Peaire A. E., Shridhar V., Smith D. I., Kelly J., Durocher Y. & Commissiong J. W. (2003) MANF: a new mesencephalic, astrocyte-derived neurotrophic factor with selectivity for dopaminergic neurons. *Journal of Molecular Neuroscience*, Vol. 20, No. 2, pp. 173-188, ISSN 0895-8696

Petzinger G. M., Walsh J. P., Akopian G., Hogg E., Abernathy A., Arevalo P., Turnquist P., Vucković M., Fisher B. E., Togasaki D. M. & Jakowec M. W. (2007) Effects of treadmill exercise on dopaminergic transmission in the 1-methyl-4-phenyl-1,2,3,6-tetrahydropyridine-lesioned mouse model of basal ganglia injury. *Journal of Neuroscience*, Vol. 27, No. 20, pp. 5291-5300. ISSN 1529-2401

Pietranera L., Lima A., Roig P. & De Nicola A. F. (2010) Involvement of brain-derived neurotrophic factor and neurogenesis in oestradiol neuroprotection of the hippocampus of hypertensive rats. *Journal of Neuroendocrinology*, Vol. 22, No. 10, pp. 1082-1092, ISSN 1365-2826

Platania P., Seminara G., Aronica E., Troost D., Vincenza Catania M. & Angela Sortino M. (2005) 17beta-estradiol rescues spinal motoneurons from AMPA-induced toxicity: a role for glial cells. *Neurobiology of Disease*, Vol. 20, No. 2, pp. 461-470, ISSN 0969-9961

Przedborski S. & Ischiropoulos H. (2005) Reactive oxygen and nitrogen species: weapons of neuronal destruction in models of Parkinson's disease. *Antioxidants & Redox Signaling*, Vol. 7, No. 5-6, pp. 685-693, ISSN 1523-0864

Rajasankar S., Manivasagam T. & Surendran S. (2009a) Ashwagandha leaf extract: a potential agent in treating oxidative damage and physiological abnormalities seen in a mouse model of Parkinson's disease. *Neuroscience Letters*, Vol. 454, No. 1, pp. 11-15, ISSN 0304-3940

Rajasankar S., Manivasagam T., Sankar V., Prakash S., Muthusamy R., Krishnamurti A. & Surendran S. (2009b) Withania somnifera root extract improves catecholamines and physiological abnormalities seen in a Parkinson's disease model mouse. *Journal of Ethnopharmacology*, Vol. 125, No. 3, pp. 369-373, ISSN 0378-8741

Ramaswamy S., Soderstrom K. E. & Kordower J. H. (2009) Trophic factors therapy in Parkinson's disease. *Progress in Brain Research*, Vol. 175, No. pp. 201-216, ISSN 0079-6123

Ramirez A. D., Liu X. & Menniti F. S. (2003) Repeated estradiol treatment prevents MPTP-induced dopamine depletion in male mice. *Neuroendocrinology*, Vol. 77, No. 4, pp. 223-231, ISSN 0028-3835

Ratan R. R., Murphy T. H. & Baraban J. M. (1994) Oxidative stress induces apoptosis in embryonic cortical neurons. *Journal of Neurochemistry*, Vol. 62, No. 1, pp. 376-379, ISSN 0022-3042

Remy S., Naveilhan P., Paille V., Brachet P. & Neveu I. (2003) Lipopolysaccharide and TNFalpha regulate the expression of GDNF, neurturin and their receptors. *Neuroreport*, Vol. 14, No. 11, pp. 1529-1534, ISSN 0022-3042

Ren X. M. (2008) Fifty cases of Parkinson's disease treated by acupuncture combined with madopar. *Journal of Traditional Chinese Medicine*, Vol. 28, No. 4, pp. 255-257, ISSN 0255-2922

Ridgel A. L., Vitek J. L. & Alberts J. L. (2009) Forced, not voluntary, exercise improves motor function in Parkinson's disease patients. *Neurorehabilitation and Neural Repair*, Vol. 23, No 6, pp. 600-608, ISSN 1552-6844

Rocha S. C. M., Cristovão A. C., Branco D. & Baltazar G. (2010) Astrocyte-derived GDNF is able to prevent the activation of midbrain microglia induced by Zymosan A. *FENS Abstr., vol. 5, 164.33*, FENS Fórum 2010, Amsterdam. The Nederlands. July 2010.

Rodriguez-Navarro J. A., Solano R. M., Casarejos M. J., Gomez A., Perucho J., de Yebenes J. G. & Mena M. A. (2008) Gender differences and estrogen effects in parkin null mice. *Journal of Neurochemistry*, Vol. 106, No. 5, pp. 2143-2157, ISSN 1471-4159

Ron D. & Janak P. H. (2005) GDNF and addiction. *Reviews in Neuroscience*, Vol. 16, No. 4, pp. 277-285, ISSN 16519005

Rosenblad C., Georgievska B. & Kirik D. (2003) Long-term striatal overexpression of GDNF selectively downregulates tyrosine hydroxylase in the intact nigrostriatal dopamine system. *European Journal of Neuroscience*, Vol. 17, No. 2, pp. 260-270, ISSN 0953-816X

Saavedra A., Baltazar G. & Duarte E. P. (2007) Interleukin-1beta mediates GDNF up-regulation upon dopaminergic injury in ventral midbrain cell cultures. *Neurobiology of Disease*, Vol. 25, No. 1, pp. 92-104, ISSN 0969-9961

Saavedra A., Baltazar G. & Duarte E. P. (2008) Driving GDNF expression: the green and the red traffic lights. *Progress in Neurobiology*, Vol. 86, No. 3, pp. 186-215, ISSN 0301-0082

Saavedra A., Baltazar G., Carvalho C. M. & Duarte E. P. (2005) GDNF modulates HO-1 expression in substantia nigra postnatal cell cultures. *Free Radical Biology & Medicine*, Vol. 39, No. 12, pp. 1611-1619, ISSN 0891-5849

Saavedra, A., Baltazar, G., Santos, P., Carvalho, C.M. & Duarte, E.P. (2006) Selective injury to dopaminergic neurons up-regulates GDNF in substantia nigra postnatal cell cultures: role of neuron-glia crosstalk. *Neurobiology of Disease*, Vol. 23, No. 3, pp. 533-542, ISSN 0969-9961

Sapkota K., Kim S., Kim M. K. & Kim S. J. (2010) A detoxified extract of Rhus verniciflua Stokes upregulated the expression of BDNF and GDNF in the rat brain and the human dopaminergic cell line SH-SY5Y. *Bioscience Biotechnology, and Biochemistry*, Vol. 74, No. 10, pp. 1997-2004, ISSN 0916-8451

Sapkota K., Kim S., Park S. E. & Kim S. J. (2011) Detoxified extract of Rhus verniciflua Stokes inhibits rotenone-induced apoptosis in human dopaminergic cells, SH-SY5Y. *Cellular and Molecular Neurobiology*, Vol. 31, No. 2, pp. 213-223, ISSN 0272-4340

Sasco A. J., Paffenbarger R. S., Jr., Gendre I. & Wing A. L. (1992) The role of physical exercise in the occurrence of Parkinson's disease. *Archives of Neurology*, Vol. 49, No. 4, pp. 360-365, ISSN 0003-9942

Satake K., Matsuyama Y., Kamiya M., Kawakami H., Iwata H., Adachi K. & Kiuchi K. (2000) Up-regulation of glial cell line-derived neurotrophic factor (GDNF) following traumatic spinal cord injury. *Neuroreport*, Vol. 11, No. 17, pp. 3877-3881, ISSN 0959-4965

Sawada H., Ibi M., Kihara T., Urushitani M., Akaike A. & Shimohama S. (1998) Estradiol protects mesencephalic dopaminergic neurons from oxidative stress-induced neuronal death. *Journal of Neuroscience Research,* Vol. 54, No. 5, pp. 707-719, ISSN 0306-4012

Sawada H., Ibi M., Kihara T., Urushitani M., Honda K., Nakanishi M., Akaike A. & Shimohama S. (2000) Mechanisms of antiapoptotic effects of estrogens in nigral dopaminergic neurons. *The FASEB Journal,* Vol. 14, No. 9, pp. 1202-1214, ISSN 0892-6638

Schreiber S. L. (1991) Chemistry and biology of the immunophilins and their immunosuppressive ligands. *Science,* Vol. 251, No. 4991, pp. 283-287, ISSN 0036-8075

Sherer T. B., Fiske B. K., Svendsen C. N., Lang A. E. & Langston J. W. (2006) Crossroads in GDNF therapy for Parkinson's disease. *Movement Disorders,* Vol. 21, No. 2, pp. 136-141, ISSN 0885-3185

Shulman L. M. (2007) Gender differences in Parkinson's disease. *Gender Medicine,* Vol. 4, No. 1, pp. 8-18, ISSN 1550-8579

Siegel G. J. & Chauhan N. B. (2000) Neurotrophic factors in Alzheimer's and Parkinson's disease brain. *Brain Research-Brain Research Reviews,* Vol. 33, No. 2-3, pp. 199-227, ISSN 0165-0173

Singer C. A., Rogers K. L. & Dorsa D. M. (1998) Modulation of Bcl-2 expression: a potential component of estrogen protection in NT2 neurons. *Neuroreport,* Vol. 9, No. 11, pp. 2565-2568, ISSN 0959-4965

Slevin J. T., Gerhardt G. A., Smith C. D., Gash D. M., Kryscio R. & Young B. (2005) Improvement of bilateral motor functions in patients with Parkinson disease through the unilateral intraputaminal infusion of glial cell line-derived neurotrophic factor. *Journal of Neurosurgery,* Vol. 102, No. 2, pp. 216-222, ISSN 0022-3085

Smith A. D. & Zigmond M. J. (2003) Can the brain be protected through exercise? Lessons from an animal model of parkinsonism. *Experimental Neurology,* Vol. 184, No. 1, pp. 31-39, ISSN 0014-4886

Smith B. A., Goldberg N. R. S. & Meshul C. K. (2011) Effects of treadmill exercise on behavioral recovery and neural changes in the substantia nigra and striatum of the 1-methyl-4-phenyl-1,2,3,6-tetrahydropyridine-lesioned mouse. *Brain Research,* Vol. 1386, pp. 70-80, ISSN 0006-8993

Smith M. P. & Cass W. A. (2007) GDNF reduces oxidative stress in a 6-hydroxydopamine model of Parkinson's disease. *Neuroscience Letters,* Vol. 412, No. 3, pp. 259-263, ISSN 0304-3940

Soderstrom K., O'Malley J., Steece-Collier K. & Kordower J. H. (2006) Neural repair strategies for Parkinson's disease: insights from primate models. *Cell Transplantation,* Vol. 15, No. 3, pp. 251-265, ISSN 0963-6897

Sriram K., Benkovic S. A., Miller D. B. & O'Callaghan J. P. (2002) Obesity exacerbates chemically induced neurodegeneration. *Neuroscience,* Vol. 115, No. 4, pp. 1335-1346, ISSN 0306-4522

Steiner B., Winter C., Hosman K., Siebert E., Kempermann G., Petrus D. S. & Kupsch A. (2006) Enriched environment induces cellular plasticity in the adult substantia nigra and improves motor behavior function in the 6-OHDA rat model of Parkinson's disease. *Experimental Neurology,* Vol. 199, No. 2, pp. 291-300, ISSN 0014-4886

Sutoo D. & Akiyama K. (2003) Regulation of brain function by exercise. *Neurobiology of Disease*, Vol. 13, No. 1, pp. 1-14, ISSN 0969-9961

Tajiri N., Yasuhara T., Shingo T., Kondo A., Yuan W., Kadota T., Wang F., Baba T., Tayra J. T., Morimoto T., Jing M., Kikuchi Y., Kuramoto S., Agari T., Miyoshi Y., Fujino H., Obata F., Takeda I., Furuta T. & Date I. (2010) Exercise exerts neuroprotective effects on Parkinson's disease model of rats. *Brain Research*, Vol. 1310, pp. 200-207, ISSN 0006-8993

Tan S., Wood M. & Maher P. (1998) Oxidative stress induces a form of programmed cell death with characteristics of both apoptosis and necrosis in neuronal cells. *Journal of Neurochemistry*, Vol. 71, No. 1, pp. 95-105, ISSN 0022-3042

Tansey M. G. & Goldberg M. S. (2010) Neuroinflammation in Parkinson's disease: Its role in neuronal death and implications for therapeutic intervention. *Neurobiology of Disease*, Vol. 37, No. 3, pp. 510-518, ISSN 1095-953X

Tatarewicz S. M., Wei X., Gupta S., Masterman D., Swanson S. J. & Moxness M. S. (2007) Development of a maturing T-cell-mediated immune response in patients with idiopathic Parkinson's disease receiving r-metHuGDNF via continuous intraputaminal infusion. *Journal of Clinical Immunology*, Vol. 27, No. 6, pp. 620-627, ISSN 0271-9142

Tian Y. Y., Jiang B., An L. J. & Bao Y. M. (2007) Neuroprotective effect of catalpol against MPP(+)-induced oxidative stress in mesencephalic neurons. *European Journal of Pharmacology*, Vol. 568, No. 1-3, pp. 142-148, ISSN 0014-2999

Tillerson J. L., Caudle W. M., Reveron M. E. & Miller G. W. (2003) Exercise induces behavioral recovery and attenuates neurochemical deficits in rodent models of Parkinson's disease. *Neuroscience*, Vol. 119, No. 3, pp. 899-911, ISSN 0306-4522

Tillerson J. L., Cohen A. D., Philhower J., Miller G. W., Zigmond M. J. & Schallert T. (2001) Forced limb-use effects on the behavioral and neurochemical effects of 6-hydroxydopamine. *Journal of Neuroscience*, Vol. 21, No. 12, pp. 4427-4435, ISSN 1529-2401

Tokugawa K., Yamamoto K., Nishiguchi M., Sekine T., Sakai M., Ueki T., Chaki S. & Okuyama S. (2003) XIB4035, a novel nonpeptidyl small molecule agonist for GFRalpha-1. *Neurochemistry International*, Vol. 42, No. 1, pp. 81-86, ISSN 0197-0186

Tripanichkul W., Sripanichkulchai K. & Finkelstein D. I. (2006) Estrogen down-regulates glial activation in male mice following 1-methyl-4-phenyl-1,2,3,6-tetrahydropyridine intoxication. *Brain Research*, Vol. 1084, No. 1, pp. 28-37, ISSN 0006-8993

Tsai C. H., Lo S. K., See L. C., Chen H. Z., Chen R. S., Weng Y. H., Chang F. C. & Lu C. S. (2002) Environmental risk factors of young onset Parkinson's disease: a case-control study. *Clinical Neurology and Neurosurgery*, Vol. 104, No. 4, pp. 328-333, ISSN 0303-8467

Turner C. A. & Lewis M. H. (2003) Environmental enrichment: effects on stereotyped behavior and neurotrophin levels. *Physiology & Behavior*, Vol. 80, No. 2-3, pp. 259-266, ISSN 0031-9384

Vastag B. (2010) Biotechnology: Crossing the barrier. *Nature*, Vol. 466, No. 7309, pp. 916-918, ISSN 0028-0836

Vegeto E., Pollio G., Pellicciari C. & Maggi A. (1999) Estrogen and progesterone induction of survival of monoblastoid cells undergoing TNF-alpha-induced apoptosis. *The FASEB Journal*, Vol. 13, No. 8, pp. 793-803, ISSN 0892-6638

Vegeto E., Bonincontro C., Pollio G., Sala A., Viappiani S., Nardi F., Brusadelli A., Viviani B., Ciana P. & Maggi A. (2001) Estrogen prevents the lipopolysaccharide-induced inflammatory response in microglia. *Journal of Neuroscience*, Vol. 21, No. 6, pp. 1809-1818, ISSN 1529-2401

Verity A. N., Wyatt T. L., Hajos B., Eglen R. M., Baecker P. A. & Johnson R. M. (1998) Regulation of glial cell line-derived neurotrophic factor release from rat C6 glioblastoma cells. *Journal of Neurochemistry*, Vol. 70, No. 2, pp. 531-539, ISSN 0042-3042

Verity A. N., Wyatt T. L., Lee W., Hajos B., Baecker P. A., Eglen R. M. & Johnson R. M. (1999) Differential regulation of glial cell line-derived neurotrophic factor (GDNF) expression in human neuroblastoma and glioblastoma cell lines. *Journal of Neuroscience Research*, Vol. 55, No. 2, pp. 187-197, ISSN 0360-4012

Visanji N. P., Orsi A., Johnston T. H., Howson P. A., Dixon K., Callizot N., Brotchie J. M. & Rees D. D. (2008) PYM50028, a novel, orally active, nonpeptide neurotrophic factor inducer, prevents and reverses neuronal damage induced by MPP+ in mesencephalic neurons and by MPTP in a mouse model of Parkinson's disease. *The FASEB Journal*, Vol. 22 No. 7 pp. 2488-2497, ISSN 1530-6860

Wang X. J., Ye M., Zhang Y. H. & Chen S. D. (2007) CD200-CD200R regulation of microglia activation in the pathogenesis of Parkinson's disease. *Journal of NeuroImmune Pharmacology*, Vol. 2, No. 3, pp. 259-264, ISSN 1557-1904

Wang Y. C., Cheng Y. H., Ma J., Gan S. Y., Wang S. J., Zhou H., Du Y. J., Yang M. & Shen F. (2010) [Effects of electroacupuncture on the expression of GDNF and Ret in Parkinson's disease model rats]. *Zhongguo ZhenJiu*, Vol. 30, No. 9, pp. 739-743, ISSN 0255-2930

Wei G., Wu G. & Cao X. (2000a) Dynamic expression of glial cell line-derived neurotrophic factor after cerebral ischemia. *Neuroreport*, Vol. 11, No. 6, pp. 1177-1183, ISSN 0959-4969

Wei G., Huang Y., Wu G. & Cao X. (2000b) Regulation of glial cell line-derived neurotrophic factor expression by electroacupuncture after transient focal cerebral ischemia. *Acupuncture and Electrotherapy Research*, Vol. 25, No. 2, pp. 81-90, ISSN 0360-1293

Widenfalk J., Olson L. & Thoren P. (1999) Deprived of habitual running, rats downregulate BDNF and TrkB messages in the brain. *Neuroscience Research*, Vol. 34, No. 3, pp. 125-132, ISSN 0168-0102

Widenfalk J., Lundstromer K., Jubran M., Brene S. & Olson L. (2001) Neurotrophic factors and receptors in the immature and adult spinal cord after mechanical injury or kainic acid. *Journal of Neuroscience*, Vol. 21, No. 10, pp. 3457-3475, ISSN 1529-2401

Wooten G. F., Currie L. J., Bovbjerg V. E., Lee J. K. & Patrie J. (2004) Are men at greater risk for Parkinson's disease than women? *Journal of Neurology, Neurosurgery & Psychiatry*, Vol. 75, No. 4, pp. 637-639, ISSN 0022-3050

Wu, A., Molteni, R., Ying, Z. & Gomez-Pinilla, F. (2003) A saturated-fat diet aggravates the outcome of traumatic brain injury on hippocampal plasticity and cognitive function by reducing brain-derived neurotrophic factor. *Neuroscience*, Vol. 119, No. 2, pp. 365-375, ISSN 0306-4522

Wu D. C., Jackson-Lewis V., Vila M., Tieu K., Teismann P., Vadseth C., Choi D. K., Ischiropoulos H. & Przedborski S. (2002) Blockade of microglial activation is neuroprotective in the 1-methyl-4-phenyl-1,2,3,6-tetrahydropyridine mouse model of Parkinson disease. *Journal of Neuroscience*, Vol. 22, No. 5, pp. 1763-1771, ISSN 1529-2401

Wu X., Chen P. S., Dallas S., Wilson B., Block M. L., Wang C. C., Kinyamu H., Lu N., Gao X., Leng Y., Chuang D. M., Zhang W., Lu R. B. & Hong J. S. (2008) Histone deacetylase inhibitors up-regulate astrocyte GDNF and BDNF gene transcription and protect dopaminergic neurons. *International Journal of Neuropsychopharmacology*, Vol. 11, No. 8, pp. 1123-1134, ISSN 1461-1457

Xia C. F., Boado R. J., Zhang Y., Chu C. & Pardridge W. M. (2008) Intravenous glial-derived neurotrophic factor gene therapy of experimental Parkinson's disease with Trojan horse liposomes and a tyrosine hydroxylase promoter. *Journal of Gene Medicine*, Vol. 10, No. 3, pp. 306-315, ISSN 1099-498X

Xing B., Xin T., Zhao L., Hunter R. L., Chen Y. & Bing G. (2010) Glial cell line-derived neurotrophic factor protects midbrain dopaminergic neurons against lipopolysaccharide neurotoxicity. *Journal of Neuroimmunology*, Vol. 225, No. 1-2, pp. 43-51, ISSN 1872-8421

Xu G., Xiong Z., Yong Y., Wang Z., Ke Z., Xia Z. & Hu Y. (2010) Catalpol attenuates MPTP induced neuronal degeneration of nigral-striatal dopaminergic pathway in mice through elevating glial cell derived neurotrophic factor in striatum. *Neuroscience*, Vol. 167, No. 1, pp. 174-184, ISSN 0306-4522

Xu Q., Park Y., Huang X., Hollenbeck A., Blair A., Schatzkin A. & Chen H. (2010) Physical activities and future risk of Parkinson disease. *Neurology*, Vol. 75, No. 4, pp. 341-348, ISSN 0028-3878

Yasuhara T., Hara K., Maki M., Matsukawa N., Fujino H., Date I. & Borlongan C. V. (2007) Lack of exercise, via hindlimb suspension, impedes endogenous neurogenesis. *Neuroscience*, Vol. 149, No. 1, pp. 182-191, ISSN 0306-4522

Yoon M. C., Shin M. S., Kim T. S., Kim B. K., Ko I. G., Sung Y. H., Kim S. E., Lee H. H., Kim Y. P. & Kim C. J. (2007) Treadmill exercise suppresses nigrostriatal dopaminergic neuronal loss in 6-hydroxydopamine-induced Parkinson's rats. *Neuroscience Letters*, Vol. 423, No. 1, pp. 12-17, ISSN 0304-3940

Young D., Lawlor P. A., Leone P., Dragunow M. & During M. J. (1999) Environmental enrichment inhibits spontaneous apoptosis, prevents seizures and is neuroprotective. *Nature Medicine*, Vol. 5, No. 4, pp. 448-453, ISSN 1078-8956

Yu H., Oh-Hashi K., Tanaka T., Sai A., Inoue M., Hirata Y. & Kiuchi K. (2006) Rehmannia glutinosa induces glial cell line-derived neurotrophic factor gene expression in astroglial cells via cPKC and ERK1/2 pathways independently. *Pharmacological Research*, Vol. 54, No. 1, pp. 39-45, ISSN 1043-6618

Yu Y. P., Ju W. P., Li Z. G., Wang D. Z., Wang Y. C. & Xie A. M. (2010) Acupuncture inhibits oxidative stress and rotational behavior in 6-hydroxydopamine lesioned rat. *Brain Research*, Vol. 1336, No. pp. 58-65, ISSN 0006-8993

Zesiewicz T. A. & Evatt M. L. (2009) Potential influences of complementary therapy on motor and non-motor complications in Parkinson's disease. *CNS Drugs*, Vol. 23, No. 10, pp. 817-835, ISSN 1172-7047

Zhang Y., Xia Z., Hu Y., Orsi A. & Rees D. (2008) Role of glial cell derived neurotrophic factor in the protective effect of smilagenin on rat mesencephalic dopaminergic neurons damaged by MPP+. *FEBS Letters*, Vol. 582, No. 6, pp. 956-960, ISSN 0014-5793

Zhang Z., Miyoshi Y., Lapchak P. A., Collins F., Hilt D., Lebel C., Kryscio R. & Gash D. M. (1997) Dose response to intraventricular glial cell line-derived neurotrophic factor administration in parkinsonian monkeys. *Journal of Pharmacology and Experimental Therapeutics*, Vol. 282, No. 3, pp. 1396-1401, ISSN 0022-3565

Zhou J., Zhang H., Cohen R. S. & Pandey S. C. (2005) Effects of estrogen treatment on expression of brain-derived neurotrophic factor and cAMP response element-binding protein expression and phosphorylation in rat amygdaloid and hippocampal structures. *Neuroendocrinology*, Vol. 81, No. 5, pp. 294-310, ISSN 0028-3835

Zhou Q. H., Boado R. J., Lu J. Z., Hui E. K. & Pardridge W. M. (2010) Monoclonal antibody-glial-derived neurotrophic factor fusion protein penetrates the blood-brain barrier in the mouse. *Drug Metabolism Disposition*, Vol. 38, No. 4, pp. 566-572, ISSN 0090-9556

Zhuang X. & Wang L. (2000) Acupuncture treatment of Parkinson's disease-a report of 29 cases. *Journal of Traditional Chinese Medicine*, Vol. 20, No. 4, pp. 265-267, ISSN 0255-2922

Zigmond M. J., Cameron J. L., Leak R. K., Mirnics K., Russell V. A., Smeyne R. J. & Smith A. D. (2009) Triggering endogenous neuroprotective processes through exercise in models of dopamine deficiency. *Parkinsonism & Related Disorders*, Vol. 15, Suppl 3, pp. S42-S45, ISSN 1353-8020

11

The Potential of Neurotrophic Factors for the Treatment of Parkinson's Disease

Aideen M. Sullivan* and André Toulouse
Department of Anatomy and Neuroscience, University College Cork, Cork Ireland

1. Introduction

Parkinson's disease (PD) is the second most common neurodegenerative disorder, with an incidence of 1.5 - 2% in the population over 60 years of age, which increases significantly with advancing age (for reviews see de Lau & Breteler, 2006; Toulouse & Sullivan, 2008). Since the Western world is experiencing significant increases in life expectancy, the incidence of PD is steadily escalating. The financial and economical burden to society of the treatment and care of PD patients is substantial and increasing. Thus, research on the causes of this debilitating disease is critical, as is the development of new treatments.

PD is caused by progressive degeneration of the nigrostriatal (A9) dopaminergic pathway, which projects from the substantia nigra in the midbrain to the caudate-putamen (striatum) in the forebrain (Braak et al., 2003; Fearnley & Lees, 1991; Hoehn & Yahr, 1967; Olanow & Tatton, 1999). The resulting loss of dopamine neurotransmission in the striatum causes the cardinal symptoms of the disease: tremor at rest, rigidity and bradykinesia. One of the pathological hallmarks of PD is the appearance of intracellular protein aggregates called Lewy bodies, which are found in the substantia nigra and other brain areas (for reviews see Forno, 1996; Gibb & Lees, 1988). Lewy bodies are abnormal aggregates composed of α-synuclein, ubiquitin and other proteins. Approximately 5% of PD cases are caused by heritable genetic mutations, of which at least twelve have been identified (for review see Toulouse & Sullivan, 2008). The remaining cases are sporadic and of unknown origin, although many theories have been proposed to explain the cause of dopaminergic neuronal death which occurs in PD, such as environmental toxins, mitochondrial dysfunction with resulting oxidative stress, and inflammatory mechanisms (for reviews see Dauer & Przedborski, 2003; Dawson & Dawson, 2003; Fahn & Cohen, 1992; Long-Smith et al., 2009).

At present there is no effective long-term therapy for PD. The most commonly-used treatment is administration of the dopamine precursor, levodopa, which replaces lost dopamine in the denervated striatum and relieves motor symptoms. Levodopa is generally administered in conjunction with an inhibitor of peripheral decarboxylase (carbide or benserazide), which has the effect of enhancing the central activity of levodopa and decreasing peripheral side-effects. Levodopa is successful in treating PD symptoms; however, it does not stop the ongoing neurodegeneration. Furthermore, about 50% of patients develop complications within the first five years of treatment, primarily severe motor fluctuations and dyskinesias (Freed et al., 2001; Hagell et al., 2002). Other current drug treatments include inhibitors of the dopamine breakdown enzymes catechol-O-methyltransferase (tolcapone or entacapone) or monoamine oxidase–B (selegiline and rasagiline), and dopamine receptor agonists (bromocriptine, pergolide, pramipexole, ropinirole and others). Surgical methods involving ablation of deep brain structures such as the thalamus or pallidum, or deep brain stimulation of the subthalamic nucleus or pallidum, have also been used with good success, but these procedures are not widely-available or applicable for all patients. In summary, none of the current treatments provide safe and long-lasting relief from the symptoms and none have any effect on the progression of the disease. Much of the current research is aimed at developing new and novel therapies that will slow, halt or reverse the neurodegenerative process, rather than simply treating the symptoms of the disease. These include the use of antioxidants, anti-apoptotic agents, cell-based therapies and neuroprotective factors. Neurotrophic factors are a class of proteins that have the potential to be used as neuroprotectants in PD therapy.

2. Dopaminergic neurotrophic factors

One novel therapeutic strategy under investigation is the use of neurotrophic factors, which have the potential to slow down or halt the ongoing neurodegeneration in PD patients. These are secreted proteins that play critical roles in the developing nervous system, in the induction, specification, survival and maturation of developing neurones. Certain neurotrophic factors also act in the adult brain, to support and protect mature neuronal populations. Several of these factors have been investigated for their neurotrophic and protective effects on dopaminergic neurones. PD, being primarily caused by the degeneration of one neuronal population, the nigrostriatal dopaminergic projection, lends itself to neurotrophic factor therapy. The goal of this therapeutic approach is to apply a factor(s) which can halt or even reverse the progressive degeneration of nigrostriatal dopaminergic neurones, and which can be administered to patients in a safe, targetted and long-lasting manner. Some of the neurotrophic factors have potent effects on dopaminergic neurones, which render them good targets for novel therapeutics for PD. These include glial cell line-derived neurotrophic factor (GDNF), neurturin, growth/differentiation factor (GDF) 5, transforming growth factor (TGF)β, mesencephalic astrocyte-derived neurotrophic factor (MANF) and cerebral dopaminergic neurotrophic factor (CDNF).

2.1 GDNF family of ligands (GFL)

GDNF is the neurotrophic factor that has attracted the most interest in the field of PD research. GDNF is the prototypical member of the GFL family, which is composed of four factors - GDNF, neurturin, persephin and artemin. This family of neurotrophic factors is a subfamily of the TGFβ superfamily of proteins. These factors are secreted as precursors, in the form preproGFL, which undergo proteolytic cleavage within the extracellular space to release the active peptide. It has been reported that the prepro form of some neurotrophic factors are biologically active (Lee et al., 2001).

GDNF was isolated from a glial cell line in 1993, due to its ability to promote the survival of cultured dopaminergic neurones (Lin et al., 1993). Although GDNF was originally identified as a dopaminergic neurotrophic factor, subsequent studies have shown that it can act on a wide variety of neuronal types, including motor, noradrenergic, enteric, parasympathetic, sympathetic and sensory neurones (for reviews, see Airaksinen & Saarma, 2002; Airaksinen et al., 1999; Aron & Klein, 2011; Baloh et al., 2000; Bespalov & Saarma, 2007). It also plays important roles in the developing kidney and in spermatogenesis. GDNF is expressed throughout the brain, as well as in peripheral tissues (Choi-Lundberg & Bohn, 1995).

2.1.1 Signalling by GFLs

Signalling by the four GFL proteins is mediated through the receptor tyrosine kinase, Ret, in combination with a second receptor that is unique to each of the four ligands (for reviews see Airaksinen & Saarma, 2002; Airaksinen et al., 1999; Aron & Klein, 2011). Each of the GFLs acts as a disulphide-linked homodimer, binding to two molecules of a specific glycosyl-phosphatidylinositol-anchored co-receptor, the GDNF family receptors α (GFRα), which are a family of transmembrane receptor proteins. GDNF binds preferentially to GFRα1, neurturin to GFRα2, persephin to GFRα3 and artemin to GFRα4. Binding of dimeric GFL to its GFRα results in recruitment of the Ret receptor, using a mechanism which involves lipid rafts. The resulting complex composed of GFL, GFRα and Ret activates the intracellular tyrosine kinase domain of Ret, triggering intracellular signalling cascades (for reviews see Airaksinen & Saarma, 2002; Airaksinen et al., 1999; Sariola & Saarma, 2003). Many signalling pathways are involved, including Ras-extracellular signal-regulated kinase (ERK), phosphoinositide 3-kinase (PI3K)-Akt, Src and phospholipaseCγ-protein kinase (PK)C. Activation of these pathways results in many diverse cellular changes, including neuronal survival. An alternative signalling pathway for GDNF and neurturin has also been identified, whereby each of these ligands can bind to the neural cell adhesion molecule (NCAM) in the absence of Ret (Cao et al., 2008; Paratcha et al., 2003; Sariola & Saarma, 2003). The GDNF-NCAM complex can subsequently bind GFRα1, which leads to the activation of intracellular signalling pathways, involving focal adhesion kinase and Fyn kinase, both of which play roles in neuronal migration during development (Paratcha & Ledda, 2008). In addition to NCAM, other cell adhesion molecules, such as integrin β1 and N-cadherin, which are expressed on nigral dopaminergic neurones, may be involved in GDNF's actions on these cells during development (see Cao et al., 2010). GDNF, neurturin and artemin, but not persephin, have also been reported to act through a heparin sulphate proteoglycan, syndecan-3, a transmembrane protein which can mediate neurite outgrowth after binding to matrix-bound GFLs (Barnett et al., 2002; Bespalov et al., 2011).

The receptors Ret and GRFα1 are expressed at high levels on dopaminergic neurones of the adult rat substantia nigra (Glazner et al., 1998; Golden et al., 1998; Horger et al., 1998; Matsuo et al., 2000; Nosrat et al., 1997; Sarabi et al., 2001; Treanor et al., 1996; Trupp et al., 1996; Trupp et al., 1997; Widenfalk et al., 1997; Yu et al., 1998), while GRFα2 has been reported to be expressed in regions adjacent to these neurones (Horger et al., 1998). In the developing brain, both Ret and GRFα1 are expressed in the midbrain from E11.5 in the rat (Nosrat et al., 1997) and E10 in the mouse (Golden et al., 1999). Transcripts for both Ret and GFRα1 have been found in cultures of E18 rat mesencephalon (Eggert et al., 1999). A recent study by Cao and colleagues found that the expression of Ret protein in the developing rat substantia nigra was evident by E16 and peaked at P21 (Cao et al., 2010).

2.1.2 Effects of GDNF *in vitro*

GDNF has consistently been shown to promote the survival of dopaminergic neurones *in vitro*. In the study that first described GDNF, the protective effects of this factor on dopaminergic neurones in cultures of embryonic rat midbrain were reported (Lin et al., 1993). Another study reported similar results, with application of GDNF improving the survival of cultured midbrain dopaminergic neurones by 1.6-fold (Krieglstein et al., 1995). GDNF was also shown to induce the expression of the dopamine synthetic enzyme, tyrosine hydroxylase (TH), in fetal human and rat cortical cultures (Theofilopoulos et al., 2001) and promotes the morphological differentiation of dopaminergic neurones *in vitro* (Widmer et al., 2000). As well as enhancing the survival and differentiation of embryonic rat dopaminergic neurones, GDNF can protect these cells from specific toxins. Hou and colleagues found that GDNF could protect cultured dopaminergic neurones from the toxic effects of 1-methyl-4-phenylpyridinium ion (MPP+), after the toxin had been removed from the cultures (Hou et al., 1996). Genetically-engineered cells overexpressing GDNF have been shown to exert dose-dependent protective effects on cultured dopaminergic neurones against MPP+ toxicity (Ma et al., 2000). GDNF treatment has also been reported to reduce apoptosis in dopaminergic neurones cultured from embryonic rat (Clarkson et al., 1995; Sawada et al., 2000) and human (Clarkson et al., 1997) midbrain. Repeated treatment with GDNF from the time of plating was found to protect cultured embryonic rat dopaminergic neurones from the toxin 6-hydroxydopamine (6-OHDA), when this toxin was applied after nine days *in vitro* (Eggert et al., 1999). However, another study applied GDNF to similar cultures after four days *in vitro*, which was a day before they received 6-OHDA treatment, and found no protective effects (Kramer et al., 1999). A study reported that the neuroprotective effects of GDNF on dopaminergic neurones *in vitro* were dependent on cAMP signalling pathways (Engele & Franke, 1996). GDNF has also been found to protect cultured dopaminergic neurones from lipopolysaccharide-induced degeneration, a model of neuroinflammation (Xing et al., 2010). Most of the above studies were conducted on embryonic day 14 (E14) rat midbrain, the time point at which dopaminergic neurones are undergoing their terminal mitotic divisions and are beginning to differentiate. An *in vitro* study showed that GDNF can also support nigrostriatal dopaminergic neurones during their period of natural developmental death, which occurs postnatally (Burke et al., 1998). Midbrain cultures may contain dopaminergic neurones of two origins, the nigrostriatal pathway, which degenerates in PD and the mesolimbic pathway, which is largely spared in this disease. Differential effects of GDNF treatment on nigrostriatal (A9) and mesolimbic (A10) dopaminergic neurones *in vitro* have been reported, whereby a single dose of GDNF selectively enhanced the survival of A9 cells, while repeated exposure to this factor only increased the survival of A10 cells (Borgal et al., 2007).

2.1.3 Effects of neurturin *in vitro*

A second factor of the GFL family, neurturin, was purified due to its survival-promoting effects on sympathetic neurones (Kotzbauer et al., 1996). It was found to have neurotrophic effects on developing dopaminergic neurones *in vitro*, similar in strength to those of GDNF (Akerud et al., 1999; Horger et al., 1998). Neurturin is expressed in the ventral midbrain and striatum during development (Horger et al., 1998). Neurturin also protects cultured motor neurones from degeneration and induces neuritic sprouting in spinal cord neurones *in vitro* (Bilak et al., 1999).

2.1.4 Effects of persephin and artemin *in vitro*

Persephin, a third member of the GFL family, has also been found to exert neurotrophic effects on midbrain dopaminergic neurones *in vitro* (Milbrandt et al., 1998) and *in vivo* (Akerud et al., 2002). This factor also has trophic effects on motor neurones (Milbrandt et al., 1998) and has not been extensively investigated for its clinical potential in PD. The fourth member of the GFL family, artemin, has survival-promoting effects on dopaminergic neurones in culture (Baloh et al., 1998) and *in vivo* (Cass et al., 2006), and also has potent actions on sensory neurones of the dorsal root ganglia (Baloh et al., 1998). Like persephin, artemin has not progressed into clinical trials for PD; however it has been tested as a therapeutic for neuropathy (Gardell et al., 2003). In contrast to GDNF and neurturin, artemin and particularly persephin appear to act primarily outside of the CNS, as their receptors are expressed at higher levels in the periphery.

2.2 TGFβ

Some members of the TGFβ superfamily have potent neurotrophic and protective effects on dopaminergic neurones. The TGFβ superfamily is a large family of secreted polypeptide growth factors, which play diverse physiological roles. They are involved in the development, differentiation and maintenance of the nervous system. There are two branches of the TGFβ superfamily - the TGFβ / activin group and the bone morphogenetic protein (BMP) / GDF group (for reviews see de Caestecker, 2004; Hogan, 1996; Krieglstein et al., 2002; Mehler et al., 1997). TGFβ3, a member of the TGFβ / activin group, has neuroprotective effects on dopaminergic neurones *in vitro* and *in vivo* (for review, see Roussa et al., 2009). Treatment with TGFβ2 or TGFβ3 has been reported to have potent neuroprotective effects on cultured embryonic rat dopaminergic neurones (Poulsen et al., 1994; Unsicker et al., 1996). It has been hypothesized that the neurotrophic effects of GDNF on many types of neurones, including dopaminergic neurones, require the presence of TGFβ3 (Krieglstein et al., 1998; Schober et al., 2007), which acts by recruiting the GFRα1 receptor to the membrane (Peterziel et al., 2002).

2.3 GDF5

Another member of the TGFβ superfamily of proteins, GDF5, is also being investigated for its therapeutic potential in PD. GDF5 (also known as BMP-14 or CDMP1) is a member of the BMP subfamily, which is the largest subgroup of the TGFβ superfamily, comprising at least 20 members. BMPs are involved in diverse physiological functions, including the development of the nervous system, where they play roles in early CNS patterning as well as in neural cell fate determination, differentiation, and survival (for reviews see Ebendal et al., 1998; Hall & Miller, 2004; Mehler et al., 1997).

GDF5 mRNA and protein expression have been found in the embryonic, neonatal and adult rat brain (Krieglstein et al., 1995; O'Keeffe et al., 2004; Storm et al., 1994). GDF5 protein expression in the rat brain peaks at E14, the time at which dopaminergic neurones in the developing midbrain are undergoing terminal differentiation (O'Keeffe et al., 2004). GDF5 protein is also expressed in several regions of the adult rat brain, including striatum and midbrain (O'Keeffe et al., 2004).

2.3.1 Signalling by GDF5 and other BMPs

BMPs such as GDF5 are synthesised as large precursor proteins of approximately 400-500 amino acids, which contain an N-terminal region which is necessary for secretion of the protein, a prodomain which directs folding of the protein, and a C-terminal mature active peptide (for reviews, see Bragdon et al., 2011; Sieber et al., 2009). The active proteins are each composed of 50-100 amino acids and generally contain seven cysteine residues. Six of these cysteines form disulphide bonds and the seventh (which is not present in GDF3, GDF9 or BMP15) forms a disulphide bond with another monomer, to form the biologically-active dimeric molecule. The BMPs generally act as homodimers, although heteromeric complexes of BMP2/6, BMP2/7 and BMP2b/7 have been described (Little & Mullins, 2009; Sieber et al., 2009). Many of the BMPs have been found to create complexes with their respective prodomains following release into the extracellular environment as active dimers (for review, see Bragdon et al., 2011). The soluble active form of each BMP is capable of diffusion away from its site of release, while the form that is complexed with its prodomain remains in the extracellular matrix, usually bound to fibrillins (Ramirez & Rifkin, 2009; Sengle et al., 2008).

BMPs signal by binding to two types of transmembrane serine-threonine kinase receptors, type I and type II receptors, and subsequently activating intracellular signalling pathways which culminate in diverse cellular changes, many of which are dependent upon Smad protein-dependent gene transcription (for reviews, see Bragdon et al., 2011; de Caestecker, 2004; Ebendal et al., 1998; Kawabata et al., 1998; Massague, 1996; Miyazono, 1999; Nohe et al., 2004; Yamashita et al., 1996). Individual BMPs can signal through any of several type I receptors and type II receptors. GDF5 signals predominantly through the type I receptor BMPR1b and the type II receptor BMPR2 (Nishitoh et al., 1996). Each of the BMP receptors is composed of a short extracellular ligand-binding portion which contains 10-12 cysteine residues, a single transmembrane region, and an intracellular part which contains the serine-threonine kinase domain. The type I receptors contain a glycine-serine rich region (a 'GS box') within their cytoplasmic domain. This GS box is necessary for their activation and is not present in the type II receptors. The various BMPs bind to type I and type II receptors with differing affinities. The presence of a prodomain within a BMP protein complex appears to decrease binding to Type II, but not to Type I, receptors (Sengle et al., 2008). Upon binding of a BMP to its specific receptors, a multimeric complex is formed, of variable composition, but usually consisting of two type I and two type II receptors. The initial binding stage is to the type I receptor, which anchors the ligand to the membrane and facilitates subsequent binding to the type II receptor. This induces phosphorylation by the constitutively-active type II receptor kinase of serine residues within the GS box of the type I receptor, which stimulates intracellular signalling cascades, generally resulting in the activation of Smad proteins. Activated Smads can then translocate into the nucleus and affect transcription.

Smad proteins are divided into three subclasses: regulatory Smads (R-Smads; Smad-1, -5 and -8), common Smad (Co-Smad; Smad 4) and inhibitory Smads (I-Smads; Smad-6 and -7). During BMP signalling, the C-terminal region of a regulatory Smad (Smads 1, 5 or 8) is phosphorylated by the type I receptor, which activates the canonical Smad signalling pathway. Phosphorylation of an R-Smad induces it to bind to Smad 4, followed by nuclear translocation of this complex (for reviews see Kawabata et al., 1998; Massague et al., 2005; Nohe et al., 2004). This complex, in co-operation with a range of co-activators and co-repressors, can affect the transcription of a wide variety of genes (for reviews see Attisano & Wrana, 2000; Miyazono et al., 2001; Shi & Massague, 2003). The I-Smads compete with the R-Smads for binding to the type I receptor, and can also bind to Smad-4 to form a complex which is non-functional and which blocks the activated R-Smads from binding to Smad-4 to affect transcription.

BMPs have recently been found to also act via Smad-independent mechanisms, which do not involve transcriptional changes. These pathways are activated by the same receptors as those used in Smad-dependent signalling, but involve the stimulation of various intracellular signalling cascades, involving proteins such as ERK, PI3K, PKA, PKC, p38 mitogen activated protein (MAP) kinase, C-jun N-terminal kinase and nuclear factor kappa B. Many of these pathways are initiated by interaction of the BMP receptor with bone morphogenetic receptor associated molecule 1 (BRAM1) or with X-linked inhibitor of apoptosis (XIAP), stimulating the activation of TGFβ-activated kinase 1 (TAK1) and TAK1-binding protein (TAB1) (for reviews see de Caestecker, 2004; Sieber et al., 2009). The MAP kinases enter the nucleus upon phosphorylation and affect transcription of target genes. BMP receptors are thought to act in such a transcription-independent manner to induce cytoskeletal changes, which may be involved in neural cell migration during development (see Sieber et al., 2009).

The physiological regulation of BMP signalling through their receptors is complex and involves a large array of modulatory molecules. For example, BMP signalling is modulated by the presence of several endogenous antagonists, which block or diminish the binding of BMPs to their specific receptors (for reviews, see Bragdon et al., 2011; de Caestecker, 2004; Kawabata et al., 1998; Rider & Mulloy, 2011; Sieber et al., 2009). At least fifteen BMP antagonist molecules have been identified, some of which also act as antagonists of other TGFβ superfamily members. Noggin is the most-studied BMP antagonist and it has been shown to block the actions of BMP2, BMP4, BMP7, GDF5 and GDF6. Furthermore, several BMP co-receptors have been identified, which can either promote or inhibit BMP signalling (for reviews, see Corradini et al., 2009; Sieber et al., 2009). The repulsive guidance molecules (RGM)-a and -c, Dragon (RGMb) and the receptor tyrosine kinase (RTK) c-Kit are examples of positive co-receptors which augment signalling by BMPs, whereas the decoy receptor, BMP and activin membrane-bound protein (BAMBI), and the RTKs Ror2 and TrkC are negative modulators. Intracellular modulation of BMP signalling also occurs, whereby several proteins can act to regulate BMP signalling by binding to the intracellular region of their receptors and forming mulicomponent signalling complexes which can enhance or inhibit both Smad-dependent and Smad-independent pathways (for review, see Sieber et al., 2009). Ligand-dependent endocytic trafficking of the BMP receptors also plays a modulatory role, and can both enhance or decrease the efficiency of BMP signalling (for review, see de Caestecker, 2004). Individual BMPs can activate multiple signalling pathways by signalling through distinct receptor oligomeric complexes, demonstrating the complexity and diversity of the biological actions of these proteins.

2.3.2 Effects of GDF5 *in vitro*

On embryonic rat dopaminergic neurones *in vitro*, GDF5 has selective trophic actions which are comparable to those of GDNF. Application of GDF5 promotes the survival of dopaminergic neurones in embryonic rat midbrain cultures and protects them against the dopaminergic neurotoxin MPP+ (Krieglstein et al., 1995) and against free radical-induced damage (Lingor et al., 1999). Another study found that application of recombinant human GDF5 induced a dramatic increase in the number of dopaminergic neurones, in cultures of embryonic rat midbrain (O'Keeffe et al., 2004). This study found that the effects of GDF5 in these cultures may be dependent on BMPR1b, since application of GDF5 at the time of plating, when BMPR1b is expressed, increases dopaminergic neuronal number, but application after six days *in vitro*, when this receptor is no longer expressed, had no effect. GDF5 treatment also induced morphological changes in cultured embryonic rat dopaminergic neurones, stimulating neurite outgrowth and branching (Clayton & Sullivan, 2007; O'Keeffe et al., 2004). Clayton and Sullivan found that the effects of GDF5 were much greater when cultures were prepared from the lateral part of the developing midbrain. Furthermore, the BMPR1b receptor was expressed at higher levels in the lateral than in the medial region, suggesting that GDF5 acts through this receptor to increase dopaminergic neuronal number. Combined application of GDF5 and GDNF have been shown to have additive neurotrophic effects on cultured embryonic rat dopaminergic neurones, indicating that these two factors may act on separate subpopulations of cells (Wood et al., 2005).

2.4 MANF and CDNF

MANF and CDNF are members of a recently-described family of evolutionarily-conserved proteins, of approximately 150-160 amino acids, which are secreted from glial cells and have potent effects on dopaminergic neurones (for review, see Lindholm & Saarma, 2010). CDNF mRNA and protein have been found in both developing (E13 to postnatal day 10) and adult mouse striatum and substantia nigra, suggesting that this factor may provide trophic support to mature dopaminergic neuronal cell bodies and their terminals, as well play a role in the development of these cells (Lindholm et al., 2007). CDNF is a paralogue of MANF, which was originally isolated from a rat mesencephalic astrocyte cell line and found to have selective trophic effects on dopaminergic neurones *in vitro* (Petrova et al., 2003). Polymorphisms of CDNF have recently been linked to an early-onset form of PD (Choi et al., 2011). *In vivo* secretion of MANF has been demonstrated (Apostolou et al., 2008). Like CDNF, MANF is expressed in the rodent nigrostriatal system during the early postnatal period, as well as in the adult (Lindholm et al., 2008). The Drosophila homologue of MANF, DmMANF, is essential for the maintenance and function of dopaminergic neurones (Palgi et al., 2009). Although the receptors for MANF and CDNF have yet to be identified, it appears that they may act by a different mechanism to the GFL family members to exert their neurotrophic effects on dopaminergic neurones. It is possible that at least part of the action of MANF is via inhibition of endoplasmic reticulum (ER) stress-induced neuronal cell death (see Lindholm & Saarma, 2010; Voutilainen et al., 2009), as MANF is located in the ER and has been shown to inhibit ER stress-induced non-neuronal cell death *in vitro* (Apostolou et al., 2008). MANF has also been found to have protective effects on cardiac myocytes in an *in vitro* model of ischemia (Tadimalla et al., 2008). Overexpression of MANF has recently been shown to block apoptotic cell death in sympathetic neurones cultured from the neonatal mouse superior cervical ganglion (Hellman et al., 2011), supporting an intracellular mechanism of action.

3. Dopaminergic neurotrophic factors in animal models of PD

3.1 Effects of GDNF *in vivo*

In normal adult rats, a single injection of GDNF into either the substantia nigra or striatum significantly increased the levels of dopamine and its metabolites in the striatum and nigra (Martin et al., 1996). Several studies have reported neuroprotective and functional (improvement of motor symptoms) effects of GDNF in adult animal models of PD (for reviews, see Balemans & Van Hul, 2002; Bjorklund et al., 2009; Bjorklund & Lindvall, 2000; Bjorklund et al., 1997; Deierborg et al., 2008; Gash et al., 1996; Ramaswamy et al., 2009). In one early study, repeated injections of recombinant rat GDNF protected against dopaminergic cell loss induced by transection of the adult rat medial forebrain bundle (MFB), the fibre bundle containing the dopaminergic projections from the substantia nigra to the striatum (Beck et al., 1995). Another study found that delivery of GDNF using polymer-encapsulated baby hamster kidney (BHK) cells at one week before axotomy of the adult rat MFB induced motor improvements and rescued nigral dopaminergic neurones, without significant protection of striatal dopamine levels (Tseng et al., 1997).

The most widely-used laboratory model of PD involves unilateral injection of the selective dopaminergic toxin, 6-OHDA, into either the MFB, the substantia nigra or the striatum of the adult rat. This results in the degeneration of nigrostriatal dopaminergic neurones and consequent depletion of striatal dopamine transmission on one side of the brain. Stereotaxic injection of 6-OHDA into the MFB or substantia nigra induces a substantial lesion of the nigrostriatal pathway (Ungerstedt & Arbuthnott, 1970), while intrastriatal injection of this toxin induces a more protracted neurodegeneration, which begins after a delay of about a week and continues for several weeks (Sauer & Oertel, 1994). Several groups have examined the effects of intracerebral injection of recombinant GDNF in rats with 6-OHDA-induced lesions of the MFB. A single dose of GDNF to the substantia nigra, given four weeks after a 6-OHDA lesion of MFB, resulted in improvements in motor deficits (drug-induced rotational asymmetry, a commonly-used motor test in rat PD models) and preservation of nigral dopaminergic neurones (Bowenkamp et al., 1995; Hoffer et al., 1994). GDNF injection just above the substantia nigra and into the lateral ventricle immediately before 6-OHDA injection into the MFB conferred significant protective effects on nigral dopaminergic neurones, on striatal dopamine release and uptake, and on motor function (Opacka-Juffry et al., 1995). In adult rats with bilateral 6-OHDA lesions of the MFB, a model of severe PD, injection of high doses of GDNF into the lateral ventricles resulted in improved motor function and sparing of nigral dopaminergic neurones (Bowenkamp et al., 1997). Although GDNF has been reported to have protective actions in 6-OHDA-lesioned rats of all ages, its effects appear to be dependent on the age of the host, as one study found that young rats displayed significantly higher levels of neuroprotection than aged rats (Fox et al., 2001). This may be relevant to clinical trials, where the age of the patient may determine the extent of neuroprotection that is achievable with GDNF treatment.

The intrastriatal lesion model has been used extensively in studies on neurotrophic factors, since in this model it is possible to administer the factors while the progressive neurodegeneration is still taking place. Supranigral administration of recombinant human GDNF for four weeks, starting at the day of a 6-OHDA-induced lesion of the rat striatum, completely prevented nigral cell death (Sauer et al., 1995). When administered one day before a 6-OHDA lesion of either the striatum or substantia nigra, intranigral injection of GDNF had protective effects on rat nigral dopaminergic cell bodies (Kearns & Gash, 1995). A series of four intrastriatal injections of GDNF was found to decrease drug-induced rotations and preserve nigrostriatal dopaminergic neurones in adult rats with 6-OHDA-induced striatal lesions (Shults et al., 1996). Long-term rescue of nigrostriatal dopaminergic neurones from intrastriatal 6-OHDA lesions was reported after short-term GDNF treatment, beginning five days after the lesion and being administered every fourth day for one month (Winkler et al., 1996). Long-term protection against rotational asymmetry, reductions in striatal dopamine levels and uptake, and death of nigral dopaminergic cell bodies induced by 6-OHDA lesions of the MFB was conferred by a single dose of GDNF, divided between the lateral ventricle and substantia nigra (Sullivan et al., 1998). GDNF injections into the striatum at one week after an intrastriatal 6-OHDA lesion resulted in reinnervation of the striatum as well as recovery of motor function (Rosenblad et al., 1998), indicating that the ability of intrastriatal GDNF injection to confer behavioural improvements may be due to its effects on the remaining striatal afferents in the partially-denervated striatum.

For application to clinical studies, the optimal injection site for production of safe and effective results is obviously an important consideration. Some studies have directly compared the sites of administration of GDNF in 6-OHDA-lesioned rats. In a study designed to compare the various sites of intracerebral injection, intrastriatal GDNF had significant protective effects on motor function and on the integrity of the nigrostriatal pathway, intranigral GDNF protected nigral cell bodies but not striatal innervation or motor function, while intraventricular GDNF had no significant effects (Kirik et al., 2000). Another study by the same group found that delayed intraventricular infusion of GDNF starting two weeks after an intrastriatal 6-OHDA lesion had profound protective effects on the integrity and function of the nigrostriatal pathway, which lasted for six weeks after cessation of GDNF infusion, whereas the effects of intrastriatal infusion stopped upon withdrawal of GDNF (Kirik et al., 2001). Another group found that delayed intrastriatal infusion of a high dose of GDNF at four weeks after an intrastriatal 6-OHDA lesion induced restorative effects on the nigrostriatal dopaminergic pathway, in terms of both motor behaviour and the integrity of dopaminergic neurones and their terminals (Aoi et al., 2000). Thus, the intrastriatal route of administration appears to be the most efficacious in this rodent model of PD. In another study, sequential application of GDNF over the nigra for two weeks, followed by injections of GDNF into the striatum for three weeks, in rats with intrastriatal 6-OHDA lesions, protected nigral dopaminergic cell bodies but did not prevent striatal denervation or improve motor function (Rosenblad et al., 2000). This suggests that the motor improvements observed in the other studies were dependent on an ability of GDNF to induce reinnervation of the lesioned striatum, perhaps by stimulating axonal sprouting from the remaining dopaminergic neurones. Thus, once the axonal retraction to the level of the nigra has occurred, application of GDNF to the striatum appears to be ineffective. This is an important consideration for clinical studies, as it suggests that there is a window of opportunity in which GDNF application may be therapeutically effective, but that this factor may not be useful at advanced stages of the disease.

In another commonly-used animal model of PD, N-methyl-4-phenyl-1,2,3,6-tetrahydropyridine (MPTP)-treated adult mice, GDNF administration induces potent effects on nigrostriatal dopaminergic neurones (Tomac et al., 1995). This study found that GDNF could be injected either before or one week after MPTP treatment, to confer significant preventative or restorative effects, respectively. Another study reported that GDNF injection into the striatum at one week after MPTP treatment of young or aged mice induced recovery of motor function (Date et al., 1998).

Another well-established animal model of PD is the MPTP-treated non-human primate brain, which has the advantage of being closer than the rodent brain to the human brain in terms of organisation and size. Gash and colleagues showed that administration of recombinant GDNF every four weeks in MPTP-treated rhesus monkeys induced motor recovery as well as a significant increase in the size of cell nigral dopaminergic neurones and in the density of their striatal projections (Gash et al., 1996). Combined application of oral levodopa and intracerebroventricular GDNF resulted in significant behavioural improvements with reduced levodopa-induced side-effects, in MPTP-treated rhesus monkeys (Miyoshi et al., 1997). Another study found that intraventricular GDNF improved motor function and reduced levodopa-induced dyskinesias in MPTP-treated monkeys (Iravani et al., 2001). Significant recovery of motor function for at least four months was reported in MPTP-treated monkeys that had received GDNF into the lateral ventricles (Zhang et al., 1997). Intraventricular injections of GDNF were found to induce increases in dopamine levels in the substantia nigra, but not the striatum, of MPTP-treated rhesus monkeys (Gerhardt et al., 1999). Infusion of GDNF into the putamen of MPTP-treated rhesus monkeys induced a gradual and significant reduction in parkinsonian symptoms (Grondin et al., 2002). This appeared to be a regenerative action, since GDNF was injected at three months after the MPTP lesion, when the nigrostriatal pathway had presumably undergone significant degeneration. Chronic intraputaminal administration of GDNF in aged rhesus monkeys had a long-lasting protective action on nigrostriatal dopaminergic neurones and on motor function, without any adverse side-effects (Maswood et al., 2002). In addition to effects on PD models, a single intranigral injection of GDNF can induce increases in nigrostriatal dopamine neurotransmission in normal rhesus monkeys, lasting for at least three weeks (Gash et al., 1995).

Like all neurotrophic proteins, GDNF is metabolised rapidly in the brain and thus single injections of this factor cannot confer permanent effects. Gene therapy approaches have been applied in attempts to achieve long-term and targeted delivery of GDNF to the injured nigrostriatal pathway. An adenoviral vector was used to deliver GDNF into or close to the substantia nigra (Choi-Lundberg et al., 1997; Mandel et al., 1997) or into the striatum (Balemans & Van Hul, 2002; Bilang-Bleuel et al., 1997; Choi-Lundberg et al., 1998) of rats with intrastriatal 6-OHDA lesions. Each of these studies reported significant motor improvements, as well as direct effects on nigral dopaminergic neurones and their terminals. When administered into the substantia nigra at ten weeks after a 6-OHDA lesion of the adult rat MFB, adenoviral vector-delivered GDNF induced significant motor improvements and recovery of nigrostriatal dopamine neuronal function (Lapchak et al., 1997). Adenoviral-delivered GDNF induced behavioural and neuroprotective effects when injected into the substantia nigra, but not when injected intrastriatally, in rats that had intrastriatal 6-OHDA lesions (Kozlowski et al., 2000). In MPTP-treated mice, adenoviral vector-mediated GDNF delivery to the striatum prevented depletion of striatal dopamine levels (Kojima et al., 1997). A study which compared the effects of intrastriatal and perinigral injection of an adenoviral vector encoding GDNF found that, while both injection routes conferred protective effects on dopaminergic cell bodies in the nigra, only the intrastriatal route reduced motor deficits in rats with intrastriatal 6-OHDA lesions (Connor et al., 1999).

Another vector system, based on adeno-associated virus (AAV) 2, has also shown efficacy in animal models of PD. Mandel and co-workers reported significant protective effects on the nigrostriatal pathway and its functioning, in adult rats with intrastriatal 6-OHDA lesions following intranigral injection of AAV2-GDNF either three weeks before (Mandel et al., 1997) or just after the lesion (Mandel et al., 1999). AAV2-mediated delivery of GDNF to the striatum, but not to the substantia nigra, induced gradual behavioural recovery and regeneration of the 6-OHDA-lesioned nigrostriatal system in adult rats (Kirik et al., 2000). AAV vectors have advantages over adenoviral vectors in that they can integrate and stably express their transgene product in non-dividing cells such as neurons. Also, they are relatively safe as there is little or no host immune response, due to the absence of viral genes in these vectors. Their disadvantage is that they can only deliver gene constructs of relatively small size compared to those that adenoviral vectors can accommodate. Furthermore, there is a delay before the transgene is expressed following intracerebral injection of an AAV vector.

A third type of vector system, based on lentiviruses, has also been used to deliver GDNF in PD animal models, with promising results. Lentiviral vectors have the capacity to deliver large transgenes and they can integrate efficiently into non-dividing cells. Delivery of the human GDNF gene using lentiviral vectors in MPTP-lesioned rhesus monkeys and in aged rhesus monkeys achieved long-term gene expression and significant functional benefits

(Kordower et al., 2000). Kordower and colleagues administered lentiviral-GDNF to the striatum and substantia nigra of nonlesioned aged monkeys and MPTP-treated young monkeys and found extensive expression of GDNF in all of the brains. Lentiviral-delivered GDNF reversed motor deficits in the aged monkeys, and prevented nigrostriatal degeneration and the development of functional deficits in the MPTP-lesioned animals. Another study used a lentiviral vector to achieve long-term delivery of GDNF to the striatum and substantia nigra of aged rhesus monkeys, and found that this treatment conferred significant protective effects on the functioning and integrity of the nigrostriatal pathway (Emborg et al., 2009). Lentiviral delivery of GDNF was also found to increase the number of intrinsic dopaminergic neurones in the primate striatum (Palfi et al., 2002). Dowd et al found that lentiviral-mediated GDNF delivery into the striatum and above the substantia nigra rescued complex motor behaviour (such as corridor, staircase, stepping and cylinder tasks), as well as drug-induced rotational asymmetry, in rats with 6-OHDA lesions of the MFB (Dowd et al., 2005). Lentiviral-mediated delivery is very effective, but there are concerns about its safety, which will have to be addressed before clinical application of this system is feasible.

Thus, gene therapy has shown great promise as a means of achieving long-term and targeted delivery of GDNF to the nigrostriatal system (for reviews see Bjorklund & Lindvall, 2000; Kordower, 2003; Manfredsson et al., 2009). Viral vector technology has also been used to deliver GDNF to the brain in models of other diseases. For example, significant neuroprotective effects were reported in a study that used adenoviral vectors to deliver GDNF to the cortex in an adult rat model of focal cortical trauma (Hermann et al., 2001). Adenoviral-mediated GDNF expression has been reported to rescue rat retinal ganglion cells after axotomy (Schmeer et al., 2002), to protect motoneurones in a transgenic mouse model of amyotrophic lateral sclerosis (Wang, et al., 2002) and to promote functional recovery in a rat model of spinal cord injury (Tai et al., 2003). AAV-2-mediated delivery of GDNF was found to confer neuroprotective effects and motor improvements in both a toxin-mediated adult rat model (McBride et al., 2003) and in a transgenic mouse model of Huntington's disease (McBride et al., 2006).

Another avenue of exploration is the co-administration of neurotrophic factors with neuronal transplants in cell replacement therapy approaches to PD. Transplantation of embryonic midbrain tissue is a promising and successful therapy for PD, but is limited by the poor survival of the transplanted dopaminergic neurones (for recent reviews, see Brundin et al., 2010; Hedlund & Perlmann, 2009; Olanow et al., 2009). GDNF has been shown by several groups to improve the survival and integration of grafted embryonic dopaminergic neurones in animal models of PD. Rosenblad and colleagues reported that repeated injections of this factor adjacent to embryonic rat ventral midbrain grafts in the 6-OHDA-lesioned rat striatum improved the survival of the grafted dopaminergic cells and induced earlier recovery of motor function than untreated grafts (Rosenblad et al., 1996). Improvements in the survival of grafted dopaminergic neurones and their integration into the host striatum were also reported after pre-incubation of the grafts with GDNF (Apostolides et al., 1998; Granholm et al., 1997; Sullivan et al., 1998; Yurek, 1998). Injection of GDNF along the nigrostriatal tract stimulated the outgrowth of dopaminergic fibres from intranigral grafts towards the striatum (Sinclair et al., 1996; Tang et al., 1998; Wang, Y. et al., 1996). Enhancement of complex motor functions, as well as improved graft survival, were found in 6-OHDA-lesioned rats that had received GDNF-pretreated grafts (Mehta et al., 1998). GDNF pretreatment has also been used to promote the survival of human fetal

midbrain tissue, prior to grafting into two PD patients (Mendez et al., 2000). These patients displayed a large increase in fluorodopa uptake after one year, an index of striatal dopaminergic transmission, as measured by positron emission tomography (PET).
Ex vivo gene therapy approaches have been applied in attempts to extend the effects of exogenous GDNF, which is rapidly metabolised *in vivo*. Genetically-modified embryonic rat midbrain cells which overexpress GDNF have been found to induce earlier functional recovery in 6-OHDA-lesioned rats than control grafts (Bauer et al., 2000). GDNF-overexpressing rat neural precursor cells also significantly increased the survival of co-grafted embryonic dopaminergic neurones (Ostenfeld et al., 2002). Human neural progenitor cells have been used to deliver GDNF, which conferred protective effects on the lesioned nigrostriatal pathway in adult rats (Behrstock et al., 2006). This cellular delivery system, which allows the release of GDNF under an inducible promoter, has also been found to provide GDNF to the aged monkey brain for at least three months (Behrstock et al., 2006). Encapsulation technology involves enclosing cells within a semi-permeable membrane composed of polymer fibres, which allows outward diffusion of any proteins secreted by the cells, while preventing the cells from proliferating extensively and forming tumours. Intrastriatal grafting of an encapsulated GDNF-expressing human (BHK) cell line has been shown to confer neuroprotective and restorative effects in 6-OHDA-lesioned rats (Date et al., 2001; Shingo et al., 2002), particularly when the GDNF-expressing cells are implanted at an early stage of the disease progression (Yasuhara et al., 2005). Encapsulated human fibroblasts genetically engineered to overexpress GDNF were found to exert regenerative effects when implanted into the rat striatum one week after an intrastriatal 6-OHDA lesion (Sajadi et al., 2006). Although the cells were removed after six weeks, the regenerative effects on motor function and on nigral dopaminergic neurones were evident for a further seven weeks, indicating that transient delivery of GDNF was sufficient to confer sustained effects. In MPTP-treated primates, encapsulated GDNF-expressing cells induced transient motor improvements and increases in striatal dopamine uptake, without any adverse side-effects (Kishima et al., 2004). Encapsulated cells expressing GDNF have also been applied in combination with embryonic rat brain grafts in 6-OHDA-lesioned rats, and were found to improve the survival of the grafted dopaminergic neurones and their functional effects (Sautter et al., 1998). Encapsulated cell technology may have great potential for future clinical studies, should the promising effects found in these animal studies be extended to show long-term and safe delivery of appropriate doses of neurotrophic proteins (for reviews see Bensadoun et al., 2003; Lindvall & Wahlberg, 2008).

3.2 Effects of neurturin *in vivo*

Neurturin has been found to exert protective and functional effects on dopaminergic nigrostriatal neurones after 6-OHDA lesions of the adult rat MFB (Akerud et al., 1999; Horger et al., 1998) or of the striatum (Oiwa et al., 2002; Rosenblad et al., 1999), and after axotomy of the MFB in adult rats (Tseng et al., 1998). The study by Rosenblad and colleagues directly compared the effects of neurturin with those of GDNF in the striatal 6-OHDA lesion model. They found that neurturin was less efficacious than GDNF after intrastriatal and especially after intraventricular delivery, which may reflect poor solubility of neurturin *in vivo* (Rosenblad et al., 1999). Another study showed that delivery of neurturin into the cerebral ventricles of adult rats using mini-pumps resulted in an increase in striatal dopamine levels (Hoane et al., 1999). A recent study reported that intranigral injection of recombinant neurturin induced increases in striatal dopamine release, which were similar in magnitude to those induced by intranigral injection of recombinant GDNF (Cass & Peters, 2010). Intracerebral delivery of recombinant neurturin has also been found to protect nigrostriatal dopaminergic neurones and induce improvements in motor function in MPTP-treated monkeys (Grondin et al., 2008; Li et al., 2003). Co-administration with recombinant neurturin protein has been reported to improve the survival of fetal rat dopaminergic neurones after intrastriatal grafting into 6-OHDA-lesioned adult rats (Rosenblad et al., 1999).

The need for sustained delivery of neurotrophic proteins to the brain led to studies using viral vector-based delivery systems, which have shown promising results in animal models of PD. Lentiviral gene delivery to the striatum of 6-OHDA-lesioned adult rats of a modified neurturin construct, which had the pro-region deleted and replaced with an immunoglobulin heavy-chain signal peptide, had protective effects on the nigrostriatal pathway (Fjord-Larsen et al., 2005). Sustained functional recovery, with minimal side-effects, was achieved following stereotaxic injection of an adeno-associated virus (AAV) 2–based vector encoding the human neurturin gene, in MPTP-treated monkeys (Kordower et al., 2006) and 6-OHDA-lesioned rats (Gasmi et al., 2007). Stable expression of neurturin using this AAV2 delivery system was achieved for at least a year in rats (Gasmi et al., 2007).

Kordower and colleagues showed that, ten months after treatment with AAV2-neurturin into the striatum and substantia nigra, MPTP-treated parkinsonian monkeys showed a large reduction in the intensity of their motor symptoms compared to buffer-injected animals, which displayed stable symptoms throughout the study. This functional recovery was accompanied by significant preservation of dopaminergic neurones (Kordower et al., 2006).

A study using the same expression system in 6-OHDA-lesioned adult rats found long-term neurturin expression in the striatum and dose-dependant protective effects on the nigrostriatal dopaminergic neurones for at least ten months (Gasmi et al., 2007). Similar results were found after application of this system in aged monkeys and no adverse effects were recorded in this study after thorough toxicological testing (Herzog et al., 2007). A further study by this group found that the expression of neurturin using this system could be sustained for a year in rhesus monkeys, as could its therapeutic effects (Herzog et al., 2009). Unlike the case with GDNF, no antibodies to neurturin or no pathological abnormalities were detected after AAV2-delivery in primates (see Bartus et al., 2007).

Neurturin has also been reported to have protective effects on striatal projection neurones in a rat model of Huntington's disease (Perez-Navarro et al., 2000). AAV-2-mediated delivery of neurturin had neuroprotective effects and induced motor improvements in a genetic mouse model of Huntington's disease (Ramaswamy et al., 2009).

3.3 Effects of GDF5 *in vivo*

Several *in vivo* studies have shown that GDF5 can protect and restore adult rat nigrostriatal dopaminergic neurones in 6-OHDA-lesioned models of PD. The first such study reported that intracerebral injection of recombinant human GDF5 just above the substantia nigra and into the lateral ventricles produced significant improvements in motor function, protected nigral dopaminergic neurones and their striatal terminals, and preserved striatal levels of dopamine, its metabolites and its uptake, in rats with 6-OHDA lesions of the MFB (Sullivan et al., 1997). A follow-up study compared three injection sites and found that application of GDF5 into either the striatum or substantia nigra, but not into the lateral ventricle, produced optimal neuroprotective effects (Sullivan et al., 1999). Delayed intrastriatal administration of recombinant human GDF5 at one or two weeks after an intrastriatal 6-OHDA lesion resulted in significant improvements in motor behaviour but only the one-week injection regimen induced sparing of nigral dopaminergic cell bodies, whereas there was no significant rescue of striatal dopaminergic terminals after either time-point of treatment (Hurley et al., 2004). This indicates that there is a window of time at which the degenerating nigrostriatal pathway can be rescued by exogenous trophic factors. This has relevance to clinical studies, as such therapies may only be effective at earlier stages of the disease. GDF5 has also been reported to improve the survival and function of grafted dopaminergic neurones to the same extent as GDNF (Sullivan et al., 1998). This study found that incubation of embryonic rat midbrain tissue in GDF5 or GDNF prior to intrastriatal grafting into rats which had 6-OHDA lesions of the MFB, produced significant improvements in the survival of the grafted cells. Furthermore, GDF5-treated grafts conferred significant motor improvements and preservation of nigral dopaminergic neurones and their striatal terminals in 6-OHDA-lesioned rats, to at least the same extent as GDNF-treated grafts (Sullivan et al., 1998). Each of these *in vivo* studies involved infusion of recombinant GDF5 protein, which can only be effective for a limited time due to its being metabolised in the brain. Future studies will examine alternative administration methods, such as viral vector-mediated delivery or the use of encapsulated cell technology. One recent study reported that GDF5-overexpressing embryonic rat midbrain transplants survived well in the 6-OHDA-lesioned adult rat striatum and had significant effects to improve motor behaviour in these animals (O'Sullivan et al., 2010).

3.4 Effects of MANF / CDNF *in vivo*

Intracerebral injection of recombinant human CDNF has been reported to have potent protective and restorative effects on the 6-OHDA-lesioned adult rat nigrostriatal pathway (Lindholm et al., 2007). Intrastriatal administration of recombinant human MANF also has protective and restorative effects on dopaminergic neurones in 6-OHDA-lesioned adult rats (Voutilainen et al., 2009). Both of these studies reported motor recovery (reductions in drug-induced rotations) and preservation of dopaminergic nigral cell bodies and their terminals in the striatum, conferred by intrastriatal injection of the neurotrophic factor six hours before or four weeks after intrastriatal injection of 6-OHDA. The same group recently reported that intrastriatal infusion of CDNF via mini-pumps for two weeks, beginning at two weeks after an intrastriatal 6-OHDA lesion, was able to confer motor improvements and partially protect dopaminergic nigral cell bodies and their striatal terminals (Voutilainen et al., 2011). It is interesting that MANF appears to be transported through the brain in a different manner to that of GDNF, as radiolabelled MANF is transported to the cortex after intrastriatal injection (Voutilainen et al., 2009), while labelled GDNF is retrogradely transported to the substantia nigra (Leitner et al., 1999; Tomac et al., 1995), as is labelled CDNF (Voutilainen et al., 2011). Recombinant human MANF has also been reported to have neuroprotective effects on cortical neurones in an adult rat model of ischemic stroke (Airavaara et al., 2009).

4. Dopaminergic neurotrophic factors in clinical trials

4.1 GDNF in clinical trials

The potent and reproducible effects of GDNF in animal models led to the initiation of clinical trials using this factor in PD patients. The clinical application of neurotrophic factors is hampered by the fact that these proteins do not cross the blood-brain barrier, and are rapidly degraded *in vivo*. The need for direct intracerebral delivery of neurotrophic factors may increase the level of complications in patients. The first clinical trial in PD patients was a randomised controlled trial involving 50 patients, and used intraventricular delivery of recombinant human GDNF (r-methionylGDNF, liatermin®, manufactured by Amgen) or placebo (Nutt et al., 2003). This study reported no significant benefits of GDNF treatment over the placebo, probably because GDNF did not reach the striatum in sufficient amounts. In addition, troublesome side-effects were observed, including pain, depression, appetite loss and l'Hermitte's sign (Kordower et al., 1999; Nutt et al., 2003); these may have been due to the intraventricular delivery mechanism that was used in this trial.

Due to the suggestion that intraventricular delivery did not achieve GDNF delivery to the target tissues in the striatum, subsequent trials used direct administration to brain parenchyma using a catheter system. Promising results emerged from two open-label trials, which used intraputaminal infusion of recombinant GDNF (Gill et al., 2003; Love et al., 2005; Patel et al., 2005; Slevin et al., 2005). These trials both reported improvements in the patients' motor symptoms and in activities of daily living, without any serious side-effects. Gill and colleagues demonstrated that direct unilateral (in one patient) or bilateral (in four patients) intraputaminal infusion of GDNF had long-lasting benefits in five patients suffering from advanced PD. After 24 months of treatment, all patients reported complete absence of akinesia and a 73% reduction in the duration of dyskinesic episodes. Motor dysfunction was reduced in both on- and off- medication phases compared to the pre-treatment level (UPDRS part III score was reported to be 57% lower off medication and 48% lower on medication). Similarly, functional deficits were reduced by 63% when off medication and 58% when on medication (UPDRS part II score) (Patel et al., 2005). The second study, by Slevin and co-workers, used unilateral intraputaminal infusion of escalating doses of GDNF in ten patients with advanced PD and reported similar results, showing bilateral motor improvements after 24 weeks (Slevin et al., 2005). In both studies, the only consistent adverse effect was a mild l'Hermitte's sign. Improvements in dopamine storage were detected in the regions surrounding the catheter which was used for infusion of GDNF (Gill et al., 2003; Love et al., 2005).

The two open-label studies demonstrated the feasibility and sustainability of GDNF treatment by intraputaminal infusion. However, a subsequent randomised placebo-controlled trial, involving 34 patients (17 received GDNF and 17 received placebo), reported no significant motor improvements in PD patients (Lang et al., 2006). After six months of bilateral intraputaminal infusion of recombinant GDNF, there were no significant differences between the motor UPDRS scores in patients that had received GDNF and in those that had received a placebo. Furthermore, safety concerns were raised, since approximately 10% of the GDNF-treated patients developed antibodies against the peptide, which could potentially counteract the therapeutic benefits (Tatarewicz et al., 2007). A similar proportion of patients who had participated in the two open-label trials also developed antibodies to GDNF (Slevin et al., 2005). PET studies showed a significant increase in 18F-dopa intake in the GDNF-infused patients compared to the placebo group, demonstrating a functional effect of GDNF infusion, although this did not translate into significant motor improvements (Lang et al., 2006). The discrepancies between the open-label and placebo-controlled trials may have been due to variations in patient selection, as well as to a placebo effect. Optimisation of surgical methodologies, catheter design and positioning, drug dosage and diffusion, and patient selection will be necessary for any future GDNF clinical studies. The development of inexplicable cerebellar pathology in a primate model of PD after administration of a high dose of GDNF has raised a further safety issue (Hovland et al., 2007). This resulted in a controversial decision by Amgen to cease all clinical trials using GDNF (see Barker, 2006; Lang et al., 2006; Penn et al., 2006). A recent study paved the way for future clinical trials by investigating GDNF distribution in the non-human primate brain following AAV2-mediated intraputaminal delivery (Richardson et al., 2011). It appears to be generally accepted that GDNF therapy for PD requires further development in pre-clinical trials and it is probable that alternative methodologies, such as viral vector-mediated expression, may prove to be more effective for achieving long-term and targeted GDNF delivery (see Evans & Barker, 2008; Morrison et al., 2007; Sherer et al., 2006).

4.2 Neurturin in clinical trials

Based on the promising results found in animal studies using AAV2-mediated gene transfer of neurturin (CERE-120®), an open-label Phase 1 clinical trial using gene therapy to deliver neurturin was initiated in PD patients by the company Ceregene (Marks et al., 2008). Twelve patients, each suffering from advanced PD, received bilateral intraputaminal injections of AAV2-neurturin (at one of two doses) and were followed for twelve months. Results showed that neurturin-treated patients displayed reductions in their off-medication UPDRS score, decreases in the time spent in the 'off' period and reductions in dyskinesias, without any adverse side-effects (Marks et al., 2008). However, a subsequent double-blind Phase 2 trial, which involved 58 PD patients, was reported to have failed. In this trial, intraputaminal AAV2-neurturin did not have superior effects on motor function than sham surgery, when assessed after twelve months, and only modest benefits were recorded after eighteen months. Serious adverse side-effects were reported in about a third of the neurturin-treated patients (Marks et al., 2010). Ceregene began to recruit PD patients for a new double-blind trial using AAV2-neurturin in September 2010 (www.ceregene.com/press_101910.asp). This multi-centre phase 2 trial will involve about 52 patients, half of whom will receive intraputaminal AAV2-neurturin and half of whom will receive sham

Neurotrophic factor	Trial type	Delivery Site	No. of patients	Age / duration of disease (years)	Benefits	Side-effects	Reference
rh-methionyl-GDNF	MC,R,DB, PC	ICV	50	58±8 / 11±6	No	LS, Nausea, Anorexia	Nutt 2003
rh-methionyl-GDNF	Open-label	IPu	5	54.2±6 / 19±9.8	Yes	LS	Gill 2003 Patel 2005
rh-methionyl-GDNF	Open-label	IPu	10	57.9±9.3 / 8.7±3.6	Yes	LS, Headaches	Slevin 2005
rh-methionyl-GDNF	MC,R,DB, PC	IPu	33	56±7.2 / 9.7±3.9	No	LS , Anti-GDNF antibodies	Lang 2006
AAV2-neurturin	Open-label	IPu	12	57±8 / 11±3	Yes	Headaches	Marks 2008
AAV2-neurturin	MC, DB, SSC	IPu	58	60±7 / 10±3	No	Headaches	Marks 2010

(rh - recombinant human, MC - multi-centre, R - randomised, DB - double-blind, PC – placebo-controlled, SSC - sham surgery-controlled, ICV - intracerebroventricular, IPu - intraputaminal, LS - l'Hermitte's sign)

Table 1. Clinical trials using neurotrophic factors

surgery. It is hoped that a new dosing regimen, designed to maximise the delivery of the neurturin gene throughout the degenerating nigrostriatal system, will be the key to a promising outcome from this trial. This hypothesis is based on a post mortem analysis on the brains of some of the patients who had received AAV2-neurturin (and who had died of unrelated causes), which found that neurturin had been retrogradely transported from the intraputaminal injection site to the substantia nigra (Bartus et al., 2011). The company subsequently administered AAV2-neurturin to both the substantia nigra and the striatum of six PD patients and, based on analysis of the safety data from these six patients, are now recruiting patients for the second phase of this trial.

5. Conclusion

Despite the recent disappointing results in clinical trials with GDNF and neurturin, there remains an optimism that neurotrophic factors will prove to be useful in PD therapy (see Aron & Klein, 2011; Deierborg et al., 2008; Manfredsson et al., 2009). Optimisation of delivery methods is needed and vital information is being gleaned in this respect from studies in animal models of PD, such as grafting of encapsulated cells expressing neurotrophic factors and viral-mediated neurotrophic factor delivery (for reviews see Bjorklund et al., 2000; Deierborg et al., 2008; Kordower, 2003; Zurn et al., 2001). It is likely that neurotrophic factors will be most applicable in the early stages of the disease, to provide neuroprotection to the remaining nigrostriatal dopaminergic neurones before extensive neuronal loss has occurred (see Bjorklund et al., 2009). For future clinical trials, optimisation of surgical and infusion protocols, as well as careful patient selection, will be critical to advance this promising therapeutic approach. Animal studies have provided signs that neurotrophic factor therapy may be more applicable in young patients than in old, and also that patients with an earlier, less severe, disease stage may be more responsive to this type of therapy than those at advanced disease stages.

Researchers are currently investigating the use of stem or progenitor cells as a possible alternative to freshly-dissected embryonic midbrain for transplantation in PD patients. The use of such cells would alleviate some of the ethical and practical concerns associated with the use of fresh embryonic tissue. It is likely that neurotrophic factors could be used to improve stem cell therapy for PD, both to enhance the survival of transplanted dopaminergic precursor cells, and to induce a dopaminergic cell fate in unspecified progenitors.

In conclusion, much research still remains to be conducted in the area of neurotrophic factor therapy for PD. In the case of those factors which have been tested in clinical trials (GDNF and neurturin) optimisation of the surgical delivery procedures and patient selection will be critical to the ongoing development of this therapeutic approach. Exploration of novel delivery mechanisms, such as viral vector-mediated delivery (as has been used in the Ceregene neurturin trials) and cell encapsulation, which has been tested in animal models of PD to deliver GDNF, will be critical. More information is needed about factors such as GDF5 and CDNF, which have shown promise in preclinical models of PD. Knowledge of the receptors and signal transduction pathways that are involved in the neurotrophic and protective effects of these factors will aid the future development of safe and targeted therapeutics.

6. References

Airaksinen, M.S. & Saarma, M. (2002). The GDNF family: signalling, biological functions and therapeutic value. Nat Rev Neurosci, Vol. 3, No. 5, pp. 383-394.

Airaksinen, M.S.; Titievsky, A. & Saarma, M. (1999). GDNF family neurotrophic factor signaling: four masters, one servant? Mol Cell Neurosci, Vol. 13, No. 5, pp. 313-325.

Airavaara, M.; Shen, H.; Kuo, C.C.; Peranen, J.; Saarma, M.; Hoffer, B. & Wang, Y. (2009). Mesencephalic astrocyte-derived neurotrophic factor reduces ischemic brain injury and promotes behavioral recovery in rats. J Comp Neurol, Vol. 515, No. 1, pp. 116-124.

Akerud, P.; Alberch, J.; Eketjall, S.; Wagner, J. & Arenas, E. (1999). Differential effects of glial cell line-derived neurotrophic factor and neurturin on developing and adult substantia nigra dopaminergic neurons. J Neurochem, Vol. 73, No. 1, pp. 70-78.

Akerud, P.; Holm, P.C.; Castelo-Branco, G.; Sousa, K.; Rodriguez, F.J. & Arenas, E. (2002). Persephin-overexpressing neural stem cells regulate the function of nigral dopaminergic neurons and prevent their degeneration in a model of Parkinson's disease. Mol Cell Neurosci, Vol. 21, No. 2, pp. 205-222.

Aoi, M.; Date, I.; Tomita, S. & Ohmoto, T. (2000). The effect of intrastriatal single injection of GDNF on the nigrostriatal dopaminergic system in hemiparkinsonian rats: behavioral and histological studies using two different dosages. Neurosci Res, Vol. 36, No. 4, pp. 319-325.

Apostolides, C.; Sanford, E.; Hong, M. & Mendez, I. (1998). Glial cell line-derived neurotrophic factor improves intrastriatal graft survival of stored dopaminergic cells. Neuroscience, Vol. 83, No. 2, pp. 363-372.

Apostolou, A.; Shen, Y.; Liang, Y.; Luo, J. & Fang, S. (2008). Armet, a UPR-upregulated protein, inhibits cell proliferation and ER stress-induced cell death. Exp Cell Res, Vol. 314, No. 13, pp. 2454-2467.

Aron, L. & Klein, R. (2011). Repairing the parkinsonian brain with neurotrophic factors. Trends Neurosci, Vol. 34, No. 2, pp. 88-100.

Attisano, L. & Wrana, J.L. (2000). Smads as transcriptional co-modulators. Curr Opin Cell Biol, Vol. 12, No. 2, pp. 235-243.

Balemans, W. & Van Hul, W. (2002). Extracellular regulation of BMP signaling in vertebrates: a cocktail of modulators. Dev Biol, Vol. 250, No. 2, pp. 231-250.

Baloh, R.H.; Enomoto, H.; Johnson, E.M., Jr. & Milbrandt, J. (2000). The GDNF family ligands and receptors - implications for neural development. Curr Opin Neurobiol, Vol. 10, No. 1, pp. 103-110.

Baloh, R.H.; Tansey, M.G.; Lampe, P.A.; Fahrner, T.J.; Enomoto, H.; Simburger, K.S.; Leitner, M.L.; Araki, T.; Johnson, E.M., Jr. & Milbrandt, J. (1998). Artemin, a novel member of the GDNF ligand family, supports peripheral and central neurons and signals through the GFRalpha3-RET receptor complex. Neuron, Vol. 21, No. 6, pp. 1291-1302.

Barker, R.A. (2006). Continuing trials of GDNF in Parkinson's disease. Lancet Neurol, Vol. 5, No. 4, pp. 285-286.

Barnett, M.W.; Fisher, C.E.; Perona-Wright, G. & Davies, J.A. (2002). Signalling by glial cell line-derived neurotrophic factor (GDNF) requires heparan sulphate glycosaminoglycan. J Cell Sci, Vol. 115, No. Pt 23, pp. 4495-4503.

Bartus, R.T.; Herzog, C.D.; Bishop, K.; Ostrove, J.M.; Tuszynski, M.; Kordower, J.H. & Gasmi, M. (2007). Issues regarding gene therapy products for Parkinson's disease: the development of CERE-120 (AAV-NTN) as one reference point. Parkinsonism Relat Disord, Vol. 13 Suppl 3, No. pp. S469-477.

Bartus, R.T.; Herzog, C.D.; Chu, Y.; Wilson, A.; Brown, L.; Siffert, J.; Johnson, E.M., Jr.; Olanow, C.W.; Mufson, E.J. & Kordower, J.H. (2011). Bioactivity of AAV2-neurturin gene therapy (CERE-120): differences between Parkinson's disease and nonhuman primate brains. Mov Disord, Vol. 26, No. 1, pp. 27-36.

Bauer, M.; Meyer, M.; Grimm, L.; Meitinger, T.; Zimmer, J.; Gasser, T.; Ueffing, M. & Widmer, H.R. (2000). Nonviral glial cell-derived neurotrophic factor gene transfer enhances survival of cultured dopaminergic neurons and improves their function after transplantation in a rat model of Parkinson's disease. Hum Gene Ther, Vol. 11, No. 11, pp. 1529-1541.

Beck, K.D.; Valverde, J.; Alexi, T.; Poulsen, K.; Moffat, B.; Vandlen, R.A.; Rosenthal, A. & Hefti, F. (1995). Mesencephalic dopaminergic neurons protected by GDNF from axotomy-induced degeneration in the adult brain. Nature, Vol. 373, No. 6512, pp. 339-341.

Behrstock, S.; Ebert, A.; McHugh, J.; Vosberg, S.; Moore, J.; Schneider, B.; Capowski, E.; Hei, D.; Kordower, J.; Aebischer, P. & Svendsen, C.N. (2006). Human neural progenitors deliver glial cell line-derived neurotrophic factor to parkinsonian rodents and aged primates. Gene Ther, Vol. 13, No. 5, pp. 379-388.

Bensadoun, J.C.; Pereira de Almeida, L.; Fine, E.G.; Tseng, J.L.; Deglon, N. & Aebischer, P. (2003). Comparative study of GDNF delivery systems for the CNS: polymer rods, encapsulated cells, and lentiviral vectors. J Control Release, Vol. 87, No. 1-3, pp. 107-115.

Bespalov, M.M. & Saarma, M. (2007). GDNF family receptor complexes are emerging drug targets. Trends Pharmacol Sci, Vol. 28, No. 2, pp. 68-74.

Bespalov, M.M.; Sidorova, Y.A.; Tumova, S.; Ahonen-Bishopp, A.; Magalhaes, A.C.; Kulesskiy, E.; Paveliev, M.; Rivera, C.; Rauvala, H. & Saarma, M. (2011). Heparan sulfate proteoglycan syndecan-3 is a novel receptor for GDNF, neurturin, and artemin. J Cell Biol, Vol. 192, No. 1, pp. 153-169.

Bilak, M.M.; Shifrin, D.A.; Corse, A.M.; Bilak, S.R. & Kuncl, R.W. (1999). Neuroprotective utility and neurotrophic action of neurturin in postnatal motor neurons: comparison with GDNF and persephin. Mol Cell Neurosci, Vol. 13, No. 5, pp. 326-336.

Bilang-Bleuel, A.; Revah, F.; Colin, P.; Locquet, I.; Robert, J.J.; Mallet, J. & Horellou, P. (1997). Intrastriatal injection of an adenoviral vector expressing glial-cell-line-derived neurotrophic factor prevents dopaminergic neuron degeneration and behavioral impairment in a rat model of Parkinson disease. Proc Natl Acad Sci U S A, Vol. 94, No. 16, pp. 8818-8823.

Bjorklund, A.; Bjorklund, T. & Kirik, D. (2009). Gene therapy for dopamine replacement in Parkinson's disease. Sci Transl Med, Vol. 1, No. 2, pp. 2ps2.

Bjorklund, A.; Kirik, D.; Rosenblad, C.; Georgievska, B.; Lundberg, C. & Mandel, R.J. (2000). Towards a neuroprotective gene therapy for Parkinson's disease: use of adenovirus, AAV and lentivirus vectors for gene transfer of GDNF to the nigrostriatal system in the rat Parkinson model. Brain Res, Vol. 886, No. 1-2, pp. 82-98.

Bjorklund, A. & Lindvall, O. (2000). Parkinson disease gene therapy moves toward the clinic. Nat Med, Vol. 6, No. 11, pp. 1207-1208.

Bjorklund, A.; Rosenblad, C.; Winkler, C. & Kirik, D. (1997). Studies on neuroprotective and regenerative effects of GDNF in a partial lesion model of Parkinson's disease. Neurobiol Dis, Vol. 4, No. 3-4, pp. 186-200.

Borgal, L.; Hong, M.; Sadi, D. & Mendez, I. (2007). Differential effects of glial cell line-derived neurotrophic factor on A9 and A10 dopamine neuron survival *in vitro*. Neuroscience, Vol. 147, No. 3, pp. 712-719.

Bowenkamp, K.E.; Hoffman, A.F.; Gerhardt, G.A.; Henry, M.A.; Biddle, P.T.; Hoffer, B.J. & Granholm, A.C. (1995). Glial cell line-derived neurotrophic factor supports survival of injured midbrain dopaminergic neurons. J Comp Neurol, Vol. 355, No. 4, pp. 479-489.

Bowenkamp, K.E.; Lapchak, P.A.; Hoffer, B.J.; Miller, P.J. & Bickford, P.C. (1997). Intracerebroventricular glial cell line-derived neurotrophic factor improves motor function and supports nigrostriatal dopamine neurons in bilaterally 6-hydroxydopamine lesioned rats. Exp Neurol, Vol. 145, No. 1, pp. 104-117.

Braak, H.; Del Tredici, K.; Rub, U.; de Vos, R.A.; Jansen Steur, E.N. & Braak, E. (2003). Staging of brain pathology related to sporadic Parkinson's disease. Neurobiol Aging, Vol. 24, No. 2, pp. 197-211.

Bragdon, B.; Moseychuk, O.; Saldanha, S.; King, D.; Julian, J. & Nohe, A. (2011). Bone morphogenetic proteins: a critical review. Cell Signal, Vol. 23, No. 4, pp. 609-620.

Brundin, P.; Barker, R.A. & Parmar, P. (2010). Neural grafting in Parkinson's disease : Problems and possibilities. Prog Brain Res, Vol. 184, pp. 265-294.

Burke, R.E.; Antonelli, M. & Sulzer, D. (1998). Glial cell line-derived neurotrophic growth factor inhibits apoptotic death of postnatal substantia nigra dopamine neurons in primary culture. J Neurochem, Vol. 71, No. 2, pp. 517-525.

Cao, J.P.; Li, F.Z.; Zhu, Y.Y.; Yuan, H.H.; Yu, Z.Q. & Gao, D.S. (2010). Expressions and possible roles of GDNF receptors in the developing dopaminergic neurons. Brain Res Bull, Vol. 83, No. 6, pp. 321-330.

Cao, J.P.; Wang, H.J.; Yu, J.K.; Yang, H.; Xiao, C.H. & Gao, D.S. (2008). Involvement of NCAM in the effects of GDNF on the neurite outgrowth in the dopamine neurons. Neurosci Res, Vol. 61, No. 4, pp. 390-397.

Cass, W.A. & Peters, L.E. (2010). Neurturin effects on nigrostriatal dopamine release and content: comparison with GDNF. Neurochem Res, Vol. 35, No. 5, pp. 727-734.

Cass, W.A.; Peters, L.E.; Harned, M.E. & Seroogy, K.B. (2006). Protection by GDNF and other trophic factors against the dopamine-depleting effects of neurotoxic doses of methamphetamine. Ann N Y Acad Sci, Vol. 1074, No. pp. 272-281.

Choi-Lundberg, D.L. & Bohn, M.C. (1995). Ontogeny and distribution of glial cell line-derived neurotrophic factor (GDNF) mRNA in rat. Brain Res Dev Brain Res, Vol. 85, No. 1, pp. 80-88.

Choi-Lundberg, D.L.; Lin, Q.; Chang, Y.N.; Chiang, Y.L.; Hay, C.M.; Mohajeri, H.; Davidson, B.L. & Bohn, M.C. (1997). Dopaminergic neurons protected from degeneration by GDNF gene therapy. Science, Vol. 275, No. 5301, pp. 838-841.

Choi-Lundberg, D.L.; Lin, Q.; Schallert, T.; Crippens, D.; Davidson, B.L.; Chang, Y.N.; Chiang, Y.L.; Qian, J.; Bardwaj, L. & Bohn, M.C. (1998). Behavioral and cellular protection of rat dopaminergic neurons by an adenoviral vector encoding glial cell line-derived neurotrophic factor. Exp Neurol, Vol. 154, No. 2, pp. 261-275.

Choi, J.M.; Hong, J.H.; Chae, M.J.; Hung, N.P.; Kang, H.S.; Ma, H.I. & Kim, Y.J. (2011). Analysis of mutations and the association between polymorphisms in the cerebral dopamine neurotrophic factor (CDNF) gene and Parkinson disease. Neurosci Lett, Vol. 493, No. 3, pp. 97-101.

Clarkson, E.D.; Zawada, W.M. & Freed, C.R. (1995). GDNF reduces apoptosis in dopaminergic neurons *in vitro*. Neuroreport, Vol. 7, No. 1, pp. 145-149.

Clarkson, E.D.; Zawada, W.M. & Freed, C.R. (1997). GDNF improves survival and reduces apoptosis in human embryonic dopaminergic neurons *in vitro*. Cell Tissue Res, Vol. 289, No. 2, pp. 207-210.

Clayton, K.B. & Sullivan, A.M. (2007). Differential effects of GDF5 on the medial and lateral rat ventral mesencephalon. Neurosci Lett, Vol. 427, No. 3, pp. 132-137.

Connor, B.; Kozlowski, D.A.; Schallert, T.; Tillerson, J.L.; Davidson, B.L. & Bohn, M.C. (1999). Differential effects of glial cell line-derived neurotrophic factor (GDNF) in the striatum and substantia nigra of the aged Parkinsonian rat. Gene Ther, Vol. 6, No. 12, pp. 1936-1951.

Corradini, E.; Babitt, J.L. & Lin, H.Y. (2009). The RGM/DRAGON family of BMP co-receptors. Cytokine Growth Factor Rev, Vol. 20, No. 5-6, pp. 389-398.

Date, I.; Aoi, M.; Tomita, S.; Collins, F. & Ohmoto, T. (1998). GDNF administration induces recovery of the nigrostriatal dopaminergic system both in young and aged parkinsonian mice. Neuroreport, Vol. 9, No. 10, pp. 2365-2369.

Date, I.; Shingo, T.; Yoshida, H.; Fujiwara, K.; Kobayashi, K.; Takeuchi, A. & Ohmoto, T. (2001). Grafting of encapsulated genetically modified cells secreting GDNF into the striatum of parkinsonian model rats. Cell Transplant, Vol. 10, No. 4-5, pp. 397-401.

Dauer, W. & Przedborski, S. (2003). Parkinson's disease: mechanisms and models. Neuron, Vol. 39, No. 6, pp. 889-909.

Dawson, T.M. & Dawson, V.L. (2003). Molecular pathways of neurodegeneration in Parkinson's disease. Science, Vol. 302, No. 5646, pp. 819-822.

de Caestecker, M. (2004). The transforming growth factor-beta superfamily of receptors. Cytokine Growth Factor Rev, Vol. 15, No. 1, pp. 1-11.

de Lau, L.M. & Breteler, M.M. (2006). Epidemiology of Parkinson's disease. Lancet Neurol, Vol. 5, No. 6, pp. 525-535.

Deierborg, T.; Soulet, D.; Roybon, L.; Hall, V. & Brundin, P. (2008). Emerging restorative treatments for Parkinson's disease. Prog Neurobiol, Vol. 85, No. 4, pp. 407-432.

Dowd, E.; Monville, C.; Torres, E.M.; Wong, L.F.; Azzouz, M.; Mazarakis, N.D. & Dunnett, S.B. (2005). Lentivector-mediated delivery of GDNF protects complex motor functions relevant to human Parkinsonism in a rat lesion model. Eur J Neurosci, Vol. 22, No. 10, pp. 2587-2595.

Ebendal, T.; Bengtsson, H. & Soderstrom, S. (1998). Bone morphogenetic proteins and their receptors: potential functions in the brain. J Neurosci Res, Vol. 51, No. 2, pp. 139-146.

Eggert, K.; Schlegel, J.; Oertel, W.; Wurz, C.; Krieg, J.C. & Vedder, H. (1999). Glial cell line-derived neurotrophic factor protects dopaminergic neurons from 6-hydroxydopamine toxicity *in vitro*. Neurosci Lett, Vol. 269, No. 3, pp. 178-182.

Emborg, M.E.; Moirano, J.; Raschke, J.; Bondarenko, V.; Zufferey, R.; Peng, S.; Ebert, A.D.; Joers, V.; Roitberg, B.; Holden, J.E.; Koprich, J.; Lipton, J.; Kordower, J.H. & Aebischer, P. (2009). Response of aged parkinsonian monkeys to *in vivo* gene transfer of GDNF. Neurobiol Dis, Vol. 36, No. 2, pp. 303-311.

Engele, J. & Franke, B. (1996). Effects of glial cell line-derived neurotrophic factor (GDNF) on dopaminergic neurons require concurrent activation of cAMP-dependent signaling pathways. Cell Tissue Res, Vol. 286, No. 2, pp. 235-240.

Evans, J.R. & Barker, R.A. (2008). Neurotrophic factors as a therapeutic target for Parkinson's disease. Expert Opin Ther Targets, Vol. 12, No. 4, pp. 437-447.

Fahn, S. & Cohen, G. (1992). The oxidant stress hypothesis in Parkinson's disease: evidence supporting it. Ann Neurol, Vol. 32, No. 6, pp. 804-812.

Fearnley, J.M. & Lees, A.J. (1991). Ageing and Parkinson's disease: substantia nigra regional selectivity. Brain, Vol. 114 (Pt 5), No. pp. 2283-2301.

Fjord-Larsen, L.; Johansen, J.L.; Kusk, P.; Tornoe, J.; Gronborg, M.; Rosenblad, C. & Wahlberg, L.U. (2005). Efficient *in vivo* protection of nigral dopaminergic neurons by lentiviral gene transfer of a modified Neurturin construct. Exp Neurol, Vol. 195, No. 1, pp. 49-60.

Forno, L.S. (1996). Neuropathology of Parkinson's disease. J Neuropathol Exp Neurol, Vol. 55, No. 3, pp. 259-272.

Fox, C.M.; Gash, D.M.; Smoot, M.K. & Cass, W.A. (2001). Neuroprotective effects of GDNF against 6-OHDA in young and aged rats. Brain Res, Vol. 896, No. 1-2, pp. 56-63.

Freed, C.R.; Greene, P.E.; Breeze, R.E.; Tsai, W.Y.; DuMouchel, W.; Kao, R.; Dillon, S.; Winfield, H.; Culver, S.; Trojanowski, J.Q.; Eidelberg, D. & Fahn, S. (2001). Transplantation of embryonic dopamine neurons for severe Parkinson's disease. N Engl J Med, Vol. 344, No. 10, pp. 710-719.

Gardell, L.R.; Wang, R.; Ehrenfels, C.; Ossipov, M.H.; Rossomando, A.J.; Miller, S.; Buckley, C.; Cai, A.K.; Tse, A.; Foley, S.F.; Gong, B.; Walus, L.; Carmillo, P.; Worley, D.; Huang, C.; Engber, T.; Pepinsky, B.; Cate, R.L.; Vanderah, T.W.; Lai, J.; Sah, D.W. & Porreca, F. (2003). Multiple actions of systemic artemin in experimental neuropathy. Nat Med, Vol. 9, No. 11, pp. 1383-1389.

Gash, D.M.; Zhang, Z.; Cass, W.A.; Ovadia, A.; Simmerman, L.; Martin, D.; Russell, D.; Collins, F.; Hoffer, B.J. & Gerhardt, G.A. (1995). Morphological and functional effects of intranigrally administered GDNF in normal rhesus monkeys. J Comp Neurol, Vol. 363, No. 3, pp. 345-358.

Gash, D.M.; Zhang, Z.; Ovadia, A.; Cass, W.A.; Yi, A.; Simmerman, L.; Russell, D.; Martin, D.; Lapchak, P.A.; Collins, F.; Hoffer, B.J. & Gerhardt, G.A. (1996). Functional recovery in parkinsonian monkeys treated with GDNF. Nature, Vol. 380, No. 6571, pp. 252-255.

Gasmi, M.; Brandon, E.P.; Herzog, C.D.; Wilson, A.; Bishop, K.M.; Hofer, E.K.; Cunningham, J.J.; Printz, M.A.; Kordower, J.H. & Bartus, R.T. (2007). AAV2-mediated delivery of human neurturin to the rat nigrostriatal system: Long-term efficacy and tolerability of CERE-120 for Parkinson's disease. Neurobiol Dis, Vol. 27, No. 1, pp. 67-76.

Gasmi, M.; Herzog, C.D.; Brandon, E.P.; Cunningham, J.J.; Ramirez, G.A.; Ketchum, E.T. & Bartus, R.T. (2007). Striatal Delivery of Neurturin by CERE-120, an AAV2 Vector for the Treatment of Dopaminergic Neuron Degeneration in Parkinson's Disease. Mol Ther, Vol. 15, No. 1, pp. 62-68.

Gerhardt, G.A.; Cass, W.A.; Huettl, P.; Brock, S.; Zhang, Z. & Gash, D.M. (1999). GDNF improves dopamine function in the substantia nigra but not the putamen of unilateral MPTP-lesioned rhesus monkeys. Brain Res, Vol. 817, No. 1-2, pp. 163-171.

Gibb, W.R. & Lees, A.J. (1988). The relevance of the Lewy body to the pathogenesis of idiopathic Parkinson's disease. J Neurol Neurosurg Psychiatry, Vol. 51, No. 6, pp. 745-752.

Gill, S.S.; Patel, N.K.; Hotton, G.R.; O'Sullivan, K.; McCarter, R.; Bunnage, M.; Brooks, D.J.; Svendsen, C.N. & Heywood, P. (2003). Direct brain infusion of glial cell line-derived neurotrophic factor in Parkinson disease. Nat Med, Vol. 9, No. 5, pp. 589-595.

Glazner, G.W.; Mu, X. & Springer, J.E. (1998). Localization of glial cell line-derived neurotrophic factor receptor alpha and c-ret mRNA in rat central nervous system. J Comp Neurol, Vol. 391, No. 1, pp. 42-49.

Golden, J.P.; Baloh, R.H.; Kotzbauer, P.T.; Lampe, P.A.; Osborne, P.A.; Milbrandt, J. & Johnson, E.M., Jr. (1998). Expression of neurturin, GDNF, and their receptors in the adult mouse CNS. J Comp Neurol, Vol. 398, No. 1, pp. 139-150.

Golden, J.P.; DeMaro, J.A.; Osborne, P.A.; Milbrandt, J. & Johnson, E.M., Jr. (1999). Expression of neurturin, GDNF, and GDNF family-receptor mRNA in the developing and mature mouse. Exp Neurol, Vol. 158, No. 2, pp. 504-528.

Granholm, A.C.; Mott, J.L.; Bowenkamp, K.; Eken, S.; Henry, S.; Hoffer, B.J.; Lapchak, P.A.; Palmer, M.R.; van Horne, C. & Gerhardt, G.A. (1997). Glial cell line-derived neurotrophic factor improves survival of ventral mesencephalic grafts to the 6-hydroxydopamine lesioned striatum. Exp Brain Res, Vol. 116, No. 1, pp. 29-38.

Grondin, R.; Zhang, Z.; Ai, Y.; Ding, F.; Walton, A.A.; Surgener, S.P.; Gerhardt, G.A. & Gash, D.M. (2008). Intraputamenal infusion of exogenous neurturin protein restores motor and dopaminergic function in the globus pallidus of MPTP-lesioned rhesus monkeys. Cell Transplant, Vol. 17, No. 4, pp. 373-381.

Grondin, R.; Zhang, Z.; Yi, A.; Cass, W.A.; Maswood, N.; Andersen, A.H.; Elsberry, D.D.; Klein, M.C.; Gerhardt, G.A. & Gash, D.M. (2002). Chronic, controlled GDNF infusion promotes structural and functional recovery in advanced parkinsonian monkeys. Brain, Vol. 125, No. Pt 10, pp. 2191-2201.

Hagell, P.; Piccini, P.; Bjorklund, A.; Brundin, P.; Rehncrona, S.; Widner, H.; Crabb, L.; Pavese, N.; Oertel, W.H.; Quinn, N.; Brooks, D.J. & Lindvall, O. (2002). Dyskinesias following neural transplantation in Parkinson's disease. Nat Neurosci, Vol. 5, No. 7, pp. 627-628.

Hall, A.K. & Miller, R.H. (2004). Emerging roles for bone morphogenetic proteins in central nervous system glial biology. J Neurosci Res, Vol. 76, No. 1, pp. 1-8.

Hedlund, E. & Perlmann, T. (2009) Neuronal cell replacement in Parkinson's disease. Intern Med. Vol. 266, No. 4, pp. 358-371.

Hellman, M.; Arumae, U.; Yu, L.Y.; Lindholm, P.; Peranen, J.; Saarma, M. & Permi, P. (2011). Mesencephalic astrocyte-derived neurotrophic factor (MANF) has a unique mechanism to rescue apoptotic neurons. J Biol Chem, Vol. 286, No. 4, pp. 2675-2680.

Hermann, D.M.; Kilic, E.; Kugler, S.; Isenmann, S. & Bahr, M. (2001). Adenovirus-mediated glial cell line-derived neurotrophic factor (GDNF) expression protects against subsequent cortical cold injury in rats. Neurobiol Dis, Vol. 8, No. 6, pp. 964-973.

Herzog, C.D.; Brown, L.; Gammon, D.; Kruegel, B.; Lin, R.; Wilson, A.; Bolton, A.; Printz, M.; Gasmi, M.; Bishop, K.M.; Kordower, J.H. & Bartus, R.T. (2009). Expression, bioactivity, and safety 1 year after adeno-associated viral vector type 2-mediated delivery of neurturin to the monkey nigrostriatal system support cere-120 for Parkinson's disease. Neurosurgery, Vol. 64, No. 4, pp. 602-612; discussion 612-603.

Herzog, C.D.; Dass, B.; Holden, J.E.; Stansell, J., 3rd; Gasmi, M.; Tuszynski, M.H.; Bartus, R.T. & Kordower, J.H. (2007). Striatal delivery of CERE-120, an AAV2 vector encoding human neurturin, enhances activity of the dopaminergic nigrostriatal system in aged monkeys. Mov Disord, Vol. 22, No. 8, pp. 1124-1132.

Hoane, M.R.; Gulwadi, A.G.; Morrison, S.; Hovanesian, G.; Lindner, M.D. & Tao, W. (1999). Differential *in vivo* effects of neurturin and glial cell-line-derived neurotrophic factor. Exp Neurol, Vol. 160, No. 1, pp. 235-243.

Hoehn, M.M. & Yahr, M.D. (1967). Parkinsonism: onset, progression and mortality. Neurology, Vol. 17, No. 5, pp. 427-442.

Hoffer, B.J.; Hoffman, A.; Bowenkamp, K.; Huettl, P.; Hudson, J.; Martin, D.; Lin, L.F. & Gerhardt, G.A. (1994). Glial cell line-derived neurotrophic factor reverses toxin-induced injury to midbrain dopaminergic neurons *in vivo*. Neurosci Lett, Vol. 182, No. 1, pp. 107-111.

Hogan, B.L. (1996). Bone morphogenetic proteins: multifunctional regulators of vertebrate development. Genes Dev, Vol. 10, No. 13, pp. 1580-1594.

Horger, B.A.; Nishimura, M.C.; Armanini, M.P.; Wang, L.C.; Poulsen, K.T.; Rosenblad, C.; Kirik, D.; Moffat, B.; Simmons, L.; Johnson, E., Jr.; Milbrandt, J.; Rosenthal, A.; Bjorklund, A.; Vandlen, R.A.; Hynes, M.A. & Phillips, H.S. (1998). Neurturin exerts potent actions on survival and function of midbrain dopaminergic neurons. J Neurosci, Vol. 18, No. 13, pp. 4929-4937.

Hou, J.G.; Lin, L.F. & Mytilineou, C. (1996). Glial cell line-derived neurotrophic factor exerts neurotrophic effects on dopaminergic neurons *in vitro* and promotes their survival and regrowth after damage by 1-methyl-4-phenylpyridinium. J Neurochem, Vol. 66, No. 1, pp. 74-82.

Hovland, D.N., Jr.; Boyd, R.B.; Butt, M.T.; Engelhardt, J.A.; Moxness, M.S.; Ma, M.H.; Emery, M.G.; Ernst, N.B.; Reed, R.P.; Zeller, J.R.; Gash, D.M.; Masterman, D.M.; Potter, B.M.; Cosenza, M.E. & Lightfoot, R.M. (2007). Six-month continuous intraputamenal infusion toxicity study of recombinant methionyl human glial cell line-derived neurotrophic factor (r-metHuGDNF) in rhesus monkeys. Toxicol Pathol, Vol. 35, No. 5, pp. 676-692.

Hurley, F.M.; Costello, D.J. & Sullivan, A.M. (2004). Neuroprotective effects of delayed administration of growth/differentiation factor-5 in the partial lesion model of Parkinson's disease. Exp Neurol, Vol. 185, No. 2, pp. 281-289.

Iravani, M.M.; Costa, S.; Jackson, M.J.; Tel, B.C.; Cannizzaro, C.; Pearce, R.K. & Jenner, P. (2001). GDNF reverses priming for dyskinesia in MPTP-treated, L-DOPA-primed common marmosets. Eur J Neurosci, Vol. 13, No. 3, pp. 597-608.

Kawabata, M.; Imamura, T. & Miyazono, K. (1998). Signal transduction by bone morphogenetic proteins. Cytokine Growth Factor Rev, Vol. 9, No. 1, pp. 49-61.

Kearns, C.M. & Gash, D.M. (1995). GDNF protects nigral dopamine neurons against 6-hydroxydopamine *in vivo*. Brain Res, Vol. 672, No. 1-2, pp. 104-111.

Kirik, D.; Rosenblad, C.; Bjorklund, A. & Mandel, R.J. (2000). Long-term rAAV-mediated gene transfer of GDNF in the rat Parkinson's model: intrastriatal but not intranigral transduction promotes functional regeneration in the lesioned nigrostriatal system. J Neurosci, Vol. 20, No. 12, pp. 4686-4700.

Kirik, D.; Winkler, C. & Bjorklund, A. (2001). Growth and functional efficacy of intrastriatal nigral transplants depend on the extent of nigrostriatal degeneration. J Neurosci, Vol. 21, No. 8, pp. 2889-2896.

Kishima, H.; Poyot, T.; Bloch, J.; Dauguet, J.; Conde, F.; Dolle, F.; Hinnen, F.; Pralong, W.; Palfi, S.; Deglon, N.; Aebischer, P. & Hantraye, P. (2004). Encapsulated GDNF-producing C2C12 cells for Parkinson's disease: a pre-clinical study in chronic MPTP-treated baboons. Neurobiol Dis, Vol. 16, No. 2, pp. 428-439.

Kojima, H.; Abiru, Y.; Sakajiri, K.; Watabe, K.; Ohishi, N.; Takamori, M.; Hatanaka, H. & Yagi, K. (1997). Adenovirus-mediated transduction with human glial cell line-derived neurotrophic factor gene prevents 1-methyl-4-phenyl-1,2,3,6-tetrahydropyridine-induced dopamine depletion in striatum of mouse brain. Biochem Biophys Res Commun, Vol. 238, No. 2, pp. 569-573.

Kordower, J.H. (2003). *In vivo* gene delivery of glial cell line--derived neurotrophic factor for Parkinson's disease. Ann Neurol, Vol. 53 Suppl 3, No. pp. S120-132; discussion S132-124.

Kordower, J.H.; Emborg, M.E.; Bloch, J.; Ma, S.Y.; Chu, Y.; Leventhal, L.; McBride, J.; Chen, E.Y.; Palfi, S.; Roitberg, B.Z.; Brown, W.D.; Holden, J.E.; Pyzalski, R.; Taylor, M.D.; Carvey, P.; Ling, Z.; Trono, D.; Hantraye, P.; Deglon, N. & Aebischer, P. (2000). Neurodegeneration prevented by lentiviral vector delivery of GDNF in primate models of Parkinson's disease. Science, Vol. 290, No. 5492, pp. 767-773.

Kordower, J.H.; Herzog, C.D.; Dass, B.; Bakay, R.A.; Stansell, J., 3rd; Gasmi, M. & Bartus, R.T. (2006). Delivery of neurturin by AAV2 (CERE-120)-mediated gene transfer provides structural and functional neuroprotection and neurorestoration in MPTP-treated monkeys. Ann Neurol, Vol. 60, No. 6, pp. 706-715.

Kordower, J.H.; Palfi, S.; Chen, E.Y.; Ma, S.Y.; Sendera, T.; Cochran, E.J.; Mufson, E.J.; Penn, R.; Goetz, C.G. & Comella, C.D. (1999). Clinicopathological findings following intraventricular glial-derived neurotrophic factor treatment in a patient with Parkinson's disease. Ann Neurol, Vol. 46, No. 3, pp. 419-424.

Kotzbauer, P.T.; Lampe, P.A.; Heuckeroth, R.O.; Golden, J.P.; Creedon, D.J.; Johnson, E.M., Jr. & Milbrandt, J. (1996). Neurturin, a relative of glial-cell-line-derived neurotrophic factor. Nature, Vol. 384, No. 6608, pp. 467-470.

Kozlowski, D.A.; Connor, B.; Tillerson, J.L.; Schallert, T. & Bohn, M.C. (2000). Delivery of a GDNF gene into the substantia nigra after a progressive 6-OHDA lesion maintains functional nigrostriatal connections. Exp Neurol, Vol. 166, No. 1, pp. 1-15.

Kramer, B.C.; Goldman, A.D. & Mytilineou, C. (1999). Glial cell line derived neurotrophic factor promotes the recovery of dopamine neurons damaged by 6-hydroxydopamine *in vitro*. Brain Res, Vol. 851, No. 1-2, pp. 221-227.

Krieglstein, K.; Henheik, P.; Farkas, L.; Jaszai, J.; Galter, D.; Krohn, K. & Unsicker, K. (1998). Glial cell line-derived neurotrophic factor requires transforming growth factor-beta for exerting its full neurotrophic potential on peripheral and CNS neurons. J Neurosci, Vol. 18, No. 23, pp. 9822-9834.

Krieglstein, K.; Strelau, J.; Schober, A.; Sullivan, A. & Unsicker, K. (2002). TGF-beta and the regulation of neuron survival and death. J Physiol Paris, Vol. 96, No. 1-2, pp. 25-30.

Krieglstein, K.; Suter-Crazzolara, C.; Fischer, W.H. & Unsicker, K. (1995). TGF-beta superfamily members promote survival of midbrain dopaminergic neurons and protect them against MPP+ toxicity. Embo J, Vol. 14, No. 4, pp. 736-742.

Krieglstein, K.; Suter-Crazzolara, C.; Hotten, G.; Pohl, J. & Unsicker, K. (1995). Trophic and protective effects of growth/differentiation factor 5, a member of the transforming growth factor-beta superfamily, on midbrain dopaminergic neurons. J Neurosci Res, Vol. 42, No. 5, pp. 724-732.

Lang, A.E.; Gill, S.; Patel, N.K.; Lozano, A.; Nutt, J.G.; Penn, R.; Brooks, D.J.; Hotton, G.; Moro, E.; Heywood, P.; Brodsky, M.A.; Burchiel, K.; Kelly, P.; Dalvi, A.; Scott, B.; Stacy, M.; Turner, D.; Wooten, V.G.; Elias, W.J.; Laws, E.R.; Dhawan, V.; Stoessl, A.J.; Matcham, J.; Coffey, R.J. & Traub, M. (2006). Randomized controlled trial of intraputamenal glial cell line-derived neurotrophic factor infusion in Parkinson disease. Ann Neurol, Vol. 59, No. 3, pp. 459-466.

Lang, A.E.; Langston, J.W.; Stoessl, A.J.; Brodsky, M.; Brooks, D.J.; Dhawan, V.; Elias, W.J.; Lozano, A.M.; Moro, E.; Nutt, J.G.; Stacy, M.; Turner, D. & Wooten, G.F. (2006). GDNF in treatment of Parkinson's disease: response to editorial. Lancet Neurol, Vol. 5, No. 3, pp. 200-202.

Lapchak, P.A.; Araujo, D.M.; Hilt, D.C.; Sheng, J. & Jiao, S. (1997). Adenoviral vector-mediated GDNF gene therapy in a rodent lesion model of late stage Parkinson's disease. Brain Res, Vol. 777, No. 1-2, pp. 153-160.

Lee, R.; Kermani, P.; Teng, K.K. & Hempstead, B.L. (2001). Regulation of cell survival by secreted proneurotrophins. Science, Vol. 294, No. 5548, pp. 1945-1948.

Leitner, M.L.; Molliver, D.C.; Osborne, P.A.; Vejsada, R.; Golden, J.P.; Lampe, P.A.; Kato, A.C.; Milbrandt, J. & Johnson, E.M., Jr. (1999). Analysis of the retrograde transport of glial cell line-derived neurotrophic factor (GDNF), neurturin, and persephin suggests that *in vivo* signaling for the GDNF family is GFRalpha coreceptor-specific. J Neurosci, Vol. 19, No. 21, pp. 9322-9331.

Li, H.; He, Z.; Su, T.; Ma, Y.; Lu, S.; Dai, C. & Sun, M. (2003). Protective action of recombinant neurturin on dopaminergic neurons in substantia nigra in a rhesus monkey model of Parkinson's disease. Neurol Res, Vol. 25, No. 3, pp. 263-267.

Lin, L.F.; Doherty, D.H.; Lile, J.D.; Bektesh, S. & Collins, F. (1993). GDNF: a glial cell line-derived neurotrophic factor for midbrain dopaminergic neurons. Science, Vol. 260, No. 5111, pp. 1130-1132.

Lindholm, P.; Peranen, J.; Andressoo, J.O.; Kalkkinen, N.; Kokaia, Z.; Lindvall, O.; Timmusk, T. & Saarma, M. (2008). MANF is widely expressed in mammalian tissues and differently regulated after ischemic and epileptic insults in rodent brain. Mol Cell Neurosci, Vol. 39, No. 3, pp. 356-371.

Lindholm, P. & Saarma, M. (2010). Novel CDNF/MANF family of neurotrophic factors. Dev Neurobiol, Vol. 70, No. 5, pp. 360-371.

Lindholm, P.; Voutilainen, M.H.; Lauren, J.; Peranen, J.; Leppanen, V.M.; Andressoo, J.O.; Lindahl, M.; Janhunen, S.; Kalkkinen, N.; Timmusk, T.; Tuominen, R.K. & Saarma, M. (2007). Novel neurotrophic factor CDNF protects and rescues midbrain dopamine neurons *in vivo*. Nature, Vol. 448, No. 7149, pp. 73-77.

Lindvall, O. & Wahlberg, L.U. (2008). Encapsulated cell biodelivery of GDNF: a novel clinical strategy for neuroprotection and neuroregeneration in Parkinson's disease? Exp Neurol, Vol. 209, No. 1, pp. 82-88.

Lingor, P.; Unsicker, K. & Krieglstein, K. (1999). Midbrain dopaminergic neurons are protected from radical induced damage by GDF-5 application. Short communication. J Neural Transm, Vol. 106, No. 2, pp. 139-144.

Little, S.C. & Mullins, M.C. (2009). Bone morphogenetic protein heterodimers assemble heteromeric type I receptor complexes to pattern the dorsoventral axis. Nat Cell Biol, Vol. 11, No. 5, pp. 637-643.

Long-Smith, C.M.; Sullivan, A.M. & Nolan, Y.M. (2009). The influence of microglia on the pathogenesis of Parkinson's disease. Prog Neurobiol, Vol. 89, No. 3, pp. 277-287.

Love, S.; Plaha, P.; Patel, N.K.; Hotton, G.R.; Brooks, D.J. & Gill, S.S. (2005). Glial cell line-derived neurotrophic factor induces neuronal sprouting in human brain. Nat Med, Vol. 11, No. 7, pp. 703-704.

Ma, D.; Wang, X. & Han, J. (2000). NIH 3T3 cells or engineered NIH 3T3 cells stably expressing GDNF can protect primary dopaminergic neurons. Neurol Res, Vol. 22, No. 6, pp. 538-544.

Mandel, R.J.; Snyder, R.O. & Leff, S.E. (1999). Recombinant adeno-associated viral vector-mediated glial cell line-derived neurotrophic factor gene transfer protects nigral dopamine neurons after onset of progressive degeneration in a rat model of Parkinson's disease. Exp Neurol, Vol. 160, No. 1, pp. 205-214.

Mandel, R.J.; Spratt, S.K.; Snyder, R.O. & Leff, S.E. (1997). Midbrain injection of recombinant adeno-associated virus encoding rat glial cell line-derived neurotrophic factor protects nigral neurons in a progressive 6-hydroxydopamine-induced degeneration model of Parkinson's disease in rats. Proc Natl Acad Sci U S A, Vol. 94, No. 25, pp. 14083-14088.

Manfredsson, F.P.; Okun, M.S. & Mandel, R.J. (2009). Gene therapy for neurological disorders: challenges and future prospects for the use of growth factors for the treatment of Parkinson's disease. Curr Gene Ther, Vol. 9, No. 5, pp. 375-388.

Marks, W.J., Jr.; Bartus, R.T.; Siffert, J.; Davis, C.S.; Lozano, A.; Boulis, N.; Vitek, J.; Stacy, M.; Turner, D.; Verhagen, L.; Bakay, R.; Watts, R.; Guthrie, B.; Jankovic, J.; Simpson, R.; Tagliati, M.; Alterman, R.; Stern, M.; Baltuch, G.; Starr, P.A.; Larson, P.S.; Ostrem, J.L.; Nutt, J.; Kieburtz, K.; Kordower, J.H. & Olanow, C.W. (2010). Gene delivery of AAV2-neurturin for Parkinson's disease: a double-blind, randomised, controlled trial. Lancet Neurol, Vol. 9, No. 12, pp. 1164-1172.

Marks, W.J., Jr.; Ostrem, J.L.; Verhagen, L.; Starr, P.A.; Larson, P.S.; Bakay, R.A.; Taylor, R.; Cahn-Weiner, D.A.; Stoessl, A.J.; Olanow, C.W. & Bartus, R.T. (2008). Safety and tolerability of intraputaminal delivery of CERE-120 (adeno-associated virus serotype 2-neurturin) to patients with idiopathic Parkinson's disease: an open-label, phase I trial. Lancet Neurol, Vol. 7, No. 5, pp. 400-408.

Martin, D.; Miller, G.; Cullen, T.; Fischer, N.; Dix, D. & Russell, D. (1996). Intranigral or intrastriatal injections of GDNF: effects on monoamine levels and behavior in rats. Eur J Pharmacol, Vol. 317, No. 2-3, pp. 247-256.

Massague, J. (1996). TGFbeta signaling: receptors, transducers, and Mad proteins. Cell, Vol. 85, No. 7, pp. 947-950.

Massague, J.; Seoane, J. & Wotton, D. (2005). Smad transcription factors. Genes Dev, Vol. 19, No. 23, pp. 2783-2810.

Maswood, N.; Grondin, R.; Zhang, Z.; Stanford, J.A.; Surgener, S.P.; Gash, D.M. & Gerhardt, G.A. (2002). Effects of chronic intraputamenal infusion of glial cell line-derived neurotrophic factor (GDNF) in aged Rhesus monkeys. Neurobiol Aging, Vol. 23, No. 5, pp. 881-889.

Matsuo, A.; Nakamura, S. & Akiguchi, I. (2000). Immunohistochemical localization of glial cell line-derived neurotrophic factor family receptor alpha-1 in the rat brain: confirmation of expression in various neuronal systems. Brain Res, Vol. 859, No. 1, pp. 57-71.

McBride, J.L.; During, M.J.; Wuu, J.; Chen, E.Y.; Leurgans, S.E. & Kordower, J.H. (2003). Structural and functional neuroprotection in a rat model of Huntington's disease by viral gene transfer of GDNF. Exp Neurol, Vol. 181, No. 2, pp. 213-223.

McBride, J.L.; Ramaswamy, S.; Gasmi, M.; Bartus, R.T.; Herzog, C.D.; Brandon, E.P.; Zhou, L.; Pitzer, M.R.; Berry-Kravis, E.M. & Kordower, J.H. (2006). Viral delivery of glial cell line-derived neurotrophic factor improves behavior and protects striatal neurons in a mouse model of Huntington's disease. Proc Natl Acad Sci U S A, Vol. 103, No. 24, pp. 9345-9350.

Mehler, M.F.; Mabie, P.C.; Zhang, D. & Kessler, J.A. (1997). Bone morphogenetic proteins in the nervous system. Trends Neurosci, Vol. 20, No. 7, pp. 309-317.

Mehta, V.; Hong, M.; Spears, J. & Mendez, I. (1998). Enhancement of graft survival and sensorimotor behavioral recovery in rats undergoing transplantation with dopaminergic cells exposed to glial cell line-derived neurotrophic factor. J Neurosurg, Vol. 88, No. 6, pp. 1088-1095.

Mendez, I.; Dagher, A.; Hong, M.; Hebb, A.; Gaudet, P.; Law, A.; Weerasinghe, S.; King, D.; Desrosiers, J.; Darvesh, S.; Acorn, T. & Robertson, H. (2000). Enhancement of survival of stored dopaminergic cells and promotion of graft survival by exposure of human fetal nigral tissue to glial cell line--derived neurotrophic factor in patients with Parkinson's disease. Report of two cases and technical considerations. J Neurosurg, Vol. 92, No. 5, pp. 863-869.

Milbrandt, J.; de Sauvage, F.J.; Fahrner, T.J.; Baloh, R.H.; Leitner, M.L.; Tansey, M.G.; Lampe, P.A.; Heuckeroth, R.O.; Kotzbauer, P.T.; Simburger, K.S.; Golden, J.P.; Davies, J.A.; Vejsada, R.; Kato, A.C.; Hynes, M.; Sherman, D.; Nishimura, M.; Wang, L.C.; Vandlen, R.; Moffat, B.; Klein, R.D.; Poulsen, K.; Gray, C.; Garces, A.; Johnson, E.M., Jr. & et al. (1998). Persephin, a novel neurotrophic factor related to GDNF and neurturin. Neuron, Vol. 20, No. 2, pp. 245-253.

Miyazono, K. (1999). Signal transduction by bone morphogenetic protein receptors: functional roles of Smad proteins. Bone, Vol. 25, No. 1, pp. 91-93.

Miyazono, K.; Kusanagi, K. & Inoue, H. (2001). Divergence and convergence of TGF-beta/BMP signaling. J Cell Physiol, Vol. 187, No. 3, pp. 265-276.

Miyoshi, Y.; Zhang, Z.; Ovadia, A.; Lapchak, P.A.; Collins, F.; Hilt, D.; Lebel, C.; Kryscio, R. & Gash, D.M. (1997). Glial cell line-derived neurotrophic factor-levodopa interactions and reduction of side effects in parkinsonian monkeys. Ann Neurol, Vol. 42, No. 2, pp. 208-214.

Morrison, P.F.; Lonser, R.R. & Oldfield, E.H. (2007). Convective delivery of glial cell line-derived neurotrophic factor in the human putamen. J Neurosurg, Vol. 107, No. 1, pp. 74-83.

Nishitoh, H.; Ichijo, H.; Kimura, M.; Matsumoto, T.; Makishima, F.; Yamaguchi, A.; Yamashita, H.; Enomoto, S. & Miyazono, K. (1996). Identification of type I and type II serine/threonine kinase receptors for growth/differentiation factor-5. J Biol Chem, Vol. 271, No. 35, pp. 21345-21352.

Nohe, A.; Keating, E.; Knaus, P. & Petersen, N.O. (2004). Signal transduction of bone morphogenetic protein receptors. Cell Signal, Vol. 16, No. 3, pp. 291-299.

Nosrat, C.A.; Tomac, A.; Hoffer, B.J. & Olson, L. (1997). Cellular and developmental patterns of expression of Ret and glial cell line-derived neurotrophic factor receptor alpha mRNAs. Exp Brain Res, Vol. 115, No. 3, pp. 410-422.

Nutt, J.G.; Burchiel, K.J.; Comella, C.L.; Jankovic, J.; Lang, A.E.; Laws, E.R., Jr.; Lozano, A.M.; Penn, R.D.; Simpson, R.K., Jr.; Stacy, M. & Wooten, G.F. (2003). Randomized, double-blind trial of glial cell line-derived neurotrophic factor (GDNF) in PD. Neurology, Vol. 60, No. 1, pp. 69-73.

O'Keeffe, G.W.; Dockery, P. & Sullivan, A.M. (2004). Effects of growth/differentiation factor 5 on the survival and morphology of embryonic rat midbrain dopaminergic neurones *in vitro*. J Neurocytol, Vol. 33, No. 5, pp. 479-488.

O'Keeffe, G.W.; Hanke, M.; Pohl, J. & Sullivan, A.M. (2004). Expression of growth differentiation factor-5 in the developing and adult rat brain. Brain Res Dev Brain Res, Vol. 151, No. 1-2, pp. 199-202.

O'Sullivan, D.B.; Harrison, P.T. & Sullivan, A.M. (2010). Effects of GDF5 overexpression on embryonic rat dopaminergic neurones *in vitro* and *in vivo*. J Neural Transm, Vol. 117, No. 5, pp. 559-572.

Oiwa, Y.; Yoshimura, R.; Nakai, K. & Itakura, T. (2002). Dopaminergic neuroprotection and regeneration by neurturin assessed by using behavioral, biochemical and histochemical measurements in a model of progressive Parkinson's disease. Brain Res, Vol. 947, No. 2, pp. 271-283.

Olanow, C.W.; Kordower, J.H.; Lang, A.E. & Obeso, J.A. (2009). Dopaminergic transplantation for Parkinson's disease: current status and future prospects. Ann Neurol. Vol. 66, No. 5, pp. 591-596.

Olanow, C.W. & Tatton, W.G. (1999). Etiology and pathogenesis of Parkinson's disease. Annu Rev Neurosci, Vol. 22, No. pp. 123-144.

Opacka-Juffry, J.; Ashworth, S.; Hume, S.P.; Martin, D.; Brooks, D.J. & Blunt, S.B. (1995). GDNF protects against 6-OHDA nigrostriatal lesion: *in vivo* study with microdialysis and PET. Neuroreport, Vol. 7, No. 1, pp. 348-352.

Ostenfeld, T.; Tai, Y.T.; Martin, P.; Deglon, N.; Aebischer, P. & Svendsen, C.N. (2002). Neurospheres modified to produce glial cell line-derived neurotrophic factor increase the survival of transplanted dopamine neurons. J Neurosci Res, Vol. 69, No. 6, pp. 955-965.

Palfi, S.; Leventhal, L.; Chu, Y.; Ma, S.Y.; Emborg, M.; Bakay, R.; Deglon, N.; Hantraye, P.; Aebischer, P. & Kordower, J.H. (2002). Lentivirally delivered glial cell line-derived neurotrophic factor increases the number of striatal dopaminergic neurons in primate models of nigrostriatal degeneration. J Neurosci, Vol. 22, No. 12, pp. 4942-4954.

Palgi, M.; Lindstrom, R.; Peranen, J.; Piepponen, T.P.; Saarma, M. & Heino, T.I. (2009). Evidence that DmMANF is an invertebrate neurotrophic factor supporting dopaminergic neurons. Proc Natl Acad Sci U S A, Vol. 106, No. 7, pp. 2429-2434.

Paratcha, G. & Ledda, F. (2008). GDNF and GFRalpha: a versatile molecular complex for developing neurons. Trends Neurosci, Vol. 31, No. 8, pp. 384-391.

Paratcha, G.; Ledda, F. & Ibanez, C.F. (2003). The neural cell adhesion molecule NCAM is an alternative signaling receptor for GDNF family ligands. Cell, Vol. 113, No. 7, pp. 867-879.

Patel, N.K.; Bunnage, M.; Plaha, P.; Svendsen, C.N.; Heywood, P. & Gill, S.S. (2005). Intraputamenal infusion of glial cell line-derived neurotrophic factor in PD: A two-year outcome study. Ann Neurol, Vol. 57, No. 2, pp. 298-302.

Penn, R.D.; Dalvi, A.; Slevin, J.; Young, B.; Gash, D.; Gerhardt, G. & Hutchinson, M. (2006). GDNF in treatment of Parkinson's disease: response to editorial. Lancet Neurol, Vol. 5, No. 3, pp. 202-203.

Perez-Navarro, E.; Akerud, P.; Marco, S.; Canals, J.M.; Tolosa, E.; Arenas, E. & Alberch, J. (2000). Neurturin protects striatal projection neurons but not interneurons in a rat model of Huntington's disease. Neuroscience, Vol. 98, No. 1, pp. 89-96.

Peterziel, H.; Unsicker, K. & Krieglstein, K. (2002). TGFbeta induces GDNF responsiveness in neurons by recruitment of GFRalpha1 to the plasma membrane. J Cell Biol, Vol. 159, No. 1, pp. 157-167.

Petrova, P.; Raibekas, A.; Pevsner, J.; Vigo, N.; Anafi, M.; Moore, M.K.; Peaire, A.E.; Shridhar, V.; Smith, D.I.; Kelly, J.; Durocher, Y. & Commissiong, J.W. (2003). MANF: a new mesencephalic, astrocyte-derived neurotrophic factor with selectivity for dopaminergic neurons. J Mol Neurosci, Vol. 20, No. 2, pp. 173-188.

Poulsen, K.T.; Armanini, M.P.; Klein, R.D.; Hynes, M.A.; Phillips, H.S. & Rosenthal, A. (1994). TGF beta 2 and TGF beta 3 are potent survival factors for midbrain dopaminergic neurons. Neuron, Vol. 13, No. 5, pp. 1245-1252.

Ramaswamy, S.; McBride, J.L.; Han, I.; Berry-Kravis, E.M.; Zhou, L.; Herzog, C.D.; Gasmi, M.; Bartus, R.T. & Kordower, J.H. (2009). Intrastriatal CERE-120 (AAV-Neurturin) protects striatal and cortical neurons and delays motor deficits in a transgenic mouse model of Huntington's disease. Neurobiol Dis, Vol. 34, No. 1, pp. 40-50.

Ramaswamy, S.; Soderstrom, K.E. & Kordower, J.H. (2009). Trophic factors therapy in Parkinson's disease. Prog Brain Res, Vol. 175, No. pp. 201-216.

Ramirez, F. & Rifkin, D.B. (2009). Extracellular microfibrils: contextual platforms for TGFbeta and BMP signaling. Curr Opin Cell Biol, Vol. 21, No. 5, pp. 616-622.

Richardson, R.M.; Kells, A.P.; Rosenbluth, K.H.; Salegio, E.A.; Fiandaca, M.S.; Larson, P.S.; Starr, P.A.; Martin, A.J.; Lonser, R.R.; Federoff, H.J.; Forsayeth, J.R. & Bankiewicz, K.S. (2011). Interventional MRI-guided Putaminal Delivery of AAV2-GDNF for a Planned Clinical Trial in Parkinson's Disease. Mol Ther, Vol. No. pp.

Rider, C.C. & Mulloy, B. (2011). Bone morphogenetic protein and growth differentiation factor cytokine families and their protein antagonists. Biochem J, Vol. 429, No. 1, pp. 1-12.

Rosenblad, C.; Kirik, D. & Bjorklund, A. (1999). Neurturin enhances the survival of intrastriatal fetal dopaminergic transplants. Neuroreport, Vol. 10, No. 8, pp. 1783-1787.

Rosenblad, C.; Kirik, D. & Bjorklund, A. (2000). Sequential administration of GDNF into the substantia nigra and striatum promotes dopamine neuron survival and axonal sprouting but not striatal reinnervation or functional recovery in the partial 6-OHDA lesion model. Exp Neurol, Vol. 161, No. 2, pp. 503-516.

Rosenblad, C.; Kirik, D.; Devaux, B.; Moffat, B.; Phillips, H.S. & Bjorklund, A. (1999). Protection and regeneration of nigral dopaminergic neurons by neurturin or GDNF in a partial lesion model of Parkinson's disease after administration into the striatum or the lateral ventricle. Eur J Neurosci, Vol. 11, No. 5, pp. 1554-1566.

Rosenblad, C.; Martinez-Serrano, A. & Bjorklund, A. (1996). Glial cell line-derived neurotrophic factor increases survival, growth and function of intrastriatal fetal nigral dopaminergic grafts. Neuroscience, Vol. 75, No. 4, pp. 979-985.

Rosenblad, C.; Martinez-Serrano, A. & Bjorklund, A. (1998). Intrastriatal glial cell line-derived neurotrophic factor promotes sprouting of spared nigrostriatal dopaminergic afferents and induces recovery of function in a rat model of Parkinson's disease. Neuroscience, Vol. 82, No. 1, pp. 129-137.

Roussa, E.; von Bohlen und Halbach, O. & Krieglstein, K. (2009). TGF-beta in dopamine neuron development, maintenance and neuroprotection. Adv Exp Med Biol, Vol. 651, No. pp. 81-90.

Sajadi, A.; Bensadoun, J.C.; Schneider, B.L.; Lo Bianco, C. & Aebischer, P. (2006). Transient striatal delivery of GDNF via encapsulated cells leads to sustained behavioral improvement in a bilateral model of Parkinson disease. Neurobiol Dis, Vol. 22, No. 1, pp. 119-129.

Sarabi, A.; Chang, C.F.; Wang, Y.; Hoffer, B.J. & Morales, M. (2001). Time course study of GFRalpha-1 expression in an animal model of stroke. Exp Neurol, Vol. 170, No. 2, pp. 283-289.

Sariola, H. & Saarma, M. (2003). Novel functions and signalling pathways for GDNF. J Cell Sci, Vol. 116, No. Pt 19, pp. 3855-3862.

Sauer, H. & Oertel, W.H. (1994). Progressive degeneration of nigrostriatal dopamine neurons following intrastriatal terminal lesions with 6-hydroxydopamine: a combined retrograde tracing and immunocytochemical study in the rat. , Neurosci, Vol. 59, No. 2, pp. 401-415.

Sauer, H.; Rosenblad, C. & Bjorklund, A. (1995). Glial cell line-derived neurotrophic factor but not transforming growth factor beta 3 prevents delayed degeneration of nigral dopaminergic neurons following striatal 6-hydroxydopamine lesion. Proc Natl Acad Sci U S A, Vol. 92, No. 19, pp. 8935-8939.

Sautter, J.; Tseng, J.L.; Braguglia, D.; Aebischer, P.; Spenger, C.; Seiler, R.W.; Widmer, H.R. & Zurn, A.D. (1998). Implants of polymer-encapsulated genetically modified cells releasing glial cell line-derived neurotrophic factor improve survival, growth, and function of fetal dopaminergic grafts. Exp Neurol, Vol. 149, No. 1, pp. 230-236.

Sawada, H.; Ibi, M.; Kihara, T.; Urushitani, M.; Nakanishi, M.; Akaike, A. & Shimohama, S. (2000). Neuroprotective mechanism of glial cell line-derived neurotrophic factor in mesencephalic neurons. J Neurochem, Vol. 74, No. 3, pp. 1175-1184.

Schmeer, C.; Straten, G.; Kugler, S.; Gravel, C.; Bahr, M. & Isenmann, S. (2002). Dose-dependent rescue of axotomized rat retinal ganglion cells by adenovirus-mediated expression of glial cell-line derived neurotrophic factor *in vivo*. Eur J Neurosci, Vol. 15, No. 4, pp. 637-643.

Schober, A.; Peterziel, H.; von Bartheld, C.S.; Simon, H.; Krieglstein, K. & Unsicker, K. (2007). GDNF applied to the MPTP-lesioned nigrostriatal system requires TGF-beta for its neuroprotective action. Neurobiol Dis, Vol. 25, No. 2, pp. 378-391.

Sengle, G.; Charbonneau, N.L.; Ono, R.N.; Sasaki, T.; Alvarez, J.; Keene, D.R.; Bachinger, H.P. & Sakai, L.Y. (2008). Targeting of bone morphogenetic protein growth factor complexes to fibrillin. J Biol Chem, Vol. 283, No. 20, pp. 13874-13888.

Sengle, G.; Ono, R.N.; Lyons, K.M.; Bachinger, H.P. & Sakai, L.Y. (2008). A new model for growth factor activation: type II receptors compete with the prodomain for BMP-7. J Mol Biol, Vol. 381, No. 4, pp. 1025-1039.

Sherer, T.B.; Fiske, B.K.; Svendsen, C.N.; Lang, A.E. & Langston, J.W. (2006). Crossroads in GDNF therapy for Parkinson's disease. Mov Disord, Vol. 21, No. 2, pp. 136-141.

Shi, Y. & Massague, J. (2003). Mechanisms of TGF-beta signaling from cell membrane to the nucleus. Cell, Vol. 113, No. 6, pp. 685-700.

Shingo, T.; Date, I.; Yoshida, H. & Ohmoto, T. (2002). Neuroprotective and restorative effects of intrastriatal grafting of encapsulated GDNF-producing cells in a rat model of Parkinson's disease. J Neurosci Res, Vol. 69, No. 6, pp. 946-954.

Shults, C.W.; Kimber, T. & Martin, D. (1996). Intrastriatal injection of GDNF attenuates the effects of 6-hydroxydopamine. Neuroreport, Vol. 7, No. 2, pp. 627-631.

Sieber, C.; Kopf, J.; Hiepen, C. & Knaus, P. (2009). Recent advances in BMP receptor signaling. Cytokine Growth Factor Rev, Vol. 20, No. 5-6, pp. 343-355.

Sinclair, S.R.; Svendsen, C.N.; Torres, E.M.; Martin, D.; Fawcett, J.W. & Dunnett, S.B. (1996). GDNF enhances dopaminergic cell survival and fibre outgrowth in embryonic nigral grafts. Neuroreport, Vol. 7, No. 15-17, pp. 2547-2552.

Slevin, J.T.; Gerhardt, G.A.; Smith, C.D.; Gash, D.M.; Kryscio, R. & Young, B. (2005). Improvement of bilateral motor functions in patients with Parkinson disease through the unilateral intraputaminal infusion of glial cell line-derived neurotrophic factor. J Neurosurg, Vol. 102, No. 2, pp. 216-222.

Storm, E.E.; Huynh, T.V.; Copeland, N.G.; Jenkins, N.A.; Kingsley, D.M. & Lee, S.J. (1994). Limb alterations in brachypodism mice due to mutations in a new member of the TGF beta-superfamily. Nature, Vol. 368, No. 6472, pp. 639-643.

Sullivan, A.M.; Opacka-Juffry, J. & Blunt, S.B. (1998). Long-term protection of the rat nigrostriatal dopaminergic system by glial cell line-derived neurotrophic factor against 6-hydroxydopamine *in vivo*. Eur J Neurosci, Vol. 10, No. 1, pp. 57-63.

Sullivan, A.M.; Opacka-Juffry, J.; Hotten, G.; Pohl, J. & Blunt, S.B. (1997). Growth/differentiation factor 5 protects nigrostriatal dopaminergic neurones in a rat model of Parkinson's disease. Neurosci Lett, Vol. 233, No. 2-3, pp. 73-76.

Sullivan, A.M.; Opacka-Juffry, J.; Pohl, J. & Blunt, S.B. (1999). Neuroprotective effects of growth/differentiation factor 5 depend on the site of administration. Brain Res, Vol. 818, No. 1, pp. 176-179.

Sullivan, A.M.; Pohl, J. & Blunt, S.B. (1998). Growth/differentiation factor 5 and glial cell line-derived neurotrophic factor enhance survival and function of dopaminergic grafts in a rat model of Parkinson's disease. Eur J Neurosci, Vol. 10, No. 12, pp. 3681-3688.

Tadimalla, A.; Belmont, P.J.; Thuerauf, D.J.; Glassy, M.S.; Martindale, J.J.; Gude, N.; Sussman, M.A. & Glembotski, C.C. (2008). Mesencephalic astrocyte-derived neurotrophic factor is an ischemia-inducible secreted endoplasmic reticulum stress response protein in the heart. Circ Res, Vol. 103, No. 11, pp. 1249-1258.

Tai, M.H.; Cheng, H.; Wu, J.P.; Liu, Y.L.; Lin, P.R.; Kuo, J.S.; Tseng, C.J. & Tzeng, S.F. (2003). Gene transfer of glial cell line-derived neurotrophic factor promotes functional recovery following spinal cord contusion. Exp Neurol, Vol. 183, No. 2, pp. 508-515.

Tang, F.I.; Tien, L.T.; Zhou, F.C.; Hoffer, B.J. & Wang, Y. (1998). Intranigral ventral mesencephalic grafts and nigrostriatal injections of glial cell line-derived neurotrophic factor restore dopamine release in the striatum of 6-hydroxydopamine-lesioned rats. Exp Brain Res, Vol. 119, No. 3, pp. 287-296.

Tatarewicz, S.M.; Wei, X.; Gupta, S.; Masterman, D.; Swanson, S.J. & Moxness, M.S. (2007). Development of a maturing T-cell-mediated immune response in patients with idiopathic Parkinson's disease receiving r-metHuGDNF via continuous intraputaminal infusion. J Clin Immunol, Vol. 27, No. 6, pp. 620-627.

Theofilopoulos, S.; Goggi, J.; Riaz, S.S.; Jauniaux, E.; Stern, G.M. & Bradford, H.F. (2001). Parallel induction of the formation of dopamine and its metabolites with induction of tyrosine hydroxylase expression in foetal rat and human cerebral cortical cells by brain-derived neurotrophic factor and glial-cell derived neurotrophic factor. Brain Res Dev Brain Res, Vol. 127, No. 2, pp. 111-122.

Tomac, A.; Lindqvist, E.; Lin, L.F.; Ogren, S.O.; Young, D.; Hoffer, B.J. & Olson, L. (1995). Protection and repair of the nigrostriatal dopaminergic system by GDNF *in vivo*. Nature, Vol. 373, No. 6512, pp. 335-339.

Tomac, A.; Widenfalk, J.; Lin, L.F.; Kohno, T.; Ebendal, T.; Hoffer, B.J. & Olson, L. (1995). Retrograde axonal transport of glial cell line-derived neurotrophic factor in the adult nigrostriatal system suggests a trophic role in the adult. Proc Natl Acad Sci U S A, Vol. 92, No. 18, pp. 8274-8278.

Toulouse, A. & Sullivan, A.M. (2008). Progress in Parkinson's disease-where do we stand? Prog Neurobiol, Vol. 85, No. 4, pp. 376-392.

Treanor, J.J.; Goodman, L.; de Sauvage, F.; Stone, D.M.; Poulsen, K.T.; Beck, C.D.; Gray, C.; Armanini, M.P.; Pollock, R.A.; Hefti, F.; Phillips, H.S.; Goddard, A.; Moore, M.W.; Buj-Bello, A.; Davies, A.M.; Asai, N.; Takahashi, M.; Vandlen, R.; Henderson, C.E. & Rosenthal, A. (1996). Characterization of a multicomponent receptor for GDNF. Nature, Vol. 382, No. 6586, pp. 80-83.

Trupp, M.; Arenas, E.; Fainzilber, M.; Nilsson, A.S.; Sieber, B.A.; Grigoriou, M.; Kilkenny, C.; Salazar-Grueso, E.; Pachnis, V. & Arumae, U. (1996). Functional receptor for GDNF encoded by the c-ret proto-oncogene. Nature, Vol. 381, No. 6585, pp. 785-789.

Trupp, M.; Belluardo, N.; Funakoshi, H. & Ibanez, C.F. (1997). Complementary and overlapping expression of glial cell line-derived neurotrophic factor (GDNF), c-ret proto-oncogene, and GDNF receptor-alpha indicates multiple mechanisms of trophic actions in the adult rat CNS. J Neurosci, Vol. 17, No. 10, pp. 3554-3567.

Tseng, J.L.; Baetge, E.E.; Zurn, A.D. & Aebischer, P. (1997). GDNF reduces drug-induced rotational behavior after medial forebrain bundle transection by a mechanism not involving striatal dopamine. J Neurosci, Vol. 17, No. 1, pp. 325-333.

Tseng, J.L.; Bruhn, S.L.; Zurn, A.D. & Aebischer, P. (1998). Neurturin protects dopaminergic neurons following medial forebrain bundle axotomy. Neuroreport, Vol. 9, No. 8, pp. 1817-1822.

Ungerstedt, U. & Arbuthnott, G.W. (1970). Quantitative recording of rotational behavior in rats after 6-hydroxydopamine lesions of the nigrostriatal dopamine system. Brain Res. Vol. 24, pp. 485-493.

Unsicker, K.; Suter-Crazzalora, C. & Krieglstein, K. (1996). Growth factor function in the development and maintenance of midbrain dopaminergic neurons: concepts, facts and prospects for TGF-beta. Ciba Found Symp, Vol. 196, No. pp. 70-80; discussion 80-74.

Voutilainen, M.H.; Back, S.; Peranen, J.; Lindholm, P.; Raasmaja, A.; Mannisto, P.T.; Saarma, M. & Tuominen, R.K. (2011). Chronic infusion of CDNF prevents 6-OHDA-induced deficits in a rat model of Parkinson's disease. Exp Neurol, Vol. 228, No. 1, pp. 99-108.

Voutilainen, M.H.; Back, S.; Porsti, E.; Toppinen, L.; Lindgren, L.; Lindholm, P.; Peranen, J.; Saarma, M. & Tuominen, R.K. (2009). Mesencephalic astrocyte-derived neurotrophic factor is neurorestorative in rat model of Parkinson's disease. J Neurosci, Vol. 29, No. 30, pp. 9651-9659.

Wang, L.J.; Lu, Y.Y.; Muramatsu, S.; Ikeguchi, K.; Fujimoto, K.; Okada, T.; Mizukami, H.; Matsushita, T.; Hanazono, Y.; Kume, A.; Nagatsu, T.; Ozawa, K. & Nakano, I. (2002). Neuroprotective effects of glial cell line-derived neurotrophic factor mediated by an adeno-associated virus vector in a transgenic animal model of amyotrophic lateral sclerosis. J Neurosci, Vol. 22, No. 16, pp. 6920-6928.

Wang, Y.; Tien, L.T.; Lapchak, P.A. & Hoffer, B.J. (1996). GDNF triggers fiber outgrowth of fetal ventral mesencephalic grafts from nigra to striatum in 6-OHDA-lesioned rats. Cell Tissue Res, Vol. 286, No. 2, pp. 225-233.

Widenfalk, J.; Nosrat, C.; Tomac, A.; Westphal, H.; Hoffer, B. & Olson, L. (1997). Neurturin and glial cell line-derived neurotrophic factor receptor-beta (GDNFR-beta), novel proteins related to GDNF and GDNFR-alpha with specific cellular patterns of expression suggesting roles in the developing and adult nervous system and in peripheral organs. J Neurosci, Vol. 17, No. 21, pp. 8506-8519.

Widmer, H.R.; Schaller, B.; Meyer, M. & Seiler, R.W. (2000). Glial cell line-derived neurotrophic factor stimulates the morphological differentiation of cultured ventral mesencephalic calbindin- and calretinin-expressing neurons. Exp Neurol, Vol. 164, No. 1, pp. 71-81.

Winkler, C.; Sauer, H.; Lee, C.S. & Bjorklund, A. (1996). Short-term GDNF treatment provides long-term rescue of lesioned nigral dopaminergic neurons in a rat model of Parkinson's disease. J Neurosci, Vol. 16, No. 22, pp. 7206-7215.

Wood, T.K.; McDermott, K.W. & Sullivan, A.M. (2005). Differential effects of growth/differentiation factor 5 and glial cell line-derived neurotrophic factor on dopaminergic neurons and astroglia in cultures of embryonic rat midbrain. J Neurosci Res, Vol. 80, No. 6, pp. 759-766.

Xing, B.; Xin, T.; Zhao, L.; Hunter, R.L.; Chen, Y. & Bing, G. (2010). Glial cell line-derived neurotrophic factor protects midbrain dopaminergic neurons against lipopolysaccharide neurotoxicity. J Neuroimmunol, Vol. 225, No. 1-2, pp. 43-51.

Yamashita, H.; Ten Dijke, P.; Heldin, C.H. & Miyazono, K. (1996). Bone morphogenetic protein receptors. Bone, Vol. 19, No. 6, pp. 569-574.

Yasuhara, T.; Shingo, T.; Muraoka, K.; Kobayashi, K.; Takeuchi, A.; Yano, A.; Wenji, Y.; Kameda, M.; Matsui, T.; Miyoshi, Y. & Date, I. (2005). Early transplantation of an encapsulated glial cell line-derived neurotrophic factor-producing cell demonstrating strong neuroprotective effects in a rat model of Parkinson disease. J Neurosurg, Vol. 102, No. 1, pp. 80-89.

Yu, T.; Scully, S.; Yu, Y.; Fox, G.M.; Jing, S. & Zhou, R. (1998). Expression of GDNF family receptor components during development: implications in the mechanisms of interaction. J Neurosci, Vol. 18, No. 12, pp. 4684-4696.

Yurek, D.M. (1998). Glial cell line-derived neurotrophic factor improves survival of dopaminergic neurons in transplants of fetal ventral mesencephalic tissue. Exp Neurol, Vol. 153, No. 2, pp. 195-202.

Zhang, Z.; Miyoshi, Y.; Lapchak, P.A.; Collins, F.; Hilt, D.; Lebel, C.; Kryscio, R. & Gash, D.M. (1997). Dose response to intraventricular glial cell line-derived neurotrophic factor administration in parkinsonian monkeys. J Pharmacol Exp Ther, Vol. 282, No. 3, pp. 1396-1401.

Zurn, A.D.; Widmer, H.R. & Aebischer, P. (2001). Sustained delivery of GDNF: towards a treatment for Parkinson's disease. Brain Res Brain Res Rev, Vol. 36, No. 2-3, pp. 222-229.

Part 4

Gene Therapies

12

Gene Therapy for Parkinson's Disease

Michael Douglas[1,2] and Jonathan Hazlehurst[2]
[1]*Department of Neurology, Dudley Group of Hospitals NHS Foundation Trust, Dudley,*
[2]*School of Clinical and Experimental Medicine, College of Medical and Dental Sciences, University of Birmingham, Birmingham*
UK

1. Introduction

Parkinson's disease (PD) is a common neurodegenerative disease, with a prevalence of around 250 per 100,000 population and becoming of growing importance in ageing populations. Patients become symptomatic when around 75% of striatal dopamine is lost, with ongoing yearly declines of 5-10% (Brooks 1998, Fearnley 1991). The use of levodopa (L-3,4-dihyroxyphenylalanine) as a symptomatic therapy was established nearly 50 years ago and continues to be an important approach in early and late disease (Fahn 2006). Although the majority of patients initially respond well to dopaminergic therapies, many eventually develop fluctuations in their therapeutic response, often with associated dyskinesias (Jenner 2000). Additional agents, including catechol *O*-methyltransferase inhibitors and/or monoamine oxidase inhibitors are often added in to existing medications, with a proportion of patients dependent on infused apomorphine. These therapies are symptomatic, with no effect on the underlying pathogenic processes, particularly the progressive loss of dopaminergic neurons. Novel therapies to either compliment existing approaches, or potentially alter the course of disease, are clearly desirable.

This neuronal loss in Parkinson's disease is associated with multiple functional abnormalities, including changes in excitatory glutamatergic and inhibitory GABAergic pathways controlling movement (Wichmann 2003). Disinhibited activity in the subthalamic nucleus (STN) correlates with increased activity in excitatory projections to the major nuclei of the basal ganglia - the internal globus pallidus (GPi) and substantia nigra pars reticularis (SNr). The resultant increased inhibitory outflow to the pallidal receiving areas or the thalamus and consequently reduced cortical activity are thought to be responsible for many of the motor features of Parkinson's disease (Brown 2001). The pathophysiological importance of this overactive subthalamic nucleus activity can be targeted using several approaches, including stereotactic lesioning (Alvarez 2001, Su 2003), high frequency deep brain stimulation (Benabid 1996, The Deep-Brain Stimulation for Parkinson's Disease Study Group 2001) and pharmacological silencing (Levy 2001), leading to marked improvement in motor function. More recently, these approaches and observations have prompted gene therapy trials to deliver therapeutic vectors into the striatum itself and these will be discussed later. Typically, gene therapy approaches have focused on the restoration or preservation of dopaminergic cell function within the striatum either with neurotrophic factors (Kordower 2000, Marks 2010) or the delivery of enzymes needed for dopamine synthesis (Eberling 2008, Azzouz 2002).

2. Gene delivery to the brain

Gene therapy as a therapeutic approach to central nervous system (CNS) disorders has been theoretically possible for over a decade now, and several recent technical advances have made this avenue increasingly attractive. The method of delivery of the synthetic nucleic acid will fall into one of two groups - nonviral and viral vectors. Nonviral vectors are usually forms of chemically synthesized particles, such as cationic lipids, mixed with recombinant DNA, typically delivered by direct injections. This method is technically relatively straightforward, but usually only produces transient gene expression. Viral vectors, in contrast, are derived from DNA or RNA viruses and can potentially lead to sustained gene expression through genomic integration or the formation of episomes. The past five years have seen major advances in the range of available viral vectors, with individual vector systems having specific advantages and disadvantages for the delivery of therapeutic genes to the CNS. The properties of individual classes of vector are presented here, with a particular focus on adeno-associated virus (AAV), although adenovirus, herpes simplex and lentivirus systems are discussed. With the exception of lentiviruses, retroviral vectors (typically based on murine leukaemia viruses) are unable to infect the post-mitotic cells of the CNS, and are not considered in this review. An additional consideration relates to the method of vector delivery - peripheral systemic injection is clearly not appropriate unless the vector can cross the blood brain barrier with some degree of tissue specificity. Fortunately, deep brain surgical approaches are well developed in the field of movement disorders, making targeted viral injection relatively straightforward.

2.1 Adeno-associated viruses

AAVs are simple, 4.7 kb single stranded DNA viruses (Srivastava 1983) of the *Parvoviridae* family and *Dependovirus* genus. Two genes (*cap* and *rep*) coding for capsid and viral replication proteins respectively, are flanked by inverted terminal repeats (ITRs). Additional genes are required for replication, potentially derived from either adenovirus or herpes simplex viruses (Atchison 1965, Hoggan 1966, Buller 1981). The AAV serotype 2 (AAV2) was the first to be sequenced, and is the most widely used AAV-based gene therapy vector. Subsequent research has isolated at least 100 AAV variants, with many having different tissue tropisms and apparent transduction efficiencies (Gao 2004). AAV usually persists as monomeric or concatameric episomes (Schnepp 2003), although viral integration can occur, at a defined site on human chromosome 19 (Muzyczka 1992), AAVs are particularly attractive as candidate vectors for gene therapy as they have a high theoretical level of safety (Monahan 2002, Tenenbaum 2003), as wild-type AAV is already replication defective and the virus has not been associated with any known human disease. The weak promoter activity of the terminal repeat sequence reduces the overall risk of insertional mutagenesis and oncogenic activation, so genomic integration is not likely to pose a major risk (McCarty 2004).

Early approaches to the production of recombinant AAVs involved the packing of foreign DNA into viral coats by infecting cells with wild-type AAV and helper adenovirus. This process left residual wild-type viruses contaminating preparations of recombinant AAV, with obvious problems for *in vivo* applications (Hermonat 1984). More recent systems use a two or three plasmid system (Samulski 1989), in which cells are co-transfected with a plasmid construct coding for the synthetic gene of interest flanked by the 125 base pair viral inverted terminal repeats (ITRs), in combination with further plasmids coding for *cap*, *rep* and appropriate adenoviral helper genes. This leads to the production of recombinant virus without the presence of contaminants, further enhancing safety. These advantages mean that AAV has been the predominant vector used in clinical trials.

Some disadvantages with using AAV include the relatively small size of the virus which limits the size of the insert to a maximum of approximately 4 kilobases of foreign DNA. Pre-existing humoral immunity to AAV is found in 80% of the human population, which may be enhanced after vector administration, potentially limiting transgene expression (Peden 2004, Sanftner 2004). The significance of this phenomenon is not clear for CNS based therapies, a site of relative immune privilege, but should prompt further studies into the significance and standardization of neutralising antibody titres during clinical trials.

2.2 Adenovirus

The earlier generations of adenoviral constructs were generally based around the Ad serotype 5 and containing E1 and/or E3 gene region deletions. These found early uses for *in vitro* work, but were associated with significant *in vivo* host immune responses and associated toxicity, with cell death leading to transient transgene expression. The deletion of further viral genes in more recent third generation ("gutless") vectors has reduced these problems significantly (Schiedner 1998), producing long-term gene expression. This class of viruses has several technical advantages, including relative ease in the production of high-titer stocks and generally strong gene expression (Verma 2005). Broader use of this class of vectors is still hampered by immune reactions induced by viral capsid proteins, which are likely to remain a persistent issue (Kafri 1998).

2.3 Herpes simplex virus

Herpes simplex virus has several obvious advantages for CNS delivery, including a large genome size, with resultant high packaging capacity, neurotropism and long lived episomal latency. The virus genome consists of 150 kb of double-stranded DNA, encoding more than 80 genes. Two broad classes of vector systems have been derived – amplicons and recombinant vectors. Amplicon vectors contain only *cis*-acting sequences (*ori* and *pac*) and require a packaging system, usually supplied in *trans*, from a *pac* deficient cosmid encoded HSV-1 genome (Cunningham 1993).Vectors with specific deletions in the infected cell polypeptide (ICP)-0 (ICP0), ICP4, ICP22 and ICP47 intermediate early genes retain long lived persistence, apparently without significant cellular toxicity (Samaniego 1998). Some safety concerns remain, however, but this class of vectors looks particularly promising when the delivery of a large DNA construct is required (Lachmann 1999). The use of specific promoters, such as the tyrosine hydroxylase promoter, increases transduction specificity (Cao 2008).

2.4 Lentivirus

Lentiviral vectors are usually considered separately from other retroviruses, as they can efficiently infect both dividing and non-dividing cells, potentially leading to long-term gene expression following chromosomal integration. Most lentiviruses are based on the human immunodeficiency virus (HIV) (Vigna 2000), with transgenes incorporated between elements known as long terminal repeats (LTR), sequences required for host genome integration. The *env* gene product is typically substituted for sequences from other RNA viruses (frequently the vesicular stomatitis virus glycoprotein VSV-G) to impart a wide cellular tropism, including neurons (Naldini 1996). Further specificity can be given through the use of the human glial fibrillary acidic promoter (hGFAP) or neuron-specific enolase promoter (rNSE), giving glial or neuronal specificities respectively (Jakobsson 2006). This class of vectors certain several advantages, including a relatively large capacity for cloned genes (approximately nine kilobases) (Zhao 2007), but concerns relate to the possibility of recombination events, producing replication-competent virus. The use of two or three plasmid based transfection systems, in which the capsid assembly genes are genetically isolated has increased the safety profile of this class of vectors (Zufferey 1997) and this class looks particularly promising for future studies.

3. Clinical trials with gene therapy vectors

Gene therapy vectors have been used in clinical trials for patients since 1990, with most experience using retroviral vectors (Verma 1997). Initial enthusiasm was tempered, however, following the death of a patient receiving an adenoviral vector as replacement for the enzyme defect ornithine transcarbamylase deficiency (Somia 2000). The patient death – from systemic inflammation and multiorgan failure - led to a temporary suspension of trials in 1999. Since then, technical advances and tighter regulatory frameworks have led to an increase in registered clinical trials using gene therapy and particularly using AAV. Prompted by favourable results in preclinical studies using animals ranging from mice to nonhuman primates, over 40 clinical trials using AAV as a therapeutic vector are currently registered with the US Food and Drug Administration (Mueller 2008).

Early trials, such as the Phase I trial of AAV encoded human factor IX in patients with haemophilia B provided useful safety information (Kay 2000). Following intramuscular vector injection, small but detectable levels of secreted factor IX were produced. No toxicity or chromosomal integration was seen during the time of the study. Unfortunately, cell mediated immunity to AAV was observed, which led to hepatocyte damage and eventual loss of therapeutic gene expression (Manno 2006). Phase I and II studies examined outcomes following intranasal or endobronchial administration of AAV encoded cystic fibrosis transmembrane conductance regulator. Antibody responses to AAV were observed, with limited biological effects. The safety profile appeared good, with no adverse events seen in the 120 patients treated (Mueller 2008).

In addition to the trials for PD there are several other ongoing clinical trials examining AAV mediated gene therapy to the CNS. These include ocular delivery of the RPE65 gene in Leber's congenital amaurosis, with no reported toxicity in a small number of treated patients despite a transient rise in neutralising antibodies (Simonelli 2009). Also in progress is a phase II trial using AAV to deliver nerve growth factor in patients with Alzheimer's Disease (Mandel 2010). A recent phase I trial of AAV mediated delivery of aspartoacylase for Canavan disease reported good safety, with detectable antibodies to AAV2 observed in the serum of a minority of patients. In this case, the vector was infused intracranially via burr holes, which may explain the absence of neutralising antibodies in the cerebrospinal fluid of patients and lack of CNS inflammation (McPhee 2006).

4. Gene therapy for Parkinson's disease

Clearly, several important issues need to be addressed when attempting therapeutic cellular transduction (gene delivery and expression) for Parkinson's disease. Most obvious is deciding on the therapeutic target – the pathological process underlying PD is widespread and involves multiple brain structures and their relevant cell signaling pathways. Great care needs to be taken with the specific design of the therapeutic gene, including relevant promoters, particularly if the construct is to be constitutively active.

The simplest approach is to restore dopaminergic levels in the basal ganglia, usually through the introduction of genes coding for enzymes important in dopamine production (Azzouz 2002, Hadaczek 2010) or relevant cell signaling proteins (Kaplitt 1994). One early series of experiments examined AAV mediated gene transfer into the CNS, with injection of a virus coding for tyrosine hydroxylase into 6-hydroxydopamine-lesioned rats, finding sustained transgene expression, with no cytopathic effects and no reactive gliosis (Kaplitt 1994). Other strategies aim to slow dopaminergic cell death, usually through the localized production of trophic factors such as brain-derived neurotrophic factor (BDNF) (Hyman 1991, Klein 1999), glial cell line-derived neurotrophic factor (GDNF) (Kordower 2000, Bjorklund 2000) or neurturin(Marks 2008) to promote cell survival and function. Finally, an alternative strategy is targeted at the abnormal activities of the basal ganglia, particularly the subthalamic nucleus and the internal and external segments of the globus pallidus.

4.1 Glutamate decarboxylase

It has been consistently observed that PD is associated with decreased inhibitory activity of the nigrostriatal projections, resulting in overactivity of the subthalamic nucleus and overinhibition of the thalamus. It was therefore hypothesized that, by increasing levels of locally produced γ-aminobutyric acid (GABA) in the subthalamic nucleus, these pathways could be restored to equilibrium and improve patient function. The synthetic pathway for GABA involves the catalytic action of glutamate decarboxylase (GAD) on glutamate, an enzyme found as two genetically distinct isoforms - GAD65 and GAD67 (Erlander 1991, Bu 1992). These have differing enzymatic properties, functional requirements and intracellular distributions. The first experimental study used recombinant AAV (rAAV) encoding the GAD65 and GAD67 isoforms of glutamic acid decarboxylase, with function initially characterized *in vitro*. Two AAV2 based constructs, AAV/rGAD65 and AAV/rGAD67 were able to productively infect cell lines, with both genes transcribed, leading to the production of enzymatically active GAD65 and GAD67 (Mi 1999).

The cDNAs were then used in a series of *in vivo* experiments, in which GAD65 or GAD67 were produced by rAAV with bi*cis*tronically encoded green fluorescent protein (GFP). Subsequent stereotactic injection of either vector into the STN resulted in prolonged transgene expression (monitored up to five months), with no inflammatory response seen. The cellular distribution of GAD was as expected for each isoform - with membrane restricted GAD65 and cytosolic GAD67. Stimulating electrodes were inserted into the STN, with microdialysis probes inserted into the SNr finding significantly increased release of GABA following STN stimulation in the GAD65 gene treated rats (Luo 2002). Parkinsonian 6-hydroxydopamine (6-OHDA)-lesioned rats were then injected with the viral vectors, leading to a four-fold increase in GABA release following STN stimulation. This was associated with a marked increase in the ratio of inhibitory to excitatory SNr responses. Importantly, controls (injected with GFP or saline) had unchanged responses, indicating that these results were not primarily due to local lesioning effects. GAD67 treated rats, in contrast, had a predominantly excitatory response. Additional effects and outcomes were examined, in particular potential neuroprotective effects of GAD gene administration. By pre-treating with the GAD65 containing construct prior to 6-OHDA lesioning, several functional outcomes (limb use and apomorphine-induced rotations) were significantly improved as compared to control infusions. A corresponding increased survival of tyrosine-hydroxylase positive cells was also seen in the GAD65 treated group, again suggesting a neuroprotective effect.

Subsequent studies examined the properties of the vector when injected in hemiparkinsonian macaques (Emborg 2007). In this model, MPTP is injected into the carotid artery, with subsequent injections of AAV-GAD or GFP control into the ipsilateral STN. Over the course of a 56 week period, 13 macaques (seven on active treatment, six control) were monitored, finding sustained transgene expression, improvement in clinical parameters (bradykinesia, tremor, motor skills) in GAD-treated animals and increased ipsilateral ^{18}F-fluorodeoxyglucose (FDG) PET motor cortical glucose activity. All animals survived to the 1 year end point without significant adverse events.

Prompted by these promising results, an open label phase I trial of unilateral subthalamic viral vector injection, using an AAV2 serotype encoding human GAD65 or GAD67 under the control of a CMV promoter was performed (Kaplitt 2007). Patients recruited for the trial – the first use of gene therapy for an adult neurodegenerative disorder - were reasonably typical for idiopathic Parkinson's disease, with a disease duration ranging from 6 to 13 years. Exclusion criteria included significant cognitive or psychiatric illness.

The protocol involved a stereotactic frame and MRI guided STN injection of a 50 μl solution of a 1 (low dose) to 10 (high dose) $x10^{11}$ genomes/ml solution. Unilateral injections were performed into the most symptomatic hemisphere, leaving the contralateral side untreated. Several outcomes were examined, including safety, tolerability, Parkinson's disease symptoms as rated by the Unified Parkinson's Disease Rating Scale (UPDRS), and ^{18}F-fluorodeoxyglucose (FDG) PET imaging was performed in a blinded manner, at baseline and 12 months post surgery. The procedure was well tolerated, with no deaths or unexpected neurological complications during the study period. Post procedure assessments found an improvement in the UPDRS motor scores from 3 months, sustained through to 12 months post surgery. The change was located primarily to the body side contralateral to the procedure. PET imaging found a significant decline in thalamic metabolism, ipsilateral to the injection. No changes in anti-AAV and GAD65/67 antibodies were seen after surgery (Kaplitt 2007).

Although the study was small and not blinded, the procedure appeared safe and clinical outcomes were encouraging. Some definite benefits over traditional deep brain stimulation procedures include the lack of implanted hardware and theoretical benefits could include a more physiological approach to restoring motor network function through activity dependent GABA release. Findings suggest that GABA release may be subject to autoregulatory pathways involving $GABA_A$ receptors of the STN. The full conclusions of the Phase II trial were published recently (LeWitt 2011), confirming a significant improvement in the UPDRS score six months post procedure for the AAV-GAD treated group (decreasing by 8.1 points $p<0.0001$), although sham treated patients also improved (decreasing by 4.7 points, $p<0.003$). The improvement seen in AAV-GAD treated subjects was significantly greater than in sham surgery subjects ($p=0.04$). No additional safety issues were observed. This important trial highlighted not just the importance of including significant patient numbers (22 and 23 in the treatment and control groups respectively) to provide a significant study difference, but also the need for meticulous study design, not least in the placebo group (which included a detailed sham surgery protocol). Several important questions and issues remain to be answered, in particular (i) whether the beneficial effects will be maintained in the medium to long-term; (ii) whether there will be longer term side effects of this therapeutic approach, particularly important in a gene therapy vector in which the agent is constitutively active and; (iii) how this approach compares to more traditional 'advanced' therapeutic options, such as deep brain surgery (DBS).

4.2 Glial cell line-derived neurotrophic factor

Glial cell line-derived neurotrophic factor (GDNF) was characterized as a selective neurotrophic factor for dopaminergic neurons from its ability to increase dopamine uptake in midbrain cultures without effect on serotonin or gamma amino butyric acid (GABA) uptake (Lin 1993). In addition, GDNF promoted dopaminergic neuron survival, dopamine uptake, cell body size and neurite outgrowth (Lin 1993), and was therefore identified a potential therapeutic agent in PD.

Early experiments in which GDNF was stereotactically injected into MPTP treated mice (i.e remove comma after mice) found that injection of GDNF into the striatum prior to MPTP treatment was associated with preservation of dopamine levels in the substantia nigra and striatum and preserved striatal TH immunoreactive cells. Treatment with GDNF at any time point was shown to improve the motor function as assessed by locomotion, motility and rearing compared to controls (Tomac 1995).

Initial approaches to delivering sustained in vivo GDNF used a replication deficient adenovirus containing human GDNF in the rat 6-hydroxydopamine (6-0HDA) model (Choi-Lundberg 1997). Adenovirus GDNF significantly increased substantia nigra dopaminergic cell survival compared to controls, although protein and mRNA levels were not sustained and all animals had host reactions around the needle site. Subsequent experiments used stereotactically Injected GDNF encoding lentivirus in MPTP treated rhesus monkeys (Kordower 2000). Again, lentivirally injected substantia nigra displayed increased levels of TH immunoreactive neurons. In a follow-up series of experiments, animals displayed improved functional scores, with a corresponding improvement on FDG PET scanning. Importantly, and in contrast to adenoviral approaches, lentivirally encoded GDNF transgene expression was sustained for up to eight months and inflammatory responses were minimal. Possible idiosyncratic reactions were hinted at, but not detailed, which is an important omission as, for example, cerebellar toxicity has been mentioned as a limiting factor in some cases (Berry 2010). However, this approach shows promise, prompting Amsterdam Molecular Therapeutics to obtain a license to use the GDNF gene delivered via an adeno-associated virus platform.

Future trials of GDNF gene therapy will need to be performed with scrupulous attention to control subjects. Fortunately, there already exists considerable experience using continuous putaminal infusions of recombinant GDNF. Initial open-label trials were encouraging (Gill 2003, Patel 2005), finding significant improvements in UPDRS III OFF and ON scores and statistically improved FDG uptake. It was observed, however, in a separate study that the initial benefits seen at one year had returned to baseline following a one year period of treatment withdrawal (Slevin 2007). Unfortunately, the subsequent randomized control double-blinded phase I/II trial (Lang 2006) did not support the open label findings, finding only improved FDG PET appearances at 6 months compared to baseline and improved mental health as measured by the SF-36 scoring system (frequently used to rate quality of life parameters) in the actively treated group. The reasons for the differences between the results are not clear, but highlight the critical importance of study design and the use of double blinded placebo subjects, including sham operative procedures.

4.3 Neurturin

Neurturin (NTN) was first identified 15 years ago (Creedon 1997), finding sequence homology to GDNF, with similar in vitro neuroprotective properties. These were confirmed by subsequent in vivo experiments, promoting TH positive neuronal survival when injected into the substantia nigra of 6-0HDA treated animals (Horger 1998), with improvements in functional parameters. Stereotactic injection of an NTN encoding AAV vector into the caudate nucleus, putamen and substantia nigra of MPTP treated monkeys found similar benefits (Kordower 2006), with no significant side effects at three months and one year (Herzog 2008, Herzog 2009).

These promising findings led to a Phase I, open-label trial of AAV2-NTN in 2008 (Marks 2008), involving 12 patients (ages 35 to 75) with moderate to severe levodopa responsive PD. In this cohort the diagnosis was established for a minimum of 5 years, patients were on stable doses of antiparkinsonian medications, but without good control with at least 3 hours of "off" time per day. The participants were divided between low and high treatment groups and received stereotactic guided injections bilaterally throughout the putamen. Participants experienced a significant improvement in UPDRS Part III motor score in the practically defined "off" period as compared to baseline, on average an improvement of 36%. Other than a presumed air embolus, which did not lead to complications, there were no clinically important operative adverse events.

This was followed up by the first double blind randomised Phase 2 trial of gene therapy for Parkinson's disease, published in late 2010 (Marks 2010). The 58 participants met similar eligibility criteria as the open-label study, with groups were divided 2:1 to receive either AAV-NTN or sham surgery respectively, with assessments at baseline and 1, 3, 6, 9 and 12 months and every 3 months thereafter until the final patient had been seen at 12 months. At each visit the patients were assessed with the UPDRS in the practically defined "off" state and the best "on" state. Home diary and quality of life questionnaires were also employed. The primary outcome - UPDRS Part III score in the "off" state was not significantly improved at 12 months. A range of secondary outcomes, including the mental score (Part I) in the "off" state and activities of daily living score (Part II) in the "on" state were significantly improved.

For the small number of patients followed up until 18 months the UPDRS Part III "off" score was significantly improved. Histological analysis of two patients' brains in the treatment group revealed only limited expression of the neurturin protein in the putamen and even more modest expression in the substantia nigra. Three patients in the active treatment group developed tumours: one glioblastoma, one adenocarcinoma of the prostate and one oesophageal adenocarcinoma. Quantitative PCR of biopsied tissue was negative for AAV-NTN and retrospective reanalysis of pre-procedure MRI suggested that the glioblastoma predated the intervention. There were two deaths in the treatment group one from myocardial infarction and one from a pulmonary embolus. Headache, nausea, post-procedural pain, dyskinesa, insomnia and worsening of PD were the most commonly reported adverse events and occurred more frequently in the active treatment compared to sham surgery groups. Serious adverse events secondary to surgery occurred in both groups without subsequent lasting neurological sequelae. Neurturin protein and antibodies were not detected in patient sera.

Although the trial failed to show a significant difference in the primary endpoint, the data gathered from the study was generally informative. The reasons underlying the therapeutic failure are not clear, potentially relating to inadequate levels of neurturin at the site of pathology. Planned future work, currently recruiting, will also include direct injection into the substantia nigra as well as increased dosing (Clinical trials.gov identifier NCT00985517).

4.4 Aromatic-L-amino decarboxylase (AADC)

Production of dopamine from either endogenous or exogenous levodopa is dependent on aromatic-L-amino decarboxylase (AADC). As PD progresses, patients typically require increasing doses of L-dopa and are therefore at increased risk of medication induced side effects. It is postulated that AADC activity is depleted in PD and that therapeutic restoration of this activity may lead to clinical improvement and allow reduced doses of levodopa (Bankiewicz 2000).

In a series of in vivo experiments using MPTP-induced hemiparkinsonian rhesus monkeys, AAV-AADC was injected throughout the caudate and putamen (Bankiewicz 2000). This led to increased in vivo AADC tracer activity and immunohistochemical staining, with partial restoration of to the ability to convert levodopa to dopamine in an ex vivo assay. Improvement on a range of functional scores was seen at 24 months and a subsequent imaging experiment found increased AADC levels up to 72 months (Bankiewicz 2006).

The work prompted an ongoing clinical trial in which five patients, with levodopa responsive Parkinson's disease and intractable motor fluctuations despite optimised medical therapy (Hoehn and Yahr stage III-IV), received bilateral putaminal infusions of 9×10^{10} vector genomes by stereotactic infusion. No adverse events were reported that were attributable to AAV-AADC infusions. FDG PET uptake was significantly increased at 6 months compared to baseline. The absence of controls in this safety study makes secondary clinical outcome interpretation difficult, although there were significant increases in 6 month total UPDRS scores on and off medication and 3 participants were able to take lower doses of levodopa (Eberling 2008).

This cohort was then compared with 5 patients who received a higher dose (3×10^{11} vector genomes) of AAV-AADC (Christine 2009). Of concern, three patients had intracranial haemorrhages, and four patients developed a transient increase in dyskinesias. In both cohorts the total UPDRS and UPDRS III scores improved at 6 months when assessed "off" medication, but no significant improvements were seen "on" medication in the UPDRS IIII score. This is odd, as the effect of AAV-AADC is thought to be dependent on levodopa therapy, although all patients in the high dose group were able to manage on lower doses of levodopa, hinting at efficacy. The study is ongoing and is expected to be completed in 2013 at which point 60 months of efficacy and safety data will be available.

4.5 Prosavin

Parkinson's disease potentially results from deficiencies in several steps of the dopaminergic synthetic pathway in which L-tyrosine is converted to levodopa by the enzyme tyrosine hydroxylase (TH). GTP cyclohydrolase 1 (CH1) is the rate-limiting enzyme for the generation of tetrahydrobiopterin which is a co-factor for TH. Levodopa is then converted to the biologically active dopamine by AADC. In an attempt to reconstitute these steps, genes coding for TH, CH1 and AADC were combined into a single lentiviral vector for administration to the striatum (Azzouz 2002).

Functional improvements were seen in stereotactically injected 6-0HDA lesioned rats, despite an apparently relatively modest increase in dopamine levels (Azzouz 2002). Subsequent *in vivo* microdialysis measurement in the MPTP macaque model demonstrated a greater increase in extracellular levels, so the therapeutic efficacy may have been greater than first thought (Jarraya 2009). Treated macaques exhibited restoration of the firing rate and pattern of neurons within the basal ganglia and reduced metabolic activity within the subthalamic nucleus, coupled with functional improvements. No safety issues were noted.

Although peer reviewed data has not yet been published, preliminary results of an ongoing Phase I/II clinical trial of Prosavin have been announced. Nine patients have now received Prosavin in three cohorts of 1x dose, 2x dose and 2x dose with an improved delivery method. The first cohort has had a 20% functional motor improvement at 24 months and the second cohort a 29% improvement at 12 months. The third cohort has had a 26% improvement at 3 months. All cohorts have had in improved "ON" time, stable or improved quality of life assessments and stable or reduced levodopa dosing. Whilst these are preliminary announcements the results are encouraging and have prompted the initiation of a 5x dose cohort commencing early in 2011.

5. Conclusions

Despite decades of research, Parkinson's disease is a chronic progressive neurodegenerative condition of unknown aetiology and the underlying pathogenesis remains unclear. Despite understandable reservations about using a gene therapy approach for the condition, several Phase I and II clinical trials have now reported their clinical findings, providing a wealth of experience and data. The use of adeno-associated vectors for gene therapy, with trials including several hundred patients, appears to be generally safe, with little procedure related morbidity.

Although there are definite concerns relating to the development of immunity to systemically administered AAV, leading to destruction of transduced tissues, this phenomenon has not been observed with CNS administration, suggesting a degree of immune privilege which may lead to more sustained therapeutic effects. Ongoing concerns relate primarily to the specific choice of therapeutic agent, site of action and levels of production. The use of non selective (particularly constitutively 'on') mammalian promoters such as CMV, do not permit adjustment of therapeutic effects. Current models suggest that autoregulation may occur through homeostatic feedback pathways, but this has not been demonstrated formally and long term effects on cellular phenotypes are unknown.

Ongoing monitoring of patients recruited into Phase I and II studies will be essential to establish whether initially observed benefits are sustained and to look for long term complications. Further randomized double blinded studies, with appropriate longitudinal follow-up will be necessary to properly evaluate the therapeutic effectiveness of this novel class of agents.

Further technological developments are likely, particularly involving the use of more sophisticated AAV-based viral vectors. These could use more neuron-specific promoters (eg neuron specific enolase or synapsin 1 gene promoters) and regulate protein production through the use of inducible systems (eg ecdysone-based) to control therapeutic activity in a more directed fashion. Although still in its infancy, this technology still shows great promise as a novel therapeutic approach for this devastating disease.

6. References

Alvarez, L. et al. (2001). Dorsal subthalamotomy for Parkinson's disease. *Movement Disorders*, 16, pp. 72-8.

Atchison, R.W., Casto, B.C. & Hammon, W.M. (1965). Adenovirus-Associated Defective Virus Particles. *Science*, 149, pp. 754-6.

Azzouz, M., et al. (2002). Multicistronic lentiviral vector-mediated striatal gene transfer of aromatic L-amino acid decarboxylase, tyrosine hydroxylase, and GTP cyclohydrolase I induces sustained transgene expression, dopamine production, and functional improvement in a rat model of Parkinson's disease. *The Journal of Neuroscience*, 22, pp. 10302-12.

Bankiewicz, K.S., et al. (2000). Convection-enhanced delivery of AAV vector in parkinsonian monkeys; in vivo detection of gene expression and restoration of dopaminergic function using pro-drug approach. *Experimental Neurology*, 164, pp. 2-14.

Bankiewicz, K.S., et al. (2006). Long-term clinical improvement in MPTP-lesioned primates after gene therapy with AAV-hAADC. *Molecular Therapeutics*, 14, pp. 564-70.

Benabid, A.L. et al. (1996). Chronic electrical stimulation of the ventralis intermedius nucleus of the thalamus as a treatment of movement disorders. *Journal of Neurosurgery*, 84, pp. 203-14.

Berry, A.L. and T. Foltynie. (2010). Gene therapy: a viable therapeutic strategy for Parkinson's disease? *Journal of Neurology*, 258, 179-88.

Bjorklund, A., et al. (2000). Towards a neuroprotective gene therapy for Parkinson's disease: use of adenovirus, AAV and lentivirus vectors for gene transfer of GDNF to the nigrostriatal system in the rat Parkinson model. *Brain Research*, 886, pp. 82-98.

Brooks, D.J. (1998). The early diagnosis of Parkinson's disease. *Annals of Neurology*, 44, pp. S10-8.

Brown, P. et al. (2001). Dopamine dependency of oscillations between subthalamic nucleus and pallidum in Parkinson's disease. *The Journal of Neuroscience*, 21, pp. 1033-8.

Bu, D.F., et al. (1992). Two human glutamate decarboxylases, 65-kDa GAD and 67-kDa GAD, are each encoded by a single gene. *Proceedings of the National Academy of Sciences (U S A)*, 89, pp. 2115-9.

Buller, R.M. et al. (1981). Herpes simplex virus types 1 and 2 completely help adenovirus-associated virus replication. *Journal of Virology*, 40, pp. 241-7.

Cao, H., et al. (2008). Enhanced nigrostriatal neuron-specific, long-term expression by using neural-specific promoters in combination with targeted gene transfer by modified helper virus-free HSV-1 vector particles. *BMC Neuroscience*, 9, pp. 37.

Choi-Lundberg, D.L. et al. (1997). Dopaminergic neurons protected from degeneration by GDNF gene therapy. *Science*, 275, pp. 838-41.

Christine, C.W., et al. (2009). Safety and tolerability of putaminal AADC gene therapy for Parkinson disease. *Neurology*, 73, pp. 1662-9.

Creedon, D.J., et al. (1997). Neurturin shares receptors and signal transduction pathways with glial cell line-derived neurotrophic factor in sympathetic neurons. *Proceedings of the National Academy of Sciences (U S A)*, 94, pp. 7018-23.

Cunningham, C. & Davison, A.J. (1993). A cosmid-based system for constructing mutants of herpes simplex virus type 1. *Virology*, 197, pp. 116-24.

Eberling, J.L. et al. (2008). Results from a phase I safety trial of hAADC gene therapy for Parkinson disease. *Neurology*, 70, pp. 1980-3.

Erlander, M.G., et al. (1991). Two genes encode distinct glutamate decarboxylases. *Neuron*, 7, pp. 91-100.

Emborg, M.E., et al. (2007). Subthalamic glutamic acid decarboxylase gene therapy: changes in motor function and cortical metabolism. *Journal of Cerebral Blood Flow & Metabolism*, 27, pp. 501-9.

Fahn, S. (2006). Levodopa in the treatment of Parkinson's disease. *Journal of Neural Transmission. Supplementum*, 71, pp. 1-15.

Fearnley, J.M., & Lees, A.J. (1991). Ageing and Parkinson's disease: substantia nigra regional selectivity. *Brain*, 114, pp. 2283-301.

Gao, G. et al. (2004). Clades of adeno-associated viruses are widely disseminated in human tissues. *Journal of Virology*, 78, pp. 6381-8.

Gill, S.S. et al. (2003). Direct brain infusion of glial cell line-derived neurotrophic factor in Parkinson disease. *Nature Medicine*, 9, pp. 589-95.

Hadaczek, P., et al. (2010). Eight years of clinical improvement in MPTP-lesioned primates after gene therapy with AAV2-hAADC. *Molecular Therapeutics*, 18, pp. 1458-61.

Hermonat, P.L. & Muzyczka, N. (1984). Use of adeno-associated virus as a mammalian DNA cloning vector: transduction of neomycin resistance into mammalian tissue culture cells. *Proceedings of the National Academy of Sciences (U S A)*, 81, pp. 6466-70.

Herzog, C.D., et al. (2008). Transgene expression, bioactivity, and safety of CERE-120 (AAV2-neurturin) following delivery to the monkey striatum. *Molecular Therapeutics*, 16, pp. 1737-44.

Herzog, C.D., et al., (2009). Expression, bioactivity, and safety 1 year after adeno-associated viral vector type 2-mediated delivery of neurturin to the monkey nigrostriatal system support cere-120 for Parkinson's disease. *Neurosurgery*, 64, pp. 602-12.

Hoggan, M.D., Blacklow, N.R. & Rowe, W.P. (1966). Studies of small DNA viruses found in various adenovirus preparations: physical, biological, and immunological characteristics. *Proceedings of the National Academy of Sciences (U S A)*, 55, pp. 1467-74.

Horger, B.A., et al. (1998). Neurturin exerts potent actions on survival and function of midbrain dopaminergic neurons. *Journal of Neuroscience*, 18, pp. 4929-37.

Hyman, C. et al., (1991). BDNF is a neurotrophic factor for dopaminergic neurons of the substantia nigra. *Nature*, 350, pp. 230-2.

Jakobsson, J. and Lundberg, C. (2006). Lentiviral vectors for use in the central nervous system. *Molecular Therapeutics*, 13, pp. 484-93.

Jarraya, B., et al. (2009). Dopamine gene therapy for Parkinson's disease in a nonhuman primate without associated dyskinesia. *Science Translational Medicine*, 1, pp. 2ra4.

Jenner, P. (2000). Factors influencing the onset and persistence of dyskinesia in MPTP-treated primates. *Annals of Neurology*, 47, pp. S90-9.

Kafri, T., et al. (1998). Cellular immune response to adenoviral vector infected cells does not require de novo viral gene expression: implications for gene therapy. *Proceedings of the National Academy of Sciences (U S A)*, 95, pp. 11377-82.

Kaplitt, M.G., et al. (1994). Long-term gene expression and phenotypic correction using adeno-associated virus vectors in the mammalian brain. *Nature Genetics*, 8, pp. 148-54.

Kaplitt, M.G., et al. (2007). Safety and tolerability of gene therapy with an adeno-associated virus (AAV) borne GAD gene for Parkinson's disease: an open label, phase I trial. *The Lancet*, 369, pp. 2097-105.

Kay, M.A., et al. (2000). Evidence for gene transfer and expression of factor IX in haemophilia B patients treated with an AAV vector. *Nature Genetics*, 24, pp. 257-61.

Klein, R.L. et al. (1999). Prevention of 6-hydroxydopamine-induced rotational behavior by BDNF somatic gene transfer. *Brain Res*earch, 847, pp. 314-20.

Kordower, J.H. et al. (2000). Neurodegeneration prevented by lentiviral vector delivery of GDNF in primate models of Parkinson's disease. *Science*. 290, pp. 767-73.

Kordower, J.H., et al. (2006). Delivery of neurturin by AAV2 (CERE-120)-mediated gene transfer provides structural and functional neuroprotection and neurorestoration in MPTP-treated monkeys. *Annals of Neurology*, 60, pp. 706-15.

Lachmann, R.H. & Efstathiou, S. (1999). Gene transfer with herpes simplex vectors. *Current Opinion in Molecular Therapeutics*, 1, pp. 622-32.

Lang, A.E., et al. (2006). Randomized controlled trial of intraputamenal glial cell line-derived neurotrophic factor infusion in Parkinson disease. *Annals of Neurology*, 59(3), pp. 459-66.

Levy, R. et al. (2001). Lidocaine and muscimol microinjections in subthalamic nucleus reverse Parkinsonian symptoms. *Brain*, 124, pp. 2105-18.

LeWitt, P.A. et al. (2011). AAV2-GAD gene therapy for advanced Parkinson's disease: a double-blind, sham-surgery controlled, randomised trial. *Lancet Neurology*, 10, 309-19.

Lin, L.F., et al. (1993). GDNF: a glial cell line-derived neurotrophic factor for midbrain dopaminergic neurons. *Science*, 260, pp. 1130-2.

Luo, J., et al. (2002). Subthalamic GAD gene therapy in a Parkinson's disease rat model. *Science* 298, pp. 425-9.

Mandel, R.J. (2010). CERE-110, an adeno-associated virus-based gene delivery vector expressing human nerve growth factor for the treatment of Alzheimer's disease. *Current Opinion in Molecular Therapeutics*, 12, pp. 240-7.

Manno, C.S., et al. (2006). Successful transduction of liver in hemophilia by AAV-Factor IX and limitations imposed by the host immune response. *Nature Medicine*, 12, pp. 342-7.

Marks, W.J., Jr., et al. (2008). Safety and tolerability of intraputaminal delivery of CERE-120 (adeno-associated virus serotype 2-neurturin) to patients with idiopathic Parkinson's disease: an open-label, phase I trial. *Lancet Neurology*, 7, pp. 400-8.

Marks, W.J., Jr. et al. (2010). Gene delivery of AAV2-neurturin for Parkinson's disease: a double-blind, randomised, controlled trial. *Lancet Neurology*, 9, pp. 1164-72.

McCarty, D.M., Young Jr, S.M. & Samulski, R.J. (2004). Integration of adeno-associated virus (AAV) and recombinant AAV vectors. *Annual Review of Genetics*, 38, pp. 819-45.

McPhee, S.W., et al. (2006). Immune responses to AAV in a phase I study for Canavan disease. *Journal of Gene Medicine*, 8, pp. 577-88.

Mi, J., et al. (1999). Recombinant adeno-associated virus (AAV) drives constitutive production of glutamate decarboxylase in neural cell lines. *The Journal of Neuroscience Research*, 57, pp. 137-48.

Monahan, P.E., Jooss, K. & Sands, M.S. (2002). Safety of adeno-associated virus gene therapy vectors: a current evaluation. *Expert Opinion on Drug Safety*, 1, pp. 79-91.

Mueller, C. & Flotte, T.R. (2008). Clinical gene therapy using recombinant adeno-associated virus vectors. *Gene Therapy*, 15, pp. 858-63.

Muzyczka, N. (1992). Use of adeno-associated virus as a general transduction vector for mammalian cells. *Current Topics in Microbiology and Immunology*, 158, pp. 97-129.

Naldini, L. et al., (1996). In vivo gene delivery and stable transduction of nondividing cells by a lentiviral vector. *Science*, 272, pp. 263-7.

Patel, N.K., et al. (2005). Intraputamenal infusion of glial cell line-derived neurotrophic factor in PD: a two-year outcome study. *Annals of Neurology*, 57, pp. 298-302.

Peden, C.S. et al. (2004). Circulating anti-wild-type adeno-associated virus type 2 (AAV2) antibodies inhibit recombinant AAV2 (rAAV2)-mediated, but not rAAV5-mediated, gene transfer in the brain. *Journal of Virology*, 78, pp. 6344-59.

Samaniego, L.A., Neiderhiser, L. & DeLuca, N.A. (1998). Persistence and expression of the herpes simplex virus genome in the absence of immediate-early proteins. *Journal of Virology*, 72, pp. 3307-20.

Samulski, R.J., Chang, L.S. & Shenk, T. (1989). Helper-free stocks of recombinant adeno-associated viruses: normal integration does not require viral gene expression. *Journal of Virology*, 63, pp. 3822-8.

Sanftner, L.M., et al. (2004). Striatal delivery of rAAV-hAADC to rats with preexisting immunity to AAV. *Molecular Therapy*, 9, pp. 403-9.

Schiedner, G., et al. (1998). Genomic DNA transfer with a high-capacity adenovirus vector results in improved in vivo gene expression and decreased toxicity. *Nature Genetics*, 18, pp. 180-3.

Schnepp, B.C. et al., (2003). Genetic fate of recombinant adeno-associated virus vector genomes in muscle. *Journal of Virology*, 77, pp. 3495-504.

Simonelli, F., et al. (2009). Gene therapy for Leber's congenital amaurosis is safe and effective through 1.5 years after vector administration. *Molecular Therapeutics*, 18, pp. 643-50.

Slevin, J.T. et al. (2007). Unilateral intraputamenal glial cell line-derived neurotrophic factor in patients with Parkinson disease: response to 1 year of treatment and 1 year of withdrawal. *Journal of Neurosurgery*, 106, pp. 614-20.

Somia, N. & Verma, I.M. 2000. Gene therapy: trials and tribulations. *Nature Reviews Genetics*, 1, pp. 91-9.

Srivastava, A., Lusby, E.W. & Berns, K.I. (1983). Nucleotide sequence and organization of the adeno-associated virus 2 genome. *Journal of Virology*, 45, pp. 555-64.

Su, P.C. et al. (2003). Treatment of advanced Parkinson's disease by subthalamotomy: one-year results. *Movement Disorders*, 18, pp. 531-8.

Tenenbaum, L., Lehtonen, E. & Monahan, P.E. (2003). Evaluation of risks related to the use of adeno-associated virus-based vectors. *Current Gene Therapy*, 3, pp. 545-65.

The Deep-Brain Stimulation for Parkinson's Disease Study Group. (2001). Deep-brain stimulation of the subthalamic nucleus or the pars interna of the globus pallidus in Parkinson's disease. *The New England Journal of Medicine*, 345, pp. 956-63.

Tomac, A. et al. (1995). Protection and repair of the nigrostriatal dopaminergic system by GDNF in vivo. *Nature*, 373, pp. 335-9.

Verma, I.M. & Somia, N. (1997). Gene therapy -- promises, problems and prospects. *Nature*, 389, pp. 239-42.

Verma, I.M. & Weitzman, M.D. (2005). Gene therapy: twenty-first century medicine. *Annual Reviews in Biochemistry*, 74, pp. 711-38.

Vigna, E. & Naldini, L. (2000). Lentiviral vectors: excellent tools for experimental gene transfer and promising candidates for gene therapy. *The Journal of Gene Medicine*, 2, pp. 308-16.

Wichmann, T. & DeLong, M.R. (2003). Pathophysiology of Parkinson's disease: the MPTP primate model of the human disorder. *Annals of the New York Academy of Sciences*, 991, pp. 199-213.

Zhao, J. & Lever, A.M. (2007). Lentivirus-mediated gene expression. *Methods in Molecular Biology*, 366, pp. 343-55.

Zufferey, R. et al. (1997). Multiply attenuated lentiviral vector achieves efficient gene delivery in vivo. *Nature Biotechnology*, 15, pp. 871-5.

13

Gene Therapy for Parkinson's Disease: Towards Non Invasive Approaches

Manuel Rodríguez, José M. Brito-Armas and Rafael Castro
Department of Physiology, School of Medicine, University of La Laguna
Spain

1. Introduction

The blood brain barrier (BBB) is one of the factors hampering the development of new therapies and in many cases limits the access of the therapeutic agent to the neural tissue. The BBB consists of a specialized vascular structure formed by the interaction between endothelial cells and numerous processes of astrocytes regulating the passage and diffusion of molecules between plasma and the central nervous system (CNS) (Pardridge, 2005). The endothelium is distinguished from other tissues by the presence of tight junctions between endothelial cells (which limit the exchange of even low molecular weight substances) and a reduced endocytic and pinocytic activity. Small molecules (usually less than 500 Da) and some lipid-soluble small peptides can pass the BBB without the mediation of specific transporters. However, in most cases, the transfer across the BBB requires receptor-mediated transcytosis or selective transporters, such as low density lipoprotein receptors (LDLR), insulin receptors, leptin receptors, transferrin receptors and insulin-like growth factor receptors (Pardridge, 2005). The number of specific transporters mediating the transfer of substances through the BBB is very high and probably accounts for a very substantial part of the more than 2,000 membrane transporters that probably function in the human cell. We present, in this review, some of the newly developed approaches to overcome this barrier and facilitate the access of therapeutic genes to the nervous system.

Parkinson's disease (PD) is considered here as being neurological diseases for which no etiopathogenic treatment is available and may be susceptible to gene therapy. Different proteins such as human glial cell line-derived neurotrophic factor (GDNF), brain-derived neurotrophic factor (BDNF)...which are able to reduce the vulnerability of dopaminergic neurons in laboratory animals have been described in the last ten years. For various reasons, the central administration of these proteins has not been effective in patients (short half-life, poor diffusion in neural tissue ...). Since the cellular and neurochemical substrate of the disease, and various proteins with neuroprotective capacity for these cells are known, gene therapy is outlined here as a future therapeutic option.

2. Gene therapy: An alternative treatment for neurodegenerative diseases

Conventional drugs of low molecular weight are designed to spread in cells with precise kinetics and, where necessary, use specific transport systems. Protein therapy is more complex, especially when act intracellularly, because there are not many cellular pathways to import proteins. Moreover, these molecules cannot be orally administered. The situation regarding the delivery of nucleic acids is complex because of their size (MDa) and the lack of systems to import them through the cell membrane, especially in the cell nucleus. Therefore, nucleic acids need to be packaged into either virus particles in a natural way to meet many of these conditions or artificial particles that can replace the virus. The treatment half life is also completely different since the transformation which is achieved with nucleic acids can mean a permanent alteration, unlike conventional drug treatment which is inherently transient.

Gene therapy is defined as the introduction of nucleic acids into cells to alter the course of a medical condition or disease. Initially proposed for the treatment of monogenic diseases, gene therapy is now recognized as ' a new form of drug delivery ' offering various strategies for the treatment of inborn and acquired diseases. If the future of gene therapy is to successfully compete with traditional drug treatment, it will be necessary to have economic, simple and effective methods of gene transfer.

The expression of exogenously administered genes in the brain has been proposed as an alternative therapy for a wide variety of inherited and acquired diseases of the CNS for which classical drug therapy is not affordable or not readily applicable. Gene transfer into the CNS has been investigated as a strategy to protect against neuronal damage and degeneration. The best candidates for gene therapy are neurotrophic factors, antioxidants- or antiapoptotic molecules, and different specific molecules of cell signaling, which are of great interest in neuroprotection in pathological conditions where, as in Parkinson's disease, there is free-radical production (Tenenbaum et al., 2002).

The choice of vehicle (vector) to carry the therapeutic gene (transgene) to the desired tissue or cell type is crucial to achieve successful gene transfer. Basically, the vectors used in gene therapy can be divided into two groups, viral and nonviral, each of which has advantages and disadvantages. Some viral vectors which have proven to be effective *in vivo* gene transfer into the CNS (especially lentivirus and adeno-associated virus) can be integrated in the chromosomes of transduced cells, favoring a lasting expression of transgene in experimental animals (Thomas et al., 2003). In several cases, some cell lines are genetically transformed to produce neurotransmitters or neurotrophic factors in large quantities, called *ex vivo* gene therapy, in order to be used as therapeutic alternatives for CNS disorders. However, viral vectors present important problems regarding their production and safety (Kaiser, 2002). In addition, some viral vectors induce an immune response which reduces the effectiveness and biosafety with repeated dosing. A further complication of the use of certain viral vectors is their tendency to integrate near promoters and transcriptional units, thereby increasing the possibility of adverse effects (Essner et al., 2005).

A significant effort has been made to develop non-viral alternative strategies of *in vivo* gene transfer in recent years. Naked DNA linked to a variety of molecular conjugates, such as liposomes, non-lipid nanoparticles, polymers and polypeptides has been used to this end. The manufacture of large-scale DNA is feasible and reproducible with these vectors, and the final product does not require sophisticated storage conditions. In addition, nonviral vectors have no restrictions regarding the size of the gene and do not cause a significant immune response (Conwell & Huang, 2005). However, with the use of a non-viral vector, the input of genetic material into the cell is limited due to the need to provide the DNA in the cell surface in sufficient concentrations for entry (Luo & Saltzman, 2000). It is also difficult for non-viral vectors to induce a lasting expression of therapeutic gene (Conwell & Huang, 2005; Pathak et al., 2009). Although this limits the time for use in gene therapy of brain diseases, it is also true that there has been spectacular growth, in recent years, in terms of diversity, properties and manufacturing.

The choice of an appropriate vector to transfer the desired gene in the affected brain area is crucial to establish a safe and efficient gene therapy for CNS. In recent years there has been much research into gene therapy, with significant progress in developing new gene transfer strategies in the CNS and in evaluating their potential in treating neurological diseases. Among the various systems developed for this purpose, viral vectors have undoubtedly been used most. However, due to the impediment of gene medicines in crossing the BBB, most of the work undertaken used adeno-associated viral vectors or lentiviral vectors (using invasive routes of administration such as intracerebral injection and craniotomy) that also produce a localized gene expression.

Although direct intracerebral injection of viral vectors expressing transgene-invasive gene therapy (iGT)-may be a reasonable alternative for localized treatment of neurodegenerative diseases, in which discrete brain structures are involved, the treatment of many neurological disorders requires the transfer of the transgene throughout the CNS. On the other hand, the small size of mice (major animal model) favors a more distributed gene expression, as only five vector injections are necessary throughout the brain. However, the larger human brain would require too many local injections, making the procedure clinically impractical. Therefore, in recent years there has been a dramatic shift in the strategies of non-invasive transfer of therapeutic genes in the CNS, non-invasive gene therapy (niGT) -. In this type of gene transfer, nucleic acids are indirectly introduced (usually via blood) in nervous tissue, in order to achieve therapeutic benefit, thus avoiding their direct injection into the brain parenchyma and damage to the BBB. The types and more important characteristics of non-viral and viral vectors that enable the realization of a niGT in the CNS will be described below.

3. Adenoassociated vectors: The most widely used in gene therapy for Parkinson's disease

The adeno-associated viruses (AAV) are small non-enveloped virus of 20-24 nm in diameter, which are not associated with any disease in humans (Blacklow et al., 1968). The 4.7-kb genome of the virus is packaged as a molecule of single- stranded DNA, it becomes double-stranded after infection. Recombinant AAV vectors (AAVr) lack 96% of the viral genome, which has been removed to leave only the two inverted terminal repeats involved in packaging and integration (Srivastava et al., 1983). The conventional method for generating viral stocks is to perform a transient cotransfection of 293T cells with plasmids containing the vector genome, rep and cap genes and adenovirus helper (Xiao et al., 1998). There have been recent improvements in vector production AAVr, resulting in higher titers (between about 100 and 10,000 times), and a higher proportion of infectious particles as well as free preparations of adenovirus (Zolotukhin, 2005). AAV vectors express stably transgenic products in dividing- and in non-dividing cells, and although the absence of viral genes theoretically minimizes the risk of activating the host immune responses, this will depend largely on the serotype used and the target tissue (Lowenstein et al., 2007; Wang et al., 2010). A small cloning capacity (3-4 kb) and a delayed expression of the transgene (2-3 weeks) can be included among the limitations of AAV vectors (Paterna and Büeler, 2002).

The human AAV was discovered in 1965 as a contaminant of adenovirus preparations. Following the description in 1982 of the first infectious clones of AAV2, this virus has been rapidly gaining popularity in gene therapy applications due to features such as the lack of pathogenicity, wide range of infectivity, and the ability to set a long-term transgene expression. As more serotypes are characterized and more capsids of different serotypes are combined to obtain new tropisms, it is possible that tissues which are difficult to infect with known serotypes of AAV are capable of gene transfer. This will help to expand the current range of AAV vectors. AAV serotypes share a common genomic structure but show variation in cell and tissue tropism due to differences in their capsid proteins. This involves recognition of different cell surface receptors.

So far we have identified nine serotypes of AAV vectors, and the studies with reporter genes have shown that these vectors efficiently infect the neurons (Cearley et al., 2008). The receptors responsible for the infection of AAV vectors in neurons are not fully characterized. The coinfusion of heparin and mannitol increases the diffusion of AAV2 vectors. In addition, the activity of coreceptors is necessary for a successful viral entry (Qing et al., 1999). Previous mannitol intravenous infusion in mice not only induces a global transduction in the CNS, facilitating the entry of AAV2 which is also injected intravenously, but also produces therapeutic benefits in models of neurological diseases in which there is a generalized affectation (McCarty et al., 2009). The cells which are permissive to AAV2 vectors express a number of factors, including the fibroblast growth factor receptor and the β5 subunit of integrin, αvβ5 (Qing et al., 1999; Summerford et al., 1999). Compared to the AAV2 vector, the AAV5 serotype produces a higher- transduction and distribution in the brain (Davidson et al., 2000). Thus, AAV transduction in any organ is closely linked to the local density of a specific receptor.

AAV infection is initiated by binding receptors that are serotype-specific to the cell surface. For example, heparin sulfate proteoglycan (HSPG) is one of the main AAV2 receptors (Summerford & Samulski, 1998). Binding to a receptor is not a sufficient stimulus for viral internalization, which also needs coreceptors, such as integrin heterodimers , fibroblast growth factor type 1 receptor and hepatocyte growth factor receptor, c-Met (Dos Santos & Beyer-Nardi, 2008). HSPG has a ubiquitous distribution in cells and tissues of various species. This partly explains the broad tropism of this virus into human, nonhuman primate, canine, murine and bird cells. Some derivatives of sialic acid act as AAV4 and AAV5 receptors, while the platelet-derived growth factor receptor is another cellular determinant involved in AAV5 infection (Di Pasquale et al., 2003). Different AAV serotypes preferentially transduce different cell types. In general, tropism is associated with the abundance of a specific receptor /coreceptor, although there are exceptions (Duan et al., 2000). This suggests that there are probably other internalization ways that are independent of known receptors (Ding et al., 2005).

In the past decade, viral gene transfer has progressed from being merely an application in animal research to become an experimental therapeutic strategy in humans. From the clinical and therapeutic standpoint it is essential to know the distribution in tissue and kinetics (onset, duration and removal of the expression) of AAV vectors. To date numerous AAV serotypes with variable tropism have been identified. The level of homology of amino acids in the capsid protein of serotypes 1 to 9 is about 45% (Chiorini et al., 1999; Gao et al., 2002), with the most divergent serotypes being AAV4 and AAV5. Many studies have conducted evaluations on the tropism of different AAV serotypes. Serotypes 1, 2 and 5 (Burger et al., 2004), 7-9, and rh10 (one serotype of primates), 1, 2, 5, 7 and 8 (Taymans et al., 2007), 2, 5, 8 and rh10 (Sondhi et al., 2007), 8, 9, and rh10 and rh43 (Klein et al., 2008) have been used in the brain.

An important limitation of previous studies was that the lack of uniformity in the design of plasmids, as in the production, purification and route of administration, made it difficult to compare the efficiencies of transduction of these serotypes in different tissues. In order to control the variability in these parameters, the design of plasmids, transfection, purification, titration, dialysis, storage and injection have been standardized for all AAV serotypes examined. These limitations are solved by the use of marker genes in which expression can be viewed at different times, via longitudinal studies in each animal. Thus, when using luciferase as a transgene one can evaluate the transgenic protein activity after intraperitoneal injection of its substrate (luciferin). This allows sequential measurements in the same animal (Lipshutz et al., 2001; Wu et al., 2001). Consequently, the differences in the efficiencies of transduction and biodistribution profiles will only reflect the differences in capsids of the virions of these serotypes.

The tropism and expression kinetics for 9 different serotypes of AAV have recently been studied, which have been packaged, produced, purified and injected by the same systemic route (Zincarelli et al., 2008). This administration route is therapeutically realistic, as it allows the specific expression in tissues, provided that specific promoters are used along with the administration of vectors. In the afore mentioned study a sequential follow up of transgene expression for 100 days, and 9 months after the intravenous administration of serotypes 1-9 of AAV that expressed the luciferase transgen (controlled by an early promoter/activator of CMV and flanked by ITR sequences of AAV) was carried out in mice. The bioluminescence image revealed three expression levels: a) serotypes AAV2, 3, 4 and 5 were in the low expression group, b) AAV1, 6 and 8 belonged to the moderate expression group, and c) and AAV7 and 9 corresponded to the high expression group. There was great variation in the kinetics of expression between these serotypes, where AAV7 and 9 induced a faster expression onset, and AAV3 and 4 induced a slower expression. It has been also shown that the primary targets for serotype 1, 2, 5, 6, 7 and 9 are liver and skeletal muscle, and was AAV9 whom induced greater gene expression in the heart. AAV8 and 9 induced a more ubiquitous transduction than other serotypes, but AAV9 generated a more robust expression. Within the high expression group, AAV9 also produced the largest number of viral genome copies in all examined tissues (especially liver, heart and skeletal muscle) except in the testes and lung. Significantly, the expression in the testes is an important safety issue for future clinical research with this serotype.

AAV particles are currently the preferred vehicle for gene transfer in the CNS, because they are not pathogenic, they can transduce postmitotic cells (neurons, astrocytes and oligodendrocytes) (Carter & Samulski, 2000; Monahan & Samulski, 2000), persist in cells without causing insertional mutagenesis, allow a long-term gene expression in the brain (important for the treatment of chronic disease) and spinal cord (Lo et al., 1999; Wu et al., 1998) as well as peripheral nervous system, with no associated immune response (Chen et al., 2007; Federici & Boulis, 2007). In addition, AAV vectors are safe, non toxic and incompetent for replication. The use of AAV vectors for trophic factor gene transfer to CNS also provides the added benefit of producing physiological levels of the protein, thereby avoiding side effects associated with large doses (Tenenbaum et al., 2000). Since the first successful application in 1984 using serotype 2 of AAVr (AAV2) as a vehicle for gene transfer, numerous AAVr serotypes have been isolated and characterized. Although many of these viruses have good transduction efficiencies in various body organs via simple administration, generalized transduction of CNS with relatively non-invasive methods is ineffective. We have commented previously that the BBB acts as a protective barrier that excludes potentially harmful molecules and organisms according to their size, charge and lipid solubility. Consequently, the BBB effectively blocks the spread of AAVr in the CNS (Manfredsson et al., 2009). Researchers then had to resort to directly injecting viral vectors into the brain. These injections produce a robust transduction, but are relatively local and require invasive neurosurgery.

There are currently AAV vectors expressing different capsid proteins with the ability to transduce different cell types of the CNS. Transduction varies depending on the AAV serotype used and the injected brain region. In the mouse brain, AAV1 and 5 can transduce neuronal cells and glial cells, while AAV2 can only transduce neurons (Davidson et al., 2000; Wang et al., 2003). AAV2 can only transduce cells of the nervous system located in the vicinity of the injection site. This implies the need for multiple injections or using agents such as mannitol or heparin to cover larger areas of the CNS (McCarty et al., 2004; Nguyen et al., 2001). After having examined the characteristics of transduction in the adult mouse brain, the following four new serotypes have recently been discovered in primates: AAV7, 8, 9 and Rh10 (Cearley & Wolfe, 2006). Some of the AAV serotypes previously characterized , such as AAV1, AAV2 and AAV5, have varying levels and specificity of transduction (depending on the site of injection) when administered directly into the brain. For example, a large proportion of dopaminergic neurons in the substantia nigra are infected with an AAV2 vector, and the transduction efficiency and diffusion is much lower in the striatum (Björklund et al., 2000).

Most information about efficiency and specificity of AAV vectors for treating CNS disorders comes from studies in animal models in which different vectors are evaluated according to their potential to ameliorate the symptoms of a disease or syndrome. The first clinical trial data in describing gene transfer mediated by AAV vectors in Parkinson's disease, Alzheimer's disease, and Canavan (an autosomal recessive degenerative disorder) are now being reported.

Although invasive strategies for gene therapy are used or proposed for neurodegenerative diseases there are now new serotypes of AAV (as AAV9) that enable non-invasive transfer of transgenes in the CNS.

4. Current gene therapy strategies for Parkinson's disease

Three strategies of gene therapy in parkinsonian patients were first tested in 2006, two were aimed at achieving direct symptomatic benefit and the other was aimed at preventing the natural course of the disease. In the first study, the gene transfer of aromatic amino acid decarboxylase (AAD, an enzyme that metabolizes levodopa to dopamine) to the striatum of PD patients was carried out, using AAV2 (Eberling et al., 2008). The aim was to optimize the symptomatic response to levodopa administration which could then be metabolized to dopamine more stably and constantly. However, the most convincing results were achieved with a triple enzyme transfer approach delivery, using the GTP cyclohydrolase 1 gene (GCH1) in addition to tyrosine hydroxylase (TH) and AAD genes (Shen et al., 2000; Azzouz et al., 2002; Muramatsu et al., 2002).

Dietary tyrosine (Tyr) passes the blood–brain barrier and is taken up and processed by the dopaminergic neuron. Tyr is converted by TH into L-3, 4-dihydroxyphenylalanine (DOPA), which is in turn converted by the aromatic amino acid decarboxylase into dopamine. TH is the rate-limiting enzyme in the dopamine synthesis pathway and its activity is highly dependent on the presence of tetrahydrobiopterin (BH4) which acts as a cofactor. BH4 itself is synthesized from GTP in a three-enzyme reaction where the activity of the GCH1 enzyme is rate limiting. A lentiviral vector of non-human origin was used in the triple enzyme transfer approach, now commercially known as Prosavin , which includes the three necessary genes for dopamine production and where the TH gene lacks the coding region for the regulatory N-terminal part of the enzyme to avoid negative feedback from cytosolic dopamine (Björklund et al., 2010). A clinical trial using this vector was started in 2007. One drawback of the two approaches that are now being used in clinical practice for enzyme replacement for treatment of PD patients is that the vectors used almost exclusively transduce the intrinsic striatal neurons, i.e., cells that do not normally produce dopamine (Björklund et al., 2010)). Therefore, it is conceivable that the accumulation of cytosolic dopamine and its end products will expose the transduced cells to excessive oxidative stress, since striatal transduced cells lack the vesicular storage and release mechanisms, possibly leading to toxic damage or neurodegeneration (Chen el al., 2008; Björklund et al. 2010). Moreover, non-regulated dopamine production induced by overexpression of aromatic amino acid decarboxylase may trigger or aggravate dyskinesias (Bankiewicz et al., 2006; Eberling et al., 2008).

The same AAV vector for gene transfer of glutamic acid decarboxylase to the subthalamic nucleus was used in the second approach. The aim was both to facilitate GABAergic transmission in this region, thereby reducing the overactivation of subthalamus-nigral glutamatergic neurons that mediate a substantial part of the characteristic PD disorders (in a manner analogous to that induced both by lesions and deep brain stimulation in that region) and to normalize output from the nucleus (by adding an inhibitory GABA outflow, thereby reducing excessive excitatory glutamate output to key targets such as the globus pallidus interna and the substantia nigra reticulata). This strategy has also reached phase I clinical trials: the unilateral injection of AAV2-GAD into subthalamic nucleus showed that this procedure was safe and was associated with improvements of parkinsonism (Kaplitt et al., 2007). Although studies of other gene, cell and biological therapies in patients with PD have also shown promise in small, open-label studies, subsequent randomised double-blind clinical trials have not substantiated their initial findings (Marks et al., 2010). A double-blind randomised trial was recently conducted at seven centres in the USA specialising in PD care and functional neurosurgery (Lewitt et al., 2011). This trial was conducted to assess the effect of bilateral delivery of AAV2-GAD into the subthalamic nucleus compared with bilateral sham surgery in patients with advanced PD. The use of this approach in this small phase 2 trial was intended to serve mainly as a proof-of-concept study, and the authors found evidence of a benefit of subthalamic nucleus AAV2-GAD surgery versus sham surgery. The authors also commented that several secondary outcome measures did not show improvement in the AAV2-GAD treatment group compared with the sham group. This result might indicate the absence of a benefit or relate to the fact that this small phase 2 trial was likely to be underpowered for some of the clinical outcomes that are more difficult to achieve, such as, improvement in function, daily living activities and quality of life measures (Lewitt et al., 2011). Subsequent larger clinical trials will be needed to assess whether this treatment is practical for more widespread clinical use.

The third approach uses CERE-120, an AAV2-based gene transfer vector designed to deliver the neurotrophic factor human neurturin (NRTN) to these degenerating neurons as a treatment for PD. Neurotrophic factors are naturally-ocurring proteins that restore function and prevent death of damaged neurons. A phase 1 trial in 12 moderately advanced PD patients did not identify any safety issues, while suggesting possible improvements in several measures of motor function (Marks et al., 2008). A subsequent double-blind-controlled Phase 2 trial in 58 subjects further supported the safety of CERE-120, but failed to discern any benefit compared to sham surgery on the primary endpoint (UPDRS-motor-"off" at 12 months) although there were hopeful signals in the subgroup with longer follow-up and in secondary measures (Marks et al., 2010). Two PD patients in the Phase 2 trial died from non-AAV2-NRTN-related events, and their brains were examined histologically. Although results showed NRTN-immunostaining in the targeted striatum, however, only scarce evidence of neurturin was seen in the substantia nigra compacta (SNc) cell bodies in PD (Bartus et al., 2011). These authors have proposed that human PD is associated with an underlying defect in axonal transport such that there is no effective delivery of NRTN from the source in the putamen to the dopaminergic neurons in the SNc. Their observations also suggest that the transport defect in PD is widespread in the brain: they not only noted deficient retrograde transport to the SNc, but also an absence of anterograde transport to the SN pars reticulata, suggesting that the disease produces defects in transport in dopaminergic and non-dopaminergic neurons (Bartus et al., 2011; Lewis and Standaert, 2011). In animals, Cere-120 not only increases the endogenous synthesis of dopamine, but also protects dopaminergic neurons from the effects of various neurotoxic agents (Kordower et al., 2006), rescuing them from the degenerative process (Herzog et al., 2007). As is the case in any experimental therapy, caution is paramount, but balanced against the potential for a transformative therapeutic breakthrough, it seems right to proceed with further clinical studies.

5. AAV9: The viral vector crossing blood brain barrier

The ability of AAV type 9 (AAV9) to cross the BBB after intravenous infusion (both newborn and adult mice) and transduce large areas of the brain and spinal cord has recently been reported (Foust et al., 2009). This finding has been subsequently corroborated by a second independent group (Duque et al., 2009). The results obtained are of great importance, given the longstanding interest in developing vectors that could cross the BBB. A single intravenous AAV9-GFP injection to newborn mice induced a wide transduction in neurons throughout the CNS; For example, transduction was observed in almost 60% of motor neurons of the spinal cord, in about 65% of Purkinje cells, and 10-20% of neurons in the cortex and hippocampus. Differential exposure of a receptor on the cell surface may explain the propensity of the virus to transduce a larger diversity of neurons in the brain after i.v. injection. However, intraparenchymal injection of the vector affected neurons located in regions that were poorly transduced after systemic injection, for example, the striatum. These results have raised some questions (Saunders et al., 2009): what the role of hemodynamics in the circulation of the virus is and if transduced neurons are simply a product of a greater blood flow reaching them.

Transduced cell types changed from neuronal to glial when AAV9-GFP was intravenously injected in adult animals. Thus, transduction of astrocytes and to a lesser extent of microglial cells was observed throughout the CNS, with nearly 60% of astrocytes in the spinal cord being transduced. It is interesting to note that the AAV9 mediated glial transduction was seen only after intravenous infusion, whereas intraparenchymal injection induced the classical neuronal pattern of transduction. Why does glial transduction depend on the route of administration? It is possible that viral receptors are only expressed in feet of astrocytes that line the brain blood vessels, therefore, restricting access to neurons (Abbott, 2005).

The AAV9 entry mechanism into cells is still to be resolved, as understanding the polarity of the astrocytic transduction can help determine AAV9 receptors. However, it was recently reported that terminal N-linked galactose is the primary receptor for AAV9 (Shen et al. 2011). In the study by Foust et al (Foust, et al., 2009), it appears that AAV9 peripheral administration in adult mouse infected astrocytes, once the virus interacts with the feet of perivascular astrocytes which are in direct contact with vascular endothelial cells. These cells may contain a population of receptors different from those exposed when making direct injections into the brain parenchyma, and the AAV9 mediated transduction properties were especially interesting. Even if the BBB were opened in the adult by the use of drugs, one would not expect that the particles which were still AAV of 80 nm to cross the BBB, thereby preventing the free access to potential AAV receptors in brain parenchyma (Manfredsson et al., 2009). However, following intravascular delivery, AAV9 and other vectors crossing BBB also target liver, heart, skeletal muscle and other tissues, which may cause untoward effects. A major challenge is to confine transgene expression to the CNS when rAAV9 is delivered systemically. Historically, CNS specific promoters have been used

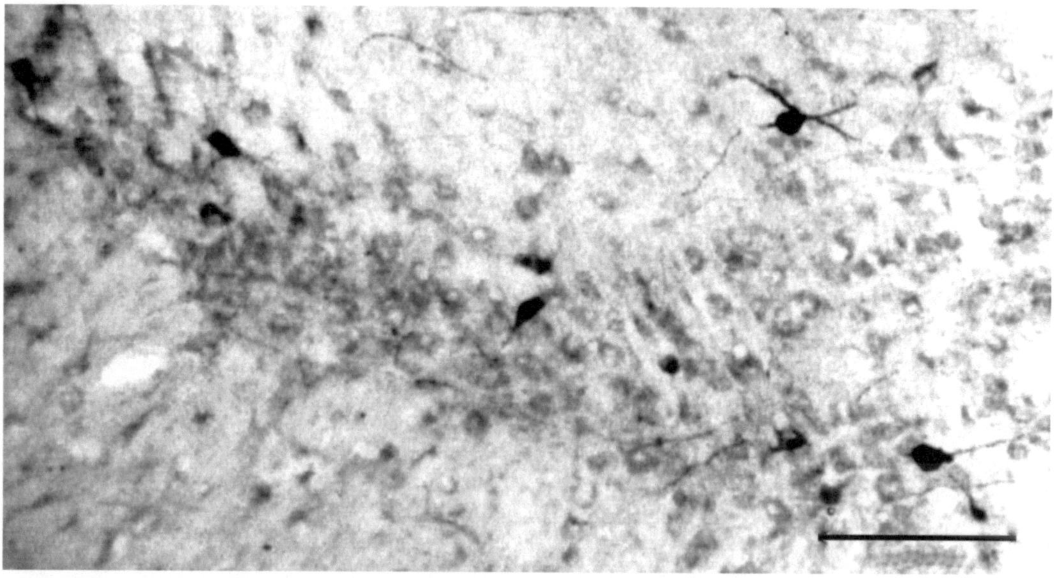

Fig.1. Intravenous injection of GFP-encoding AAV9 mediates substantia nigra transduction in old C57BL/6J mice (twenty months old). A substantia nigra anti-GFP immunohistochemistry staining was carried out after 6 weeks of AAV9 i.v. injection ($4x10^{11}$ vg in 200 µl). GFP^{+} cells can be observed with different intensities of expression. Scale bar 500 µm.

to limit transgene expression to the CNS. However, tissue-specific, strong CNS promoters are often too large to be packaged into the rAAV genome. Several potential challenges remain to using rAAV9 to treat CNS disorders. The first challenge is to deliver rAAV specifically to the CNS. As an alternative, tissue-specific endogenous microRNAs (miRNAs) were recently used to repress rAAV expression outside the CNS, by engineering perfectly complementary miRNA-binding sites into the rAAV9 genome (Xie et al., 2011). MicroRNAs (miRNAs) are a unique class of short, non-coding RNAs that mediate post-transcriptional

regulation of gene expression ranging from developmental processes to disease induction or amelioration. The authors reported the use of miRNAs to detarget rAAV9 expression both separately and concurrently in the liver, heart and skeletal muscle which are the three tissues that are most efficiently targeted by intravenously delivered rAAV9 (Zincarelli et al., 2008; Xie et al., 2011).These are promising findings which could facilitate the development of miRNA-regulated rAAV for CNS-targeted gene delivery and other applications.
AAV9 employment may have important implications for the treatment of PD (Fig.1).
Neurotrophic factors that are secreted, such as GDNF and Neurturin, are important therapeutic agents which have been proposed for the treatment of PD. Since most of these factors are secreted by glia it is easy to imagine that overexpression of trophic factors AAV9 mediated in these cells should produce a significant improvement in cell rescue, similar to or better than that found when the same neurons are therapeutic targets.

6. Nanoparticles-based vectors crossing blood brain barrier

Almost 70% of current clinical trials use viral vectors as vehicles for delivering DNA into cells to repair defective genes. Although viral vectors are effective and are widely used, it is also true that there are still some important safety aspects to be considered when viral particles are used in a therapeutic program (Thomas et al., 2003). The real goal is to achieve an efficient, non-invasive and non-viral gene therapy for the brain because of the obvious side effects of the viral vectors. This will require multidisciplinary approaches from different fields such as engineering, chemistry, cell biology, physiology, pharmacology and medicine. Although this ideal scenario has not been reached yet, a considerable amount of work on nanotechnological gene-delivery strategies to cross the BBB has been done.
The last fifteen years have seen the beginning of another scientific revolution, other than gene therapy, based on the ability to measure, manipulate and organize matter on the nanometer scale. Nanotechnology is defined as the set of knowledge and methodologies to study, manufacture and characterize functional structures with dimensions of less than a few tens of nanometers. The application of nanotechnology in biomedical research is having a significant impact on the development of new types of diagnostic and therapeutic tools. A key focus is the development and use of non-viral vector-based nanoparticles to bring about safe and efficient gene transfer. Among the major advantages of nanoscale vehicles for transfer of drugs is their ability to cross membrane barriers, particularly in the CNS.
The term "nanoparticle" refers to a structure with a diameter in the range of 1 to 100 nm, and was among the first nanoscale materials to have been directly used in biological systems. They must be functionalized in some way to be effective, which means the ability to be filled with, or attached to, therapeutic molecules (such as drugs, nucleic acids ...) or labeled with antibodies or nucleic acids to facilitate detection of a target of interest. They can be made by way of nanocrystals, drug-polymer complexes, or by creating nanoscale spheres (liposomes) able to catch molecules of drugs or other agents (LaVan et al., 2003).
Polymeric nanoparticles have been effective in gene transfer studies (Cohen et al., 2000). They are colloidal particles carrying drugs or genes of interest within a biodegradable polymer matrix. Depending on the method of preparation, nanoparticles, nanospheres or nanocapsules may be obtained. Nanospheres consist of a polymer matrix in which the drug or gene are physically and uniformly dispersed, while nanocapsules represent vesicular transport systems in which the drug or gene is confined in a cavity surrounded by a matrix polymer. Polymeric nanoparticles are more efficient in terms of transport of drugs /genes

compared with traditional oral and intravenous methods (Soppimath et al., 2001). These advantages stem from two basic properties: 1) their small size favors penetration through small capillaries, allowing a greater accumulation of the drug /gene at the target site (Soppimath et al., 2001), this is particularly relevant in the CNS, in which the transport of some drugs is limited because of their inability to cross the BBB and 2) the application of nanoparticles as vehicles for transport of drugs / genes may help overcome this obstacle. In fact, it has recently been shown that polymeric nanoparticles are effective for the transport of peptides and other agents through the BBB (Kreuter et al., 2003; Nahar et al., 2006). The use of biodegradable polymers favors the sustained release of drugs / genes into the target site over a long period (Tang et al., 2009).

Dendrimers are highly branched three-dimensional macromolecules surrounding a central core, which can be designed at the nanoscale with remarkable precision. Dendrimers have a number of free ends, to which molecules of different nature, from therapeutic agents to fluorescent molecules can be attached and transported. Different drugs or DNA molecules can be incorporated at the core, and because of its branched structure, a single dendrimer can carry a high number of molecules compared to other transport systems based on nanoparticles. Multiple terminal groups which are predominantly located on the surface may control the interaction of the macromolecules of dendrimer with their molecular environment. In fact, dendrimers tend to contain more than 100 end-groups, with diverse reactive sites to allow conjugation with different types of molecules (Jain & Gupta, 2008). Moreover, these end groups can be modified to make their interior hydrophilic and to keep their exterior hydrophobic, or vice versa (Sahoo &Labhasetwar, 2003). It has recently been shown that dendrimers can be promising gene transfer vectors for Parkinson's disease. Examples will be included later.

Fullerenes are small spheres of a few nanometers in size (nanospheres), consisting of carbon atoms located in such a way as to form nanoscale hexagonal and pentagonal structures. The best known fullerene is the carbon 60 (C-60), which consists of 60 carbon atoms forming a structure similar to that of a soccer ball. A water-soluble fullerene, derived from the C-60, capable of crossing the cell membrane and that it mainly located in mitochondria has been reported (Foley et al., 2002). This opens up great possibilities for mitochondrial gene therapy, for example, in Parkinson's disease, bearing in mind the important role of mitochondria in this disorder. The carbon nanospheres derived from glucose are an emerging class of intracellular vectors. The surfaces of these spheres are highly functionalized and require no further modification. The *in vivo* experiments have shown that these nanospheres can cross the BBB and are identified in the brain as well as in the liver and spleen (Selvi et al., 2008; Wong-Ekkabut et al., 2008). There is also evidence that nanospheres are continually being removed from these tissues over time.

Although non-viral vectors based on nanoparticles are easily produced and have low immunogenicity, there are issues about toxicity, specificity, regulation of transgene expression and transfection efficiency which need to be resolved before clinical application.

7. Application of nanoparticles in gene therapy for Parkinson's disease

The preferred strategy, in gene therapy of diseases affecting large areas of the brain, would be to administer vectors systemically. The human brain contains around 100 million capillaries covering a surface of approximately 12 m^2 (Bickel et al., 2001). Virtually every neuron in the brain has its own capillary, with an average distance of capillary to neuron of

8-20 microns (Schlageter et al., 1999). The administration of a therapeutic gene to neurons through the capillary membrane would then be the method of choice. However, we have previously seen that the BBB is a serious obstacle to the entry of macromolecules in the brain.

The basic mechanism, coined by Pardridge as molecular Trojan horses, is that a protein or DNA that is going to cross the BBB is coupled /conjugated to a ligand that is recognized by a receptor which is present on the luminal side of capillary endothelial cells of the brain. Once in the blood, the complex protein / DNA-ligand bind to the receptor, performing a process of endocytosis. This complex then moves through the endothelial cytoplasm, thereby avoiding the endosomal / lysosomal system, where it is then left on the abluminal side (brain). This system of transporting proteins across the BBB has been successfully used for vasoactive intestinal peptide, BDNF, epidermal growth factor, but also as pegylated immunoliposomes (ILP) containing plasmid DNA expressing β-galactosidase, tyrosine hydroxylase and GDNF , among others (Zhang &Pardridge, 2009).

We have previously mentioned that the BBB has specific receptor-mediated transport mechanisms, which can be used as a transport pathway of drugs/genes to the brain. The transferrin receptor is particularly interesting because its expression is restricted to the brain capillaries and to neuronal membranes (Jefferies et al, 1984). ILP have been used to deliver genes for the targeting of the brain with colloidal carriers. The transfer of pegylated immunoliposomes from the blood to the brain is achieved by monoclonal antibodies targeted against the transferrin receptor or insulin, which, by binding to their respective ligands induce receptor-mediated endocytosis (transcytosis), then subsequently incorporate foreign genes into the brain parenchyma without damaging the BBB. The gene for tyrosine hydroxylase (TH) has been expressed with intravenous administration of pegylated immunoliposomes in a PD model with 6-hydroxydopamine, which revealed the normalization of expression levels of TH in the striatum (Zhang et al., 2003).

Compared with liposomes, pegylated nanoparticles are physically and chemically more stable and can be lyophilized for long term storage. The pegylated nanoparticles conjugated with cationic albumin (CBSA-NP) may also be used for the transfer of genes to the brain (Lu et al., 2005). Therefore, more CBSA-NP marked with a fluorescent probe are accumulated in mouse brain cells (after being injected intravenously) than when using pegylated nanoparticles conjugated with native albumin. CBSA-NP incorporating plasmid expressing cytotoxic genes have been used for non-invasive experimental gene therapy of gliomas (Lu et al., 2006). Thus, for the first time, the transfer of a cytotoxic gene using a noninvasive route in the mouse brain to treat a malignant glioma has been demonstrated. The current findings encourage further studies into the application of CBSA-NP for noninvasive gene therapy of PD.

Polyamidoamine dendrimers (PAMAM) have recently emerged as a new class of nanoscale spherical polymers to have caught the eye of researchers from various scientific disciplines. It is increasingly clear that PAMAM is a multifunctional polymer with many applications, such as transfer vehicles for antisense oligonucleotides and siRNA (Kang et al., 2005). Moreover, in itself, PAMAM can behave as an efficient gene carrier. PAMAM possessing primary amino surface groups have the inherent ability to associate with and condense DNA, and have been used efficiently in biocompatible DNA transfer (Kim et al., 2004). Good efficiency of transfection is also achieved by modifying the surface of PAMAM with L-arginine. The primary amines located on the surface of these dendrimers allow conjugation with some ligands such as transferrin, to achieve efficient gene transfer to the brain. A vector for gene transfer in the brain was recently developed with this in mind. Remember that the transferrin receptor is expressed in the BBB and the neuronal membrane (Jefferies et al, 1984). Intravenous injection in mice of a nanoscale highly branched dendrimer modified with transferrin and PEG (a hydrophilic polymer that increases the biocompatibility of the vector) (PAMAM-PEG-Tf), induces a higher brain expression (almost double compared to other dendrimeric vectors) of an exogenous gene encapsulated in the vector (Huang et al., 2007a).

Intravenous administration of PAMAM dendrimers conjugated to lactoferrin (Lf) using bifunctional PEG allows the efficient expression of exogenous genes in the brain. As a ligand targeting the brain, the Lf can bind specifically with Lf receptors of brain cells. The Lf is an iron-binding glycoprotein belonging to the transferrin family. One of the advantages of Lf as a ligand for gene therapy in brain is the low plasma concentration of endogenous Lf (5 nM). Its plasma concentration is much lower than the kd of Lf receptors in the BBB (Huang et al., 2007b). This efficiently prevents the competitive inhibition of endogenous Lf with exogenously transference systems of genes/drugs cojugated to Lf. In addition, Lf transport across the BBB monolayer model appears to be unidirectional i.e. from apical to basolateral side. This unidirectional transport could result in a greater neuronal accumulation of such systems of Lf conjugates when compared to conjugates of transferrin. These advantages are partially reflected in a recent study showing that exogenous gene expression in the brain, mediated by nanoparticles conjugated to Lf is almost 5.2 times that obtained with unconjugated nanoparticles (Huang et al., 2008). *In vivo* image analysis has shown that Lf-nanoparticles accumulation was higher in the brain (but lower in other organs) than their unmodified counterparts (Huang et al., 2010a). A recent study has reported significant neuroprotective effects with Lf-nanoparticles carrying the GDNF gene, after being administered intravenously in a rat model of PD induced by the pesticide substance rotenone (Huang et al., 2010b).

However, the application of different transfer protocols has been limited by the lifetime of the protein in circulation, the need for repeated injections or low transference yields achieved in the brain. The recently published paper by Spencer and Verma gives a possible solution to the first two issues (Spencer & Verma, 2007).

The low-density lipoprotein (LDL) receptor (LDLR) family consists of a cell-surface receptors group that binds lipoprotein complexes for internalization to the lysosomes. This family consists of about 10 different receptors that are expressed in a tissue-specific manner and primarily bind apolipoprotein complexes (Brown & Goldstein, 1986). The apolipoproteins, whose more representative members are apolipoprotein B and apolipoprotein E, are attached to blood lipids in order to direct them to lysosomal degradation. Apolipoproteins bind to the LDLR on the cell surface of the targeted cell, and thereby the complex is endocytosed. In contrast, when LDLR binds to apolipoproteins in BBB it induces transcytosis to the abluminal side of the BBB and, presumably, the apolipoprotein is released and taken up by neurons and/or astrocytes (Hussain et al., 1999). Spencer and Verma used a lentivirus vector system to deliver the lysosomal enzyme glucocerebrosidase and a secreted form of GFP to the neurons and astrocytes in the CNS. These authors fused the LDLR-binding domain of the apolipoprotein B to the targeted protein, moreover adding a secretory leader sequence to allow its release. It took a single intraperitoneal injection of lentiviral vector for the protein could be detected two weeks later in the CNS, showing that it had entered through transcytosis by binding to the LDLR (Spencer & Verma, 2007).

The interesting thing about this therapeutic approach is that the lentiviral vector can also deliver genes to a peripheral organ (liver or spleen), which now serve as a source for the prolonged and continuous expression, and secretion of a therapeutic protein which has the ability to cross the BBB. This technique could be used to facilitate the passage of neuroprotective molecules, of interest in Parkinson's disease, through BBB. But there are still some unresolved issues, for example, the immunogenicity of the fusion protein and the restricted cerebral distribution of LDLR, as only a minority of brain cells are transfected. The first problem will be difficult to address while the latter may possibly be solved using other receptors that activate transcytosis, such as the diphtheria toxin receptor (De Boer & Gaillard, 2007).

8. Towards a non invasive gene therapy for Parkinson's Disease

Direct administration of transgenes in neural tissue (iGT) has advantages for the treatment of certain neurological diseases because it avoids the peripheral expression of the transgene (and related immune activation), and widespread central expression (unnecessary in focal neurological diseases). However, iGT also has significant drawbacks, most notably the use of surgical procedures (with BBB damage, nonspecific reactive gliosis, risk of infection ...) that cannot be repeated many times in the case of chronic diseases. In addition, this mode of administration usually induces intense effects on the injected brain regions, but does not diffuse well in the surrounding tissue (exponential decrease of transgene expression with distance from the injection point), and making it difficult to adjust the therapeutic dose. In contrast, non-invasive gene therapy (niGT) allows greater distribution of the transgene in the brain (particularly useful in diseases with diffuse brain affectation) and does not require surgery, thus allowing repeated administration in chronic neurological diseases (the most enduring expression of the transgene has been reported for AAV and has always been less than 10-15 months).

All gene therapy clinical trials for the treatment of PD have used the iGT, which makes sense when the therapeutic objective is aimed at preventing the degeneration of dopaminergic neurons or treating the primary symptoms associated with a specific motor area. However, it is becoming increasingly clear that from its initial stage, PD does affect non dopaminergic neuronal populations of different brain centres (brain cortex, olfactory bulb, *pedunculopontine nucleus, locus coeruleus* ...), inducing symptoms that go far beyond the original motor disorders associated with dopaminergic transmission (autonomic disorders, dementia, attentional disorders, sleep disorders, depression ...). For example, the anatomical substrate of depression has been associated with changes in either noradrenaline, serotonin and dopamine transmission in various centers such as the locus coeruleus, raphe nuclei, or various centers of the basal ganglia and the limbic system (Levy & Dubois, 2006; Remy et al., 2005). While in PD without dementia, cognitive impairments are associated with abnormalities in dopamine transmission in the cerebral cortex and ventral striatum (Owen et al., 1995), PD with dementia also includes disorders in cortical cholinergic transmission (Klein et al., 2010). Therefore, future gene therapy for this disease should target not only the dopamine centres associated with motor disorders, but also other centres and other neurotransmitters. From this perspective, the greatest extension of the effects of niGT (compared with iGT) might be particularly useful in patients with widespread central affectation; such therapeutic actions would be difficult to achieve using iGT.

9. Towards a regulatable gene therapy for Parkinson's Disease

All current gene therapy approaches for Parkinson's disease use non-adjustable constituent vectors, so that in all cases the transgene expression, once introduced in the body, escapes any external-non-adjustable gene therapy (nrGT). It is often true that animal studies show that therapeutic responses induced by nrGT are achieved with significantly lower doses than those capable of inducing undesirable side effects. In fact, in the three annotated gene therapies for PD, the dose which is intended to produce therapeutic responses is significantly lower than that for which undesirable side effects would be expected, suggesting an acceptable safety profile even when using non adjustable constituent vectors (although the available evidence in humans comes from only relatively small samples of patients who have only been followed for short periods after treatment).

Bearing in mind these considerations and taking into account the extensive AAV2 information evidencing either its low toxicity, lack of regulated promoters shown to be safe and effective in patients, and urgent clinical need in numerous neurological diseases (particularly PD), some authors have suggested that the use of adjustable vectors for human gene therapy is unnecessary and could even be inappropriate and potentially dangerous (Kordower & Olanow, 2008). Other authors, however, defend the need for regulatable promoters whenever possible, because they allow continuous monitoring of transgene expression and impede the occurrence of incidents (Cress, 2008). There is little information on the effects of sustained overexpression (months to years) or nonspecific (neurons and glia) of particular genes, which is especially relevant in the case of proteins such as neurotrophic factors whose receptors are widely distributed throughout the CNS. Therefore, it is foreseeable that in the coming years gene therapy clinical trials will start using regulatable gene therapy (rGT) with regulatable vectors (Cress, 2008), which would adjust transgene expression to its maximum biological efficiency with minimum risk of adverse effects.

Transgene expression is coupled to a transcriptional switch in the regulatable vectors (instead of being under the control of a constitutive promoter) whose activity can be regulated by an exogenous chemical. Several regulatable promoter systems by agents such as tetracycline (tet), rapamycin, mifepristone and ecdysone have been tested in animals. The best known regulatory systems are tet systems, which have shown to be efficient and safe in controlling the expression of transgenes in experimental models of various neurological diseases (Régulier et al., 2003; Blesch et al., 2005; Nuber et al., 2008). Tet systems have been developed that can promote activation (tet-ON) or inactivation (tet-OFF) of gene expression, systems that have been incorporated in lentivirus, adeno-associated virus, first-generation adenovirus or high capacity, and retrovirus. The tet system choice depends on the timing of transgene activation which is preferable in each case. It is better to use tet-off for a sustained expression of the transgene, while the tet-ON might be more suitable for transgene expression in shorter time windows, which would minimize the time of exposure of patients to chemicals not without toxicity.

Besides being a safety mechanism against uncontrolled overexpression, regulation of transgene activity could allow flexibility in the control of the therapeutic response, which is difficult to achieve by other methods. The patients' clinical conditions usually change over the course of the disease (Collier et al., 2007); thereby adjusting the dose of rGT could be key to its long-term usefulness. Since the degree of injury is specific for each patient, the response to gene therapy may vary considerably among different patients, so the inclusion

of a failsafe mechanism (in this case of a regulatable vector) could be critical for the treatment of some patients. Neurodegenerative diseases, with the development of biomarkers, could begin to be treated before the onset of symptoms. A regulated system would enable the development of a single gene construct, whose expression could be adjusted to the changing needs of each patient. In addition, advanced systems are being developed that allow the regulation of multiple transgenes introduced into the same vector and are independently controlled by different inducers (Kumar et al., 2004; Goverdhana et al., 2005). This could lead to the development of a complex rGT, in which multiple transgenes (eg, for several neurotrophic factors) may act synergistically on different therapeutic targets.
Despite the many potential benefits of rGT, its clinical use requires further detailed basic studies. There are challenges to be resolved before rGT can be considered as a safe and efficient therapeutic tool. This is the case of regulatable transgene expression inhibition in off (as tet-OFF), which may have toxic effects even at low sustained expression. The penetration would also have to be optimized in terms of the modulating agent in the target tissue /organ. Finally, more studies are needed to determine whether the immune system can recognize components of the system for regulating transgene expression, which may be particularly relevant in cases in which, as with tet-ON, the expression must be maintained for long periods (as would be the case in the treatment of chronic neurological diseases.)

10. Conclusions

Gene therapy is considered to be one of the most promising approaches to develop an effective treatment for PD, and clinical studies using such technology have progressed rapidly in less than a decade. However, the existence of BBB significantly limits its development, so all gene therapy clinical trials for the treatment of PD have used iGT, which has significant drawbacks. It is becoming increasingly clear that from its initial stage, PD does affect non dopaminergic neuronal populations of different brain centres, inducing symptoms that go far beyond the original motor disorders associated with dopaminergic transmission.
The development of new serotypes of adenoassociated vectors, such as AAV9, and of functionalized nanoparticles, such as pegylated immunoliposomes, polymeric nanoparticles, pegylated nanoparticles, dendrimers, fullerenes, as well as specific transporters specific to the low density lipoprotein receptor family, means that it is now possible to introduce and express gene material in nerve tissue following peripherical administration of the above mentioned vectors (niGT). From this perspective, the greatest extension of the effects of niGT might be particularly useful in patients with widespread central affectation, such therapeutic actions are difficult to achieve with iGT. Current gene therapy approaches for PD use non-adjustable constituent vectors, so that in all cases the transgene expression, once introduced it in the body, escapes any external-non-adjustable gene therapy. Therefore, it is foreseeable that in coming years gene therapy clinical trials for PD will start to use regulatable gene therapy (rGT) which would adjust transgene expression to its maximum biological efficiency with minimum risk of adverse effects.
Having crossed the Rubicon, one can then expect the following challenges, for example, to produce efficient vectors with regulatable promoters, to reduce the transduction of peripheral organs, to target vectors to specific neuronal and glial populations, and to demonstrate the reversal of the disease in animal models of PD. The administration of

therapeutic drugs to treat CNS disorders is a common problem shared by pharmacologists and gene therapists, but the field of noninvasive gene transfer in the CNS is on the verge of an exciting step forward. Animal studies are highly promising and it is likely that, in the future, gene therapy procedures will be useful and safe for use in patients.

11. References

Abbott, N.J. Dynamics of CNS barriers: evolution, differentiation, and modulation. (2005). *Cell Mol Neurobiol,* Vol. 25, No. 1, (February 2005), pp. 5-23, ISSN 0272-4340

Azzouz, M.; Martin-Rendon, E., Barber, R.D., Mitrophanous, K.A., Carter, E.E., Rohll, J.B., Kingsman, S.M., Kingsman, A.J., & Mazarakis, N.D. (2002). Multicistronic lentiviral vector-mediated striatal gene transfer of aromatic L- amino acid decarboxylase, tyrosine hydroxylase, and GTP cyclohydrolase I induces sustained transgene expression, dopamine production, and functional improvement in a rat model of Parkinson's disease. *J Neurosci,* Vol. 22, No. 23, (December 2002), pp. 10302–10312, ISSN 0270-6474

Bankiewicz, K.S.; Daadi, M., Pivirotto, P., Bringas, J., Sanftner, L.M., Cunningham, J., Forsayeth, J.R., & Eberling, J.L. (2006). Focal striatal dopamine may potentiate dyskinesias in parkinsonian monkeys. *Experimental Neurology,* Vol. 197, No. 2, (December 2005), pp. 363–372. ISSN 0014-4886

Bartus, R.T.; Herzog, C.D., Chu, Y., Wilson, A., Brown, L., Siffert, J., Johnson, E.M. Jr., Olanow, C.W., Mufson, E.J., & Kordower, J.H. (2011). Bioactivity of AAV2-neurturin gene therapy (CERE-120): differences between Parkinson's disease and nonhuman primate brains. *Mov Disord,* Vol. 26, No. 1, (November 2010), pp. 27-36, ISSN 0885-3185

Bickel, U.; Yoshikawa, T., & Pardridge, W.M. (2001). Delivery of peptides and proteins through the blood-brain barrier. *Adv Drug Deliv Rev,* Vol. 46, No. 1-3, (March 2001), pp. 247-279, ISSN 0169-409X

Björklund, A.; Kirik, D., Rosenblad, C., Georgievska, B., Lundberg, C., & Mandel, R.J. (2000). Towards a neuroprotective gene therapy for Parkinson's disease: use of adenovirus, AAV and lentivirus vectors for gene transfer of GDNF to the nigrostriatal system in the rat Parkinson model. *Brain Res,* Vol. 886, No.1-2 (December 2000), pp. 82-98, ISSN 00068993

Björklund, T.; Cederfjäll, E.A., & Kirik, D. (2010). Gene therapy for dopamine replacement. *Prog Brain Res,* Vol. 184, (September 2010), pp. 221-235, ISSN 0079-6123

Blacklow, N.R.; Hoggan, M.D., Kapikian, A.Z., Austin, J.B., & Rowe, W. P. (1968). Epidemiology of adenovirus- associated virus infection in a nursery population. *Am J Epidemiol,* Vol. 88, No. 3, (November 1968), pp. 368-378, ISSN 0002-9262

Blesch, A.; Conner, J., Pfeifer, A., Gasmi, M., Ramírez, A., Britton, W., Alfa, R., Verma, I., & Tuszynski, M.H. (2005). Regulated lentiviral NGF gene transfer controls rescue of medial septal cholinergic neurons. *Mol Ther,* Vol. 11, No. 6, (June 2005), pp. 916-925, ISSN 1525-0016

Brown, M.S.; & Goldstein, J.L. (1986). A receptor-mediated pathway for cholesterol homeostasis. *Science,* Vol. 232, No. 4746, (April 1986), pp. 34-47, ISSN 0036-8075

Burger, C.; Gorbatyuk, O.S., Velardo, M.J., Peden, C.S., Williams, P., Zolotukhin, S., Reier, P.J., Mandel, R.J., & Muzyczka, N. (2004). Recombinant AAV viral vectors pseudotyped with viral capsids from serotypes 1,2, and 5 display differential efficiency and cell tropism after delivery to different regions of the central nervous system. *Mol Ther*, Vol. 10, No.2, (August 2004), pp. 302-317, ISSN 1525-0016

Carter, P.J.; & Samulski, R.J. (2000). Adeno-associated viral vectors as gene delivery vehicles. *Int J Mol Med*, Vol. 6, No. 1 (July 2000), pp. 17-27, ISSN 1107-3756

Cearley, C.N.; & Wolfe, J.H. (2006).Transduction characteristics of adeno-associated virus vectors expressing cap serotypes 7, 8, 9, and Rh10 in the mouse brain. *Mol Ther*, Vol. 13, No. 3, (March 2006), pp. 528-537, ISSN 1525- 0016

Cearley, C.N.; Vandenberghe, L.H., Parente, M.K., Carnish, E.R., Wilson, J.M., & Wolfe, J.H. (2008). Expanded repertoire of AAV vector serotypes mediate unique patterns of transduction in mouse brain. *Mol Ther*, Vol. 16, No. 10, (October 2008), pp. 1710-1718, ISSN 1525-0016

Chen, J.; Wu, J., Apostolova, I., Skup, M., Irintchev, A., Kugler, S., & Schachner, M. (2007). Adenoassociated virus- mediated L1 expression promotes functional recovery after spinal cord injury. *Brain*, Vol. 130 (Pt 4), (April 2007), pp. 954-969, ISSN 0006-8950

Chen, L.; Ding, Y., Cagniard, B., Van Laar, A.D., Mortimer, A., Chi, W., Hastings, T.G., Kang, U.J., & Zhuang, X. (2008). Unregulated cytosolic dopamine causes neurodegeneration associated with oxidative stress in mice. *J Neurosci*, Vol. 28, No. 2, (January 2008), pp. 425–433, ISSN 0270-6474

Chiorini, J.A.; Kim, F.,Yang, L. & Kotin, R.M. (1999). Cloning and characterization of adenoassociated virus type 5. *J Virol*, Vol. 73, No. 2, (February 1999), pp. 1309–1319, ISSN 0022-538X

Cohen, H.; Levy, R.J., Gao, J., Fishbein, I., Kousaev, V., Sosnowski, S., Slomkowski, S., & Golomb, G. (2000). Sustained delivery and expression of DNA encapsulated in polymeric nanoparticles. *Gene Ther*, Vol. 7, No. 22, (November 2000), pp. 1896-1905, ISSN 0969- 7128

Collier, T.J.; Lipton, J., Daley, B.F., Palfi, S., Chu, Y., Sortwell, C., Bakay, R.A., Sladek, J.R. Jr, & Kordower, J.H. (2007). Aging-related changes in the nigrostriatal dopamine system and the response to MPTP in nonhuman primates: diminished compensatory mechanisms as a prelude to parkinsonism. *Neurobiol Dis*, Vol. 26, No. 1, (January 2007), pp. 56-65, ISSN 0969-9961

Conwell, C.C., & Huang L. (2005). Recent advances in non-viral gene delivery. *Adv Genet*, Vol. 53, Part. 1, (October 2005), pp. 1-18, ISBN 978-0-12-374621-4

Cress, D.E. (2008). The need for regulatable vectors for gene therapy for Parkinson's disease. *Exp Neurol*, Vol. 209, No. 1, (September 2007), pp. 30-33, ISSN 0014-4886

Davidson, B.L.; Stein, C.S., Heth, J.A., Martins, I., Kotin, R.M., Derksen, T.A., Zabner, J., Ghodsi, A., & Chiorini, J.A. (2000). Recombinant adeno-associated virus type 2, 4, and 5 vectors: transduction of variant cell types and regions in the mammalian central nervous system. *Proc Natl Acad Sci USA*, Vol. 97, No. 7, (March 2000), pp. 3428-3432, ISSN 1091-6490

De Boer, A.G.; & Gaillard, P.J. (2007). Drug targeting to the brain. *Annu Rev Pharmacol Toxicol*, Vol. 47, (September 2006), pp. 323-355, ISSN 0362-1642

Di Pasquale, G.; Davidson, B.L., Stein, C.S., Martins, I., Scudiero, D., Monks, A., & Chiorini, J. (2003). Identification of PDGFR as a receptor for AAV-5 transduction. *Nat Med,* Vol. 9, No. 10, (October 2003), pp. 1306-1312, ISSN 1078-8956

Ding, W.; Zhang, L.,Yan, Z, & Engelhardt, J.F. (2005). Intracellular trafficking of adeno-associated viral vectors. *Gene Ther,* Vol. 12, No. 11, (June 2005), pp. 873-880, ISSN 0969-7128

Dos Santos, R.; & Beyer-Nardi, N. (2008). A role for adeno-associated viral vectors in gene therapy. *Genet. Mol. Biol,* Vol. 31, No. 1, (November 2007), pp. 1-11, ISSN 1415-4757

Duan, D.; Yue, Y., Yan, Z.,Yang, J. & Engelhardt, J.F. (2000). Endosomal processing limits gene transfer to polarized airway epithelia by adeno-associated virus. *J Clin Invest,* Vol. 105, No. 11, (January 2000), pp.1573-1587, ISSN 0021-9738

Duque, S.; Joussemet, B., Riviere, C., Marais, T., Dubreil, L., Douar, A.M., Fyfe, J., Moullier, P., Colle, M.A., & Barkats, M. (2009). Intravenous administration of self-complementary AAV9 enables transgene delivery to adult motor neurons. *Mol Ther,* Vol. 17, No. 7, (April 2009), pp. 1187-1196, ISSN 1525-0016

Eberling, J.L.; Jagust, W.J., Christine, C.W., Starr, P., Larson, P., Bankiewicz, K.S., & Aminoff, M.J. (2008). Results from a phase I safety trial of hAADC gene therapy for Parkinson disease. *Neurology,* Vol. 70, No. 21, (May 2008), pp. 1980-1983, ISSN 0028-3878

Essner, J.J.; McIvor, R.S., & Hackett, P.B. (2005). Awakening gene therapy with sleeping beauty transposons. *Curr Opin Pharmacol,* Vol. 5, No. 5, (October 2005), pp. 513-519, ISSN 1471-4892

Federici, T.; & Boulis, N. (2007). Gene therapy for peripheral nervous system diseases. *Curr Gene Ther,* Vol. 7, No. 4, (August 2007), pp. 239-248, ISSN 1566-5232

Foley, S.; Crowley, C., Smaihi, M., Bonfils, C., Erlanger, B.F., Seta, P., & Larroque, C. (2002). Cellular localisation of awater-soluble fullerene derivative. *Biochem Biophys Res Commun,* Vol. 294, No. 1, (May 2002), pp. 116-119, ISSN 0006-291X

Foust, K.D.; Nurre, E., Montgomery, C.L., Hernández, A., Chan, C.M., & Kaspar, B.K. (2009). Intravascular AAV9 preferentially targets neonatal neurons and adult astrocytes. *Nat Biotechnol,* Vol. 27, No. 1, (January 2009), pp. 59-65, ISSN 1087-0156

Gao, G.; Alvira, M.,Wang, L., Calcedo, R., Johnston, J. & Wilson, J. (2002). Novel adeno-associated viruses from rhesus monkeys as vectors for human gene therapy. *Proc Natl Acad Sci USA,* Vol. 99, No. 18, (September 2002), pp. 11854–11859, ISSN 1091-6490

Goverdhana, S.; Puntel, M., Xiong, W., Zirger, J.M., Barcia, C., Curtin, J.F., Soffer, E.B., Mondkar, S., King, G.D., Hu, J., Sciascia, S.A., Candolfi, M., Greengold, D.S., Lowenstein, P.R., & Castro, M.G. (2005). Regulatable gene expression systems for gene therapy applications: progress and future challenges. *Mol Ther,* Vol. 12, No. 2, (August 2005), pp. 189-211, ISSN 1525-0016

Herzog, C.D.; Dass, B., Holden, J.E., Stansell, J 3rd., Gasmi, M., Tuszynski, M.H., Bartus, R.T., & Kordower, J.H. (2007). Striatal delivery of CERE-120, an AAV2 vector encoding human neurturina, enhances activity of the dopaminergic nigrostriatal system in aged monkeys. *Mov Disord,* Vol. 22, No. 8, (June 2007), pp. 1124-1132, ISSN 0885-3185

Huang, R., Ke, W., Han, L., Liu, Y., Shao, K., Jiang, C., & Pei, Y. (2010a). Lactoferrin modified nanoparticles could mediate efficient gene delivery to the brain in vivo. *Brain Res Bull*, Vol. 81, No. 6, (December 2009), pp. 600-604, ISSN 0361-9230

Huang, R.; Ke, W., Liu, Y., Jiang, C., & Pei, Y. (2008). The use of lactoferrina as a ligand for targeting the polyamidoamine-based gene delivery system to the brain. *Biomaterials*, Vol. 29, No. 2, (January 2008), pp. 238- 246, ISSN 0142-9612

Huang, R.; Ke, W., Liu, Y., Wu, D., Feng, L., Jiang, C., & Pei, Y. (2010b). Gene therapy using lactoferrin-modified nanoparticles in a rotenone-induced chronic Parkinson model. *J Neurol Sci*, Vol. 290, No. 1-2, (November 2009), pp. 123-130, ISSN 0022-510X

Huang, R.Q.; Ke, W.L., Qu, Y.H., Zhu, J.H., Pei, Y.Y., & Jiang, C. (2007b). Characterization of lactoferrin receptor in brain endothelial capillary cells and mouse brain. *J Biomed Sci*, Vol. 14, No. 1, (October 2006), pp. 121-128, ISSN 1423- 0127

Huang, R.Q.; Qu, Y.H., Ke, W.L., Zhu, J.H., Pei, Y.Y., & Jiang, C. (2007a). Efficient gene delivery targeted to the brain using a transferrinconjugated polyethyleneglycol-modifi ed polyamidoamine dendrimer. *FASEB J*, Vol. 21, No. 4, (January 2007), pp. 1117-1125, ISSN 0892-6638

Hussain, M.M.; Strickland, D.K., & Bakillah, A. (1999). The mammalian low-density lipoprotein receptor family. *Ann Rev Nutr*, Vol. 19, (July 1999), pp. 141-172, ISSN 0199-9885

J., Pichon, B., Velu, T., & Levivier, M. (2000). Tropism of AAV-2 vectors for neurons of the globus pallidus. *Neuroreport*, Vol. 11, No. 10, (July 2000), pp. 2277–2283, ISSN 0959-4965

Jain, N.K.; & Gupta, U. (2008). Application of dendrimer-drug complexation in the enhancement of drug solubility and bioavailability. *Expert Opin Drug Metab Toxicol*, Vol. 4, No. 8, (August 2008), pp. 1035-1052, ISSN 1742-5255

Jefferies, W.A.; Brandon, M.R., Hunt, S.V., Williams, A.F., Gatter, K.C., & Mason, D.Y. (1984). Transferrin receptor on endothelium of brain capillaries. *Nature*, Vol. 312, No. 5990, (November 1984), pp. 162-163, ISSN 0028-0836

Kaiser, J. (2002). Gene therapy. RAC's advice: proceed with caution. *Science*, Vol. 298, No. 5601, (December 2002), pp. 2113-2115, ISSN 0036-8075

Kang, H.; DeLong, R., Fisher, M.H., & Juliano, R.L. (2005). Tat-conjugated PAMAM dendrimers as delivery agents for antisense and siRNA oligonucleotides. *Pharm Res*, Vol. 22, No. 12, (October 2005), pp. 2099-2106, ISSN 0724-8741

Kaplitt, M.G.; Feigin, A., Tang, C., Fitzsimons, H.L., Mattis, P., Lawlor, P.A., Bland, R.J., Young, D., Strybing, K., Eidelberg, D., & During, M.J. (2007). Safety and tolerability of gene therapy with an adenoassociated virus (AAV) borne GAD gene for Parkinson's disease: an open label, phase I trial. *Lancet*, Vol. 369, No. 9579, (June 2007), pp. 2097-2105, ISSN 0140-6736

Kim, T.I;, Seo, H.J., Choi, J.S., Jang, H.S., Baek, J.U., Kim, K., & Park, J.S. (2004). PAMAM-PEG-PAMAM: novel triblock copolymer as a biocompatible and efficient gene delivery carrier. *Biomacromolecules*, Vol. 5, No. 6, (November 2004), pp. 2487-2492, ISSN 1525-7797

Klein, J.C.; Eggers, C., Kalbe, E., Weisenbach, S., Hohmann, C., Vollmar, S., Baudrexel, S., Diederich, N.J., Heiss, W.D., & Hilker, R. (2010). Neurotransmitter changes in dementia with Lewy bodies and Parkinson disease dementia in vivo. *Neurology*, Vol. 74, No. 11, (February 2010). pp. 885-892, ISSN 0028-3878

Klein, R.L.; Dayton, R.D.,Tatom, J.B., Henderson, K.M. &Henning, P.P. (2008). AAV8, 9, Rh10, Rh43 vector gene transfer in the rat brain: effects of serotype, promoter and purification method. *Mol Ther*, Vol. 16, No. 1, (January 2007), pp. 89–96, ISSN 1525-0016

Kordower, J.H.; & Olanow, C.W. (2008). Regulatable promoters and gene therapy for Parkinson's disease: is the only thing to fear, fear itself? *Exp Neurol*, Vol. 209, No. 1, (August 2007), pp. 34-40, ISSN 0014-4886

Kordower, J.H.; Herzog, C.D., Dass, B., Bakay, R.A., Stansell III, J., Gasmi, M., & Bartus, R.T. (2006). Delivery of neurturin by AAV2 (AAV2-NEURTURIN)-mediated gene transfer provides structural and functional neuroprotection and neurorestoration in MPTP-treated monkeys. *Ann Neurol*, Vol. 60, No. 6, (December 2006), pp. 706-715, ISSN 0364-5134

Kreuter, J.; Ramge, P., Petrov, V., Hamm, S., Gelperina, S.E., Engelhardt. B., Alyautdin, R., von Briesen, H., & Begley, D.J. (2003). Direct evidence that polysorbate-80-coated poly(butylcyanoacrylate) nanoparticles deliver drugs to the CNS via specific mechanisms requiring prior binding of drug to the nanoparticles. *Pharm Res*, Vol. 20, No. 3, (March 2003), pp. 409-416, ISSN 0724-8741

Kumar, M.B., Potter, D.W., Hormann, R.E., Edwards, A., Tice, C.M., Smith, H.C., Dipietro, M.A., Polley, M., Lawless, M., Wolohan, P.R., Kethidi, D.R., & Palli, S.R. (2004). Highly flexible ligand binding pocket of ecdysone receptor: a single amino acid change leads to discrimination between two groups of nonsteroidal ecdysone agonists. *J Biol Chem*, Vol. 279, No. 26, (April 2004), pp. 27211-27218, ISSN 0021-9258

LaVan, D.A.; McGuire, T., & Langer, R. (2003). Small-scale systems for in vivo drug delivery. *Nat Biotechnol*, Vol. 21, No. 10, (October 2003), pp. 1184-1191, ISSN 1087-0156

Levy, R.; & Dubois, B. (2006). Apathy and the functional anatomy of the prefrontal cortex-basal ganglia circuits. *Cereb Cortex*, Vol. 16, No. 7, (October 2005), pp. 916-928, ISSN 1047- 3211

Lewis, T.B.; & Standaert, D.G. (2011). Parkinson's disease, primates, and gene therapy: vive la difference? *Mov Disord*, Vol. 26, No. 1, (January 2011), pp. 2-3, ISSN 0885-3185

Lewitt, P.A.; Rezai, A.R., Leehey, M.A., Ojemann, S.G., Flaherty, A.W., Eskandar, E.N., Kostyk, S.K., Thomas, K., Sarkar, A., Siddiqui, M.S., Tatter, S.B., Schwalb, J.M., Poston, K.L., Henderson, J.M., Kurlan, R.M., Richard, I.H., Van Meter, L., Sapan, C.V., During, M.J., Kaplitt, M.G., & Feigin, A. (20011). AAV2-GAD gene therapy for advanced Parkinson's disease: a double-blind, sham-surgery controlled, randomised trial. *Lancet Neurol*, Vol. 10, No. 4, (April 2011), pp. 309-319, ISSN 1474-4422

Lipshutz, G.S.; Gruber, C.A., Cao, Y., Hardy, J., Contag, C.H. & Gaensler, K.M. (2001). *In utero* delivery of adeno- associated viral vectors: intraperitoneal gene transfer produces long-term expression. *Mol Ther*, Vol. 3, No. 3, (March 2001), pp. 284–292, ISSN 1525-0016

Lo, W.D.; Qu, G., Sferra, T.J., Clark, R., Chen, R., & Johnson, P.R. (1999). Adeno-associated virus-mediated gene transfer to the brain: duration and modulation of expression. *Hum Gene Ther*, Vol. 10, No. 2 (January1999), pp. 201-213, ISSN 1043-0342

Lowenstein, P.R.; Mandel, R.J., Xiong, W.D., Kroeger, K., & Castro, M.G. (2007). Immune responses to adenovirus and adeno-associated vectors used for gene therapy of brain diseases: the role of immunological synapses in understanding the cell biology of neuroimmune interactions. *Curr Gene Ther*, Vol. 7, No. 5, (October 2007), pp. 347-360, ISSN 1566-5232

Lu, W.; Sun, Q., Wan, J., She, Z., & Jiang, X.G. (2006). Cationic albumin conjugated pegylated nanoparticles allow gene delivery into brain tumors via intravenous administration. *Cancer Res*, Vol. 66, No. 24, (December 2006), pp. 11878-11887, ISSN 0008-5472

Lu, W.; Tan, Y.Z., Hu, K.L., & Jiang, X.G. (2005). Cationic albumin conjugated pegylated nanoparticle with its transcytosis ability and little toxicity against blood-brain barrier. *Int J Pharm*, Vol. 295, No. 1-2, (May 2005), pp. 247-260, ISSN 0378-5173

Luo, D.; & Saltzman, W. M. (2000). Enhancement of transfection by physical concentration of DNA at the cell surface. *Nat Biotechnol*, Vol. 18, No. 8, (August 2000), pp. 893-895, ISSN 1087-0156

Manfredsson, F.P.; Rising, A.C., & Mandel, R.J. (2009). AAV9: a potential blood-brain barrier buster. *Mol Ther*, Vol. 17, No. 3, (March 2009), pp. 403-405, ISSN 1525-0016

Marks, W.J. Jr.; Bartus, R.T., Siffert, J., Davis, C.S., Lozano, A., Boulis, N., Vitek, J., Stacy, M., Turner, D., Verhagen, L., Bakay, R., Watts, R., Guthrie, B., Jankovic, J., Simpson, R., Tagliati, M., Alterman, R., Stern, M., Baltuch, G., Starr, P.A., Larson, P.S., Ostrem, J.L., Nutt, J., Kieburtz, K., Kordower, J.H., & Olanow, C.W. (2010). Gene delivery of AAV2-neurturin for Parkinson's disease: a double-blind, randomised, controlled trial. *Lancet Neurol*, Vol. 9, No. 12, (October 2010), pp. 1164-1172, ISSN 1474-4422

Marks, W.J. Jr.; Ostrem, J.L., Verhagen, L., Starr, P.A., Larson, P.S., Bakay, R.A., Taylor, R., Cahn-Weiner, D.A., Stoessl, A.J., Olanow, C.W., & Bartus, R.T. (2008). Safety and tolerability of intraputaminal delivery of CERE-120 (adeno-associated virus serotype 2-neurturin) to patients with idiopathic Parkinson's disease: an open-label, phase I trial. *Lancet Neurol*, Vol. 7, No. 5, (May 2008), pp. 400-408, ISSN 1474-4422

McCarty, D.M.; DiRosario, J., Gulaid, K., Muenzer, J., & Fu, H. (2009). Mannitol-facilitated CNS entry of rAAV2 vector significantly delayed the neurological disease progression in MPS IIIB mice. *Gene Ther*, Vol. 16, No. 11, (November 2009), pp. 1340-1352, ISSN 0969-7128

McCarty, D.M.; Young, S.M. Jr., & Samulski, R. (2004). Integration of adenoassociated virus (AAV) and recombinant AAV vectors. *Annu Rev Genet*, Vol. 38, (December 2004), pp. 819-845, ISSN 0066-4197

Monahan, P.E.; & Samulski, R.J. (2000). Adeno-associated virus vectors for gene therapy: more pros than cons? *Mol Med Today*, Vol. 6, No. 11, (November 2000), pp. 433-440, ISSN 1357-4310

Muramatsu, S.-I.; Fujimoto, K.-I., Ikeguchi, K., Shizuma, N., Kawasaki, K., Ono, F., Shen, Y., Wang, L., Mizukami, H., Kume, A., Matsumura, M., Nagatsu, I., Urano, F.,

Ichinose, H., Nagatsu, T., Terao, K., Nakano, I., & Ozawa, K. (2002). Behavioral recovery in a primate model of Parkinson's disease by triple transduction of striatal cells with adeno-associated viral vectors expressing dopamine-synthesizing enzymes. *Human Gene Therapy*, Vol. 13, No. 3, (February 2002), pp. 345-354, ISSN 1043-0342

Nahar, M.; Dutta, T., Murugesan, S., Asthana, A., Mishra, D., Rajkumar, V., Tare, M., Saraf, S., & Jain, N.K. (2006). Functional polymeric nanoparticles: an efficient and promising tool for active delivery of bioactives. *Crit Rev Ther Drug Carrier Syst*, Vol. 23, No. 4, (July 2006), pp. 259-318. ISSN 0743-4863

Nguyen, J.B.; Sanchez- Pernaute, R., Cunningham, J., & Bankiewicz, K.S. (2001). Convection-enhanced delivery of AAV-2 combined with heparin increases TK gene transfer in the rat brain. *Neuroreport*, Vol. 12, No. 9, (July 2001), pp. 1961-1964, ISSN 0959-4965

Nuber, S.; Petrasch-Parwez, E., Winner, B., Winkler, J., Von Horsten, S., Schmidt, T., Boy, J., Kuhn, M., Nguyen, H.P., Teismann, P., Schulz, J.B., Neumann, M., Pichler, B.J., Reischl, G., Holzmann, C., Schmitt, I., Bornemann, A., Kuhn, W., Zimmermann, F., Servadio, A., & Riess, O. (2008). Neurodegeneration and motor dysfunction in a conditional model of Parkinson's disease. *J Neurosci*, Vol. 28, No. 10, (March 2008), pp. 2471-2484, ISSN 0270- 6474

Owen, A.M.; Sahakian, B.J., Semple, J., Polkey, C.E., & Robbins, T.W. (1995). Visuo-spatial short-term recognition memory and learning after temporal lobe excisions, frontal lobe excisions or amygdalo-hippocampectomy in man. *Neuropsychologia*, Vol. 33, No. 1, (January 1995), pp. 1-24, ISSN 0028-3932

Pardridge, W.M. (2005). Molecular Biology of the Blood-Brain Barrier. *Mol Biotechnol*, Vol. 30, No.1, (May 2005), pp. 57- 70, ISSN 1073-6085

Paterna, J.C., & Büeler, H. (2002). Recombinant adeno-associated virus vector design and gene expression in the mammalian brain. *Methods*, Vol. 28, No. 2, (October 2002), pp. 208-218, ISSN 1046-2023

Pathak, A.; Patnaik, S., & Gupta, K.C. (2009). Recent trends in non-viral vector-mediated gene delivery. *Biotechnol J*, Vol. 4, No. 11, (November 2009); pp. 1559-1572, ISSN 1860-7314

Qing, K.; Mah, C., Hansen, J., Zhou. S., Dwarki, V., & Srivastava, A. (1999). Human fi broblast growth factor receptor 1 is a co-receptor for infection by adeno-associated virus 2. *Nat Med*, Vol. 5, No. 1, (January 1999), pp. 71-77, ISSN 1078-8956

Régulier, E.; Trottier, Y., Perrin, V., Aebischer, P., & Déglon, N. (2003). Early and reversible neuropathology induced by tetracycline-regulated lentiviral overexpression of mutant huntingtin in rat striatum. *Hum Mol Genet*, Vol. 12, No. 21, (September 2003), pp. 2827-2836, ISSN 0964-6906

Remy, P.; Doder, M., Lees, A., Turjanski, N., & Brooks, D. (2005). Depression in Parkinson's disease: loss of dopamine and noradrenaline innervation in the limbic system. *Brain*, Vol. 128, No. 6, (February 2005), pp. 1314-1322, ISSN 0006-8950

Sahoo, S.K.; & Labhasetwar, V. (2003). Nanotech approaches to drug delivery and imaging. *Drug Discov Today*, Vol. 8, No. 24, (December 2003), pp. 1112-1120, ISSN 1359-6446

Saunders, N.R.; Joakim, E.K.C., & Dziegielewska, K.M. (2009). The neonatal blood-brain barrier is functionally effective, and immaturity does not explain differential targeting of AAV9. *Nat Biotechnol*, Vol. 27, No. 9, (September 2009), pp. 804-805, ISSN 1087-0156

Schlageter, K.E.; Molnar, P., Lapin, G.D., & Groothuis, D.R. (1999). Microvessel organization and structure in experimental brain tumors: microvessel populations with distinctive structural and functional properties. *Microvasc Res*, Vol. 58, No. 3, (November 1999), pp. 312-328, ISSN 0026-2862

Selvi, B.R.; Jagadeesan, D., Suma, B.S., Nagashankar, G., Arif, M., Balasubramanyam, K., Eswaramoorthy, M., & Kundu, T.K. (2008). Intrinsically fluorescent carbon nanospheres as a nuclear targeting vector: delivery of membrane impermeable molecule to modulate gene expression in vivo. *Nano Lett*, Vol. 8, No. 10, (September 2008), pp. 3182-3188, ISSN 1530-6984

Shen, S.; Bryant, K.D., Brown, S.M., Randell, S.H., & Asokan, A. (2011). Terminal N-linked galactose is the primary receptor for Adeno-associated virus 9. *J Biol Chem*, Vol. 286, No. 15, (February 2011), pp. 13532-13540, ISSN 0021- 9258

Shen, Y.; Muramatsu, S.I., Ikeguchi, K., Fujimoto, K.I., Fan, D.S., Ogawa, M., Mizukami, H., Urabe, M., Kume, A., Nagatsu, I., Urano, F., Suzuki, T., Ichinose, H., Nagatsu, T., Monahan, J., Nakano, I., & Ozawa, K. (2000). Triple transduction with adeno-associated virus vectors expressing tyrosine hydroxylase, aromatic-L-amino-acid decarboxylase, and GTP cyclohydrolase I for gene therapy of Parkinson's disease. *Human Gene Therapy*, Vol. 11, No. 11, (July 2000), pp. 1509–1519, ISSN 1043-0342

Sondhi, D.; Hackett, N.R., Peterson, D.A., Stratton, J., Baad, M., Travis, K.M., Wilson, J.M., & Crystal, R.G. (2007). Enhanced survival of the LINCL mouse following CLN2 gene transfer using the rh.10 rhesus macaque-derived adeno-associated virus vector. *Mol Ther*, Vol. 15, No. 3, (2006), pp. 481–491, ISSN 1525-0016

Soppimath, K.S.; Aminabhavi, T.M., Kulkarni, A.R., Rudzinski, W.E. (2001). Biodegradable polymeric nanoparticles as drug delivery devices. *J Control Release*, Vol. 70, No. 1-2, (January 2001), pp. 1-20, ISSN 0168-3659

Spencer, B.J.; & Verma, I.M. (2007). Targeted delivery of proteins across the blood-brain barrier. *Proc Natl Acad Sci USA*, Vol. 104, No. 18, (April 2007), pp. 7594-7599, ISSN 1091-6490

Srivastava, A.; Lusby, E.W., & Berns, K.I. (1983). Nucleotide sequence and organization of the adeno-associated virus 2 genome. *J* Virol, Vol. 45, No. 2, (February 1983), pp. 555-564, ISSN 0022-538X

Summerford, C.; & Samulski, R.J. (1998). Membrane associated heparin sulfate proteoglycan is a receptor for adeno- associated virus type 2 virions. *J Virol*, Vol. 72, No. 2, (February 1998), pp. 1438-1445, ISSN 0022-538X

Summerford, C.; Bartlett, J.S., & Samulski, R.J. (1999). AlphaVbeta5 integrin: a co-receptor for adeno-associated virus type 2 infection. *Nat Med*, Vol. 5, No. 1, (January 1999), pp. 78-82, ISSN 1078-8956

Tang, B.C.; Dawson, M., Lai, S.K., Wang, Y.Y., Suk, J.S., Yang, M., Zeitlin, P., Boyle, M.P., Fu, J., & Hanes, J. (2009). Biodegradable polymer nanoparticles that rapidly penetrate the human mucus barrier. *Proc Natl Acad Sci USA*, Vol. 106, No. 46, (November 2009), pp. 19268-19273, ISSN 1091-6490

Taymans, J.M.; Vandenberghe, L.H., Haute, C.V., Thiry, I., Deroose, C.M., Mortelmans, L., Wilson, J.M., Debyser, Z., & Baekelandt, V. (2007). Comparative analysis of adeno-associated viral vector serotypes 1, 2, 5, 7, and 8 in mouse brain. *Hum Gene Ther*, Vol. 18, No. 3, (March 2007), pp. 195–206, ISSN 1043-0342

Tenenbaum, L.; Chtarto, A., Lehtonen, E., Blum, D., Baekelandt, V., Velu, T., Brotchi, J., & Levivier, M. (2002). Neuroprotective gene therapy for Parkinson disease. *Curr Gene Ther*, Vol. 2, No. 4, (December 2002), pp. 451- 483, ISSN 1566-5232

Tenenbaum, L.; Jurysta, F., Stathopoulos, A., Puschban, Z., Melas, C., Hermens, W.T., Verhaagen, Thomas, C.E.; Ehrhardt, A., & Kay, M. A. (2003). Progress and problems with the use of viral vectors for gene therapy. *Nat Rev Genet*, Vol. 4, No. 5, (May 2003), pp. 346-358, ISSN 1471-0056

Thomas, C.E.; Ehrhardt, A., Kay, M.A. (2003). Progress and problems with the use of viral vectors for gene therapy. *Nat Rev Genet*, Vol. 4, No. 5, (May 2003), pp. 346-358, ISSN 1471-0056

Wang, C.; Wang, C.M., Clark, K.R., & Sferra, T.J. (2003). Recombinant AAV serotype 1 transduction efficiency and tropism in the murine brain. *Gene Ther*, Vol. 10, No. 17, (August 2003), pp. 1528-1534, ISSN 0969-7128

Wang, Z.; Storb, R., Lee, D., Kushmerick, M.J., Chu, B., Berger, C., Arnett, A., Allen, J., Chamberlain, J.S., Riddell, S.R., & Tapscott, S.J. (2010). Immune responses to AAV in canine muscle monitored by cellular assays and noninvasive imaging. *Mol Ther*, Vol. 18, No. 3, (March 2010), pp. 617-624, ISSN 1525-0016

Wong-Ekkabut, J.; Baoukina, S., Triampo, W., Tang, I.M., Tieleman, D.P., & Monticelli, L. (2008). Computer simulation study of fullerene translocation through lipid membranes. *Nat Nanotechnol*, Vol. 3, No. 6, (May 2008), pp. 363- 368, ISSN 1748-3387

Wu, J.C.; Sundaresan, G., Iyer, M, & Gambhir, S.S. (2001). Noninvasive optical imaging of firefly luciferase reporter gene expression in skeletal muscles of living mice. *Mol Ther*, Vol. 4, No. 4, (October 2001), pp. 297–306, ISSN 1525- 0016

Wu, P.; Phillips, M.I., Bui, J., & Terwilliger, E.F. (1998). Adeno-associated virus vector-mediated transgene integration into neurons and other nondividing cell targets. *J Virol*, Vol. 72, No. 7, (July 1998). pp. 5919-5926, ISSN 0022- 538X

Xiao, X.; Li, J., & Samulski, R.J. (1998). Production of high-titer recombinant adeno-associated virus vectors in the absence of helper adenovirus. *J Virol*, Vol. 72, No. 3, (March 1998), pp. 2224-2232, ISSN 0022-538X

Xie, J.; Xie, Q., Zhang, H., Ameres, S.L., Hung, J.H., Su, Q., He, R., Mu, X., Seher Ahmed, S., Park, S., Kato, H., Li, C., Mueller, C., Mello, C.C., Weng, Z., Flotte, T.R., Zamore, P.D., & Gao, G. (2011). MicroRNA-regulated, systemically delivered rAAV9: a step closer to CNS-restricted transgene expression. *Mol Ther*, Vol. 19, No. 3, (December 2010), pp. 526-535, ISSN 1525-0016

Zhang, Y.; & Pardridge, W.M. (2009). Near complete rescue of experimental Parkinson's disease with intravenous, non- viral GDNF gene therapy. *Pharm Res*, Vol. 26, No. 5, (December 2008), pp. 1059-1063, ISSN 0724-8741

Zhang, Y.; Calon, F., Zhu, C., Boado, R.J., & Pardridge, W.M. (2003). Intravenous nonviral gene therapy causes normalization of striatal tyrosine hydroxylase and reversal of motor impairment in experimental parkinsonism. *Hum Gene Ther*, Vol. 14, No. 1, (January 2003), pp. 1-12, ISSN 1043-0342

Zincarelli, C.; Soltys, S., Rengo, G., & Rabinowitz, J. (2008). Analysis of AAV serotypes 1-9 mediated gene expression and tropism in mice after systemic injection. *Mol Ther*, Vol. 16, No. 6, (June 2008), pp. 1073-1080, ISSN 1525-0016

Zolotukhin, S. (2005). Production of recombinant adeno-associated virus vectors. *Hum Gene Ther*, Vol. 16, No. 5, (May 2005), pp. 551-557, ISSN 1043-0342

14

Epigenetic Modulation of Adenosine A_{2A} Receptor: A Putative Therapeutical Tool for the Treatment of Parkinson's Disease

Marta Barrachina[1,2], Mairena Martín[3],
Francisco Ciruela[4] and Isidre Ferrer[1,2,5]
[1]*Institute of Neuropathology, Bellvitge University Hospital-ICS, (Bellvitge Biomedical Research Institute-) IDIBELL, L'Hospitalet de Llobregat,*
[2]*Centro de Investigación Biomédica en Red sobre Enfermedades Neurodegenerativas, CIBERNED, Barcelona,*
[3]*Departamento de Química Inorgánica, Orgánica y Bioquímica, Facultad de Químicas, Centro Regional de Investigaciones Biomédicas, Universidad de Castilla-La Mancha, Ciudad Real,*
[4]*University of Barcelona, Unit of Pharmacology, Department of Pathology and Experimental Therapeutics, L'Hospitalet de Llobregat,*
[5]*University of Barcelona, Department of Pathology and Experimental Therapeutics, L'Hospitalet de Llobregat,*
Spain

1. Introduction

Adenosine is a nucleoside distributed throughout the entire organism as an intermediary metabolite. At the extracellular level, adenosine plays multiple physiologic roles, interacting with specific receptors: A_1, A_{2A}, A_{2B} and A_3 (Fredholm et al., 2001). While the A_1Rs and A_3Rs are coupled in an inhibitory way to adenylate cyclase through the $G_{\alpha i/o}$ protein, the A_2Rs are coupled in a stimulatory way to this enzymatic activity through $G_{\alpha s}$ protein (Ralevic & Burnstock, 1998).

Adenosine levels are increased after ischemia, hypoxia, excitotoxicity, inflammation and cerebral lesions. In these situations, it is considered that high adenosine levels play a neuroprotective role (Ribeiro et al., 2002). Interestingly, adenosine regulates the release of glutamate, the main excitatory neurotransmitter of the nervous system (Sebastiao & Ribeiro, 1996). A_1Rs are widely expressed in the brain and have been shown to modulate neuronal excitability by decreasing pre-synaptic release of various neurotransmitters (Fredholm & Dunwiddie, 1988). The most dramatic inhibitory actions are on the glutamatergic system (Masino et al., 2002). In the central nervous system (CNS), A_1Rs are associated with neuroprotective processes (Angulo et al., 2003; Dunwiddie and Masino, 2001). Moreover, they are upregulated in human neurodegenerative diseases with abnormal protein aggregates and it is related to compensatory mechanisms (Albasanz et al., 2007, 2008; Angulo et al., 2003; Perez-Buira et al., 2007; Rodríguez et al., 2006). Regarding A_{2A}Rs, these receptors are concentrated in the striatum, modulating dopaminergic activity, but they are also present in the hippocampus and cerebral cortex, modulating the glutamate release in the brain. Adenosine activity through A_2 receptors (A_{2A}Rs) can eventually give rise to neurotoxicity, neuronal damage and cellular death (de Mendoça et al., 2000). In fact, A_{2A}Rs activity is associated with the outcome of cerebral injury as well as the development of Aβ-induced synaptotoxicity (Canas et al., 2009; Cunha, 2005; Stone et al., 2009).

2. Human brain A_{2A}R localization and implications in PD pathophysiology

As mentioned in the previous section, A_{2A}Rs are G protein-coupled receptors that stimulate adenylyl cyclase through $G_{\alpha s}$ proteins, promoting accumulation of intracellular cAMP (Van Calker et al., 1979). The activation of these receptors mediates multiple physiological effects of adenosine, both in the CNS and in peripheral tissues (Fredholm et al., 2001). Pharmacological activation of A_{2A}Rs promotes vasodilatation, immunosuppression, tissue protection, sleep promotion and depression (Cerqueira, 2004; El Yacoubi et al., 2003; Linden, 2001; Satoh et al., 1998).

A_{2A}Rs are widely expressed, but they are highly concentrated in spleen, thymus, leukocytes and blood platelets. A_{2A}Rs levels in immune cells play a critical role in the protection of normal tissues by attenuating inflammation and tissue damage *in vivo* (Ohta and Sitkovsky, 2001). In the CNS, A_{2A}Rs are highly expressed in the striatum (Peterfreund et al., 1996; Schiffmann et al., 1991). Most striatal neurons (95%) are GABAergic medium spiny neurons (MSNs) which can be divided into two subtypes. One subpopulation projects to the globus pallidus and contains enkephalin. The other subpopulation projects to the substantia nigra and contains substance P and dynorphin. These neurons receive inputs from glutamatergic afferents from cortical, thalamic and limbic areas and dopaminergic afferents from the substantia nigra pars compacta and the ventral tegmental area. MSNs promote two striatal efferent pathways, the "direct" and "indirect", affecting motor activation and inhibition, respectively. The MSNs of the direct pathway correspond to the subpopulation containing dynorphin and they also express dopamine D_1 receptors, whereas indirect MSNs express enkephalin, dopamine D_2 receptors (D_2Rs) and A_{2A}Rs (Schiffmann et al., 2007). In these cells, A_{2A}Rs physically interact (oligomerize) with D_2R, and this receptor-receptor interaction results in a tidy adenosine/dopamine functional interaction controlled by the A_{2A}R/D_2R oligomer. Consequently, two reciprocal antagonistic A_{2A}R/D_2R interactions have been described, namely an intermembrane interaction in which A_{2A}R mediates the inhibition of D_2R, thus modulating neuronal excitability and neurotransmitter release, and an interaction at the level of adenylyl-cyclase in which D_2R inhibits A_{2A}R-mediated protein phosphorylation and gene expression (for review see Ciruela et al., 2011). As a result of this interaction, antagonists of A_{2A}Rs have recently emerged as a leading candidate class of non-dopaminergic anti-parkinsonian agents, based in part on the unique CNS distribution of A_{2A}Rs and A_{2A}R/D_2R oligomers (Fuxe et al., 2003). Moreover, the metabotropic glutamate receptors 5 (mGluR$_5$s) are co-localized in the same GABAergic striatal output neurons and in glutamatergic nerve terminals in the striatum, and they form heteromeric complexes with A_{2A}Rs (Ferré et al., 2002; Rodrigues et al., 2005). This co-localization provides a morphological framework for the existence of multiple mGlu$_5$/A_{2A}/D_2 receptor interactions (Cabello et al., 2009). Thus, it is proposed that the increase in glutamate and adenosine extracellular levels activates A_{2A}R and mGluR$_5$, both synergizing and promoting the inhibition of D_2Rs (Ferré et al., 2007).

Of note is the characterization of A_1R-$A_{2A}R$ heteromers with antagonistic activities between the two receptors, preferentially at presynaptically level in glutamatergic terminals of cortico-striatal afferents to the MSNs (Ciruela et al., 2006; Quiroz et al., 2009). Under baseline conditions, reduced levels of extracellular adenosine stimulate the activity of A_1Rs while glutamatergic neurotransmission is inhibited. Under conditions of neuronal excitability, the extracellular adenosine levels are increased, showing $A_{2A}Rs$ affinity and inhibiting A_1R activity, and promoting the release of glutamate, which in turn also increases activation of $mGluR_5$ synergizing with $A_{2A}Rs$ and thereby facilitating more glutamate release (Rodrigues et al., 2005).
Interestingly, striatal $A_{2A}Rs$ expression levels have been found to be increased in PD patients with dyskinesias; this upregulation is attributed to the effect of levodopa (L-dopa) treatment (Calon et al., 2004). Recently, it has been proven that high $A_{2A}Rs$ levels in the striatum and in lymphocytes correlate with motor symptoms in PD patients who were previously either not pharmacologically treated or were treated with a wide spectrum of drugs and not restricted to only L-dopa (Varani et al., 2010). Therefore, $A_{2A}R$ upregulation in PD, which tonically inhibits D_2R (see above), together with the low dopamine content in the striatum, a consequence of the death of dopaminergic neurons from the substantia nigra, contribute to a synergistic impairment of D_2R function.
It remains to be clarified whether upregulation of $A_{2A}Rs$ levels in PD is a hallmark of the disease or is a consequence of dopaminergic terminal drop-off in the striatum. This issue has been quite controversial, as increased striatal levels of $A_{2A}Rs$ were shown in 6-hydroxidopamine (6-OHDA)-treated rats, as a consequence of dopamine denervation (Pinna et al., 2002), and also in 6-OHDA-treated rats with intermittent L-dopa treatment (Tomiyama et al., 2004).

3. Clinical trials with $A_{2A}R$ antagonists in PD

L-dopa remains the most effective treatment for symptomatic relief of PD, although its pharmacological administration over time induces motor dysfunctions such as dyskinesias (Obeso et al., 2000). One of the strategies to reduce these is the administration of non-dopaminergic drugs that modulate dopaminergic neurotransmission. Indeed, $A_{2A}R$ has emerged as a potential pharmacological target in PD, as its relationship with the dopaminergic system has been clearly demonstrated (Ferré et al., 2002). There have been several clinical trials with $A_{2A}R$ antagonists, such as istradefylline (also known as KW-6002), confirming that their administration to PD patients reduces the "OFF" time and dyskinesias induced by L-dopa treatment (Bara-Jimenez et al., 2003; Factor et al., 2010; Hauser et al., 2003, 2008; LeWitt et al., 2008b; Mizuno et al., 2010; Stacy et al., 2008). As $A_{2A}Rs$ expression levels are nearly exclusive of the striatum, the use of specific antagonists for these receptors could promote a specific brain-area effect (Brooks et al., 2008). Interestingly, it has recently been described how KW-6002 preferentially targets the $A_{2A}R$ within the postsynaptic $A_{2A}R/D_2R$ oligomer located at the MSNs, thus potentiating D_2R-mediated motor activation (Orru et al., 2011). Therefore, although the use of istradefylline as a monotheraphy in PD has not been statistically demonstrated (Fernandez et al., 2010), its administration as a coadjuvant seems to allow a reduction in the L-dopa dose.
As mentioned before, there are heteromers formed by $A_{2A}R$, D_2R and $mGluR_5$ in striatal GABAergic neurons or MSNs (Cabello et al., 2009). It is proposed that the increase in glutamate and adenosine extracellular levels activates $A_{2A}R$ and $mGluR_5$, both synergizing

and promoting the inhibition of D_2Rs (Ferré et al., 2007). Interestingly, it has been demonstrated in a rat model of PD that the simultaneous inhibition of $A_{2A}R$ and $mGluR_5$ synergistically reverses the parkinsonian deficits in these animals (Coccurello et al., 2004). In this line, the use of mGluR type I antagonists as a therapy for PD has been proposed (Bonsi et al., 2007). Overall, this explains why pharmaceutical companies are going after either single compounds or combinations of drugs that will simultaneously antagonize $A_{2A}R$ and $mGluR_5$.

4. Brain DNA methylation

Studies in mice deficient in enzymes that control DNA methylation and the results of folate-free diets have established an important role for methylation in the development of the nervous system (Waterland & Jirtle, 2003). In fact, the manipulation of methylation and acetylation affects neuronal vulnerability in experimental models of neurodegenerative diseases (El-Maarri, 2003). It has also been proposed that memory processes are highly related with the level of neuronal methylation (Day & Sweatt, 2010; Liu et al., 2009).
DNA methylation is a normal process that occurs during mammal embryo development, and it is also implicated in X-chromosome inactivation and repression of proviral genes and endogenous transposons. This chemical modification is one of the most important epigenetic mechanisms in gene silencing in mammals. It is characterized by the methylation of cytosines that precede guanines in the well-known CpG sites. Those genome CpG-rich regions are called CpG islands (CGIs); they present a size between 200 bp and several kilobases. In general, these active gene promoter regions are not methylated, while the inactive gene promoter regions are fully methylated. Most CGIs are found in 5' UTR regions and in the first exon, although they can be found in regions distal to the transcription start site and in intronic regions. In normal tissues, CGIs are usually non-methylated, while they are methylated in tumorous cells, especially in tumor repressor genes (Illingworth & Bird, 2009; Jones, 1999).
Methylation of CpG sites is achieved by the action of DNA metyltransferases (Dnmt) which catalyze the transfer of a methyl group from S-adenosyl-L-methionine (SAM) to DNA. The human DNA Methylome map has recently been published, annotating those genes found methylated in normal tissues and in human diseases such as Alzheimer's disease (AD) and schizophrenia (SZ) (Ballestar & Esteller, 2008). DNA methylation in the CpG sites interferes with gene expression in two ways. The first is interference with the binding of transcription factors to DNA through the methyl group. The second is caused by the binding of specific proteins, such as $MeCP_2$, MBD1 and MBD2, to methyl CpG sites (methyl-CpG-binding proteins, MBDs). These MBDs recruit histone-modifying and chromatin-remodeling complexes to methylated sites (Portela & Esteller, 2010). The importance of these proteins is demonstrated by Rett syndrome, a disease causing severe mental dysfunction and brought on by $MeCP_2$ mutations (Amir et al., 1999).
The role of DNA methylation in the brain is an emerging field of research. Neuronal DNA methylation is modified with lifespan, and the analysis of 12 loci related with AD has revealed an age-specific epigenetic drift in the percentage of DNA methylation (Siegmund et al. 2007; Wang et al., 2008). Moreover, the degree of gene methylation varies among the different cerebral regions, and it has been reported that DNA methyltransferase 1 (Dnmt1) expression levels are different in the various cerebral regions (Ladd-Acosta et al., 2007).

Interestingly, Dnmt 1 is increased in the cortical interneurons where the GAD67 gene is suppressed in SZ patients (Veldic et al., 2004, 2005).

Finally, epigenetic therapies such as the use of demethylating agents are widely established in the treatment of tumors (Herranz & Esteller, 2006), but their use in neurodegeneration is poorly studied. In this line, S-adenosylmethionine (SAM) is a methyl group donor molecule necessary for DNA methylation which is reduced in AD (Linnebank et al., 2010; Morrison et al., 1996). There have been proposals to use it as a therapy for AD (Scarpa et al., 2003). Its administration to cell lines down-regulates PSEN1 and reduces β-amyloid production. In contrast, deprivation of SAM up-regulates PSEN1, increasing β-amyloid deposits in APP transgenic mice (Fuso et al., 2005, 2008). Interestingly, mice treated with L-methionine downregulate GAD67 and reelin levels by increasing DNA methylation of their respective gene promoter regions (Tremolizzo et al., 2002).

5. Endogenous SAM biosynthesis cycle and alterations in PD

SAM is the main biological methyl donor molecule in the methionine metabolic cycle, which is involved in the methylation of DNA, and protein, lipid and polyamine synthesis. Moreover, it is a precursor of glutathione in the liver and also perhaps in the brain (Vitvitsky et al, 2006). When SAM is demethylated, it is transformed into S-adenosylhomocysteine (SAH) which in turn is hydrolysed into homocysteine (HCY) and adenosine. To prevent the accumulation of HCY, it is remethylated to form methionine (Chiang et al., 1996; Lu, 2000) (see Figure 1). The SAM/SAH ratio is also known as methylation potential and its endogenous maintenance is very important.

L-dopa is the conventional drug used in the treatment of PD to minimize the lack of endogenous dopamine in these patients (Lewitt, 2008a; Tolosa et al., 1998). However, chronic treatment with L-dopa has been associated with hyperhomocysteinemia in plasma, peripheral tissues and brain of PD patients, as L-dopa metabolism requires S-adenosylmethionine (SAM) as a methyl donor (Lu, 2000; Müller et al., 2009a; Nutt, 2008; O'Suilleabhain et al, 2004; Zoccolella et al., 2006, 2009, 2010). Interestingly, it has been shown that L-dopa treatment in mice depletes the brain SAM content (Liu et al., 2000). In addition, elevated plasma homocysteine (Hcy) levels have been related to cognitive and motor impairment and have also been associated with the pathogenesis of other neurological diseases such as stroke and AD (Morris, 2003; Quadri et al., 2004; Seshadri et al., 2002). Interestingly, some polymorphisms described in *MTHFR* gene (methylenetetrahydrofolate reductase) have been associated with a reduction in its enzymatic activity, promoting an increase in the Hcy levels in L-dopa-treated PD patients (Frosst et al., 1995; Yasui et al., 2000). Vitamin B_6 enhances the direct flow of Hcy to cysteine, the precursor of gutathione. Deficits in vitamin B_6 induce oxidative stress and, in turn, enhance Hcy (Obeid et al., 2009). Therefore, several factors have been related with hyperhomocysteinemia and a concomitant reduction in the SAM levels in blood and cerebrospinal fluid of L-dopa-treated PD patients (Cheng et al., 1997). These include the following: 1. An excessive production of S-adenosylhomocysteine (SAH) when L-dopa is metabolized by catechol-O-methyltransferase (COMT), depleting the SAM levels an in turn decreasing the SAM/SAH ratio; 2. Reduced MTHFR enzymatic activity; and 3. Vitamin B_{12} or folic acid deficits (Dos Santos et al., 2009; Miller et al., 2003; Müller et al., 2001, 2009b; Woitalla et al., 2004). In this context, some clinical trials have been carried out using decarboxylase and COMT inhibitors (for instance, carbidopa and entacapone/tolcapone, respectively) or vitamin B_{12} and folate supplementation to reduce Hcy levels in PD patients (Müller et al., 2003, 2006; Zoccolella et al., 2007).

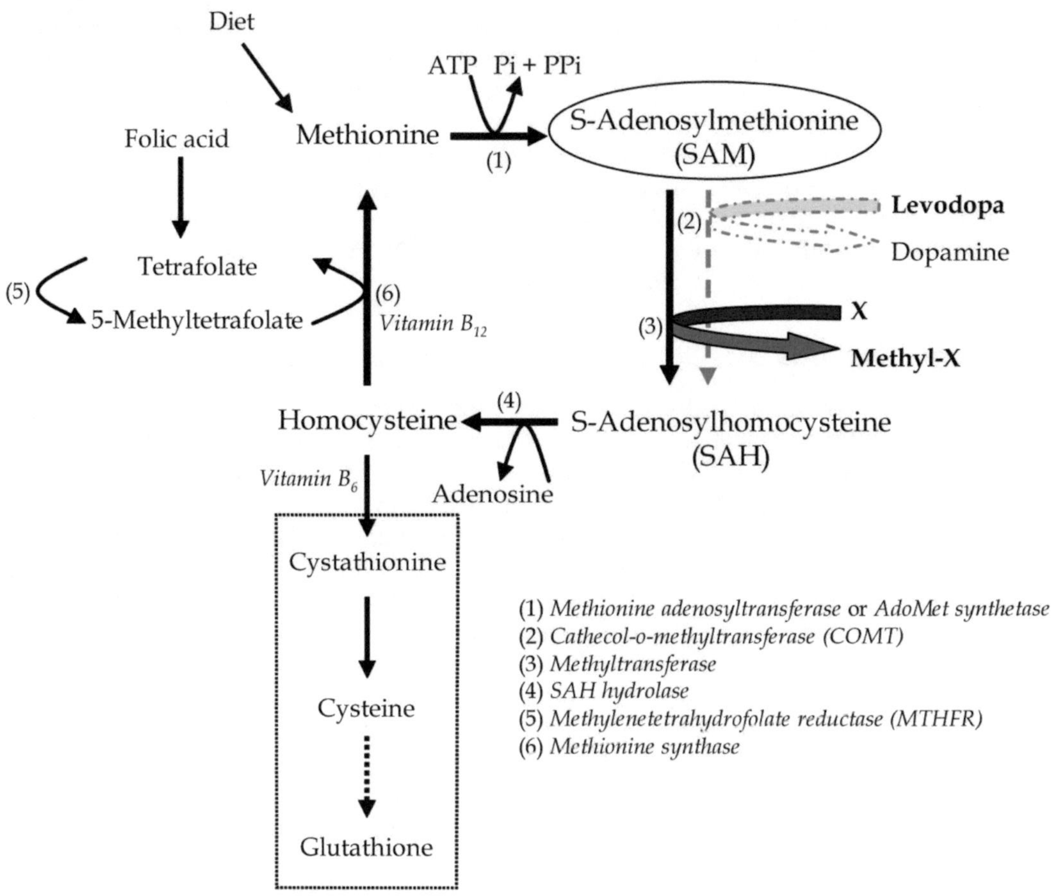

Fig. 1. SAM biosynthesis cycle

6. Epigenetic study of *ADORA2A*

$A_{2A}R$ gene (ADORA2A) is localized to chromosome 22 (Le et al., 1996; MacCollin et al., 1994; Peterfreund et al., 1996). It consists of two coding exons (exon 2 and 3) separated by a single intron of nearly 7 Kb. The exon 1 is a non-coding exon which is located at 5′ upstream exon 2 and presents 6 tissue-specific isoforms: h1A-h1F (Yu et al., 2004) (Figure 2A). Interestingly, differential expression of these isoforms has been reported in granulocytes of patients suffering from sepsis, indicating that 5′ UTR plays an important regulatory role in $A_{2A}R$ expression (Kreth et al., 2008). We recently identified a functional CGI surrounding the h1E isoform, demonstrating that DNA methylation controls basal *ADORA2A* expression in several cell lines and that it is one of the molecular mechanisms responsible for $A_{2A}Rs'$ differential expression levels in specific human brain areas, such as the putamen and the cerebellum (Buira et al., 2010a, 2010b). Interestingly, we showed that $A_{2A}R$ expression levels can be modulated by SAM treatment in SH-SY5Y (human neuroblastoma) and U87MG (human glioblastoma) cell lines. In this context, A_{2A}Rs levels have been reported to be upregulated in PD patients (Calon et al., 2004; Varani et al., 2010). Therefore, we postulated that SAM treatment could represent a therapeutical tool to reduce A_{2A}Rs levels in these patients. This is based on the fact that the DNA methylation profile of striatal *ADORA2A* in PD patients is lower than the one found in SH-SY5Y and U87MG cells (Figure 2B). Therefore, as A_{2A}Rs cell surface levels are reduced in these cells after SAM treatment, due to an increase in the DNA methylation profile of *ADORA2A* (Buira et al., 2010a), it is also plausible that the same mechanism of action could play a role in the striatum of PD patients.

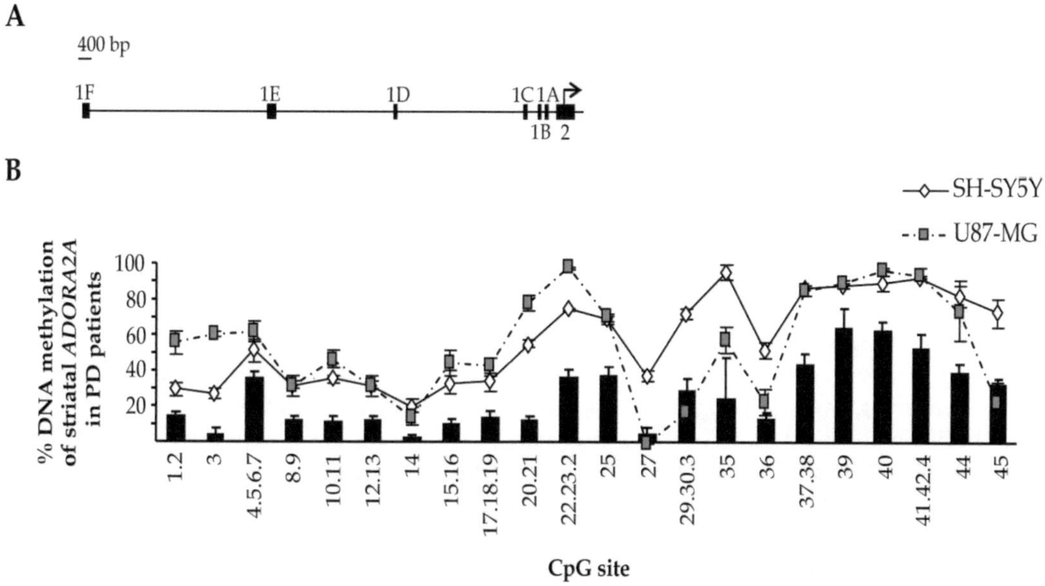

Fig. 2. A, Scaled representation of 5′ UTR region of human *ADORA2A* gene, containing 6 isoforms of non-coding exon 1 (1A-1F). Two CGIs surrounding exon 1E were recently described (Buira et al., 2010b). The translational start site (ATG) is indicated with an arrow. B, DNA methylation percentage (mean ± SD) of a locus located in the CGIs of exon 1E of 8 human post-mortem putamens of PD (black bars) and in two cell lines (black line, SH-SY5Y, n=3; dotted lines, U87-MG, n=3).

7. Clinical trials with SAM

SAM has been widely used for the treatment of liver diseases, as it increases the glutathione content (Friedel et al. 1989). Interestingly, SAM has antidepressant properties and its long term tolerability is excellent, presenting few side effects (Bell et al., 1988; Bottiglieri & Hyland, 1994; Delle Chiaie et al., 2002; Kagan et al., 1990; Lipinski et al., 1984; Papakostas, 2009, 2010). Moreover, SAM administration in patients with depression and dementia, intravenously or orally, has shown that it crosses the blood-brain barrier, and as a result, it is detected at increased levels in the cerebrospinal fluid (Bottiglieri et al., 1990).

Impaired transmethylation potential in L-dopa-treated PD patients has been proposed (De Bonis et al., 2010). The authors argue that a possible global DNA hypomethylation in hyperhomocysteinemic PD patients could be responsible for a generalized gene expression dysregulation and for playing a role in the outcome of the pathology. In accordance with this, another study has shown improved cognitive function in PD patients with a higher SAM/SAH ratio and higher plasma vitamin B_6 (Obeid et al., 2009). It is noteworthy that SAM treatment improved depression of PD patients in an open-label clinical trial (Di Rocco et al., 2000). In fact, vitamin dietary supplementation, including SAM, has been shown to be effective in patients with early and moderate stages of AD (Chan et al., 2008; Panza et al., 2009; Remington et al., 2009; Shea and Chan, 2008). Moreover, SAM supplementation also presented antioxidant properties in an AD animal model (Cavallaro et al., 2010). In line with this, oxidative stress is also present in early-stages of PD (Ferrer et al., 2010), which points up the benefits of SAM administration in this pathology as an adjunctive treatment.

8. Conclusions and proposals for future PD interventions

As mentioned in the introduction, it is noteworthy that inactivation of A_{2A}Rs enhances the affinity of D_2Rs for dopamine, this being the probable mechanism underlying the prodopaminergic effect of A_{2A}Rs antagonists in several clinical trials with PD patients. In this chapter, we have examined the literature which, in combination with our studies based on *ADORA2A* transcriptional regulation, has led us to propose SAM treatment as an epigenetic tool to modulate the increased expression of A_{2A}Rs in PD.

It is obvious that SAM treatment presents a broad spectrum of gene targets, and not only tumor supressor genes. However, it has been reported that SAM treatment promotes a decrease in the growth of hepatocellular carcinoma cells and liver cancer in animal models, hypothesising the methylation and repression of oncogenic gene promoters by this drug (Cai et al., 1998; Pascale et al., 1992). However, the existence of several clinical trials with SAM and the reduced number of side-effects in its administration must be taken into account. Based on our studies, and bearing in mind the restrictive expression of A_{2A}Rs in the brain (mainly in 95% of striatal neurons), we postulate that SAM treatment would have a "specific" effect on A_{2A}Rs in the brain. This would be especially true in a cerebral region where it colocalizes with D_2Rs, which in turn present reduced activity due to the low dopamine content in PD. Then, although SAM treatment would reduce the expression of hypomethylated genes, its effect on A_{2A}Rs might represent significant activation of D_2Rs.

Thus, the possible beneficial role of SAM in these patients should be examined in randomized controlled studies, examining supplementation to L-dopa (allowing a reduction of its dose) and to A_{2A}Rs antagonists (such as istradefylline), or in triple administration with both current therapies.

9. Acknowledgments

We are very grateful to Dr. Sandra Pérez Buira, Dr. José Luis Albasanz, Guido Dentesano and Jesús Moreno for their contributions to the study of *ADORA2A* transcriptional regulation. We thank T. Yohannan for editorial help. The experimental work described in the present chapter was funded by grants from the Ministerio de Ciencia e Innovación, (PI05/1631, CP08/00095, BFU2008-00138), the European Union through the Marie-Curie Research Training Network PRAIRIES (Contract MRTN-CT-2006-035810), the Consejería de Educación y Ciencia (PCI08-0125), the Consejería de Sanidad-FISCAM (PI-2007/50 and G-2007-C/13) of the Junta de Comunidades de Castilla-La Mancha and the Fundació La Marató de TV3 (092330, 090331).

10. References

Albasanz, J.L.; Rodríguez, A.; Ferrer, I. & Martín, M. (2007). Up-regulation of adenosine A1 receptors in frontal cortex from Pick's disease cases. *The European journal of neuroscience*, Vol.26, No.12, pp. 3501-3508

Albasanz, J.L.; Perez, S.; Barrachina, M.; Ferrer, I. & Martín, M. (2008). Up-regulation of adenosine receptors in the frontal cortex in Alzheimer's disease. *Brain pathology*, Vol.18, No.2, pp. 211-219

Amir, R.E.; Van den Veyver, I.B.; Wan, M.; Tran, C.Q.; Francke, U. & Zoghbi, H.Y. (1999). Rett syndrome is caused by mutations in X-linked MECP2, encoding methyl-CpG-binding protein 2. *Nature Genetics*, Vol.23, No.2, pp. 185-188

Angulo, E.; Casadó, V.; Mallol, J., Canela, E.I., Viñals, F., Ferrer, I., Lluis, C. & Franco, R. (2003). A1 adenosine receptors accumulate in neurodegenerative structures in Alzheimer disease and mediate both amyloid precursor protein processing and tau phosphorylation and translocation. *Brain pathology*, Vol.13, No.4, pp. 440-451

Ballestar, E. & Esteller, M. (2008). SnapShot: the human DNA methylome in health and disease. *Cell*, Vol.135, No.6, pp. 1144-1144

Bara-Jimenez, W.; Sherzai, A.; Dimitrova, T.; Favit, A.; Bibbiani, F.; Gillespie, M.; Morris, M.J.; Mouradian, M.M. & Chase, T.N. (2003). Adenosine A(2A) receptor antagonist treatment of Parkinson's disease. *Neurology*, Vol.61, No.3, pp. 293-296

Bell, K.M.; Plon, L.; Bunney, W.E. Jr. & Potkin, S.G. (1988). S-adenosylmethionine treatment of depression: a controlled clinical trial. *The American journal of psychiatry*, Vol.145, No.9, pp. 1110-1114

Bonsi, P.; Cuomo, D.; Picconi, B.; Sciamanna, G.; Tscherter, A.; Tolu, M.; Bernardi, G.; Calabresi, P. & Pisani, A. (2007). Striatal metabotropic glutamate receptors as a target for pharmacotherapy in Parkinson's disease. *Amino acids*, Vol.32, No.2, pp. 189-195

Bottiglieri, T.; Godfrey, P.; Flynn, T.; Carney, M.W.; Toone, B.K. & Reynolds, E.H. (1990). Cerebrospinal fluid S-adenosylmethionine in depression and dementia: effects of treatment with parenteral and oral S-adenosylmethionine. *Journal of neurology, neurosurgery, and psychiatry*, Vol.53, No.12, pp. 1096-1098

Bottiglieri, T. & Hyland, K. (1994). S-adenosylmethionine levels in psychiatric and neurological disorders: a review. *Acta neurologica Scandinavica. Supplementum*, Vol. 154, pp. 19-26

Brooks, D.J.; Doder, M.; Osman, S.; Luthra, S.K.; Hirani, E.; Hume, S.; Kase, H.; Kilborn, J.; Martindill, S. & Mori, A. (2008). Positron emission tomography analysis of [11C]KW-6002 binding to human and rat adenosine A2A receptors in the brain. *Synapse*, Vol.62, No.9, pp. 671-681

Buira, S.P.; Albasanz, J.L.; Dentesano, G.; Moreno, J.; Martín, M.; Ferrer, I. & Barrachina, M. (2010a). DNA methylation regulates adenosine A(2A) receptor cell surface expression levels. *Journal of neurochemistry*, Vol.112, No.5, pp. 1273-1285

Buira, S.P.; Dentesano, G.; Albasanz, J.L.; Moreno, J.; Martín, M.; Ferrer, I. & Barrachina, M. (2010b). DNA methylation and Yin Yang-1 repress adenosine A2A receptor levels in human brain. *Journal of neurochemistry*, Vol.115, No.1, pp. 283-295

Cabello, N.; Gandía, J.; Bertarelli, D.C.; Watanabe, M.; Lluís, C.; Franco, R.; Ferré, S.; Luján, R. & Ciruela, F. (2009). Metabotropic glutamate type 5, dopamine D2 and adenosine A2a receptors form higher-order oligomers in living cells. *Journal of neurochemistry*, Vol. 109, No.5, pp. 1497-1507

Cai, J.; Mao, Z.; Hwang, J.J. & Lu, S.C. (1998). Differential expression of methionine adenosyltransferase genes influences the rate of growth of human hepatocellular carcinoma cells. *Cancer research*, Vol.58, No.7, pp. 1444-1450

Calon, F.; Dridi, M.; Hornykiewicz, O.; Bédard, P.J.; Rajput, A.H. & Di Paolo, T. (2004). Increased adenosine A2A receptors in the brain of Parkinson's disease patients with dyskinesias. *Brain*, Vol.127, No.Pt 5, pp. 1075-1084

Canas, P.M.; Porciúncula, L.O.; Cunha, G.M.; Silva, C.G.; Machado, N.J.; Oliveira, J.M.; Oliveira, C.R. & Cunha, R.A. (2009). Adenosine A2A receptor blockade prevents synaptotoxicity and memory dysfunction caused by beta-amyloid peptides via p38 mitogen-activated protein kinase pathway. *The Journal of neuroscience*, Vol.29, No.47, pp. 14741-14751

Cavallaro, R.A.; Fuso, A.; Nicolia, V. & Scarpa, S. (2010). S-adenosylmethionine prevents oxidative stress and modulates glutathione metabolism in TgCRND8 mice fed a B-vitamin deficient diet. *Journal of Alzheimer's disease*, Vol.20, No.4, pp. 997-1002

Cerqueira, M.D. (2004). The future of pharmacologic stress: selective A2A adenosine receptor agonists. *The American journal of cardiology*, Vol.94, No.2A, pp. 33D-40D

Chan, A.; Paskavitz, J.; Remington, R.; Rasmussen, S. & Shea, T.B. (2008). Efficacy of a vitamin/nutriceutical formulation for early-stage Alzheimer's disease: a 1-year, open-label pilot study with a 16-month caregiver extension. *American journal of Alzheimer's disease and other dementias*, Vol.23, No.6, pp. 571-585

Cheng, H.; Gomes-Trolin, C.; Aquilonius, S.M.; Steinberg, A.; Löfberg, C.; Ekblom, J. & Oreland, L. (1997). Levels of L-methionine S-adenosyltransferase activity in erythrocytes and concentrations of S-adenosylmethionine and S-adenosylhomocysteine in whole blood of patients with Parkinson's disease. *Experimental neurology*, Vol.145, No.2Pt1, pp. 580-585

Chiang, P.K.; Gordon, R.K.; Tal, J.; Zeng, G.C.; Doctor, B.P.; Pardhasaradhi, K. & McCann P.P. (1996). S-Adenosylmethionine and methylation. *The FASEB journal*, Vol.10, No.4, pp. 471-480

Ciruela, F.; Casadó, V.; Rodrigues, R.J.; Luján, R.; Burgueño, J.; Canals, M.; Borycz, J.; Rebola, N.; Goldberg, S.R.; Mallol, J.; Cortés, A.; Canela, E.I.; López-Giménez, J.F.; Milligan, G.; Lluis, C.; Cunha, R.A.; Ferré, S. & Franco, R. (2006). Presynaptic control of striatal glutamatergic neurotransmission by adenosine A1-A2A receptor heteromers. *The Journal of neuroscience*, Vol.26, No.7 pp. 2080-2087

Ciruela, F.; Gómez-Soler, M.; Guidolin, D.; Borroto-Escuela, D.O.; Agnati, L.F.; Fuxe, K. & Fernández-Dueñas, V. (2011). Adenosine receptor containing oligomers: Their role in the control of dopamine and glutamate neurotransmission in the brain. *Biochimica et biophysica acta*, Vol.1808, No.5, pp. 1245-1255

Coccurello, R.; Breysse, N. & Amalric, M. (2004). Simultaneous blockade of adenosine A2A and metabotropic glutamate mGlu5 receptors increase their efficacy in reversing Parkinsonian deficits in rats. *Neuropsychopharmacology*, Vol.29, No.8, pp. 1451-1461

Cunha, R.A. (2005). Neuroprotection by adenosine in the brain: From A(1) receptor activation to A (2A) receptor blockade. *Purinergic signalling*, Vol.1, No.2, pp. 111-134

Day, J.J. & Sweatt, J.D. (2010). DNA methylation and memory formation. *Nature neuroscience*, Vol.13, No.11, pp. 1319-1323

De Bonis, M.L., Tessitore, A., Pellecchia, M.T., Longo, K., Salvatore, A., Russo, A., Ingrosso, D., Zappia, V., Barone, P., Galletti, P. & Tedeschi, G. (2010). Impaired transmethylation potential in Parkinson's disease patients treated with L-Dopa. *Neuroscience letters*, Vol.468, No.3, pp. 287-291

Delle Chiaie, R.; Pancheri, P. & Scapicchio, P. (2002). Efficacy and tolerability of oral and intramuscular S-adenosyl-L-methionine 1,4-butanedisulfonate (SAMe) in the treatment of major depression: comparison with imipramine in 2 multicenter studies. *The American journal of clinical nutrition*, Vol.76, No.5, pp. 1172S-1176S

Di Rocco, A.; Rogers, J.D.; Brown, R.; Werner, P. & Bottiglieri, T. (2000). S-Adenosyl-Methionine improves depression in patients with Parkinson's disease in an open-label clinical trial. *Movement disorders*, Vol.15, No.6, pp. 1225-1229

de Mendonça, A.; Sebastião, A.M. & Ribeiro, J.A. (2000). Adenosine: does it have a neuroprotective role after all? *Brain research. Brain research reviews*, Vol.33, No.2-3, pp. 258-274

Dos Santos, E.F.; Busanello, E.N.; Miglioranza, A.; Zanatta, A.; Barchak, A.G.; Vargas, C.R.; Saute, J.; Rosa, C.; Carrion, M.J.; Camargo, D.; Dalbem, A.; da Costa, J.C.; de Sousa Miguel, S.R.; de Mello Rieder, C.R. & Wajner, M. (2009). Evidence that folic acid deficiency is a major determinant of hyperhomocysteinemia in Parkinson's disease. *Metabolic brain disease*, Vol.4, No.2, pp. 257-269

Dunwiddie, T.V. & Masino, S.A. (2001). The role and regulation of adenosine in the central nervous system. *Annual review of neuroscience*, Vol. 24, pp. 31-55

El-Maarri, O. (2003). DNA methylation and human diseases. *Advances in experimental medicine and biology*, Vol.544, pp. 135-144

El Yacoubi, M.; Costentin, J. & Vaugeois, J.M. (2003). Adenosine A2A receptors and depression. *Neurology*, Vol.61, No.11 Suppl 6, pp. S82-S87

Factor, S.; Mark, M.H.; Watts, R.; Struck, L.; Mori, A.; Ballerini, R.; Sussman, N.M. & Istradefylline 6002-US-007 Study Group. (2010). A long-term study of istradefylline in subjects with fluctuating Parkinson's disease. *Parkinsonism & related disorders*, Vol.16, No.6, pp. 423-426

Fernandez, H.H.; Greeley, D.R.; Zweig, R.M.; Wojcieszek, J.; Mori, A.; Sussman, N.M. & 6002-US-051 Study Group. (2010). Istradefylline as monotherapy for Parkinson disease: results of the 6002-US-051 trial. *Parkinsonism & related disorders*, Vol.16, No.1, pp. 16-20

Ferré, S.; Karcz-Kubicha, M.; Hope, B.T.; Popoli, P.; Burgueño, J.; Gutiérrez, M.A.; Casadó, V.; Fuxe, K.; Goldberg, S.R.; Lluis, C.; Franco, R. & Ciruela, F. (2002). Synergistic interaction between adenosine A2A and glutamate mGlu5 receptors: implications for striatal neuronal function. *Proceeding of the National Academy of Sciences of the United States of America*, Vol.99, No.18, pp.11940-11945

Ferré, S.; Ciruela, F.; Woods, A.S.; Lluis, C. & Franco, R. (2007). Functional relevance of neurotransmitter receptor heteromers in the central nervous system. *Trends in Neuroscience*, Vol.30, No.9, pp. 440-446

Ferrer, I.; Martinez, A.; Blanco, R.; Dalfó, E. & Carmona, M. (2010) Neuropathology of sporadic Parkinson disease before the appearance of parkinsonism: preclinical Parkinson disease. *Journal of neural transmission*, 2010 Sep 23. [Epub ahead of print]

Fredholm, B.B. & Dunwiddie, T.V. (1988). How does adenosine inhibit transmitter release? *Trends in pharmacological sciences*, Vol.9, No.4, pp. 130-134

Fredholm, B.B.; IJzerman, A.P.; Jacobson, K.A.; Klotz, K.N. & Linden, J. (2001). International Union of Pharmacology. XXV. Nomenclature and classification of adenosine receptors. *Pharmacological reviews*, Vol.53, No.4, pp. 527-552

Friedel, H.A.; Goa, K.L. & Benfield, P. (1989). S-adenosyl-L-methionine. A review of its pharmacological properties and therapeutic potential in liver dysfunction and affective disorders in relation to its physiological role in cell metabolism. *Drugs*, Vol.38, No.3, pp. 389-416

Frosst, P.; Blom, H.J.; Milos, R.; Goyette, P.; Sheppard, C.A.; Matthews, R.G.; Boers, G.J.; den Heijer, M.; Kluijtmans, L.A.; van den Heuvel, L.P.; et al. (1995). A candidate genetic risk factor for vascular disease: a common mutation in methylenetetrahydrofolate reductase. *Nature genetics*, Vol.10, No.1, pp. 111-113

Fuso, A.; Seminara, L.; Cavallaro, R.A.; D'Anselmi, F. & Scarpa, S. (2005). S-adenosylmethionine/homocysteine cycle alterations modify DNA methylation status with consequent deregulation of PS1 and BACE and beta-amyloid production. *Molecular and cellular neurosciences*, Vol.28, No.1, pp. 195-204

Fuso, A.; Nicolia, V.; Cavallaro, R.A.; Ricceri, L.; D'Anselmi, F.; Coluccia, P.; Calamandrei, G. & Scarpa, S. (2008). B-vitamin deprivation induces hyperhomocysteinemia and brain S-adenosylhomocysteine, depletes brain S-adenosylmethionine, and enhances PS1 and BACE expression and amyloid-beta deposition in mice. *Molecular and cellular neurosciences*, Vol.37, No.4, pp. 731-746

Fuxe, K.; Agnati, L.F.; Jacobsen, K.; Hillion, J.; Canals, M.; Torvinen, M.; Tinner-Staines, B.; Staines, W.; Rosin, D.; Terasmaa, A.; Popoli, P.; Leo, G.; Vergoni, V.; Lluis, C.; Ciruela, F.; Franco, R. & Ferré, S. (2003). Receptor heteromerization in adenosine A2A receptor signaling: relevance for striatal function and Parkinson's disease. *Neurology*, Vol.61, No.11, pp. S19-S23

Hauser, R.A.; Hubble, J.P.; Truong, D.D. & Istradefylline US-001 Study Group. (2003). Randomized trial of the adenosine A(2A) receptor antagonist istradefylline in advanced PD. *Neurology*, Vol.61, No.3, pp. 297-303

Hauser, R.A.; Shulman, L.M.; Trugman, J.M.; Roberts, J.W.; Mori, A.; Ballerini, R.; Sussman, N.M. & Istradefylline 6002-US-013 Study Group. (2008). Study of istradefylline in patients with Parkinson's disease on levodopa with motor fluctuations. *Movement disorders*, Vol.23, No.15, pp. 2177-2185

Herranz, M. & Esteller, M. (2006). New therapeutic targets in cancer: the epigenetic connection. *Clinical & translational oncology*, Vol.8, No.4, pp. 242-249

Illingworth, R.S. & Bird, A.P. (2009). CpG islands--'a rough guide'. *FEBS letters*, Vol.583, No.11, pp. 1713-1720

Jones, P.A. (1999). The DNA methylation paradox. *Trends in genetics*, Vol.15, No.1, pp.34-37

Kagan, B.L.; Sultzer, D.L.; Rosenlicht, N. & Gerner, R.H. (1990). Oral S-adenosylmethionine in depression: a randomized, double-blind, placebo-controlled trial. *The American journal of psychiatry*, Vol.147, No.5, pp. 591-595

Kreth, S.; Ledderose, C.; Kaufmann, I.; Groeger, G. & Thiel, M. (2008). Differential expression of 5'-UTR splice variants of the adenosine A2A receptor gene in human granulocytes: identification, characterization, and functional impact on activation. *The FASEB journal*, Vol.22, No.9, pp. 3276-3286

Ladd-Acosta, C.; Pevsner, J.; Sabunciyan, S.; Yolken, R.H.; Webster, M.J.; Dinkins, T.; Callinan, P.A.; Fan, J.B.; Potash, J.B. & Feinberg, A.P. (2007). DNA methylation signatures within the human brain. *American journal of human genetics*, Vol.81, No.6, pp. 1304-1315

Le, F.; Townsend-Nicholson, A.; Baker, E.; Sutherland, G.R. & Schofield, P.R. (1996). Characterization and chromosomal localization of the human A2a adenosine receptor gene: ADORA2A. *Biochemical and biophysical research communications*, Vol.223, No.2, pp. 461-467

Lewitt, P.A. (2008a). Levodopa for the treatment of Parkinson's disease. *The New England journal of medicine*, Vol.359, No.23, pp. 2468-2476

LeWitt, P.A.; Guttman, M.; Tetrud, J.W.; Tuite, P.J.; Mori, A.; Chaikin, P.; Sussman, N.M. & 6002-US-005 Study Group. (2008b). Adenosine A2A receptor antagonist istradefylline (KW-6002) reduces "off" time in Parkinson's disease: a double-blind, randomized, multicenter clinical trial (6002-US-005). *Annals of neurology*, Vol.63, No.3, pp. 295-302

Linden, J. (2001). Molecular approach to adenosine receptors: receptor-mediated mechanisms of tissue protection. *Annual review of pharmacology and toxicology*, Vol.41, pp. 775-787

Linnebank, M.; Popp, J.; Smulders, Y.; Smith, D.; Semmler, A.; Farkas, M.; Kulic, L.; Cvetanovska, G.; Blom, H.; Stoffel-Wagner, B.; Kölsch, H.; Weller, M. & Jessen, F. (2010). S-adenosylmethionine is decreased in the cerebrospinal fluid of patients with Alzheimer's disease. *Neuro-degenerative diseases*, Vol.7, No.6, pp. 373-378

Lipinski, J.F.; Cohen, B.M.; Frankenburg, F.; Tohen, M.; Waternaux, C.; Altesman, R.; Jones, B. & Harris, P. (1984). Open trial of S-adenosylmethionine for treatment of depression. *The American journal of psychiatry*, Vol.141, No.3, pp. 448-450

Liu, L.; van Groen, T.; Kadish, I. & Tollefsbol, T.O. (2009). DNA methylation impacts on learning and memory in aging. *Neurobiology of aging*, Vol.30, No.4, pp.549-560

Liu, X.X.; Wilson, K. & Charlton, C.G. (2000). Effects of L-dopa treatment on methylation in mouse brain: implications for the side effects of L-dopa. *Life sciences*, Vol.66, No.23, pp. 2277-2288

Lu, S.C. (2000). S-Adenosylmethionine. *The international journal of biochemistry & cell biology*, Vol.32, No.4, pp. 391-395

MacCollin, M.; Peterfreund, R.; MacDonald, M.; Fink, J.S. & Gusella, J. (1994). Mapping of a human A2a adenosine receptor (ADORA2) to chromosome 22. *Genomics*, Vol.20, No.2, pp. 332-333

Masino, S.A.; Diao, L.; Illes, P.; Zahniser, N.R.; Larson, G.A.; Johansson, B.; Fredholm, B.B. & Dunwiddie, T.V. (2002). Modulation of hippocampal glutamatergic transmission by ATP is dependent on adenosine a(1) receptors. *The Journal of pharmacological and experimental therapeutics*, Vol.303, No.1, pp. 356-363

Miller, J.W.; Selhub, J.; Nadeau, M.R.; Thomas, C.A.; Feldman, R.G. & Wolf, P.A. (2003). Effect of L-dopa on plasma homocysteine in PD patients: relationship to B-vitamin status. *Neurology*, Vol.60, No.7, pp. 1125-1129

Mizuno, Y.; Hasegawa, K.; Kondo, T.; Kuno, S.; Yamamoto, M. & Japanese Istradefylline Study Group. (2010). Clinical efficacy of istradefylline (KW-6002) in Parkinson's disease: a randomized, controlled study. *Movement disorders*, Vol.25, No.10, pp. 1437-1443

Morris, M.S. (2003). Homocysteine and Alzheimer's disease. *Lancet neurology*, Vol.2, No.7, pp. 425-428

Morrison, L.D.; Smith, D.D. & Kish, S.J. (1996). Brain S-adenosylmethionine levels are severely decreased in Alzheimer's disease. *Journal of neurochemistry*, Vol.67, No.3, pp. 1328-1331

Müller, T.; Woitalla, D.; Hauptmann, B.; Fowler, B. & Kuhn, W. (2001). Decrease of methionine and S-adenosylmethionine and increase of homocysteine in treated patients with Parkinson's disease. *Neuroscience letters*, Vol.308, No.1, pp. 54-56

Müller, T.; Woitalla, D. & Kuhn, W. (2003). Benefit of folic acid supplementation in parkinsonian patients treated with levodopa. *Journal of neurology, neurosurgery, and psychiatry*, Vol.74, No.4, pp. 549

Müller, T. & Kuhn, W. (2006). Tolcapone decreases plasma levels of S-adenosyl-L-homocysteine and homocysteine in treated Parkinson's disease patients. *European journal of clinical pharmacology*, Vol.62, No.6, pp. 447-450

Müller, T. & Kuhn, W. (2009a). Homocysteine levels after acute levodopa intake in patients with Parkinson's disease. *Movement disorders*, Vol.24, No.9, pp. 1339-1343

Müller, T. & Muhlack, S. (2009b) Peripheral COMT inhibition prevents levodopa associated homocysteine increase. *Journal of neural transmission*, Vol.116, No.10, pp. 1253-1256

Nutt, J.G. (2008). Pharmacokinetics and pharmacodynamics of levodopa. *Movement disorders*, Vol.23, No.3, pp. S580-S584

Obeid, R.; Schadt, A.; Dillmann, U.; Kostopoulos, P.; Fassbender, K. & Herrmann, W. (2009). Methylation status and neurodegenerative markers in Parkinson disease. *Clinical chemistry*, Vol.55, No.10, pp. 1852-1860

Obeso, J.A.; Olanow, C.W. & Nutt, J.G. (2000). Levodopa motor complications in Parkinson's disease. *Trends in neurosciences*, Vol.23, No.10, pp. S2-S7

Orru, M.; Bakešová, J.; Brugarolas, M.; Quiroz, C.; Beaumont, V.; Goldberg, S.R.; Lluís, C.; Cortés, A.; Franco, R.; Casadó, V.; Canela, E.I. & Ferré, S. (2011) Striatal pre- and post-synaptic profile of adenosine A(2A) receptor antagonists. *PLoS One*, Vol.6, No.1, pp. e16088

O'Suilleabhain, P.E.; Sung, V.; Hernandez, C.; Lacritz, L.; Dewey, R.B. Jr; Bottiglieri, T. & Diaz-Arrastia, R. (2004). Elevated plasma homocysteine level in patients with Parkinson disease: motor, affective, and cognitive associations. *Archives of neurology*, Vol.61, No.6, pp. 865-868

Ohta, A. & Sitkovsky, M. (2001). Role of G-protein-coupled adenosine receptors in downregulation of inflammation and protection from tissue damage. Nature, Vol.414, No.6866, pp. 916-920

Panza, F.; Frisardi, V.; Capurso, C.; D'Introno, A.; Colacicco, A.M.; Vendemiale, G.; Capurso, A. & Solfrizzi, V. (2009). Possible role of S-adenosylmethionine, S-adenosylhomocysteine, and polyunsaturated fatty acids in predementia syndromes and Alzheimer's disease. *Journal of Alzheimer's disease*, Vol.16, No.3, pp. 467-470

Papakostas, G.I. (2009). Evidence for S-adenosyl-L-methionine (SAM-e) for the treatment of major depressive disorder. *The Journal of clinical psychiatry*, Vol.70, No.5, pp. 18-22

Papakostas, G.I.; Mischoulon, D.; Shyu, I.; Alpert, J.E. & Fava, M. (2010). S-adenosyl methionine (SAMe) augmentation of serotonin reuptake inhibitors for antidepressant nonresponders with major depressive disorder: a double-blind, randomized clinical trial. *The American journal of psychiatry*, Vol.167, No.8, pp. 942-948

Pascale, R.M.; Marras, V.; Simile, M.M.; Daino, L.; Pinna, G.; Bennati, S.; Carta, M.; Seddaiu, M.A.; Massarelli, G. & Feo, F. (1992). Chemoprevention of rat liver carcinogenesis by S-adenosyl-L-methionine: a long-term study. *Cancer research*, Vol.52, No.18, pp. 4979-4986

Peterfreund, R.A.; MacCollin, M.; Gusella, J. & Fink, J.S. (1996). Characterization and expression of the human A2a adenosine receptor gene. *Journal of neurochemistry*, Vol.66, No.1, pp. 362-368

Pinna, A.; Corsi, C.; Carta, A.R.; Valentini, V.; Pedata, F. & Morelli, M. (2002). Modification of adenosine extracellular levels and adenosine A(2A) receptor mRNA by dopamine denervation. *European journal of pharmacology*, Vol.446, No.1-3, pp. 75-82

Perez-Buira, S.; Barrachina, M.; Rodriguez, A.; Albasanz, J.L.; Martín, M. & Ferrer, I. (2007). Expression levels of adenosine receptors in hippocampus and frontal cortex in argyrophilic grain disease. *Neuroscience letters*, Vol.423, Vol.3, pp.194-199

Portela, A. & Esteller, M. (2010). Epigenetic modifications and human disease. *Nature biotechnology*, Vol.28, No.10, pp.1057-1068

Quadri, P.; Fragiacomo, C.; Pezzati, R.; Zanda, E.; Forloni, G.; Tettamanti, M. & Lucca, U. (2004). Homocysteine, folate, and vitamin B-12 in mild cognitive impairment, Alzheimer disease, and vascular dementia. The *American journal of clinical nutrition*, Vol.80, No.1, pp. 114-122

Quiroz, C.; Luján, R.; Uchigashima, M.; Simoes, A.P.; Lerner, T.N.; Borycz, J.; Kachroo, A.; Canas, P.M.; Orru, M.; Schwarzschild, M.A.; Rosin, D.L.; Kreitzer, A.C.; Cunha, R.A.; Watanabe, M. & Ferré, S. (2009). Key modulatory role of presynaptic adenosine A2A receptors in cortical neurotransmission to the striatal direct pathway. *ScientificWorldJournal*, No.9, pp. 1321-1344

Ralevic, V. & Burnstock, G. (1998). Receptors for purines and pyrimidines. *Pharmacological reviews*, Vol.50, No.3, pp. 413-492

Remington, R.; Chan, A.; Paskavitz, J. & Shea, T.B. (2009). Efficacy of a vitamin/nutriceutical formulation for moderate-stage to later-stage Alzheimer's disease: a placebo-controlled pilot study. *American journal of Alzheimer's disease and other dementias*, Vol.24, No.1, pp. 27-33

Ribeiro, J.A.; Sebastião, A.M. & de Mendonça, A. (2002). Adenosine receptors in the nervous system: pathophysiological implications. *Progress in neurobiology*, Vol.68, No.6, pp. 377-392

Rodrigues, R.J.; Alfaro, T.M.; Rebola, N.; Oliveira, C.R. & Cunha, R.A. (2005). Co-localization and functional interaction between adenosine A(2A) and metabotropic group 5 receptors in glutamatergic nerve terminals of the rat striatum. *Journal of neurochemistry*, Vol.92, No.3, pp. 433-441

Rodríguez, A.; Martín, M.; Albasanz, J.L.; Barrachina, M.; Espinosa, J.C.; Torres, J.M. & Ferrer, I. (2006). Adenosine A1 receptor protein levels and activity is increased in the cerebral cortex in Creutzfeldt-Jakob disease and in bovine spongiform encephalopathy-infected bovine-PrP mice. *Journal of neuropathology and experimental neurology*, Vol.65, No.10, pp. 964-975

Satoh, S.; Matsumura, H. & Hayaishi, O. (1998). Involvement of adenosine A2A receptor in sleep promotion. European journal of pharmacology, Vol.351, No.2, pp. 155-162

Scarpa, S.; Fuso, A.; D'Anselmi, F. & Cavallaro, R.A. (2003). Presenilin 1 gene silencing by S-adenosylmethionine: a treatment for Alzheimer disease? *FEBS letters*, Vol.541, No.1-3, pp. 145-148

Schiffmann, S.N.; Libert, F.; Vassart, G. & Vanderhaeghen, J.J. (1991). Distribution of adenosine A2 receptor mRNA in the human brain. *Neuroscience letters*, Vol.130, No.2, pp. 177-181

Schiffmann, S.N.; Fisone, G.; Moresco, R.; Cunha, R.A. & Ferré, S. (2007). Adenosine A2A receptors and basal ganglia physiology. *Progress in neurobiology*, Vol.83, No.5, pp. 277-292

Sebastião, A.M. & Ribeiro, J.A. (1996). Adenosine A2 receptor-mediated excitatory actions on the nervous system. *Progress in neurobiology*, Vol.48, No.3, pp. 167-189

Seshadri, S.; Beiser, A.; Selhub, J.; Jacques, P.F.; Rosenberg, I.H.; D'Agostino, R.B.; Wilson, P.W. & Wolf, P.A. (2002). Plasma homocysteine as a risk factor for dementia and Alzheimer's disease. *The New England journal of medicine*, Vol.346, No.7, pp. 476-483

Shea, T.B. & Chan, A. (2008). S-adenosyl methionine: a natural therapeutic agent effective against multiple hallmarks and risk factors associated with Alzheimer's disease. *Journal of Alzheimer's disease*, Vol.13, No.1, pp.67-70

Siegmund, K.D.; Connor, C.M.; Campan, M.; Long, T.I.; Weisenberger, D.J.; Biniszkiewicz, D.; Jaenisch, R.; Laird, P.W. & Akbarian, S. (2007). DNA methylation in the human cerebral cortex is dynamically regulated throughout the life span and involves differentiated neurons. *PLoS One*, Vol.2, No.9, pp. e895

Stacy, M.; Silver, D.; Mendis, T.; Sutton, J.; Mori, A.; Chaikin, P. & Sussman, N.M. (2008). A 12-week, placebo-controlled study (6002-US-006) of istradefylline in Parkinson disease. *Neurology*, Vol.70, No.23, pp. 2233-2240

Stone, T.W.; Ceruti, S. & Abbracchio, M.P. (2009). Adenosine receptors and neurological disease: neuroprotection and neurodegeneration. *Handbook of experimental pharmacology*, Vol.193, pp.535-587

Tolosa, E.; Martí, M.J.; Valldeoriola, F. & Molinuevo, J.L. (1998). History of levodopa and dopamine agonists in Parkinson's disease treatment. *Neurology*, Vol.50, No.6 Suppl 6, pp. S2-S10

Tomiyama, M.; Kimura, T.; Maeda, T.; Tanaka, H.; Kannari, K. & Baba, M. (2004). Upregulation of striatal adenosine A2A receptor mRNA in 6-hydroxydopamine-lesioned rats intermittently treated with L-DOPA. *Synapse*, Vol.52, No.3, pp. 218-222

Tremolizzo, L.; Carboni, G.; Ruzicka, W.B.; Mitchell, C.P.; Sugaya, I.; Tueting, P.; Sharma, R.; Grayson, D.R.; Costa, E. & Guidotti, A. (2002). An epigenetic mouse model for molecular and behavioral neuropathologies related to schizophrenia vulnerability. *Proceeding of the National Academy of Sciences of the United States of America*, Vol.99, No.26, pp. 17095-17100

Van Calker, D.; Müller, M. & Hamprecht, B. (1979). Adenosine regulates via two different types of receptors, the accumulation of cyclic AMP in cultured brain cells. *Journal of neurochemistry*, Vol.33, No.5, pp. 999-1005

Varani, K.; Vincenzi, F.; Tosi, A.; Gessi, S.; Casetta, I.; Granieri, G.; Fazio, P.; Leung, E.; MacLennan, S.; Granieri, E. & Borea, P.A. (2010). A2A adenosine receptor overexpression and functionality, as well as TNF-alpha levels, correlate with motor symptoms in Parkinson's disease. *The FASEB journal*, Vol.24, No.2, pp.587-598

Veldic, M.; Caruncho, H.J.; Liu, W.S.; Davis, J.; Satta, R.; Grayson, D.R.; Guidotti, A. & Costa, E. (2004) DNA-methyltransferase 1 mRNA is selectively overexpressed in telencephalic GABAergic interneurons of schizophrenia brains. *Proceeding of the National Academy of Sciences of the United States of America*, Vol.101, No.1, pp. 348-353

Veldic, M.; Guidotti, A.; Maloku, E.; Davis, J.M. & Costa, E. (2005). In psychosis, cortical interneurons overexpress DNA-methyltransferase 1. *Proceeding of the National Academy of Sciences of the United States of America*, Vol.102, No.6, pp. 2152-2157

Vitvitsky, V.; Thomas, M.; Ghorpade, A.; Gendelman, H.E. & Banerjee, R. (2006). A functional transsulfuration pathway in the brain links to glutathione homeostasis. *The Journal of biological chemistry*, Vol. 281, No.47, pp. 35785-35793

Wang, S.C.; Oelze, B. & Schumacher, A. (2008). Age-specific epigenetic drift in late-onset Alzheimer's disease. *PLoS One*, Vol.3, No.7, pp. e2698

Waterland, R.A. & Jirtle, R.L. (2003). Transposable elements: targets for early nutritional effects on epigenetic gene regulation. *Molecular and cellular biology*, Vol.23, No.15, pp. 5293-5300

Woitalla, D.; Kuhn, W. & Müller, T. (2004). MTHFR C677T polymorphism, folic acid and hyperhomocysteinemia in levodopa treated patients with Parkinson's disease. *Journal of neural transmission*, Vol.68, pp. 15-20

Yasui, K.; Kowa, H.; Nakaso, K.; Takeshima, T. & Nakashima, K. (2000). Plasma homocysteine and MTHFR C677T genotype in levodopa-treated patients with PD. *Neurology*, Vol.55, No.3, pp. 437-440

Yu, L.; Frith, M.C.; Suzuki, Y.; Peterfreund, R.A.; Gearan, T.; Sugano, S.; Schwarzschild, M.A.; Weng, Z.; Fink, J.S. & Chen, J.F. (2004). Characterization of genomic organization of the adenosine A2A receptor gene by molecular and bioinformatics analyses. *Brain research*, Vol.1000, No.1-2, pp. 156-173

Zoccolella, S.; Lamberti, P.; Iliceto, G.; Dell'Aquila, C.; Diroma, C.; Fraddosio, A.; Lamberti, S.V.; Armenise, E.; Defazio, G.; de Mari, M. & Livrea, P. (2006). Elevated plasma homocysteine levels in L-dopa-treated Parkinson's disease patients with dyskinesias. *Clinical chemistry and laboratory medicine*, Vol.44, No.7, pp. 863-866

Zoccolella, S.; Iliceto, G.; deMari, M.; Livrea, P. & Lamberti, P. (2007). Management of L-Dopa related hyperhomocysteinemia: catechol-O-methyltransferase (COMT) inhibitors or B vitamins? Results from a review. *Clinical chemistry and laboratory medicine*, Vol.45, No.12, pp. 1607-1613

Zoccolella, S.; dell'Aquila, C.; Abruzzese, G.; Antonini, A.; Bonuccelli, U.; Canesi, M.; Cristina, S.; Marchese, R.; Pacchetti, C.; Zagaglia, R.; Logroscino, G.; Defazio, G.; Lamberti, P. & Livrea, P. (2009). Hyperhomocysteinemia in levodopa-treated patients with Parkinson's disease dementia. *Movement disorders*, Vol.24, No.7, pp. 1028-1033

Zoccolella, S.; Lamberti, S.V.; Iliceto, G.; Santamato, A.; Lamberti, P. & Logroscino, G. (2010). Hyperhomocysteinemia in L-dopa treated patients with Parkinson's disease: potential implications in cognitive dysfunction and dementia? *Current medicinal chemistry*, Vol.17, No.28, pp. 3253-3261

Part 5

Cell Therapies

15

1980-2011: Parkinson's Disease and Advance in Stem Cell Research

Lidia Cova[1] and Marie-Therese Armentero[2]
[1]*Department of Neurology, Laboratory of Neuroscience, IRCCS Istituto Auxologico Italiano, Milan*
[2]*Laboratory of Functional Neurochemistry, Interdepartmental Research Centre for Parkinson's Disease, IRCCS National Institute of Neurology C. Mondino, Pavia, Italy*

1. Introduction

Replenishing the depleted striatal dopamine stores with its immediate precursor, L-3,4-dihydroxyphenylalanine (L-DOPA), to mimic dopamine-mediated neurotransmission still represents the gold standard for treating Parkinson's disease (PD). This pharmacological therapy offers immediate and effective symptomatic relief, especially at the early stages of the disease; it has, however, no influence on underlying neurodegenerative processes (Dass et al., 2006) that continue to evolve with time and are paralleled by a gradual loss of drug efficacy. As the disease progresses, steady adaptation, mostly continuous increase, of dopaminergic drug dosage is necessary, thereby favoring the emergence of considerable side effects, such as dyskinesia and psychiatric disturbances. The development of new treatments, or combination of treatments, able to relief motor symptoms and also delay or even halt the loss of dopaminergic neurons, has been and remains a fundamental issue for the development of innovative clinical strategies in PD. Transplantation of dopamine-secreting cells directly providing dopamine in the striatum, in particular, has been considered an adequate substitute to pharmacotherapy. However, although efficacy of this approach has now been asserted in numerous pre-clinical studies utilizing animal models of PD, positive outcomes in clinical trials involving PD patients have been very variable and rather modest, and have been plagued by graft-induced dyskinesias. New sources for cell replacement and particularly stem cells (including induced patient-derived cells) may now provide advantages for future clinical therapies (Wakeman et al., 2011).

This chapter will briefly introduce rodent and nonhuman primate PD-like models commonly used in pre-clinical studies, which represent a fundamental platform for the pre-clinical evaluation of innovative interventions. We will then evidence the progresses accomplished since the first intracerebral transplantation of fetal neural tissue in PD patients describing the subsequent novel discoveries for the application of stem cell to pre-clinical PD models, and give an overview of ongoing cell-based therapeutic strategies. Thereafter, multiple issues connected to stem transplantation to efficiently contrast adverse effects of increased age will be reviewed including decrease of apoptosis related to tissue degeneration, requirement of correct graft integration in the host vascular and neural circuits, reduction of diffuse inflammatory response/oxidative stress and correct release of key growth factors. In addition we will discuss the emergence of novel biotechnologies that will, most likely, help unravel the complex interrelationship between transplanted stem cells and the host environment and will favor the development of novel therapeutic procedures readily applicable in PD patients.

2. Animal models: A necessary pre-clinical tool for the development of innovative cellular therapy in PD

Animal models represent a fundamental step in the attempt to elucidate gene-environment interactions and to define pathogenic mechanisms involved in the aetiology and progression of the neurodegenerative diseases. Most of the current knowledge on pathophysiology of PD originates from studies conducted on animal models of the disease, since animals and humans share several anatomical features (as shown in Figure 1). In addition, they represent the first essential pre-clinical platform for the evaluation of any targeted therapeutic intervention. Notably, subsequent clinical trials in small human cohorts remain essential for the development of efficient therapies able also to alleviate disability related non-motor symptoms (Meissner et al., 2011) which are currently underestimated in animal models (Dunnett and Lelos, 2010).

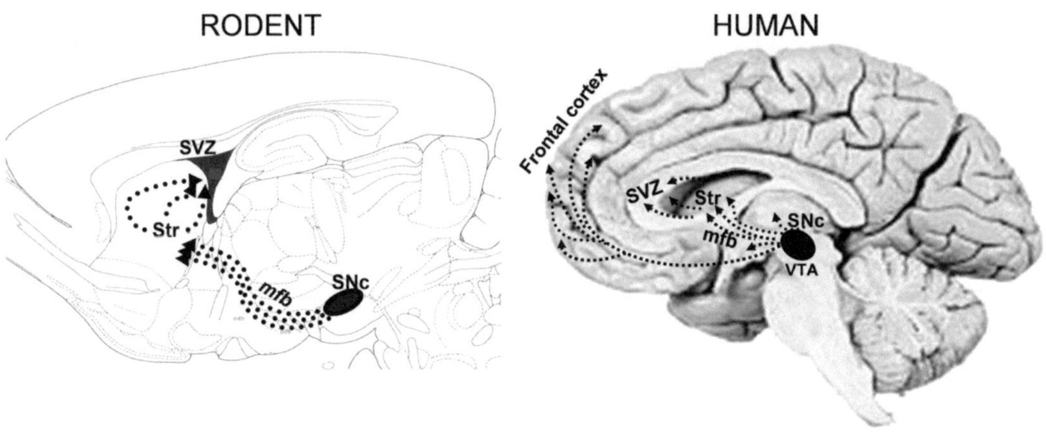

Str=striatum; SVZ=subventricular zone; mfb=median forbrain bundle; SNc=Substantia nigra; VTA= ventral tegmental area

Fig. 1. Anatomical comparison between mouse and human brains
The comparison between rodent (A) and human brain (B) enlightens their anatomical similarities and physiology. The connections between striatum, SNc, and cerebral cortex in the human brain are indicated by dotted black lines and may correlate the simultaneous degeneration of these areas during disease onset and progression. Moreover, dopaminergic innervations of the striatum/SVZ (black dotted lines) could also explain reduction of adult brain neurogenesis both in PD patients and animal models.

PD models have been classically based on the administration of neurotoxins able to replicate some of the pathological and phenotypic features of the human disease both in rodents and primates. Toxins can be given systemically or intra-cerebrally, depending on the type of toxin used and animal specie involved, and mimic the selective degeneration of nigrostriatal neurons characteristic of the human disorder.

The classical systemic model is based on the injection of 1-methyl-4-phenyl-1,2,3,6-tetrahydropyridine (MPTP), a toxin that selectively affects dopaminergic neurons and first recognized in the mid-1980's as the cause of marked parkinsonism in young drug users of Northern California (Langston et al., 1983). MPTP crosses the blood brain barrier and is transformed in its active metabolite, 1-methyl-4-phenylpyridinium ion (MPP+) that is then actively taken up by dopaminergic neurons of the substantia nigra pars compacta (SNc). Systemic administration of MPTP to nonhuman primates induces a parkinsonian phenotype closely resembling the human pathology. MPTP-treated monkeys have an excellent anti-symptomatic response to dopaminergic drug treatment and develop motor complications linked to long term L-DOPA therapy (Kim et al., 2009). Concordantly, several pharmacological drugs currently applied to treated PD patients (i.e. dopamine agonists, amantadine, etc..) have been developed in this MPTP model (Fox et al., 2006). Alternative cell replacement strategies using various cell sources have been successfully performed indicating the technical feasibility of the model for future studies (Redmond et al., 2010; Serra et al., 2008). The large related costs and the difficulty to reliably standardize acute toxin administration to replicate most of the underlying mechanisms of a chronic progressive disorder form still represent major drawbacks and limit the use of this PD model in large scale studies (Fox and Brotchie, 2010). MPTP can also be systemically administered to mice but not rat, which are resistant, and several different experimental paradigms have been developed and used over time.

The prototypical intracerebral model is based on the local injection of 6-hydroxydopamine (6-OHDA) and was the first PD animal model ever generated (Ungerstedt, 1968). Six-OHDA is a hydroxylated analogue of dopamine and, similarly to MPTP, is actively taken up by dopaminergic neurons. The neurotoxin can be injected in the SNc, or into the medial forebrain bundle (mfb) that conveys efferent fibers from the nigral cell bodies to the striatum (as shown in Figure 1) and causes massive and rapid anterograde degeneration of the nigrostriatal pathway. This procedure induces large nigral cell loss and striatal dopamine depletion (90-100%). The neurotoxin can also be injected into the striatum; in this case rapid damage to striatal dopaminergic terminals is observed followed by a progressive loss of SNc neurons (50-70% neuronal loss), which are secondarily affected through a "dying back" mechanism. This procedure has a slower time course compared to the intra-mfb injection and provides a progressive model of nigrostriatal degeneration, more similar to the gradual evolution of the neurodegenerative process of human PD. Importantly, injection of 6-OHDA is commonly carried out unilaterally, with the contralateral hemisphere serving as control, because of the high mortality rate associated with bilateral injection. The rat 6-OHDA model is commonly used in neuroprotective studies, both involving administration of novel pharmaceutical compounds or cell transplantation because it is i) cost-effective, ii) highly reproducible and iii) opened to articulate behavioural analyses (Redmond et al., 2010; Serra et al., 2008).

Numerous transgenic mouse models, that reproduce monogenic mutations observed in familiar forms of PD, have also been developed over the years. These models have not been discussed in this chapter as they typically display very low degree or even no nigrostriatal degeneration (for review see (Dawson et al., 2010)) and are not commonly used in stem cell transplantation experiments.

3. Neural tissue transplantation

In 1987, the first clinical trials involving transplantation of human fetal mesencephalic tissues or xenotransplantation of fetal pig neural cells in humans were performed with the clear scope of replacing dopaminergic neurons lost during PD progression. Since then and overall, contradictory results have been observed, even among patient groups treated within the same centers (Bjorklund et al., 2003). Along with the observed poor graft survival (around 10%; (Hagell and Brundin, 2001), a substantial subset of patients (15-56%) developed dyskinesias (Freed et al., 2001; Hagell and Brundin, 2001; Olanow et al., 2003), while the presence of Lewy bodies in long-term implants, recently reported, suggests the possibility of a *host-to-graft* disease propagation (Kordower et al., 2008; Li et al., 2008; Mendez et al., 2008). Functional improvements, represented by reduction of symptoms (30%-40% improvement of the unified Parkinson's disease rating scale, motor score in the drug-free phase) have been clearly observed (Hagell and Brundin, 2001) even in the long term (Mendez et al., 2008; Piccini et al., 1999). Positive outcomes were dampened by enhanced microglial activation and disruption of blood brain barrier linked to surgical procedures (Olanow et al., 2003). Failures were also related to the scarcity, as well as heterogeneous composition of the donor tissue itself (Carlsson et al., 2009; Freed et al., 2001). Nonetheless, these first trials supported the feasibility of transplantation procedures as an alternative therapeutic approach in PD (Brundin et al., 2010; Olanow et al., 2003). Moreover, these first trials have enlightened critical parameters mandatory for successful tranplantations including: a) purity of cell preparation; b) correct localization of the graft in the host brain c) preference for reduced age of donor/host cells (whenever possible), d) limited extension of brain injury at the time of transplantation (early pathological phases), and e) appropriate time of grafting (in relation to disease onset) to maximize survival of endogenous dopaminergic neurons (Lindvall and Kokaia, 2009). Altogether, these observations have encouraged the search for alternative cell sources that need to be efficient, safe, and ethically acceptable (additional details on this debated/controversial topic can be found in (Kimmelman et al., 2009)).

4. Stem cell therapy

The scientific progresses in biological and cellular technologies have allowed a better conception of the mechanisms involved in cell development, and in particular of factors/conditions ruling Stem Cells (SCs) proliferation and differentiation. Essentially, SCs are undifferentiated multipotent cells capable of both self-renewal and generation of several differentiated functional cell types to preserve tissue homeostasis throughout the entire life span of an organism. Multiple properties of SCs, including their the ability to potentially generate an unlimited number of dopaminergic neurons under physiological conditions, make them attractive candidates for regenerative therapy (Dass et al., 2006).

Therefore, SCs have been increasingly recognized as a valuable replacement and/or supporting tool for PD wherein a well-characterized cell type is mainly affected. Cell therapy may be performed using either autologous (ideal from an immunologic perspective) or allogeneic tissue-specific differentiated cells. Transplantation of healthy SCs that have been collected, expanded and eventually pre-differentiated *in vitro* have been originally proposed as a feasible appealing neural-replacement strategy. To date, several fetal and adult SC lineages have been directly differentiated into multiple cellular types, including neural cells and dopaminergic phenotypes. These naïve SCs, or their induced neuronal progeny, have been successfully transplanted in animal models of PD granting significant behavioral improvements. Ideally, however, new therapies should not only aim at replenishing the depleted dopamine store, but should also allow rescue of neuronal terminals and soma both in striatum and SNc.

Innovative therapeutic strategy should also take advantage and enhance the plastic property of the adult Central Nervous System (CNS) to regenerate affected brain areas through the activation of endogenous neurogenesis following cell transplantation. To reach these targets, other known intrinsic properties of SCs have already been exploited. Indeed, the potential of SCs to restore injured tissues is not only related to their direct differentiation but also to their capacity to produce and release trophic factors that may in turn inhibit apoptosis, promote angiogenesis and even direct stimulation of host regeneration (Lindvall and Kokaia, 2009; Lindvall and Kokaia, 2010). Neuroprotection can also be enhanced by transplanting SCs engineered to express either tyrosine hydroxylase (TH), the rate-limiting enzyme of dopamine synthesis, or neurotrophic factors, such as glial cell-line derived neurotrophic factor (GDNF), the most potent survival factor for degenerating dopaminergic neurons. Grafting of engineered SCs in this case provides a substantial reservoir allowing the unlimited supply of the required substance without the requirement of invasive injection pumps, as detailed below. Several SC types have already been transplanted in PD animal models yielding interesting but variable results (Wakeman et al., 2011).

SCs can be efficiently derived from early stage embryos (pluripotent SCs with unlimited potential to differentiate) or from committed resident tissues (multipotent SCs with restricted potential to differentiate). Interestingly almost all organs arising from endodermal, mesodermal and ectodermal germ layers can originate both fetal and adult SCs (i.e. amniotic/cord blood and tissue derived SCs). Regardless of their origin SCs could physiologically repair damaged tissues after intense injuries also promoting angiogenesis and neurogenesis processes, essential for CNS development and regeneration (Lindvall and Kokaia, 2010).

4.1 Embryonic stem cells

Embryonic Stem cells (ES) are derived from the inner cell mass of pre-implantation embryos and are a source of pluripotent cells, as they are able to differentiate into all adult cell types. Once established, the pluripotent ES cells can be maintained under defined culture conditions, but can also be induced to terminally differentiate into a specific lineage (Bibikova et al., 2008). ES cells may potentially give rise to an infinite number of dopaminergic neurons that may be subsequently transplanted in depleted brain areas either in animal models of PD or even in patients (Lindvall and Kokaia, 2009). A particular emphasis has been posted on the validation of reliable methods for differentiation of ES cells towards midbrain dopaminergic neurons with a high survival index following transplantation (Hwang et al., 2010). Several protocols, characterized by presence of different feeder cell layers (i.e. bone marrow stromal cells, (Perrier et al., 2004) or astrocytes (Roy et al., 2006)) coupled to morphogen/growth factor exposition, have been developed. Transplantation of these *in vitro*-differentiated cells has produced variable results and often gave rise to tissue overgrowth with formation of neuroepithelial tumors, probably linked to the presence of residual immature cells in the original grafts. To overcome uncontrolled proliferation within transplants, cell-sorting protocols have been applied to specifically isolate pure populations of ES-derived dopaminergic neurons. These procedures, however, selectively impaired neuron survival indicating that fundamental factors were lost in the negative fraction (Friling et al., 2009).

Recently, epigenetic manipulation to force dopaminergic gene expression has been also exploited (Andersson et al., 2006). Following transplantation in parkinsonian rats, these differentiated cells integrated in the brain of the animals and significantly improved PD-related behavioral stereotypies (Yang et al., 2010). Application of this methodology to clinical practice, however, remains unrealistic until well-standardized, tumor-free samples will be available. Additional protocols for induction of dopaminergic phenotypes in ES cells have been recently developed (Chambers et al., 2009; Cooper et al., 2010), but functional efficacy of these cells has not been tested in PD animal models yet. Moreover, their use is still limited by our scarce knowledge of the development and specification of midbrain dopaminergic neurons (Pruszak and Isacson, 2009). Altogether, all experimental studies performed so far, demonstrate that ES-derived dopaminergic neurons are still unable to efficiently survive in and innervate lesioned brain areas in animal models of PD without inducing the formation of tumors (Arenas, 2010). In addition, ES cells frequently carry aberrant chromosome content in relation to growth advantage (Meisner and Johnson, 2008). Finally, the therapeutic application of ES cells will necessarily require both animal cell- and serum-free conditions (Klimanskaya et al., 2005), still substantially limiting their standardized application in clinic (Gruen and Grabel, 2006).

4.2 Induced pluripotent SCs

Recently, induced Pluripotent SCs (iPS) have been derived from primary fibroblast cultures obtained from cutaneous biopsies of patients affected by neurodegenerative diseases (Kriks and Studer, 2009; Lindvall and Kokaia, 2009). This complex reprogramming sequence was performed by exogenous expression of specific transcription factors that allowed a cellular switch from an epigenome of reduced potency to one of pluripotency (Kiskinis and Eggan, 2010). The resulting iPS cells could then be differentiated into autologous, patient-specific non-mitotic cells, such dopaminergic neurons and glial cells, normally present only in the CNS, and generally only available post-mortem.

iPS cells present several advantages when compare to ES cells: 1) their possible autologous derivation (Park et al., 2008b), 2) the consequent lack of mandatory immunosuppressant therapy following transplantation, and 3) the absence of ethical concerns related to embryo disruption (Arenas, 2010). These derived and/or differentiated cells can be used as donor cells in transplantation paradigms and represent a valuable tool to dissect intrinsic pathological mechanisms or test new pharmacological approaches in samples not readily available from live patients (Abeliovich and Doege, 2009; Gunaseeli et al., 2011; Xu et al., 2010a). However, the use of oncogenes or retrovirus in the current iPS cell establishment protocol raises considerable safety concerns (Pasi et al., 2011). Indeed, iPS progenies show high propensity to form teratomas considerably restricting their potential use in cell therapy (Miura et al., 2009). Heterogeneity of iPS cell composition with variable levels of transgene expression overtime suggests a prudent approach for iPS application to clinical trials (Kiskinis and Eggan, 2010). Recently, alternative protocols that allow direct fibroblast reprogramming towards neurons without generation of pluripotent cells have been developed (Vierbuchen et al., 2010). An additional notable potential risk of autologous therapeutic reprogramming is linked to the possibility that unknown genetic factors, involved in the patient's disease, could also potentially lead to disease-related alterations of the transplanted cells in the long term (Hwang et al., 2010). Transplantation of committed neural cells selected from differentiated PD patient-derived iPS cells has been tested in a lesional rodent model of PD with some overall beneficial effects. Transplanted cells integrated into the striatum of parkinsonian rats and improved behavioral deficits for up to 8 weeks, although no noticeable dopaminergic innervation from grafted cells to the surrounding striatum was observed (Wernig et al., 2008). Recently, Hargus et al, showed that iPS–derived dopaminergic neurons can be implanted and survive, without signs of neurodegeneration or tumor formation, both in healthy and 6-OHDA lesioned rats (Hargus et al., 2010). Although the grafted cells sent proper projections to close and remote target areas, acquisition of the appropriate regional identity is still argued. A significant behavioral improvement related to high survival of the transplanted dopaminergic neurons was also reported in simple, but not in complex motor functions, that rely on functional connections between grafted and host cells. Therefore, whether these preliminary results can be successfully translated into human clinical studies still awaits more experimental data (Hanna et al., 2010). Additional long-term studies will be necessary to recreate the correct pathophysiological conditions before validation of this model as an alternative cell-based therapy in PD (Kiskinis and Eggan, 2010). It has been hypothesized that an effective therapeutic effect following transplantation requires the survival of at least 10^5 electrophysiologically active dopaminergic cells, appropriately contacting and reinnnervating striatum, without tumor formation (Arenas, 2010). Nevertheless, iPS cells could still be exploited for drug screening or as disease model to unravel pathological cascades in PD (Xu et al., 2010a). An important draw back in the clinical application of iPS cells also resides in the elevated production costs of personalized iPS. The establishment of centralized iPS cell bank(s) has been proposed to insure that fibroblast-derived dopaminergic neurons for transplantation are obtained following the Good Manufacturing Practice (GMP) guidelines for clinical trial materials.

4.3 Patient-derived Neural SCs

An innovative cellular approach is based on patient-derived neural stem cells (NSC) obtained from biopsies of their olfactory mucosa biopsies. This procedure allows the derivation of large quantities of NSC that can be grown *in vitro* as floating differentiable neurospheres. The cells bear significant pathological, disease-specific alterations in gene and protein expression, as well as cell function, such as dysregulated mitochondrial function, oxidative stress and xenobiotic metabolism (Matigian et al., 2010). Direct exploitation of these patient-derived neural cells will help obtain new insights in specific candidate genes and cell pathways for future studies of brain disease. These SCs could partially overcome the lack of appropriate animal models, faithfully recapitulating all of the clinical and pathological phenotypes of the disease, to study the mechanisms underlying PD as well as to develop translational drug development (Schule et al., 2009). In addition, these cells have a considerable advantage over ES and iPS cells, as they do not require reprogramming, and represent an important tool, with a considerable translational impact to all complex diseases. Moreover, biopsies easily obtained from neural tissues could supply new biomarkers for monitoring disease progression in PD patients. Development of such biomarkers represents a necessary step for the accomplishment essential for quality research and clinical trials (Lebouvier Thibaud et al., 2010). Derivation of patient NSC encompasses all the specific gene-environment interactions which appear fundamental along ageing process in sporadic neurological as well as psychiatric disorders (Matigian et al., 2010). Patient derived SCs are particularly intriguing for their potential in cell therapy and regenerative medicine: they may provide novel insights for the development of therapeutic strategies, aiming to contrast the neurodegenerative processes of PD. The discovery of the

specific molecules involved in these biological events could also shed light on new pharmacological disease-modifying treatments and novel potential targets, readily applicable to patients (Schule et al., 2009).
Anyway, a cautionary approach is required, since this invasive methodology still requires development of standardized, validated protocols able to reach a structure (olfactory mucosa) not accessible to routine biopsies (Parkkinen et al., 2009)].

4.4 Multipotent adult stem cells

Multipotent SCs have been identified within specific niches in most adult tissues including bone marrow, muscle, brain, heart and liver. Adult SCs that comprise fetal, amniotic, umbilical cord blood, placental, as well as tissue derived SCs (i.e. hematopoietic, neural, mesenchymal, skin SCs) are less abundant and proliferative, and possess limited potential to differentiate compared to ES cells. A key added value of adult SCs, however, is their potential use in autologous therapies, in which cells can be harvested and used within the same patient, thus avoiding the ethical concerns and risks linked to ES cells (Fricker-Gates and Gates, 2010). The ideal procedure involves isolation of SCs from tissues and their preservation in standardized stocks at centralized unit banks for long term storage and subsequent transplantation into patients upon request (Arenas, 2010) (see Figure 2). In this section we will summarize the actual state of the art and deadlocks regarding three main SC lineages: hematopoietic (HSC), mesenchymal (MSC) and neural (NSC).
Bone marrow resident HSC and MSC constitute two important cell sources for pre-clinical transplantation. HSC can be easily derived from autologous/allogeneic bone marrow or peripheral blood, and are routinely used in transplantation procedures for the treatment of several immuno-deficient/autoimmune diseases, as well as hematopoietic disorders, to reconstitute peripheral cell lineages (i.e. leukocytes, erythrocytes, etc). Recently, transplantation of HSC, engineered to release TH, has been reported to produce significant therapeutic effects in PD rats (Zhang et al., 2008).
A large body of data on the application of MSC in cell therapy can be found in literature; MSC are non-hematopoietic, multipotent cells which arise from the stromal structures of the bone marrow and are preserved in adults (Picinich et al., 2007). MSC can generate mature endothelial cells and several mesenchymal cell lineages including osteoblasts, chondrocytes, adipocytes and myoblasts (Liu et al., 2009). Several publications report efficient and multi-disciplinary protocols for their differentiation, *in vitro,* towards dopaminergic neurons (Heinrich et al., 2009; Kitada and Dezawa, 2009) even including the use of lentiviral vectors to induce TH expression (Barzilay et al., 2009). Positive outcomes in acute hypoxic-ischemic damages have been obtained utilizing MSC isolated from several stem sources, such as human placenta and amniotic fluid, either naïve (Cipriani et al., 2007) or following neural differentiation (Park et al., 2011). Positive results, such as stability and physiology of the correct phenotype *in vitro* (Thomas et al., 2011) and *in vivo* after transplantation of MSC in animal models of PD (Shetty et al., 2009), as well as in PD patients (Venkataramana et al., 2010) have been reported. The long-term fate of grafted cells is still, however, matter of debate (Schwarz and Storch, 2010; Schwarz and Schwarz, 2011) and application of cell therapy to a chronic degenerative disease like PD appears rather complex. Successful outcomes of transplantation can be influenced by multiple factors largely dependent on the source and type of SCs adopted. For example, it has been reported that neural differentiation of MSC is required before intrastriatal transplantation in PD rats to observe a graft-dependent improvement of motor deficits (Levy et al., 2008). Transplantation of naïve

human umbilical vein-derived dopaminergic-like cell in a rat model of PD did not improve motor dysfunction, and required administration of a neurotrophin, nerve growth factor, to induce substantial recovery (Li et al., 2010a). Lineage negative cells from umbilical cord blood efficiently gave rise to neuronal cells and oligodendrocytes *in vitro* (Chua et al., 2009) while lineage specific (cKit+) amniotic-derived SCs fail to acquire a dopaminergic phenotype after epigenetic stimuli both *in vitro* and in an animal model of PD (Donaldson et al., 2009). Concordantly, upon neuronal induction bone marrow-derived MSC down-regulate markers of other lineages, but fail to differentiate into functional neurons (Thomas et al., 2011). The functional positive effects exerted by transplanted MSC in PD animal models, are still controversial on the basis of technical criticisms, strength of trial design or inconsistent experimental approaches (Meyer et al., 2010). MSC have a significant protective effect against dopaminergic cell loss both *in vitro* and *in vivo* (Park et al., 2008a), but whether this results from true dopaminergic neuron replacement and how the cells actually induced functional improvement are still far from being clarified (White, 2011). Thus, before MSC can be considered a reliable source for clinical replacement of dopaminergic cells, their ability to transdifferentiate terminally towards a neuronal lineage needs to be resolved and their mechanism of action following transplantation needs to be elucidated (Schwarz and Storch, 2010).

Another promising source of SC is represented by NSC, that can be derived from various source including the subventricular zone (SVZ), ES, umbilical cord blood, MSC, fetal brain as well as spinal cord, and grown in suspension as floating clusters (neurospheres) (Meyer et al., 2010). NSC can restore functions lost during ageing, and both migrate towards and repair neurological damages, exerting positive influence on the surrounding cells, including dysfunctional neurons (Ourednik et al., 2002). Autologous transplantation of *in vitro*-expanded cortical and subcortical tissue samples, obtained from a PD patient during a neurosurgical procedure, produced long lasting motor improvements (Lévesque et al., 2009). Interestingly, fetal and adult NSC possess comparable intrinsic therapeutic potential in terms of cell survival, integration and functional outcomes in a rat model of PD (Muraoka et al., 2008). However, albeit feasible, harvesting samples from patient remains an invasive procedure and is difficult to translate into a routine therapy. NSC do not give rise to dopaminergic neurons under physiological conditions, but several protocols have been optimized for their forced differentiation towards this lineage. Mimicking the procedures for dopaminergic differentiation from ES cells, a group has reported the differentiation of immature NSC into forebrain, but not midbrain (area A9), dopaminergic cells (Papanikolaou et al., 2008), while forced expression of Nurr1, a transcriptional factor specific for midbrain dopamine neuron development, induced dopaminergic neuron phenotype in NSC isolated both from SVZ and the white matter (Shim et al., 2007). The appearance of specific neuronal subtypes is not solely a direct consequence of external cues or the expression of neurotrophins but likely depends on the integrated temporal sequence of multiple factors that finally results in the correct neuronal phenotype. Regionalization and specification of the midbrain territory rely on a defined pattern of transcription factor expression and secretion of soluble molecules within the neuroectoderm in physiological conditions. This pattern is a composite process difficult to correctly recapitulate *in vitro* and has been only partially unraveled (Fricker-Gates and Gates, 2010). Interestingly, transplantation of NSC derived from MSC, using a complex protocol based on TH transfection and culture in media for differentiation, in 6-OHDA lesioned rats has been recently reported. Cell grafting induced significant behavioral improvements that were associated with partial preservation of dopamine content (Zou et al., 2010). A similar approach was applied to MPTP-lesioned parkinsonian rhesus monkeys; transplantation of TH- transfected bone marrow cells in the caudate nucleus and SNc improved both PD-related alterations in glucose metabolism and dopamine transport with an overall recovery of behavioral symptoms (Xu et al., 2010b). Similarly, allogeneic NSC modified to stably express and release the neurotrophic factor Neurotrophin-3 (NT-3), displayed enhanced dopaminergic neuron differentiation as well as migration distance, and induced the reinnervation in the neural circuitry coupled to functional recovery upon transplantation in 6-OHDA-treated rats (Gu et al., 2009). Recently, Murrell and colleagues proposed that dopaminergic neurons may be generated directly from adult olfactory SC of PD patients, similarly to Matigian et al (Matigian et al., 2010): in this paper the authors further demonstrated that differentiation of neural progenitor cells in dopaminergic-like neurons was able to correct behavioral asymmetry in the rat model of PD (Murrell et al., 2008).

Albeit these overall positive data, additional long term trials on the safety, efficacy, as well as further understanding of the biological mechanisms activated by graft procedures still need to be accomplished. So far, real functional integration between ectopically grafted SC-derived dopaminergic neurons in the denervated striatum has been demonstrated only in organotypic cultures of wild type mouse striatum (Tonnesen et al., 2011). Therefore, studies aimed at the characterization of the molecular basis of the integration in/differentiation of (genetically modified) NSC, and their progeny, within the dopaminergic network deserve further extensive development. Finally, the invasive intracerebral procedure required for the isolation of NSC as a possible SC source in the treatment of neurodegenerative diseases still remains a major draw back for their clinical application.

It is also important to notice that all the three SC lineages (HSC, MSC and NSC) can be obtained from bank-stored umbilical cord blood and amniotic/placenta cells, while only HSC and MSC can be easily isolated from autologous peripheral blood, thus amplifying the potential SC pool for clinical or experimental settings without ethical concerns (Figure 2).

5. Stem Cell & Neuroinflammation

Recent discoveries regarding the role of the immune system in brain damage coupled to the development of new technologies to manipulate the immune response make immunotherapies an attractive target to treat neurological diseases (Tansey and Goldberg, 2010). In the past decade, neuroinflammation has emerged as an important substrate for PD (Brochard et al., 2009). Several epidemiologic studies have reported an inverse correlation between the chronic assumption of non-steroidal anti-inflammatory drugs and the risk of developing PD (Chen et al., 2003). Unrestrained widespread neuroinflammation emerges during the early phases of the neurodegenerative process both in PD patients and in animal models of the disease (Whitton, 2010) and significant evidence demonstrates that neuroinflammatory processes participate in PD pathophysiology. Gliosis and lymphocyte infiltration associated with production of soluble factors - potentially protective or toxic - are consistently reported in parkinsonian animals and PD patients (McGeer et al., 1988; McGeer and McGeer, 2004; McGeer and McGeer, 2008) Most studies in animal models of PD have demonstrated that efficient neuroprotective strategies that decrease nigrostriatal degeneration also consistently reduce associated neuroinflammatory processes, and *vice-versa*, underlying the fundamental link between neuroinflammation and neurodegeneration. Recent data have also supported the idea that a reduction in the levels of anti-inflammatory factors itself can further enhance vulnerability of dopaminergic neurons to apoptosis in a neurodegenerative environment (Barnum and Tansey, 2010; Lu et al., 2010; Maguire-Zeiss and Federoff, 2010). Furthermore, it has been recently suggested that pro-inflammatory cytokines exert a negative impact on neuronal differentiation, while anti-inflammatory cytokines facilitate neurogenesis (Mathieu et al., 2010) and neuronal migration towards appropriate targets (Das and Basu, 2008). These data clearly indicate that pro- and anti-inflammatory responses must be strictly balanced to prevent the potential detrimental effects of prolonged or unregulated inflammation on vulnerable neuronal populations (Lee and Park, 2009). It has been shown that outcome of the transplantation of ES-derived TH-positive cells in an MPTP mouse model of PD is strictly dependent on the concomitant administration immunosuppressive treatment (Toriumi et al., 2009) that significantly improved survival and integration of grafted SC overtime.

Noteworthy, inflammation, which has long been considered as thoroughly disastrous for brain repair, is now known to produce some positive effects on stem/progenitor cell recruitment/survival by growth factor signalling and the secretion of chemoattractant cytokines (Cayre et al., 2009; Mathieu et al., 2010). Conversely, inflammatory mediators, such as nitric oxide (NO) and reactive oxygen species (ROS), can contribute to neurodegeneration by triggering aberrant protein modifications with consequent misfolding and loss of function (Vicente Miranda and Outeiro, 2010). Application of MSC, a particular SC lineage described above (section 4.4), that knowingly possess significant inherent immunomodulatory properties, opens new perspective for cell transplantation in PD. MSC can interactively act on their environment through the local/distal release of trophic factors, as well as on the activation of immune response by means of cell contact-dependent mechanism and modulation of noxious inflammatory components (Lee and Park, 2009). MSC were proven to effectively protect dopaminergic neurons from lipopolysaccharide (LPS)-induced neurotoxicity, both *in vitro* and *in vivo*, via anti-inflammatory mechanisms involving the modulation of microglial activation (Kim et al., 2009). Microglia, in turn are responsible for the correct phagocytic clearance following injury, thus facilitating the reorganization of neuronal circuits and triggering repair (Neumann et al., 2009). Notably, aside from immunomodulation, the complex network of biological mechanisms activated by MSC transplantation includes their homing to the SNc, substitution of dopaminergic neurons, modulation of apoptosis and modification of ubiquitin-proteasome function. Concordantly, at the moment, MSC constitute the most attractive and autologous candidate disease modifying strategy for PD and other neurodegenerative disorders (Karussis et al., 2008).

6. Neurorepair/Neurogenesis

The nigrostriatal network is highly organized and finely regulated in relation to specific functions and circumstances. As a consequence, restoring lost dopaminergic neurons does not necessarily coincide with correct reconstruction the pathway (Obeso et al., 2008). Partial maintenance of neuron survival and function in the SNc within the neurodegenerative environment, following transplantation of SCs could, *per se*, potentially translate in significant therapeutic outcomes. Substantial neuroprotective effects against dopaminergic depletion have been observed, for example, after transplantations of naïve, undifferentiated SCs such as adult adipose-derived adult stromal cells (McCoy et al., 2008), human NSC (Yasuhara et al., 2006) or human MSC (Blandini et al., 2010) in 6-OHDA lesioned rats.

Similarly, neuroprotection was evident following grafting of human MSC in an animal model of progressive parkinsonism (Park et al., 2010; Park et al., 2008a). In an interesting approach, transplantation of genetically engineered NSC, in animal models of brain tumor or injury, could served as incessant sources of secreted therapeutic agents (neuroprotective or tumoricidal) playing the role of biological minipumps (Chen et al., 2007). This procedure could readily be applicable to neurodegenerative diseases, including PD. As already described for neuroinflammation, the complex interactions between grafted SCs and endogenous surrounding cells can reciprocally influence outcome of transplantation both through direct interconnections (adherent junctions) or long distance mediations (release of soluble factors) (Boucherie and Hermans, 2009). In Amyotrophic Lateral Sclerosis for example, non-neuronal neighboring cells, including astrocytes, can drastically enhance neuronal survival (Nagai et al., 2007). Concordantly, in PD, glial cells play a critical role in homeostatic mechanisms that promote neuronal survival through release of an array of pro- and anti-inflammatory cytokines, anti-oxidants and neurotrophic factors within the microenvironment of the brain (L' Episcopo et al., 2010). Interestingly, grafting of MSC differentiated towards astrocyte-like phenotypes resulted in relevant improvements of motor impairment in 6-OHDA lesioned rats in the absence of dopaminergic differentiation (Bahat-Stroomza et al., 2009). Similarly, naïve MSC transplanted in the striatum of 6-OHDA lesioned animals acquired a glial-like phenotype and significantly reduced the toxin-induced neurodegeneration (Blandini et al., 2010).

Recent innovative approaches also include the use viral vectors to induce selected SC to produce/release specific neurotrophins possibly active in repairing/rescuing the degenerating nigrostriatal system. New protocols for efficient transduction of MSC allowing enhanced delivery of GDNF have been developed. Transplantation of the transduced cells in experimental PD resulted in the preservation of striatal TH immunoreactivity around the graft (Moloney et al., 2010). Similarly, GDNF- and Brain Derived Neurotrophic Factor (BDNF)-secreting MSC transplanted in 6-OHDA lesion rats improved behavioral deficits, typically detected in these animals (Sadan et al., 2009). Human neural progenitor cells that had been genetically modified to release GDNF, readily survived without tumor formation, following the intrastriatal transplantation into the brain of aged monkeys (Behrstock et al., 2006). A comparative study with non human primate has evidenced that the striato-nigral axon-transport is also compromised in advanced PD patient potentially limiting the regular retrograde transport of factors towards affected neuronal bodies in the SNc (Bartus et al., 2011). These therapeutic strategies may, therefore, be applicable mainly to patients at an early stage of the disease when part of the nigrostriatal network is still spared and may be rescued. Different clinical approaches may be required as disease proceeds with the wide loss of dopaminergic neurons (Rascol, 2009).

Donor cells, to physiologically repair damaged neural circuitry using SC transplantation, must be able to survive in sufficient number, to differentiate into the appropriate cell type and to adequately support the host brain environment. To optimize functional recovery and minimize side effects, grafted SCs should be able to functionally integrate in and be regulated by the host brain. Outcome of transplantation may be directly affected by time of grafting and cell number (Darsalia et al., 2011). Correlation between cell amount and therapeutic effects has, for example, been demonstrated for naive MSC that dose-dependently and regionally sustained the survival of striatal/nigral dopaminergic terminals and enhanced neurogenesis, following intrastriatal transplantation in parkinsonian rats (Blandini et al., 2010; Cova et al., 2010). Among the pathogenetic mechanisms involved in

PD a role of reduced neurogenesis has been suggested (Geraerts et al., 2007). The SVZ, one of the two neurogenic zones region located in the lateral wall of the ventricles that maintains the largest pool of proliferating cells in the mature mammalian CNS, receives organized projections from the SNc. These efferent projections can influence precursor cell proliferation in both adult animal (Baker et al., 2004; O'Keeffe et al., 2009a) and primate models (Freundlieb et al., 2006), probably through dopamine-induced release of Epidermal Growth Factor in the SVZ (O'Keeffe et al., 2009b). Dopaminergic denervation within SVZ causes a reduced rate of neural precursor mitosis and abridged neuronal maturation in the long term, a phenomenon common among PD patients (Hoglinger et al., 2004) and toxin-induced animal models of PD (Aponso et al., 2008; He et al., 2006; He et al., 2008; Winner et al., 2009; Winner et al., 2006).

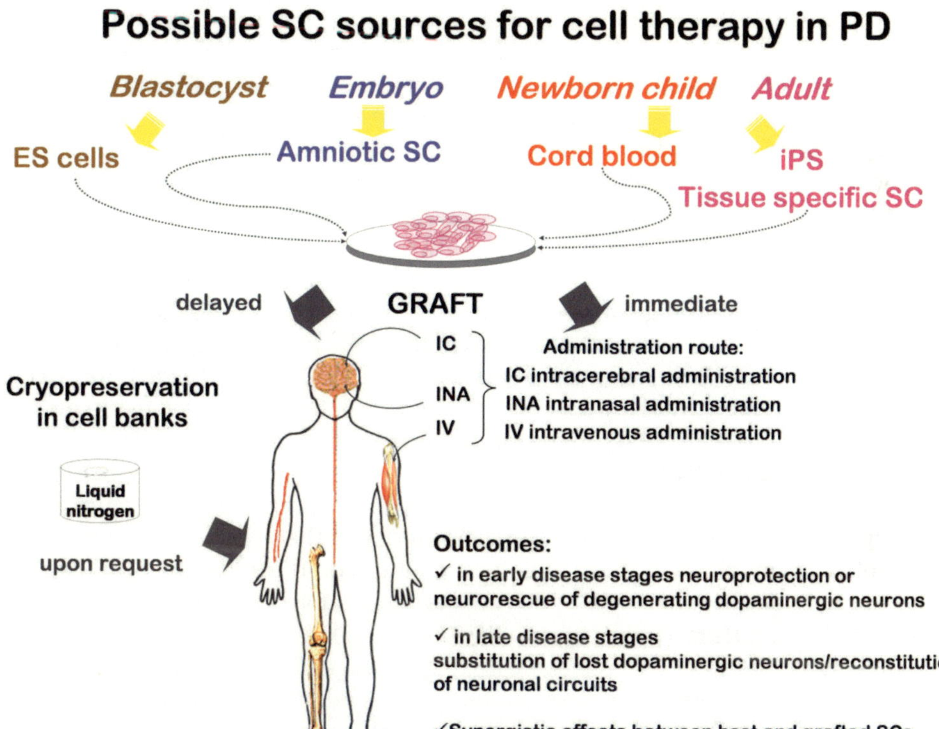

Fig. 2. Schematic flow chart for cell therapy in PD
A clinical approach to PD therapy will require 1) SC isolation (possible from different sources) 2) their expansion *in vitro* 3) direct or delayed transplantation through alternative or multiple administration routes. Independently from SC type and injection site, the therapeutic outcomes will depend upon donor and host ages, extension of the neuronal degeneration and graft size. The possible reparative mechanisms exerted by SC transplantation comprise neuronal replacement, neuroprotection of residual dopaminergic neurons and stimulation of endogenous neurogenesis, which may variably contribute to observed behavioral and physiological improvements. In PD cell therapy all the manipulations involving SCs should be conducted following the GMP guidelines in the absence of serum or other animal components.

Release of growth factor by grafted SC may influence adult neurogenesis and up-regulate self renewal and/or differentiation of adult host cells both under physiological and pathological conditions. Pre-clinical data suggest that modulation of endogenous neurogenesis may represent an alternative ways to slow down neuronal cell loss and possibly regenerate affected brain areas by modulation of endogenous neurogenesis (Geraerts et al., 2007; Okano et al., 2007). Administration of several growth factors (i.e. Transforming Growth Factor-α, BDNF and Fibroblast Growth Factor) in striatum enhanced neuronal differentiation within SVZ with overall improvements in murine behavior (Chiocco et al., 2007). Moreover, in the SNc pharmacological activation of dopamine receptor D3 with a selective agonist -7-hydroxy-N,N-di-n-propyl-2aminotetralin- induced cell proliferation and maturation towards dopaminergic phenotype (Van Kampen and Eckman, 2006), thus suggesting the possible occurrence of adult neurogenesis in this region under the pathological conditions in PD (Arias-Carrion et al., 2009). Presence of neurogenesis in the SNc suggests that disease progression may rely on the loss of dopaminergic neurons as well as on the malfunctioning in their turnover. Possible efficacy of orthotopic dopaminergic neurogenesis in PD has been questioned for a long time (Hermann and Storch, 2008), but transplantation experiments have indicated that several SC types, including neural precursors (Arias-Carrion et al., 2006; Madhavan et al., 2009) and MSC (Cova et al., 2010), can significantly support endogenous neurogenesis during the degenerative process in animal models of PD (Hess and Borlongan, 2008). Neurogenesis has been confirmed in SVZ of human brains (Curtis et al., 2007), but its physiological role is still uncertain (Zhao et al., 2008). Similarly, the existence of an improved neuronal reconstruction in the basal ganglia of the human PD brain (Yoshimi et al., 2005) is still a matter of debate. The reasons for decreased neurogenesis observed with aging and in pathological states may be related to an intrinsic inability to respond to the proliferative stimulation in the neurogenic niche, a reduction in the number of proliferative SC number, or the presence of activated microglia and neuroinflammation (Russo et al., 2011). Therefore, unraveling the localization as well as the degree of neurogenesis rate in human brains, together with the discovery of the specific molecules involved in these biological events, could lead to the discovery of new pharmacological disease-modifying treatments and novel potential targets, readily applicable to PD patients (Lindvall and Kokaia, 2010). Finally, it appears realistic to combine the synergistic effects between exogenous and endogenous SC actions to obtain cues on potential mechanisms involved in the noxious effects of neurodegeneration in PD as possible targets for clinical therapy (see Figure 2) (Madhavan and Collier, 2010).

7. Stem cell transplantation: Delivery method and timing

To date different SC types, as well as route of cell administration have shown efficacy in animal models. Two main routes have been generally used for SC delivery: intracerebral and intravascular. The first one is a stereotaxic transplantation of cells into the brain. Given, in PD, that brain damage principally occurs in both striatum (dopaminergic terminals) and SNc (neuronal soma), the best transplantation site, that would provide the most efficient and widest SC engraftment, is unknown. Nowadays, striatal administration of SCs is the most common approach for pre-clinical trials in PD (Blandini et al., 2010; Yasuhara et al., 2006; Zhu et al., 2009), although SC transplantation in mfb is also feasible (Gu et al., 2009). Gu and colleagues showed that double injection of NT-3 transfected NSC in mfb and ventral tegmental area of parkinsonian rats generates new TH positive cells in these areas with relevant behavioral and functional recovery (Gu et al., 2009).

Although the intracerebral route has provided a large panel of positive results in animal models and has allowed a better understanding of mechanisms underlying disease pathology, independently of the graft site, an outsized dilemma still resides in its invasive nature. To bypass this concern intravascular administration has also been undertaken. Intravenous administration of MSC after in 6-OHDA lesioned rats yields preservation of dopaminergic system and relevant behavioral improvements, although no transplanted SCs were observed in brain one month after injection (Wang et al., 2010). The intravenous administration route has obvious clinical advantages compared to intracerebral injection, yet evident efficient therapeutic benefits are fully dependent on the appropriate number of cells reaching the lesion sites. Concordantly, Wang et al have reported that the majority of SCs injected intravenously mostly dispersed in pulmonary tissue (Wang et al., 2010). This is in high contrast with the intracerebral route in which a large amount of cells are injected directly in or may easily migrate within the nearer lesion site. In 6-OHDA lesioned rats, the number of SCs still present at the site of injection, 4 weeks after transplantation, was proportional to the number of cells initially injected (Cova et al., 2010). Regardless of the delivery route adopted for transplantation, the biological mechanisms activated by SC graft rely both on cellular replacement and activation of the endogenous repair mechanisms coupled to neurorescue effects exerted on degenerating neurons (Lindvall and Kokaia, 2010). To date, no data from comparative studies between several administration routes (e.g., intrastriatal, intraventricular, and intravenous injections) of SC delivery in PD patients are available, although open labeled clinical trials with stereotaxic surgery have been already conducted (Venkataramana et al., 2010). An interesting clinical approach by multiple administration routes for the treatment of spinal cord injuries has just been developed. Such strategy induces noteworthy with improvements of the life quality for patients (Geffner et al., 2008) and could be very positively applied to chronic degenerative diseases such as PD.

Recently, an innovative alternative route for SC administration via a intranasal drop has been developed in an animal model of PD. MSC delivered into rat nostrils were found to migrate to lesion brain areas where they survived for at least 6 months (Danielyan et al., 2011). In these animals striatal dopamine levels were increased and motor functions improved up to 68% of values observed in control animals (Danielyan et al., 2011). This administration route appears safe and could potentially be repeated overtime in a given patients. The intranasal procedure could avoid problems related to surgical implantation of SCs, although the positive outcomes need to be further confirmed before any clinical applications.

Future therapeutic trials should also evaluate how the time point at which SC transplantation is performed, with respect to the cerebral insult, may influence efficacy of the procedure: earlier cell grafts may provide effective neuroprotection to degenerating neurons but the hostile environment may endanger their long-term survival by spreading disease hallmarks (Kordower et al., 2008; Li et al., 2008; Mendez et al., 2008). In principle, a time interval sufficient to allow *in vitro* expansion of autologous SCs, would obviously be desirable both from a practical and clinical perspective. On the other hand, transplantation at later disease stages, when cell loss is almost complete, will mainly aim at replacing lost dopaminergic neurons and will certainly be affected by the reduced expression of homing signals secreted in degenerative brain tissues. Conversely, transplantation at early stage will mostly rely on rescue and regeneration of surviving neurons. For CNS repair,

transplantation of proliferating progenitors cells, whose fate is less predictable since they are more proliferative than neurons, would face difficulties in sorting from stray pluripotent SCs, in the absence of specific markers. A clear trial design will necessarily need to take in account all these different biological mechanisms and, most importantly, will require the development of the appropriate biomarkers (Rascol, 2009) to follow disease progression.
The choice of a specific SC type and its state of differentiation, as well as the amount of cells and route of administration will depend on the experimental endpoints, keeping in mind that each one faces inherent problems connected to local control of immune rejection, final differentiation towards dopaminergic neurons and cytokine release distally. For example transplantation of ES cells can lead to tumor formation and systemic injection of SCs may result in dispersion of the cells in non-target tissues. Circulating HSC could participate in the regeneration of peripheral tissues/organs, but only if a sufficient number of SCs is activated. Finally, as clearly pointed out by Irving Weissman, any future SC clinical application in neurodegenerative diseases will need to respect the four thresholds of clinical effectiveness: 1) cell homing to the diseased or injured tissue 2) effective engraftment, not just fusion with host cells 3) physiological effectiveness 4) permanence overtime (Weissman, 2000).

8. *In vivo* imaging and transplantation

As mentioned above animal models of PD are fundamental tools to evaluate feasibility and potential of a given SC population. To date translation of results obtained in pre-clinical animal models of PD has been difficult. In particular, the effect and long-term survival of transplanted cells remains an open issue. The development of innovative imaging techniques, combined with the creation of reporter transgenic mice, has widen our understanding of some pathological mechanisms of the disease and allowed the identification of specific pharmacological targets (van Nuenen et al., 2009). Precise tracking of transplanted SCs through novel imaging techniques, as well as monitoring of engraftment efficiency directly *in vivo* allows the immediate correlation between beneficial effects and SC localization/amount (Lee et al., 2008). Genetic tags have and continue to help researchers and bioethicists to track transplanted cells overtime following their behavior and dispersion in tissues in animals. The simplest tag uses genetic recombination to introduce a fluorescent marker, such as green fluorescent protein, into a cell, but magnetic nanoparticles have also been proven to be helpful (Ferreira et al., 2008). Since cell therapy relies on SC involvement in physiological circuits their upshots could persist over a long time and should, therefore, be devoid of side effects. Homing, engraftment, cell fate, persistence and tumor formation of labeled SCs and their progeny needs to be carefully evaluated and could potentially be assessed using *in vivo* imaging. In complex neurodegenerative diseases, such as PD, grafted SCs or derived progenitor cells may protect residual neurons rather than replacing the degenerated ones. Therefore, tagged grafts could be easily characterized to determine if transplanted cells trigger endogenous mechanisms of repair or whether they directly replace lost cell populations. Successful application of magnetically-labeled mouse embryonic SCs to a rat model of PD coupled to the study of their diffusion up to 6 months post transplant has already demonstrated the feasibility and safety of this approach (Stroh et al., 2009). Imaging techniques are already used to study early and presymptomatic stages of PD (Wu et al., 2011) and effectively measures outcomes in clinical trials of neuroprotection demonstrate that it is a practical non invasive method extensible to all PD patients (Pavese et al., 2009). PET measurements of 6-(18F) fluorodopa (18F-FDOPA) uptake indicate nigrostriatal neuronal integrity and may provide a useful endophenotype for PD linkage studies (Kumakura and Cumming, 2009). Clinical benefits and graft viability of embryonic dopamine cell implantation have been followed by functional imaging for up to 4 years after graft in 33 patients, thus correlating motor improvements with increased 18F-FDOPA uptake (Ma et al., 2010).

9. Conclusions

Gaining more information about the pathology of the disease, the probable behavior of the grafted cells, as well as the reciprocal interconnections between the transplants and the host environment in animal models will be useful to predict possible complications and undesirable side effects readily translatable to future clinical trials for PD patients (Li et al., 2010b). Caution needs to be adapted since xenograft models of disease in animals may not accurately predict the same response in humans due to inherent differences. However, pre-clinical data will help improve patient selection for future clinical trials, assess restoration of brain connectivity, and monitor inflammatory processes in the continuous search of novel therapeutic targets (Politis and Piccini, 2010). Moreover, targeted delivery of SCs through alternative routes could be easily compared in animal models. Concordantly, one objective of modern neuroimaging is to identify markers for clinical diagnosis, monitor the disease progression, define the exact SC placement and analyze the impact of long-term drug/cell therapy through the direct spatio-temporal visualization of SCs as well as their effect on disease progression in patients, using non invasive techniques (Lee et al., 2008). A successful SC therapy requires extensive knowledge on SC properties, appropriate harvesting, manipulation and apt implantation, but also subsequent graft monitoring in the long time to verify the permanence of reparative mechanisms (Nikolic et al., 2009). On the basis of these data, it may be possible to properly select SC type, administration timing and delivery route for specific disease entities, anatomic areas, and physiologic circumstances to obtain reproducible experimental results for the creation of effective clinical protocols (Lindvall and Kokaia, 2010).

Additionally, cell transplantation in animal is often performed before or contemporaneously to neurotoxin lesion. Further development of experimental models that more accurately recreate neurodegenerative conditions present in patients, in which treatment can only intervene when the degenerative process is overt and motor symptoms are manifest, is required. In particular, the creation of genetic animal models is becoming increasingly important to elucidate gene-environment interactions, define pathogenic mechanisms, and provide a platform for testing cell therapeutic interventions (Magen and Chesselet, 2010).

The development and validation of conventional pharmacological therapy for clinical use is a long process that usually requires at least a decade. Cell transplantation, which represents an advanced therapeutic strategy far more complex than any pharmaceutical compound, was introduced surprisingly early into the clinic. Although some positive effects have been observed in the pioneering clinical studies sufficient caution should be taken before this strategy can be "routinely" applied to PD patients in order to avoid complications that may set back the field. In particular, defining and validating a specific cell type that may be consistently used in transplantation procedures is still a milestone that needs to be achieved. Extensive interactions and communication between clinicians and pre-clinical scientists is mandatory to allow the constant fine-tuning of the design of therapeutic strategies for PD patients.

10. References

Abeliovich A, Doege CA. Reprogramming therapeutics: iPS cell prospects for neurodegenerative disease. Neuron 2009; 61: 337-9.

Andersson E, Tryggvason U, Deng Q, Friling S, Alekseenko Z, Robert B, et al. Identification of intrinsic determinants of midbrain dopamine neurons. Cell 2006; 124: 393-405.

Aponso PM, Faull RL, Connor B. Increased progenitor cell proliferation and astrogenesis in the partial progressive 6-hydroxydopamine model of Parkinson's disease. Neuroscience 2008; 151: 1142-53.

Arenas E. Towards stem cell replacement therapies for Parkinson's disease. Biochem Biophys Res Commun 2010; 396: 152-6.

Arias-Carrion O, Hernandez-Lopez S, Ibanez-Sandoval O, Bargas J, Hernandez-Cruz A, Drucker-Colin R. Neuronal precursors within the adult rat subventricular zone differentiate into dopaminergic neurons after substantia nigra lesion and chromaffin cell transplant. J Neurosci Res 2006; 84: 1425-37.

Arias-Carrion O, Yamada E, Freundlieb N, Djufri M, Maurer L, Hermanns G, et al. Neurogenesis in substantia nigra of parkinsonian brains? J Neural Transm Suppl 2009: 279-85.

Bahat-Stroomza M, Barhum Y, Levy YS, Karpov O, Bulvik S, Melamed E, et al. Induction of adult human bone marrow mesenchymal stromal cells into functional astrocyte-like cells: potential for restorative treatment in Parkinson's disease. J Mol Neurosci 2009; 39: 199-210.

Baker SA, Baker KA, Hagg T. Dopaminergic nigrostriatal projections regulate neural precursor proliferation in the adult mouse subventricular zone. Eur J Neurosci 2004; 20: 575-9.

Barnum CJ, Tansey MG. Modeling neuroinflammatory pathogenesis of Parkinson's disease. Prog Brain Res 2010; 184: 113-32.

Bartus RT, Herzog CD, Chu Y, Wilson A, Brown L, Siffert J, et al. Bioactivity of AAV2-neurturin gene therapy (CERE-120): Differences between Parkinson's disease and nonhuman primate brains. Mov Disord 2011; 26: 27-36.

Barzilay R, Ben-Zur T, Bulvik S, Melamed E, Offen D. Lentiviral delivery of LMX1a enhances dopaminergic phenotype in differentiated human bone marrow mesenchymal stem cells. Stem Cells Dev 2009; 18: 591-601.

Behrstock S, Ebert A, McHugh J, Vosberg S, Moore J, Schneider B, et al. Human neural progenitors deliver glial cell line-derived neurotrophic factor to parkinsonian rodents and aged primates. Gene Ther 2006; 13: 379-88.

Bibikova M, Laurent LC, Ren B, Loring JF, Fan JB. Unraveling epigenetic regulation in embryonic stem cells. Cell Stem Cell 2008; 2: 123-34.

Bjorklund A, Dunnett SB, Brundin P, Stoessl AJ, Freed CR, Breeze RE, et al. Neural transplantation for the treatment of Parkinson's disease. Lancet Neurol 2003; 2: 437-45.

Blandini F, Cova L, Armentero MT, Zennaro E, Levandis G, Bossolasco P, et al. Transplantation of undifferentiated human mesenchymal stem cells protects against 6-hydroxydopamine neurotoxicity in the rat. Cell Transplant 2010; 19: 203-17.

Boucherie C, Hermans E. Adult stem cell therapies for neurological disorders: benefits beyond neuronal replacement? J Neurosci Res 2009; 87: 1509-21.

Brochard V, Combadiere B, Prigent A, Laouar Y, Perrin A, Beray-Berthat V, et al. Infiltration of CD4+ lymphocytes into the brain contributes to neurodegeneration in a mouse model of Parkinson disease. J Clin Invest 2009; 119: 182-92.

Brundin P, Barker RA, Parmar M. Neural grafting in Parkinson's disease Problems and possibilities. Prog Brain Res 2010; 184: 265-94.

Carlsson T, Carta M, Munoz A, Mattsson B, Winkler C, Kirik D, et al. Impact of grafted serotonin and dopamine neurons on development of L-DOPA-induced dyskinesias in parkinsonian rats is determined by the extent of dopamine neuron degeneration. Brain 2009; 132: 319-35.

Cayre M, Canoll P, Goldman JE. Cell migration in the normal and pathological postnatal mammalian brain. Prog Neurobiol 2009; 88: 41-63.

Chambers SM, Fasano CA, Papapetrou EP, Tomishima M, Sadelain M, Studer L. Highly efficient neural conversion of human ES and iPS cells by dual inhibition of SMAD signaling. Nat Biotechnol 2009; 27: 275-80.

Chen H, Zhang SM, Hernan MA, Schwarzschild MA, Willett WC, Colditz GA, et al. Nonsteroidal anti-inflammatory drugs and the risk of Parkinson disease. Arch Neurol 2003; 60: 1059-64.

Chen HI, Bakshi A, Royo NC, Magge SN, Watson DJ. Neural stem cells as biological minipumps: a faster route to cell therapy for the CNS? Curr Stem Cell Res Ther 2007; 2: 13-22.

Chiocco MJ, Harvey BK, Wang Y, Hoffer BJ. Neurotrophic factors for the treatment of Parkinson's disease. Parkinsonism Relat Disord 2007; 13 Suppl 3: S321-8.

Chua SJ, Bielecki R, Wong CJ, Yamanaka N, Rogers IM, Casper RF. Neural progenitors, neurons and oligodendrocytes from human umbilical cord blood cells in a serum-free, feeder-free cell culture. Biochem Biophys Res Commun 2009; 379: 217-21.

Cipriani S, Bonini D, Marchina E, Balgkouranidou I, Caimi L, Grassi Zucconi G, et al. Mesenchymal cells from human amniotic fluid survive and migrate after transplantation into adult rat brain. Cell Biol Int 2007; 31: 845-50.

Cooper O, Hargus G, Deleidi M, Blak A, Osborn T, Marlow E, et al. Differentiation of human ES and Parkinson's disease iPS cells into ventral midbrain dopaminergic neurons requires a high activity form of SHH, FGF8a and specific regionalization by retinoic acid. Mol Cell Neurosci 2010; 45: 258-66.

Cova L, Armentero MT, Zennaro E, Calzarossa C, Bossolasco P, Busca G, et al. Multiple neurogenic and neurorescue effects of human mesenchymal stem cell after transplantation in an experimental model of Parkinson's disease. Brain Res 2010; 1311: 12-27.

Curtis MA, Eriksson PS, Faull RL. Progenitor cells and adult neurogenesis in neurodegenerative diseases and injuries of the basal ganglia. Clin Exp Pharmacol Physiol 2007; 34: 528-32.

Danielyan L, Schafer R, von Ameln-Mayerhofer A, Bernhard F, Verleysdonk S, Buadze M, et al. Therapeutic efficacy of intranasally delivered mesenchymal stem cells in a rat model of Parkinson disease. Rejuvenation Res 2011; 14: 3-16.

Darsalia V, Allison SJ, Cusulin C, Monni E, Kuzdas D, Kallur T, et al. Cell number and timing of transplantation determine survival of human neural stem cell grafts in stroke-damaged rat brain. J Cereb Blood Flow Metab 2011; 31: 235-42.

Das S, Basu A. Inflammation: a new candidate in modulating adult neurogenesis. J Neurosci Res 2008; 86: 1199-208.

Dass B, Olanow CW, Kordower JH. Gene transfer of trophic factors and stem cell grafting as treatments for Parkinson's disease. Neurology 2006; 66: S89-103.

Dawson TM, Ko HS, Dawson VL. Genetic animal models of Parkinson's disease. Neuron 2010; 66: 646-61.

Donaldson AE, Cai J, Yang M, Iacovitti L. Human amniotic fluid stem cells do not differentiate into dopamine neurons in vitro or after transplantation in vivo. Stem Cells Dev 2009; 18: 1003-12.

Dunnett SB, Lelos M. Behavioral analysis of motor and non-motor symptoms in rodent models of Parkinson's disease. Prog Brain Res 2010; 184: 35-51.

Ferreira L, Karp JM, Nobre L, Langer R. New opportunities: the use of nanotechnologies to manipulate and track stem cells. Cell Stem Cell 2008; 3: 136-46.

Fox SH, Brotchie JM. The MPTP-lesioned non-human primate models of Parkinson's disease. Past, present, and future. Prog Brain Res 2010; 184: 133-57.

Fox SH, Lang AE, Brotchie JM. Translation of nondopaminergic treatments for levodopa-induced dyskinesia from MPTP-lesioned nonhuman primates to phase IIa clinical studies: keys to success and roads to failure. Mov Disord 2006; 21: 1578-94.

Freed CR, Greene PE, Breeze RE, Tsai WY, DuMouchel W, Kao R, et al. Transplantation of embryonic dopamine neurons for severe Parkinson's disease. N Engl J Med 2001; 344: 710-9.

Freundlieb N, Francois C, Tande D, Oertel WH, Hirsch EC, Hoglinger GU. Dopaminergic substantia nigra neurons project topographically organized to the subventricular zone and stimulate precursor cell proliferation in aged primates. J Neurosci 2006; 26: 2321-5.

Fricker-Gates RA, Gates MA. Stem cell-derived dopamine neurons for brain repair in Parkinson's disease. Regen Med 2010; 5: 267-78.

Friling S, Andersson E, Thompson LH, Jonsson ME, Hebsgaard JB, Nanou E, et al. Efficient production of mesencephalic dopamine neurons by Lmx1a expression in embryonic stem cells. Proc Natl Acad Sci U S A 2009; 106: 7613-8.

Geffner LF, Santacruz P, Izurieta M, Flor L, Maldonado B, Auad AH, et al. Administration of autologous bone marrow stem cells into spinal cord injury patients via multiple routes is safe and improves their quality of life: comprehensive case studies. Cell Transplant 2008; 17: 1277-93.

Geraerts M, Krylyshkina O, Debyser Z, Baekelandt V. Concise review: therapeutic strategies for Parkinson disease based on the modulation of adult neurogenesis. Stem Cells 2007; 25: 263-70.

Gruen L, Grabel L. Concise review: scientific and ethical roadblocks to human embryonic stem cell therapy. Stem Cells 2006; 24: 2162-9.

Gu S, Huang H, Bi J, Yao Y, Wen T. Combined treatment of neurotrophin-3 gene and neural stem cells is ameliorative to behavior recovery of Parkinson's disease rat model. Brain Res 2009; 1257: 1-9.

Gunaseeli I, Doss MX, Antzelevitch C, Hescheler J, Sachinidis A. Induced pluripotent stem cells as a model for accelerated patient- and disease-specific drug discovery. Curr Med Chem 2011; 17: 759-66.

Hagell P, Brundin P. Cell survival and clinical outcome following intrastriatal transplantation in Parkinson disease. J Neuropathol Exp Neurol 2001; 60: 741-52.

Hanna JH, Saha K, Jaenisch R. Pluripotency and cellular reprogramming: facts, hypotheses, unresolved issues. Cell 2010; 143: 508-25.

Hargus G, Cooper O, Deleidi M, Levy A, Lee K, Marlow E, et al. Differentiated Parkinson patient-derived induced pluripotent stem cells grow in the adult rodent brain and reduce motor asymmetry in Parkinsonian rats. Proc Natl Acad Sci U S A 2010; 107: 15921-6.

He XJ, Nakayama H, Dong M, Yamauchi H, Ueno M, Uetsuka K, et al. Evidence of apoptosis in the subventricular zone and rostral migratory stream in the MPTP mouse model of Parkinson disease. J Neuropathol Exp Neurol 2006; 65: 873-82.

He XJ, Yamauchi H, Uetsuka K, Nakayama H. Neurotoxicity of MPTP to migrating neuroblasts: studies in acute and subacute mouse models of Parkinson's disease. Neurotoxicology 2008; 29: 413-20.

Heinrich AC, Patel SA, Reddy BY, Milton R, Rameshwar P. Multi- and inter-disciplinary science in personalized delivery of stem cells for tissue repair. Curr Stem Cell Res Ther 2009; 4: 16-22.

Hermann A, Storch A. Endogenous regeneration in Parkinson's disease: do we need orthotopic dopaminergic neurogenesis? Stem Cells 2008; 26: 2749-52.

Hess DC, Borlongan CV. Stem cells and neurological diseases. Cell Prolif 2008; 41 Suppl 1: 94-114.

Hoglinger GU, Rizk P, Muriel MP, Duyckaerts C, Oertel WH, Caille I, et al. Dopamine depletion impairs precursor cell proliferation in Parkinson disease. Nat Neurosci 2004; 7: 726-35.

Hwang DY, Kim DS, Kim DW. Human ES and iPS cells as cell sources for the treatment of Parkinson's disease: current state and problems. J Cell Biochem 2010; 109: 292-301.

Karussis D, Kassis I, Kurkalli BG, Slavin S. Immunomodulation and neuroprotection with mesenchymal bone marrow stem cells (MSCs): a proposed treatment for multiple sclerosis and other neuroimmunological/neurodegenerative diseases. J Neurol Sci 2008; 265: 131-5.

Kim YJ, Park HJ, Lee G, Bang OY, Ahn YH, Joe E, et al. Neuroprotective effects of human mesenchymal stem cells on dopaminergic neurons through anti-inflammatory action. Glia 2009; 57: 13-23.

Kimmelman J, London AJ, Ravina B, Ramsay T, Bernstein M, Fine A, et al. Launching invasive, first-in-human trials against Parkinson's disease: ethical considerations. Mov Disord 2009; 24: 1893-901.

Kiskinis E, Eggan K. Progress toward the clinical application of patient-specific pluripotent stem cells. J Clin Invest 2010; 120: 51-9.

Kitada M, Dezawa M. Induction system of neural and muscle lineage cells from bone marrow stromal cells; a new strategy for tissue reconstruction in degenerative diseases. Histol Histopathol 2009; 24: 631-42.

Klimanskaya I, Chung Y, Meisner L, Johnson J, West MD, Lanza R. Human embryonic stem cells derived without feeder cells. Lancet 2005; 365: 1636-41.

Kordower JH, Chu Y, Hauser RA, Freeman TB, Olanow CW. Lewy body-like pathology in long-term embryonic nigral transplants in Parkinson's disease. Nat Med 2008; 14: 504-6.

Kriks S, Studer L. Protocols for generating ES cell-derived dopamine neurons. Adv Exp Med Biol 2009; 651: 101-11.

Kumakura Y, Cumming P. PET studies of cerebral levodopa metabolism: a review of clinical findings and modeling approaches. Neuroscientist 2009; 15: 635-50.

L' Episcopo F, Tirolo C, Testa N, Caniglia S, Morale M, Marchetti B. Glia as a turning point in the therapeutic strategy of Parkinson's disease. CNS Neurol Disord Drug Targets 2010; 9: 349-72.

Langston JW, Ballard P, Tetrud JW, Irwin I. Chronic Parkinsonism in humans due to a product of meperidine-analog synthesis. Science 1983; 219: 979-80.

Lebouvier Thibaud, Maddalena Tasselli, Sébastien Paillusson, Hélène Pouclet, Neunlist M, Derkindere aP. Biopsable neural tissues: toward new biomarkers for Parkinson's disease? . Frontiers in Psychiatry 2010; 1: doi: 10.3389/fpsyt.2010.00128

Lee PH, Park HJ. Bone marrow-derived mesenchymal stem cell therapy as a candidate disease-modifying strategy in Parkinson's disease and multiple system atrophy. J Clin Neurol 2009; 5: 1-10.

Lee Z, Dennis JE, Gerson SL. Imaging stem cell implant for cellular-based therapies. Exp Biol Med (Maywood) 2008; 233: 930-40.

Lévesque MF, Neuman T, Rezak M. Therapeutic Microinjection of Autologous Adult Human Neural Stem Cells and Differentiated Neurons for Parkinson's Disease: Five-Year Post-Operative Outcome. The Open Stem Cell Journal 2009; 1: 20-29.

Levy YS, Bahat-Stroomza M, Barzilay R, Burshtein A, Bulvik S, Barhum Y, et al. Regenerative effect of neural-induced human mesenchymal stromal cells in rat models of Parkinson's disease. Cytotherapy 2008; 10: 340-52.

Li JY, Englund E, Holton JL, Soulet D, Hagell P, Lees AJ, et al. Lewy bodies in grafted neurons in subjects with Parkinson's disease suggest host-to-graft disease propagation. Nat Med 2008; 14: 501-3.

Li M, Zhang SZ, Guo YW, Cai YQ, Yan ZJ, Zou Z, et al. Human umbilical vein-derived dopaminergic-like cell transplantation with nerve growth factor ameliorates motor dysfunction in a rat model of Parkinson's disease. Neurochem Res 2010a; 35: 1522-9.

Li SC, Tachiki LM, Luo J, Dethlefs BA, Chen Z, Loudon WG. A biological global positioning system: considerations for tracking stem cell behaviors in the whole body. Stem Cell Rev 2010b; 6: 317-33.

Lindvall O, Kokaia Z. Prospects of stem cell therapy for replacing dopamine neurons in Parkinson's disease. Trends Pharmacol Sci 2009; 30: 260-7.

Lindvall O, Kokaia Z. Stem cells in human neurodegenerative disorders--time for clinical translation? J Clin Invest 2010; 120: 29-40.

Liu ZJ, Zhuge Y, Velazquez OC. Trafficking and differentiation of mesenchymal stem cells. J Cell Biochem 2009; 106: 984-91.

Lu L, Li F, Wang X. Novel anti-inflammatory and neuroprotective agents for Parkinson's disease. CNS Neurol Disord Drug Targets 2010; 9: 232-40.

Ma Y, Tang C, Chaly T, Greene P, Breeze R, Fahn S, et al. Dopamine cell implantation in Parkinson's disease: long-term clinical and (18)F-FDOPA PET outcomes. J Nucl Med 2010; 51: 7-15.

Madhavan L, Collier TJ. A synergistic approach for neural repair: cell transplantation and induction of endogenous precursor cell activity. Neuropharmacology 2010; 58: 835-44.

Madhavan L, Daley BF, Paumier KL, Collier TJ. Transplantation of subventricular zone neural precursors induces an endogenous precursor cell response in a rat model of Parkinson's disease. J Comp Neurol 2009; 515: 102-15.

Magen I, Chesselet MF. Genetic mouse models of Parkinson's disease The state of the art. Prog Brain Res 2010; 184: 53-87.

Maguire-Zeiss KA, Federoff HJ. Future directions for immune modulation in neurodegenerative disorders: focus on Parkinson's disease. J Neural Transm 2010; 117: 1019-25.

Mathieu P, Battista D, Depino A, Roca V, Graciarena M, Pitossi F. The more you have, the less you get: the functional role of inflammation on neuronal differentiation of endogenous and transplanted neural stem cells in the adult brain. J Neurochem 2010; 112: 1368-85.

Matigian N, Abrahamsen G, Sutharsan R, Cook AL, Vitale AM, Nouwens A, et al. Disease-specific, neurosphere-derived cells as models for brain disorders. Dis Model Mech 2010; 3: 785-98.

McCoy MK, Martinez TN, Ruhn KA, Wrage PC, Keefer EW, Botterman BR, et al. Autologous transplants of Adipose-Derived Adult Stromal (ADAS) cells afford dopaminergic neuroprotection in a model of Parkinson's disease. Exp Neurol 2008; 210: 14-29.

McGeer PL, Itagaki S, Boyes BE, McGeer EG. Reactive microglia are positive for HLA-DR in the substantia nigra of Parkinson's and Alzheimer's disease brains. Neurology 1988; 38: 1285-91.

McGeer PL, McGeer EG. Inflammation and the degenerative diseases of aging. Ann N Y Acad Sci 2004; 1035: 104-16.

McGeer PL, McGeer EG. Glial reactions in Parkinson's disease. Mov Disord 2008; 23: 474-83.

Meisner LF, Johnson JA. Protocols for cytogenetic studies of human embryonic stem cells. Methods 2008; 45: 133-41.

Meissner WG, Frasier M, Gasser T, Goetz CG, Lozano A, Piccini P, et al. Priorities in Parkinson's disease research. Nat Rev Drug Discov 2011; 10: 377-93.

Mendez I, Vinuela A, Astradsson A, Mukhida K, Hallett P, Robertson H, et al. Dopamine neurons implanted into people with Parkinson's disease survive without pathology for 14 years. Nat Med 2008; 14: 507-9.

Meyer AK, Maisel M, Hermann A, Stirl K, Storch A. Restorative approaches in Parkinson's Disease: which cell type wins the race? J Neurol Sci 2010; 289: 93-103.

Miura K, Okada Y, Aoi T, Okada A, Takahashi K, Okita K, et al. Variation in the safety of induced pluripotent stem cell lines. Nat Biotechnol 2009; 27: 743-5.

Moloney TC, Rooney GE, Barry FP, Howard L, Dowd E. Potential of rat bone marrow-derived mesenchymal stem cells as vehicles for delivery of neurotrophins to the Parkinsonian rat brain. Brain Res 2010; 1359: 33-43.

Muraoka K, Shingo T, Yasuhara T, Kameda M, Yuen WJ, Uozumi T, et al. Comparison of the therapeutic potential of adult and embryonic neural precursor cells in a rat model of Parkinson disease. J Neurosurg 2008; 108: 149-59.

Murrell W, Wetzig A, Donnellan M, Feron F, Burne T, Meedeniya A, et al. Olfactory mucosa is a potential source for autologous stem cell therapy for Parkinson's disease. Stem Cells 2008; 26: 2183-92.

Nagai M, Re DB, Nagata T, Chalazonitis A, Jessell TM, Wichterle H, et al. Astrocytes expressing ALS-linked mutated SOD1 release factors selectively toxic to motor neurons. Nat Neurosci 2007; 10: 615-22.

Neumann H, Kotter MR, Franklin RJ. Debris clearance by microglia: an essential link between degeneration and regeneration. Brain 2009; 132: 288-95.

Nikolic B, Faintuch S, Goldberg SN, Kuo MD, Cardella JF. Stem cell therapy: a primer for interventionalists and imagers. J Vasc Interv Radiol 2009; 20: 999-1012.

O'Keeffe GC, Barker RA, Caldwell MA. Dopaminergic modulation of neurogenesis in the subventricular zone of the adult brain. Cell Cycle 2009a; 8: 2888-94.

O'Keeffe GC, Tyers P, Aarsland D, Dalley JW, Barker RA, Caldwell MA. Dopamine-induced proliferation of adult neural precursor cells in the mammalian subventricular zone is mediated through EGF. Proc Natl Acad Sci U S A 2009b; 106: 8754-9.

Obeso JA, Rodriguez-Oroz MC, Benitez-Temino B, Blesa FJ, Guridi J, Marin C, et al. Functional organization of the basal ganglia: therapeutic implications for Parkinson's disease. Mov Disord 2008; 23 Suppl 3: S548-59.

Okano H, Sakaguchi M, Ohki K, Suzuki N, Sawamoto K. Regeneration of the central nervous system using endogenous repair mechanisms. J Neurochem 2007; 102: 1459-65.

Olanow CW, Goetz CG, Kordower JH, Stoessl AJ, Sossi V, Brin MF, et al. A double-blind controlled trial of bilateral fetal nigral transplantation in Parkinson's disease. Ann Neurol 2003; 54: 403-14.

Ourednik J, Ourednik V, Lynch WP, Schachner M, Snyder EY. Neural stem cells display an inherent mechanism for rescuing dysfunctional neurons. Nat Biotechnol 2002; 20: 1103-10.

Papanikolaou T, Lennington JB, Betz A, Figueiredo C, Salamone JD, Conover JC. In vitro generation of dopaminergic neurons from adult subventricular zone neural progenitor cells. Stem Cells Dev 2008; 17: 157-72.

Park HJ, Bang G, Lee BR, Kim HO, Lee PH. Neuroprotective effect of human mesenchymal stem cells in an animal model of double toxin-induced multiple system atrophy-parkinsonism. Cell Transplant 2010.

Park HJ, Lee PH, Bang OY, Lee G, Ahn YH. Mesenchymal stem cells therapy exerts neuroprotection in a progressive animal model of Parkinson's disease. J Neurochem 2008a; 107: 141-51.

Park IH, Arora N, Huo H, Maherali N, Ahfeldt T, Shimamura A, et al. Disease-specific induced pluripotent stem cells. Cell 2008b; 134: 877-86.

Park S, Koh SE, Maeng S, Lee WD, Lim J, Lee YJ. Neural progenitors generated from the mesenchymal stem cells of first-trimester human placenta matured in the hypoxic-ischemic rat brain and mediated restoration of locomotor activity. Placenta 2011; 32: 269-76.

Parkkinen L, Silveira-Moriyama L, Holton JL, Lees AJ, Revesz T. Can olfactory bulb biopsy be justified for the diagnosis of Parkinson's disease? Comments on "olfactory bulb alpha-synucleinopathy has high specificity and sensitivity for Lewy body disorders". Acta Neuropathol 2009; 117: 213-4; author reply 217-8.

Pasi CE, Dereli-Oz A, Negrini S, Friedli M, Fragola G, Lombardo A, et al. Genomic instability in induced stem cells. Cell Death Differ 2011.

Pavese N, Kiferle L, Piccini P. Neuroprotection and imaging studies in Parkinson's disease. Parkinsonism Relat Disord 2009; 15 Suppl 4: S33-7.

Perrier AL, Tabar V, Barberi T, Rubio ME, Bruses J, Topf N, et al. Derivation of midbrain dopamine neurons from human embryonic stem cells. Proc Natl Acad Sci U S A 2004; 101: 12543-8.

Piccini P, Brooks DJ, Bjorklund A, Gunn RN, Grasby PM, Rimoldi O, et al. Dopamine release from nigral transplants visualized in vivo in a Parkinson's patient. Nat Neurosci 1999; 2: 1137-40.

Picinich SC, Mishra PJ, Mishra PJ, Glod J, Banerjee D. The therapeutic potential of mesenchymal stem cells. Cell- & tissue-based therapy. Expert Opin Biol Ther 2007; 7: 965-73.

Politis M, Piccini P. Brain imaging after neural transplantation. Prog Brain Res 2010; 184: 193-203.

Pruszak J, Isacson O. Molecular and cellular determinants for generating ES-cell derived dopamine neurons for cell therapy. Adv Exp Med Biol 2009; 651: 112-23.

Rascol O. "Disease-modification" trials in Parkinson disease: target populations, endpoints and study design. Neurology 2009; 72: S51-8.

Redmond DE, Jr., Weiss S, Elsworth JD, Roth RH, Wakeman DR, Bjugstad KB, et al. Cellular repair in the parkinsonian nonhuman primate brain. Rejuvenation Res 2010; 13: 188-94.

Roy NS, Cleren C, Singh SK, Yang L, Beal MF, Goldman SA. Functional engraftment of human ES cell-derived dopaminergic neurons enriched by coculture with telomerase-immortalized midbrain astrocytes. Nat Med 2006; 12: 1259-68.

Russo I, Barlati S, Bosetti F. Effects of neuroinflammation on the regenerative capacity of brain stem cells. J Neurochem 2011; 116: 947-56.

Sadan O, Bahat-Stromza M, Barhum Y, Levy YS, Pisnevsky A, Peretz H, et al. Protective effects of neurotrophic factor-secreting cells in a 6-OHDA rat model of Parkinson disease. Stem Cells Dev 2009; 18: 1179-90.

Schule B, Pera RA, Langston JW. Can cellular models revolutionize drug discovery in Parkinson's disease? Biochim Biophys Acta 2009; 1792: 1043-51.

Schwarz J, Storch A. Transplantation in Parkinson's disease: will mesenchymal stem cells help to reenter the clinical arena? Transl Res 2010; 155: 55-6.

Schwarz SC, Schwarz J. Translation of stem cell therapy for neurological diseases. Transl Res 2011; 156: 155-60.

Serra PA, Pluchino S, Marchetti B, Desole MS, Miele E. The MPTP mouse model: cues on DA release and neural stem cell restorative role. Parkinsonism Relat Disord 2008; 14 Suppl 2: S189-93.

Shetty P, Ravindran G, Sarang S, Thakur AM, Rao HS, Viswanathan C. Clinical grade mesenchymal stem cells transdifferentiated under xenofree conditions alleviates motor deficiencies in a rat model of Parkinson's disease. Cell Biol Int 2009; 33: 830-8.

Shim JW, Park CH, Bae YC, Bae JY, Chung S, Chang MY, et al. Generation of functional dopamine neurons from neural precursor cells isolated from the subventricular zone and white matter of the adult rat brain using Nurr1 overexpression. Stem Cells 2007; 25: 1252-62.

Stroh A, Boltze J, Sieland K, Hild K, Gutzeit C, Jung T, et al. Impact of magnetic labeling on human and mouse stem cells and their long-term magnetic resonance tracking in a rat model of Parkinson disease. Mol Imaging 2009; 8: 166-78.

Tansey MG, Goldberg MS. Neuroinflammation in Parkinson's disease: its role in neuronal death and implications for therapeutic intervention. Neurobiol Dis 2010; 37: 510-8.

Thomas MG, Stone L, Evill L, Ong S, Ziman M, Hool L. Bone marrow stromal cells as replacement cells for Parkinson's disease: generation of an anatomical but not functional neuronal phenotype. Transl Res 2011; 157: 56-63.

Tonnesen J, Parish CL, Sorensen AT, Andersson A, Lundberg C, Deisseroth K, et al. Functional integration of grafted neural stem cell-derived dopaminergic neurons monitored by optogenetics in an in vitro Parkinson model. PLoS One 2011; 6: e17560.

Toriumi H, Yoshikawa M, Matsuda R, Nishimura F, Yamada S, Hirabayashi H, et al. Treatment of Parkinson's disease model mice with allogeneic embryonic stem cells: necessity of immunosuppressive treatment for sustained improvement. Neurol Res 2009; 31: 220-7.

Ungerstedt U. 6-Hydroxy-dopamine induced degeneration of central monoamine neurons. Eur J Pharmacol 1968; 5: 107-10.

Van Kampen JM, Eckman CB. Dopamine D3 receptor agonist delivery to a model of Parkinson's disease restores the nigrostriatal pathway and improves locomotor behavior. J Neurosci 2006; 26: 7272-80.

van Nuenen BF, van Eimeren T, van der Vegt JP, Buhmann C, Klein C, Bloem BR, et al. Mapping preclinical compensation in Parkinson's disease: an imaging genomics approach. Mov Disord 2009; 24 Suppl 2: S703-10.

Venkataramana NK, Kumar SK, Balaraju S, Radhakrishnan RC, Bansal A, Dixit A, et al. Open-labeled study of unilateral autologous bone-marrow-derived mesenchymal stem cell transplantation in Parkinson's disease. Transl Res 2010; 155: 62-70.

Vicente Miranda H, Outeiro TF. The sour side of neurodegenerative disorders: the effects of protein glycation. J Pathol 2010; 221: 13-25.

Vierbuchen T, Ostermeier A, Pang ZP, Kokubu Y, Sudhof TC, Wernig M. Direct conversion of fibroblasts to functional neurons by defined factors. Nature 2010; 463: 1035-41.

Wakeman DR, Dodiya HB, Kordower JH. Cell transplantation and gene therapy in Parkinson's disease. Mt Sinai J Med 2011; 78: 126-58.

Wang F, Yasuhara T, Shingo T, Kameda M, Tajiri N, Yuan WJ, et al. Intravenous administration of mesenchymal stem cells exerts therapeutic effects on parkinsonian model of rats: focusing on neuroprotective effects of stromal cell-derived factor-1alpha. BMC Neurosci 2010; 11: 52.

Weissman IL. Translating stem and progenitor cell biology to the clinic: barriers and opportunities. Science 2000; 287: 1442-6.

Wernig M, Zhao JP, Pruszak J, Hedlund E, Fu D, Soldner F, et al. Neurons derived from reprogrammed fibroblasts functionally integrate into the fetal brain and improve symptoms of rats with Parkinson's disease. Proc Natl Acad Sci U S A 2008; 105: 5856-61.

White RB. Looks like a duck, quacks like a duck ... still behaves like a bone marrow stromal cell. Transl Res 2011; 157: 53-5.

Whitton PS. Neuroinflammation and the prospects for anti-inflammatory treatment of Parkinson's disease. Curr Opin Investig Drugs 2010; 11: 788-94.

Winner B, Desplats P, Hagl C, Klucken J, Aigner R, Ploetz S, et al. Dopamine receptor activation promotes adult neurogenesis in an acute Parkinson model. Exp Neurol 2009; 219: 543-52.

Winner B, Geyer M, Couillard-Despres S, Aigner R, Bogdahn U, Aigner L, et al. Striatal deafferentation increases dopaminergic neurogenesis in the adult olfactory bulb. Exp Neurol 2006; 197: 113-21.

Wu Y, Le W, Jankovic J. Preclinical biomarkers of Parkinson disease. Arch Neurol 2011; 68: 22-30.

Xu L, Tan YY, Ding JQ, Chen SD. The iPS technique provides hope for Parkinson's disease treatment. Stem Cell Rev 2010a; 6: 398-404.

Xu Q, Jiang X, Ke Y, Zhang S, Xu R, Zeng Y. Gene therapy in hemiparkinsonian rhesus monkeys: long-term survival and behavioral recovery by transplantation of autologous human tyrosine hydroxylase-expressing neural stem cells. Cytotherapy 2010b; 12: 226-37.

Yang JR, Liao CH, Pang CY, Huang LL, Lin YT, Chen YL, et al. Directed differentiation into neural lineages and therapeutic potential of porcine embryonic stem cells in rat Parkinson's disease model. Cell Reprogram 2010; 12: 447-61.

Yasuhara T, Matsukawa N, Hara K, Yu G, Xu L, Maki M, et al. Transplantation of human neural stem cells exerts neuroprotection in a rat model of Parkinson's disease. J Neurosci 2006; 26: 12497-511.

Yoshimi K, Ren YR, Seki T, Yamada M, Ooizumi H, Onodera M, et al. Possibility for neurogenesis in substantia nigra of parkinsonian brain. Ann Neurol 2005; 58: 31-40.

Zhang S, Zou Z, Jiang X, Xu R, Zhang W, Zhou Y, et al. The therapeutic effects of tyrosine hydroxylase gene transfected hematopoetic stem cells in a rat model of Parkinson's disease. Cell Mol Neurobiol 2008; 28: 529-43.

Zhao C, Deng W, Gage FH. Mechanisms and functional implications of adult neurogenesis. Cell 2008; 132: 645-60.

Zhu Q, Ma J, Yu L, Yuan C. Grafted neural stem cells migrate to substantia nigra and improve behavior in Parkinsonian rats. Neurosci Lett 2009; 462: 213-8.

Zou Z, Jiang X, Zhang W, Zhou Y, Ke Y, Zhang S, et al. Efficacy of Tyrosine Hydroxylase gene modified neural stem cells derived from bone marrow on Parkinson's disease--a rat model study. Brain Res 2010; 1346: 279-86.

16

Cell Therapy for Parkinson's Disease: Status and Perspectives

Pia Jensen, Christina Krabbe and Morten Meyer
Department of Neurobiology Research, Institute of Molecular Medicine, University of Southern Denmark, Odense C Denmark

1. Introduction

Idiopathic Parkinson's disease (PD) is caused by progressive degeneration of melanin containing dopaminergic neurons in substantia nigra pars compacta in the upper brain stem. The loss of dopaminergic neurons results in a gradual decrease of dopaminergic input to the striatum leading to the cardinal symptoms rigidity, tremor, hypokinesia and occasionally postural instability.

One of the prospects for a curative treatment for PD is to replace the lost dopaminergic neurons by intracerebral transplantation. Grafting of fetal midbrain dopaminergic neurons into the dopamine-depleted striatum has thus emerged as an experimental therapeutic approach for PD. Preclinical and clinical trials have demonstrated that such fetal dopaminergic neurons have the potential to markedly improve motor function in animal models and PD patients. Over the last decades, approximately 400 PD patients have been grafted, and graft survival in the dopamine-depleted striatum, with substantial motor improvements, has been reported particularly in younger patients. However, looking across all the studies, where several different protocols and donor ages have been used, the symptomatic relief is inconsistent and not yet of a magnitude that would justify treatment at a large scale. Ethical concerns related to the use of human fetal brain tissue, shortage of suitable donor tissue and a poor survival of grafted dopaminergic neurons has stimulated the search for other reliable sources of donor material and development of applicable gene technological techniques for improving graft survival, differentiation and functional integration.

Expanded midbrain precursor cells, predifferentiated human embryonic stem cells or induced pluripotent stem cells as well as human neural stem cells and mesenchymal stem cells have been proposed as promising alternative sources of donor cells. In this chapter we will review current status and discuss crucial issues that remain to be resolved to develop cell replacement into an effective and safe therapy.

2. Treatment strategies for Parkinson's disease

Conventional treatment of PD is symptomatic and includes pharmacotherapy, possibly combined with surgical deep brain stimulation (DBS). These symptomatic treatments are highly effective at managing the motor symptoms, especially in the early stages of the disease. However, they have limited capability to improve symptoms at more advanced stages, thus new therapeutic and restorative strategies, including the use of neuroprotective agents, *in vivo* gene therapy, genetically engineered cell lines ("cell factories") and stem cells, are in development. Providing a continuous supply of dopamine to the striatum using viral delivery of enzymes in the dopamine synthesis is one approach. Other experimental strategies aim at protecting and stimulating sprouting of remaining dopaminergic neurons using neurotrophic factors or directly replacing lost innervation by transplantation of primary dopaminergic tissue or stem cell-derived dopaminergic neurons. Here we focus on the perspectives of recent developments in the latter approach and provide a historical review of neural transplantation as potential future therapy for PD.

2.1 Symptomatic treatment strategies

The observation of dopamine depletion in the striatum of PD patients (Carlsson, Lindqvist, and Magnusson 1957), led to development of the now classical L-dopa replacement therapy, with subsequent dramatic clinical benefit to virtually all patients. Medication with the dopamine precursor L-dopa results in effective improvements of motor symptoms, and it is still the most commonly used drug for treatment of PD - alone or in combination with other drugs acting primarily on the dopaminergic system. Unfortunately, L-dopa gradually loses its effect (typically after 5-7 years of L-dopa treatment) as the remaining dopaminergic neurons continue to degenerate and patients experience end-of-dose deterioration and start to fluctuate between states, where they are immobile called "off"-periods" and states where they are able to move called "on"-periods". In addition, the treatment is coupled to further motor complications such as L-dopa-induced dyskinesias and often also psychiatric symptoms (Fahn 2006). This clearly underlines the need for development of new systemic pharmacological therapies or alternative treatment strategies.

In addition to L-dopa treatment, other drugs are used to stimulate the deteriorated dopaminergic neurotransmission, such as dopamine agonists and inhibitors of monoamine oxidase B and catechol-*O*-methyl transferase, both enzymes which prevent the breakdown of dopamine (Hauser and Zesiewicz 2007). So far, no medication has been shown to slow the loss of dopaminergic neurons in PD, but there are some indications from preclinical studies that the monoamine oxidase B inhibitor, rasagiline, might have neuroprotective effects. Recently, a large, double-blind placebo-controlled clinical trial showed that patients receiving a rasagiline dose of 1 mg per day experienced benefits that were consistent with a possible disease modifying effect, whereas treatment with a dose of 2 mg per day had no such effect (Olanow et al. 2009). Thus, these results must be further evaluated and additional studies performed in order to draw valid conclusions. A problem in studies of neuroprotection by medicaments known for symptomatic relief is the use of clinical measures, such as a change in score on the Unified Parkinson's Disease Rating Scale (UPDRS), as primary outcome measures. This makes it difficult to distinguish pure symptomatic benefit from real neuroprotection, as both would be reflected in improved scores. Thus, the possibilities of using independent and objective biomarkers in future trials, such as Positron Emmision Tomography (PET) imaging of nigrostriatal dopamine terminals are being investigated (Lohle and Reichmann 2010).

Surgical procedures, such as thalamotomy or pallidotomy, and circuit inhibition by high-frequency DBS through electrodes implanted in the globus pallidus or the subthalamic nucleus have gained considerably attention as therapies for PD. In general, DBS is preferable to the prior ablative surgical methods since electrical stimulation is both reversible and programmable. Especially, stimulation in the subthalamic nucleus has shown to improve motor function and reduce dyskinesias and need for medication (Pahwa et al. 2006). Although ablative surgery and DBS eliminate or ameliorate certain symptoms of the disease, the long-term effect is not well known. DBS has been increasingly established in several clinical trials, but questions remain regarding the best timing of the procedure, the best anatomical target for stimulation, ways to avoid preoperative and postoperative adverse effects as well as which patients should be selected for the treatment (Morley and Hurtig 2010). Unfortunately, this treatment is also not restorative and cannot slow down or prevent disease progression, and most patients experience progressive worsening over time. Furthermore, DBS only treat a fairly specific set of symptoms (mostly, L-dopa induced dyskinesias and/or tremor) and has no effect on other clinical manifestations, such as postural instability.

2.2 Intracerebral transplantation – a historical perspective

Cell replacement therapy for treatment of PD is based on the idea that immature dopaminergic neurons, following transplantation and functional integration, can restore dopaminergic neurotransmission and exert long-lasting effects on motor symptoms. Based on data from animal experimentation, the current main focus is on elevating striatal dopamine levels rather than trying to reconstruct the relatively long nigrostriatal pathway.
Here we provide an overview of different cell types and tissues that have been used for grafting in PD - with emphasis on fetal ventral mesencephalic tissue, which has resulted in the greatest clinical benefits. This is followed by a discussion of future perspectives of cell replacement for PD, with particular focus on stem cell based strategies.

2.2.1 Autografts

Ethical and immunological issues can be avoided by use of autografts for treatment of any disorder, including PD, making this strategy very attractive. The first clinical experiments with grafting to the brains of PD patients involved autografts of adrenal medullary tissue, which secretes dopamine among other catecholamines (Backlund et al. 1985; Lindvall et al. 1987; Drucker-Colin et al. 1988; Freed, Poltorak, and Becker 1990). These small open-label clinical trials caused initial enthusiasm, but have largely been abandoned since 1989 after failure in a number of clinical trials (Allen et al. 1989; Goetz et al. 1991). Some patients experienced modest effects for a limited period of time, and post-mortem studies showed poor survival of the grafted tissue (Hurtig et al. 1989; Kordower et al. 1991). A recent follow-up study, performed 16 years after adrenal medulla transplantation showed few surviving chromaffin cells and a complete absence of tyrosine hydroxylase (TH)-positive cells at the graft site, providing evidence of no long-term survival of adrenal medullary transplants (Kompoliti et al. 2007).
Autografts of sympathetic ganglion neurons, collected from the cervical or thoracic sympathetic chain, have also been considered as a source of donor cells for PD patients. Sympathetic ganglion neurons have been shown to express the enzymes aromatic amino acid decarboxylase and vesicular monoamine transporter 2, which are involved in production and transport of dopamine, both *in vitro* and after transplantation to a rat model of PD (Nakao et al. 2001; Nakao et al. 2004). Thus, their ability to convert exogenous L-dopa to dopamine and to store the synthesized dopamine was thought to be a potential action. Accordingly, some patients experienced increased duration of L-dopa-induced "on"-periods

with consequent reduction of time spent in "off" phase with overall improvement in bradykinesia, but no significant change in the UPDRS scores (Itakura et al. 1997; Nakao et al. 2004). Overall, these limited clinical benefits along with the rather invasive techniques for obtaining the ganglionic tissue make this an unsuitable approach.

A third approach has been autografts of carotid body cells, which normally secrete dopamine and divide in response to hypoxic stimuli (Espejo et al. 1998). Striatal transplantation of carotid body cells resulted in partial functional recovery in rat and primate models of PD (Espejo et al. 1998; Luquin et al. 1999). This led to a small clinical study (Arjona et al. 2003), where most patients experienced motor improvement seen as a reduction in their UPDRS "off"-score, however, there was no increase in [^{18}F]-fluorodopa uptake in the transplanted striatum as seen by PET imaging. Furthermore, it was shown that the surviving number of dopaminergic neurons in the transplants was very low (Arjona et al. 2003). Thus, the reason for the motor improvements remains unclear.

2.2.2 Fetal ventral mesencephalic grafts

In 1979, the first two successful attempts of transplantation with fetal ventral mesencephalic cells in animal models were reported (Perlow et al. 1979; Bjorklund and Stenevi 1979). These studies showed that rat fetal ventral mesencephalic tissue transplanted into rats with unilateral 6-hydroxydopamine (6-OHDA) lesions could reverse lesion-induced behavioral deficits. Furthermore, the grafted dopaminergic neurons innervated the striatum and were found to form synapses with host neurons. These initial and pioneering results initiated a series of studies in rodents examining the survival and functional capacity of dopaminergic neurons following grafting into different brain regions (Dunnett et al. 1983; Dunnett et al. 1981; Freund et al. 1985). Improvements were clearly seen when grafts were placed in the striatum, whereas attempts to graft into the substantia nigra, the ventral mesencephalic sub-region with dopaminergic cell body degeneration, showed survival of cells, but they did not innervate the striatum and had no significant functional effects (Dunnett et al. 1983). In 1986, human fetal ventral mesencephalic tissue was reported to survive transplantation into immunosuppressed, 6-OHDA lesioned rats and exert functional effects on motor behavior (Brundin et al. 1986; Stromberg et al. 1986). The best outcomes were seen for tissue derived from human fetuses, obtained at 5.5-8 weeks postconception. The results of these studies paved the way for the first systematic clinical transplantation trials with dopaminergic neurons to PD patients.

Since 1987, several so-called open-label trials (trials where small groups of patients receive transplants without the use of any control group or blinding procedure) have been performed. These initial trials have revealed that fetal human nigral neurons, taken at a stage of development when they have started to express their dopaminergic phenotype, can survive, integrate and function in the human brain. In 1990, the first study demonstrating survival and functional effects of grafted human ventral mesencephalic tissue in an immunosuppressed PD patient was published (Lindvall et al. 1990) and during the following years a wide number of open-label trials reported improved motor functions in the absence of medication and reduced time spend in the "off" phase (Madrazo et al. 1990; Brundin et al. 2000; Freed et al. 1992; Freed, Breeze, Rosenberg, Schneck, Wells, Barrett, Grafton, Huang et al. 1990; Freed, Breeze, Rosenberg, Schneck, Wells, Barrett, Grafton, Mazziotta et al. 1990; Lindvall et al. 1989; Lindvall et al. 1994; Peschanski et al. 1994). Furthermore, in some cases even reduced dyskinesias in the "on" state were seen (Freed, Breeze, Rosenberg, Schneck, Wells, Barrett, Grafton, Huang et al. 1990; Freed, Breeze,

Rosenberg, Schneck, Wells, Barrett, Grafton, Mazziotta et al. 1990; Madrazo et al. 1990) and some patients were able to stop their antiparkinsonian medication. Imaging studies showed that the grafts gradually gave rise to improved striatal [^{18}F]-fluorodopa uptake and few patients, who died of unrelated courses long time after surgery, had several thousand surviving dopaminergic neurons that innervated their striatum (Mendez et al. 2005; Kordower et al. 1995).

A major problem with transplantation of mesencephalic dopaminergic neurons in PD is that the outcome has varied dramatically between transplantation centers and also between patients treated at the same center essentially using the same procedure. Two main parameters are likely to be responsible for the mixed outcomes. First, differences between the PD patients regarding age, genetic background, stage of their disease, prior medication and precise neuropathological profile. The second issue is related to the surgery and post-grafting treatment such as numbers of cells being grafted, number and sites of injection, variation in surgical technique as well as tissue preparation (fresh versus stored tissue) and immunosuppression treatment (Bjorklund et al. 2003).

2.2.2.1 Double-blind placebo-controlled trials

The greatest setback for the neural transplantation field in PD was the outcome of two double-blind placebo-controlled trials in the late 1990s (Olanow et al. 2003; Freed et al. 2001). The objective of these trials, funded by the National Institute of Health (USA), was to properly support the clinical benefits of the transplantation procedure seen in the open label trials. The first trial involved 40 PD patients between 34 and 75 years of age and with average disease duration of 14 years (Freed et al. 2001). Patients were randomly assigned to receive a transplant or undergo sham surgery. The human ventral mesencephalic donor tissue, obtained from 7-8 week old fetuses, was cultured for up to 4 weeks as "tissue strands". Cultured tissue from two embryos was transplanted into the putamen on each side and no immunosuppression was used. Control patients received a sham-surgery with burr holes, but without penetration of the meninges. One year after transplantation there was no significant improvement in the transplant group (20% reduction in the motor part of the UPDRS as compared to the placebo group). However, when looking at the subgroup of younger patients (<60 years) a significant reduction of 30-35% was found. Though, subsequent analysis have suggested that the main determinant of this correlation was the preoperative L-dopa responsiveness rather than the age of the patient, as even older patients with good preoperative L-dopa responsiveness showed similar improvements (Bjorklund et al. 2003). Although the clinical benefits were modest and variable, PET scannings showed significant increase in [^{18}F]-fluorodopa uptake in the putamen of the transplant as compared to the placebo group, and postmortem analysis showed dopaminergic neuronal survival and fiber outgrowth in the graft. However, the number of surviving dopaminergic neurons was lower than that reported for other patients with good clinical response to their transplants (Freed et al. 2001).

Another outcome and concern from this trial was the appearance of L-dopa-independent, graft-induced dyskinesias in 15% of the patients more than 1 year after surgery. The reasons for the limited clinical outcome and the induction of graft-induced dyskinesias remain largely unknown, but various factors have been suggested to be of critical relevance. For instance, the amount of grafted tissue was smaller than that of other more successful trials, which may explain the low recovery of dopaminergic neurons seen by postmortem analysis. Furthermore, the absence of immunosuppressive treatment may have compromised dopaminergic cell survival, as may the storage of the fetal tissue up to 4 weeks prior to transplantation.

The second double-blind placebo-controlled trial involved 34 patients with advanced PD, aged between 30 and 75 years (Olanow et al. 2003). Patients were randomly assigned to receive bilateral transplantation with either 1 or 4 donors per side or sham surgery. Solid ventral mesencephalic tissue was obtained from 6-9 week old fetuses and stored for 2 days prior to transplantation. All patients received immunosuppression (cyclosporine A) starting 2 weeks before the transplantation and continuing for up to 6 month after surgery. Two years after transplantation, no significant treatment effects were assessed by the motor component of the UPDRS in the "off" medication, but there was a tendency for an improved motor score for the 4-donor group. Moreover, no differences between groups in terms of the change in time spend in "on" without dyskinesias and in required L-dopa dose was found. However, subsequent analysis based on disease severity showed that patients in the 4-donor group with preoperative less severe disease did display significant improvements in their UPDRS motor scores. Also patients both in the 1 and 4-donor groups showed significant motor improvements compared to placebo at 6 and 9 month after transplantation, but this effect declined thereafter, which may be related to the withdrawal of the immunosuppressive therapy at this time point. In fact, the initial improvements were similar to that reported for some of the previous open label trials. PET scannings showed significant bilateral increase in striatal [^{18}F]-fluorodopa uptake in both transplant groups as compared to the placebo group, with the 4-donor group displaying the greatest increase. Postmortem analysis also revealed good survival of dopaminergic neurons with relatively good innervations of the striatum, again with the 4-donor group showing the best results. However, as in the study by Freed et al. (2001), development of significant off-medication graft-induced dyskinesias were observed in 56% of the grafted patients 6 to 12 month after transplantation.

Thus, the results of these two double-blind placebo-controlled trials raised serious concerns about the utility and safety of fetal ventral mesencephalic transplants in PD patients. The main concerns related to the moderate efficacy of the transplants compared to previous open-label trials and to the development of graft-induced dyskinesias in a significant number of patients. The differences in the study design between the open-label trials and the placebo-controlled trials may contribute the the poor outcome of the placebo-controlled studies. However, the specific reasons remain largely unresolved as further discussed in the next section.

2.2.2.2 Lessons from the clinical trials and the TRANSEURO project

Several issues have been suggested as explanations for the inconsistencies of the transplantation trials using fetal ventral mesencephalic tissue, such as patient selection, tissue preparation, graft placement and the need for immunosuppressive treatment. So far there is no clear consensus as to whether one or all of these factors contribute. As a consequence of all these possible confounders a re-evaluation of the field of neural grafting for PD has been undertaken. First, the indications that patient selection may be an important factor come from the observations that the best results in the double-blind placebo-controlled trials were seen for patients with less severe disease and good preoperative response to L-dopa. Furthermore, there is also some evidence that older patients generally do less well (Winkler, Kirik, and Bjorklund 2005). Second, parameters such as the number and age of donor fetuses, surgical techniques applied and graft placement may all have affected the survival and functional integration of the grafted dopaminergic neurons. In the study by Freed et al. (2001) the method involved less tissue, stored for longer times, while the Olanow et al. (2003) study used tissue pieces, stored for a short period of time. Several studies have shown that a variety of issues in the preparation process are critical for the optimization of dopaminergic cell survival in the transplants and some of the factors used in the protocols from these trials may have had harmful effects on dopaminergic cell survival after transplantation. Third, immunosuppression is an issue. Even though the brain is considered an immunologically privileged site, the host immunesystem can respond to the graft. Previous animal experiments have shown that intracerebral allografts of fetal ventral mesencephalic tissue can survive for prolonged periods in the absence of any immunosuppression (Head and Griffin 1985). However, in cases where the donor and host differ immunologically on both major and minor histocompatibility antigens, the graft is likely to induce a long-lasting inflammatory response, accompanied by upregulation of class I and class II antigens on the grafted cells, sustained expression of immunological markers, and macrophage and microglial activation at the graft site (Hudson et al. 1994; Shinoda et al. 1995, 1996). The intensity of the immune reaction can increase over time, indicating that the immune cells observed in the brain after grafting are not stationary and inactive but rather provide an ongoing inflammatory process (Shinoda et al. 1995). Nonetheless, the major clinical transplantation centers have in some cases chosen not to immunosuppres the PD patients (Freed et al. 2001) or to use a mild treatment for only 6 month (Olanow et al. 2003). Lastly, the mechanisms behind the development of graft-induced dyskinesias are not fully understood. These dyskinesias differ in nature compared to the typical L-dopa-induced dyskinesias. The severity tend to correlate negatively with the [^{18}F]-fluorodopa uptake in the striatum prior to transplantation, but it does not correlate with improvement in the UPDSC scores or daily medication needs after transplantation. Moreover, their appearance does not seem to relate to the severity of the preoperative L-dopa induced dyskinesias or the change in these after transplantation. Several factors have been suggested to cause the graft induced dyskinesias, such as inhomogeneous dopaminergic reinnervation of the host putamen (Ma et al. 2002), the presence of cells other than A9 dopaminergic neurons within the grafts, especially serotonergic neurons included in the grafts (Carlsson et al. 2007; Carta et al. 2007) and the graft size and placement in the striatum (Lane et al. 2006).

Thus, increased understanding of possible mechanism behind the disappointing results of the two double-blind placebo-controlled trials has led to initiation of a new clinical trial using fetal transplants for PD. This exciting project, called TRANSEURO, is funded by the 7th Framework Program of the European Commission and is a major collaboration between leading experts as clinicians, scientists, industrial partners, ethicists and patients' representative in this field (http://www.transeuro.org.uk/index.html). The main goals of the project are to show that consistency and efficacy of dopaminergic cell replacement in PD can be improved by careful attention to tissue preparation and delivery, patient selection and immunosuppressive treatment as discussed above. Moreover, to show that dopaminergic cell replacement can be clinically efficacious in the absence of any troublesome graft induced dyskinesias in patients with mild PD and to develop a protocol that can serve as a template for all future clinical trials in the cell therapy field, including expected future stem cell-based therapies. The first patients are to be transplanted in the beginning of 2012. After that, a double-blind placebo-controlled trial will be performed at several centers in Europe and USA. The general idea is to try to push the field ahead, while techniques for development of suitable cells from human stem cells are being conducted (Holden 2009).

2.2.2.3 Long-term post-mortem studies of fetal mesencephalic grafts

Recent post-mortem studies have shown that grafted dopaminergic neurons survive for up to 16 years in the brains of PD patients after transplantation (Mendez et al. 2008; Li et al. 2008; Kordower et al. 2008). These studies include in total 6 patients with long-term survival (9-16 years) after transplantation and all had experienced clinical benefits, though to a variable degree. In general, the grafts contained numerous TH-positive dopaminergic neurons with fibers innervating the host striatum. The grafts largely resembled those in patients who died 1.5-4 years after transplantation (Mendez et al. 2005; Kordower et al. 1996), though with lower numbers of TH-positive cells. Thus, these studies provide the first evidence of long-term survival of grafted dopaminergic neurons in PD. However, in two of these studies Lewy bodies and α-synuclein aggregates were found in few of the grafted cells (Kordower et al. 2008; Li et al. 2008). Low levels of dopamine transporter was also found in some of the grafted cells, which had not been seen for patients who died 1.5 year after transplantation (Kordower et al. 2008). Thus, these observations suggest that the pathogenetic process in PD can affect the transplanted neurons. At the moment, it is unclear what the functional significance of these findings is, but it is important to note that the majority of the grafted cells appeared normal and healthy and even if the graft may start to degenerate after 10 years or more due to host to graft disease propagation, the therapeutic window for cell transplantation would still be wide enough to allow a significant clinical intervention.

2.2.3 Xenografts

Xenografting is transplantation of tissue between different species. Fetal porcine neural tissue has been considered the most suitable alternative source for transplantation into the human brain due to the ease of breeding and the similarity in brain size combined with a protracted gestational period, which may provide the basis for long-distance axonal growth after grafting. Another interesting perspective has been the potential development of non-immunogenic transgenic donor pigs. The ability of xenografted ventral mesencephalic tissue to survive and mediate functional benefits in animal models of PD (Brevig et al. 2001; Galpern et al. 1996; Huffaker et al. 1989) led to a clinical safety trial, where 12 PD patients received unilateral striatal transplants of porcine ventral mesencephalic tissue suspensions (Schumacher et al. 2000; Deacon et al. 1997). A significant reduction in UPDRS was reported for some patients, but there was no increase in [^{18}F]-fluorodopa uptake at the transplant site, and a postmortem study of a patient who died of unrelated causes 8 month after transplantation showed that only around 650 TH-positive neurons out of 12 million transplanted cells had survived. This finding suggests a lack of trophic support of the grafted tissue. Furthermore, some lymphocyte infiltration into and around the graft was found even though the patient was immunosupressed with cyclosporine A (Deacon et al. 1997). A second double-blind placebo controlled trial involving 18 patients caused only moderate improvements in UPDRS scores in both transplant and sham surgery groups. However, these results have only been published in a press release in March 2001 (Wijeyekoon and Barker 2009).

Due to these disappointing results the clinical use of this approach is considered doubtful, especially as the use of xenogenic tissue deals with some additional issues as compared to allogenic grafts. First, there are the problems of increased graft rejection and second, there is the risk of spreading infection across the species barrier by porcine endogenous retroviruses

(Sayles, Jain, and Barker 2004). Thus, further work will be required to decide if fetal porcine tissue is of clinical relevance.

3. Stem cells

Stem cells are defined as undifferentiated cells without mature, tissue-specific characteristics that are able to reproduce themselves by division into identical daughter cells. Moreover, in response to proper stimuli stem cells are able to produce more specific progenitor cells that can further differentiate into one or more functional cell types. Stem cells are considered to represent a very promising source of cells cell replacement therapy in a number of diseases, including PD, due to these key properties, namely, self-renewal and multipotentiality as well as the possibility to manipulate these cells *in vitro*.

Dopaminergic neurons can be generated from stem cells of different sources (Fig. 1). Embryonic stem cells (ESCs) are isolated from the inner cell mass of the preimplantation blastocyst, and they have unlimited self-renewal capacity and are pluripotent, since they are

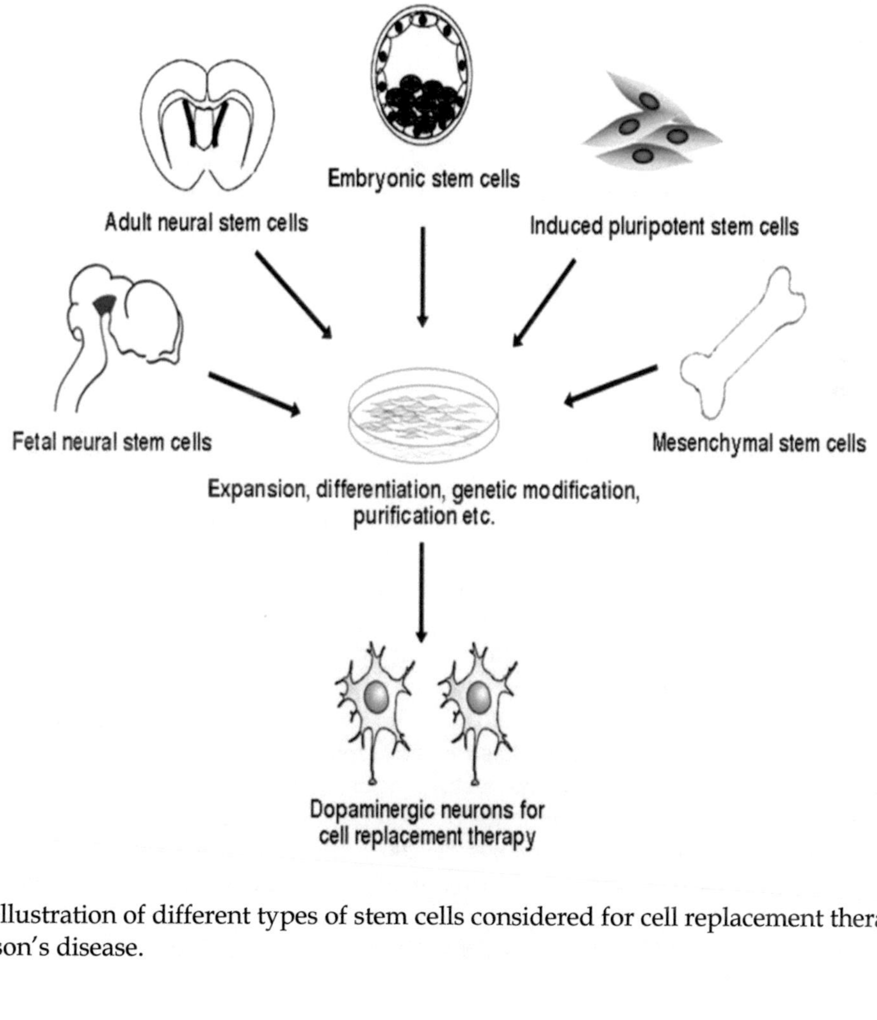

Fig. 1. Illustration of different types of stem cells considered for cell replacement therapy in Parkinson's disease.

able to generate cells of all three germ layers. Somatic or tissue-derived stem cells can be isolated from developing tissues of the fetus or in the newborn, juvenile or adult organism. Somatic stem cells have a more limited proliferation capacity than ESCs and are termed multipotent, typically being able to differentiate into the different cell types of one germ layer. Potential groups of stem cells for cell therapy for PD include ESCs, neural stem cells (NSCs), mesenchymal stem cells (MSCs) and more recently induced pluripotent stem (iPS) cells, which all will be discussed separately in this section.
The most important question, using stem cells as a therapy for PD, remains whether it is possible to generate a large number of cells with the capacity to survive and function as dopaminergic neurons following transplantation and to be sure that these stem cell derived grafts do not show adverse effects such as tumor formation or immune rejection (Table 1).

3.1 Embryonic stem cells

Generally, human ESCs are considered the most promising source of stem cells for cell therapy in PD as well as other diseases, since they have several advantages to somatic stem cells. First, most somatic stem cells are difficult to isolate and propagate, whereas ESCs are easily derived and are able to grow almost indefinitely in culture. Second, ESCs can be genetically manipulated by homologous recombination to correct a genetic defect, whereas somatic stem cells only can be genetically manipulated through the introduction of viral transgenes. Third, ESCs can be guided into becoming any type of cell in the body through specific culture conditions, whereas the differentiation potential of somatic stem cells is much more restricted. The major limitation is ethical issues regarding the use of fertilized eggs for derivation of ESCs. The challenges in providing cells for replacement therapy for PD both lie in stimulating ESCs to form neurons and, afterwards to make these neurons differentiate into functional dopaminergic cells. Thus, several strategies have been used to differentiate ESCs into dopaminergic neurons in vitro. In 2000, two reports for the first time described the generation of midbrain dopaminergic neurons from mouse ESCs (Kawasaki et al. 2000; Lee et al. 2000). Kawasaki et al. (2000) used a co-culture strategy in which the ESCs were grown on a layer of bone marrow stromal cells (PA6) to induce neural differentiation and the generation of dopaminergic neurons. They named this neural inducing effect as stromal cell-derived inducing activity (SDIA). The study by Lee et al. (2000) was based on a five-stage protocol, based on the generation, and later differentiation of spherical aggregate structures called embryoid bodies and addition of different combinations of factors known to promote dopaminergic differentiation such as fibroblast growth factor 8 (FGF8), sonic hedgehog (Shh) and ascorbic acid. The co-culture system resulted in a yield of approximately 16% TH-positive cells (Kawasaki et al. 2000), whereas the five-stage protocol only resulted in around 5% TH-positive cells (Lee et al. 2000). In 2002, Kim et al. reported that 78% TH-positive cells could be generated *in vitro* by using the five-stage protocol if the mouse ESCs overexpressed the midbrain precursor transcription factor Nurr1 (Kim et al. 2002). Since then, several studies using non-genetic modification approaches for differentiation of mouse ESCs have followed by the co-culturing strategy, the five-stage strategy, or a combination of both, however the number of neurons adopting a dopaminergic phenotype has varied considerably (Barberi et al. 2003; Inden et al. 2004; Rodriguez-Gomez et al. 2007; Morizane et al. 2006). In order to deal with this inefficiency several groups have followed the example by Kim et al. (2002) and manipulated mouse ESCs to overexpressed genes know to promote the dopaminergic phenotype, such as Nurr1 (Sonntag et al. 2004; Chung et al. 2002), Pitx3 (Chung et al. 2005;

Hedlund et al. 2008) and Lmx1a (Friling et al. 2009; Andersson et al. 2007), which have resulted in much higher yields of dopaminergic neurons. However, these transgenic approaches have limitations towards clinic use until the safety of such manipulations has been addressed.

In vivo studies have shown that it is possible to transplant ESCs into rodent models of PD and form dopaminergic neurons with a midbrain morphology that can ameliorate some of the motor symptoms (Rodriguez-Gomez et al. 2007; Barberi et al. 2003; Bjorklund et al. 2002; Kim et al. 2002; Hedlund et al. 2008). In 2002, Bjorklund et al. grafted undifferentiated mouse ESCs into the striatum of 6-OHDA-lesioned rats. Results showed that the grafted cells survived for 14-16 weeks and developed into midbrain-like dopaminergic neurons, thus the local inductive environment was indeed sufficient to induce dopaminergic differentiation of the undifferentiated ESCs. However, 20% of the grafted animals showed teratoma formation (Bjorklund et al. 2002). Several other studies have used different protocols for pre-differentiation of ESCs before transplantation (Shim et al. 2004; Nishimura et al. 2003; Kim et al. 2002) and prolonged *in vitro* differentiation seems to diminish the risk of tumor formation, but at the same time reduces survival of grafted cells as well as their the ability to integrate into the host tissue (Chung et al. 2002). In another approach, several groups focus on using fluorescence activated cell sorting (FACS) to select and purify midbrain dopaminergic neurons in the cell suspension before transplantation in order to minimize the risk of tumor formation (Hedlund et al. 2008; Chung et al. 2006).

Human ESCs can also be induced to become dopaminergic neurons both in vitro and in vivo. As for the mouse ESCs the most promising strategy for the generation of dopaminergic neurons has been co-culture systems (Perrier et al. 2004; Zeng et al. 2004) as compared to the multiple-stage method (Carpenter et al. 2001; Zhang et al. 2001). In 2004, Perrier et al. reported a very successful protocol for the generation of dopaminergic neurons from human ESCs. In this protocol the human ESCs were co-cultured with bone marrow stromal cells and treated in a sequential manner with patterning and differentiation molecules, including FGF8, Shh, FGF2, brain-derived neurotrophic factor (BDNF), glial cell line derived neuroptrophic factor (GDNF), transforming growth factor (TGF)-β3, dibutyryl-cAMP, and ascorbic acid. This treatment resulted in a yield of 65-80% TH-positive cells out of total neurons. Moreover, the dopaminergic neurons expressed several midbrain dopaminergic markers, released dopamine, had TH-positive synaptic terminals, and showed the presence of depolarization-induced and tetrodotoxin sensitive actions potentials, indicating that these cells were truly functional midbrain dopaminergic neurons (Perrier et al. 2004). More recently, great efforts have been put into defining chemical conditions that enhance dopaminergic differentiation in order to get rid of feeder layers and co-culture that compromise clinical use (Iacovitti et al. 2007; Song et al. 2008). Interestingly, a study by Vazin et al. (2009) identified four factors secreted from mouse stromal PA6 cells that are often used as feeder cells in the co-culture system, and these factors greatly enhanced the generation of neurons including the dopaminergic phenotype from human ESCs when added to the medium.

Dopaminergic neurons derived from human ESCs have also been transplanted into rodent models of PD, but the number of surviving TH-positive cells has been very low, and many of the transplants have shown evidence of proliferating cells and teratoma formation (Ben-Hur et al. 2004; Park et al. 2005; Zeng et al. 2004). Hence, improving the survival of the grafted human ESCs is a major challenge that has to be overcome before clinical application of the cells is possible. Interestingly, Roy et al. 2006 found a significant improved generation of TH-positive cells (up to 67% of total cells counted), when the human ESCs were cultured according to a feeder-based protocol in which human midbrain astrocytes were used to induce dopaminergic differentiation. These cells induced a significant behavioural recovery when transplanted into the striatum of parkinsonian rats. The dopaminergic neurons were reported to survive for 8 weeks, however neural tissue overgrowth and neuroepithelial tumors were found (Roy et al. 2006). More recent studies, using longer differentiation periods have produced larger numbers of dopaminergic neurons in the transplants (Yang et al. 2008).

As described above, the use, growth and differentiation of ESCs are not without disadvantages, and the use of fertilized eggs raise ethical concerns and limitations. In order to use human ESCs in the clinic it is important to culture the ESCs in xeno-free systems, which have not been the case for several existing protocols. However, as discussed above this issue has started to be resolved by production of chemically defined medias. Other problems that need to be solved before clinical use are the low survival and maintenance of the transplanted human ESC-derived dopaminergic neurons, and in addition the high risk of teratoma formations or other kinds of uncontrolled cell growth such as tumors by residual undifferentiated cells. Moreover, the risk of immune rejection questions the safety of clinical application of human ESCs.

3.2 Neural stem cells

NSCs are multipotent stem cells derived from neural tissues, which have the ability to self-renew and give rise to cells restricted to the neuronal and glial lineages, namely neurons, astrocytes and oligodendrocytes. Such NSCs are found in the developing nervous system and in certain regions of the adult brain. One advantage of NSCs as compared to ESCs is that they are less likely to form tumors after transplantation, since they are not pluripotent and capable of unlimited proliferation, and they seem to be more genomically stable than ESCs (Maitra et al. 2005; Draper et al. 2004). Both ESCs and fetal or adult NSCs represent potential cell sources for therapy, which and will be described and discussed in the following paragraphs (Fig. 2).

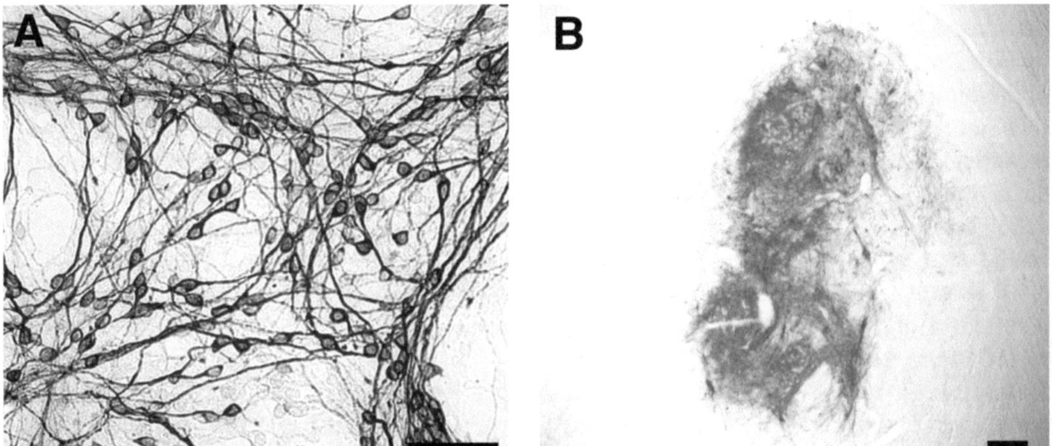

Fig. 2. A) *In vitro* differentiated TH-positive dopaminergic neurons generated from human neural stem cells. B) Intrastriatal porcine neural tissue graft containing TH-positive dopaminergic neurons in a rat model of Parkinson's disease. Scale bars 200 μm.

3.2.1 NSCs cells in the embryonic brain

NSCs from the developing central nervous system proliferate in response to similar growth factors regardless of which part of the brain they originate. However, they are not equivalent to each other and seem to maintain certain region-specific properties, even after they have been cultured *in vitro* for prolonged periods (Ostenfeld et al. 2002; Hitoshi et al. 2002; Schwarz et al. 2006). Hence, the most obvious place to look for stem cells able to generate dopaminergic neurons for PD is in the developing midbrain. Stem cells from this area are more likely to show a similar phenotype, and should have a straightforward differentiation pathway to form midbrain specific dopaminergic neurons (Ostenfeld et al. 2002; Horiguchi et al. 2004).

As previously described (section 2.2.2), PD patients have been successfully transplanted with ventral mesencephalic tissue from embryos at different stages. However, tissue from several human embryos is required for each patient due to the poor survival of the grafted neurons, thus resulting in practical-logistic problems. To overcome this problem several groups have focused on the idea of expanding ventral mesencephalic tissue to reduce the number of fetuses required for transplantation of one patient. In 1998, Studer et al. isolated neural precursor cells from the rat ventral mesecephalon and successfully expanded these cells by use of the mitogen FGF2, resulting in a 10-fold increase in the total number of cells and a 3-fold increase in the number of dopaminergic neurons. When transplanted into the striatum of 6-OHDA-lesioned rats the cells induced functional recovery. However, despite these promising results the general survival of grafted dopaminergic neurons was only around 3-5% (Studer, Tabar, and McKay 1998). Subsequently, the proportion of TH-positive cells generated by this method was further increased by culturing the cells at physiologically low oxygen tension (Studer et al. 2000). Carvey et al. 2001 reported a generation of 20-25% TH-positive cells from rat embryonic ventral mesencephalic precursor cells by using a combination of the cytokines IL-1 and IL-11, leukemia inhibitory factor and GDNF. They further expanded these cells and found clones containing up to 98% TH-positive cells and these were selected for transplantation into the striatum of 6-OHDA lesioned rats. The grafts completely reversed the rotational asymmetry, however, as seen in the study by Studer et al. (1998), the survival of the differentiated cells was very poor (Carvey et al. 2001).

In order to enhance the generation of midbrain specific dopaminergic neurons as well as increase the survival of these cells after transplantation genetic modification is an attractive strategy. In an early study, overexpression of Nurr1 in an immortalized NSC line originally derived from the mouse cerebellum showed a robust generation of dopaminergic neurons when these cells were co-cultured with astrocytes of mesencephalic origin (Wagner et al. 1999). Rat forebrain precursors have been reported to differentiate into dopaminergic neurons after genetic modification to co-express Nurr1, Shh and Bcl-xL or Nurr1 and Mash1, and these cells also showed behavioral benefits after transplantation into 6-OHDA- lesioned rats (Park et al. 2006). Overexpression of Nurr1 in NSCs derived from the rat ventral mesencephalon have been shown to result in 5% TH-positive neurons (Kim et al. 2007), whereas co-expression of Nurr1 and Neurogenin 2, another transcription factor important for development of mesencephalic dopaminergic neurons, did not mediate additional positive effect on the yield of TH-positive cells, but increased maturation of the dopaminergic phenotype (Andersson et al. 2007). In contrast, another study did not find increased generation of dopaminergic neurons after retroviral induction of rat mesencephalic derived NSCs with Lmx1a, Msx1, Neurogenin 2 and Pitx3 (Roybon et al. 2008). Single expression of each of these genes was not enough to promote dopaminergic differentiation and dual overexpression of Lmx1a and one of the other transcription factors also failed to generate dopaminergic neurons. The authors suggest that NSC harvested from this rather late (embryonic day 14.5) stage of development have lost their potential to be driven into a specific neuronal phenotype, thus NSC from a earlier time point or ESC may be better candidates for generation of dopaminergic neurons (Roybon et al. 2008).

Initial attempts to expand human NSCs from the developing mesencephalon only generated low numbers of dopaminergic neurons, which was also seen after transplantation into 6-OHDA-lesioned rats (Svendsen et al. 1997). Subsequently, an increased yield of dopaminergic neurons was found by culturing the human NSCs at low oxygen tension with further induction of differentiation by IL-1, IL-11, leukemia inhibitory factor and GDNF, but survival and possible *in vivo* functional effects were not addressed (Storch et al. 2001). Interestingly, Wang et al. (2004) showed that pre-differentiation of human mesencephalic NSCs with FGF8, GDNF and forskolin resulted in 26% TH-positive cells as compared to 1.4% in non-differentiated cultures *in vitro* and furthermore, the pre-differentiated cells showed increased functional recovery after transplantation (Wang et al. 2004). The yields of TH-positive cells (up to 60%) have been further improved by using a combination of BDNF, dopamine and forskolin with either retinoic acid or GDNF (Riaz et al. 2004), whereas other studies only have managed to generate 4-25% TH-positive neurons using a combination of different differentiation factors (Christophersen et al. 2006; Yang et al. 2004). These two studies also found very low numbers of surviving TH-positive cells following transplantation into 6-OHDA-lesioned rats, and it remains unclear if this is due to loss of TH expression or death of TH-positive cells after transplantation.

Another approach to obtain large numbers of human dopaminergic neurons for transplantation is to generate immortalized cell lines by genetic modification, thus such cell lines offer a theoretically unlimited source of specific NSCs. Some NSC lines have shown to generate around 20% TH-positive cells (Paul et al. 2007; Lotharius et al. 2002), but when these cells were transplanted into immunosuppressed 6-OHDA-lesioned rats they either died or loose TH expression (Paul et al. 2007). In order to enhance dopaminergic survival further genetic modifications can be added, such as overexpression of Bcl-xL, an anti-apoptotic protein stimulating commitment and survival of dopaminergic neurons (Liste, Garcia-Garcia, and Martinez-Serrano 2004; Krabbe et al. 2009). Such immortalized cells serve as important model cell lines or tools for basic stem cell research, but several safety issues have to be resolved if such cell lines should be considered for clinical use.

3.2.2 NSCs in the adult brain

The human brain is traditionally classified as a non-renewable organ unable to replace damaged or degenerated cells. Neurogenesis in the adult rat brain was first described in the early 1960s by Joseph Altman (Altman and Das 1965), but general acceptance of this neurogenesis was not made until the early 1990s (Reynolds and Weiss 1992). One major advantage of using NSCs from the adult brain compared to those from the embryonic brain is that it would abolish all ethical concerns regarding the use of embryonic tissue.

In the adult mammalian brain NSCs are mainly found in the subventricular zone (SVZ) of the lateral ventricles (Lois and Alvarez-Buylla 1994; Morshead et al. 1994) and the subgranular zone of the hippocampal dentate gyrus (Bayer, Yackel, and Puri 1982; Palmer, Ray, and Gage 1995). From the SVZ, neuroblasts migrate a long distance anteriorly, through the rostral migratory stream, to their final destination in the olfactory bulb, where they mature into local interneurons as reported both in rodents (Lois and Alvarez-Buylla 1994) and in humans (Curtis et al. 2007). Newly generated cells in the subgranular zone migrate to the granular layer of the dentate gyrus, where they replace degenerated neurons and extend projections to the CA3 area of the hippocampus (Bayer, Yackel, and Puri 1982). Several studies have shown that neurogenesis also occur, although at much lower levels, in other areas of the adult mammalian nervous system, such as the cerebral cortex (Palmer et al. 1999), hypothalamus (Markakis et al. 2004), septum (Palmer, Ray, and Gage 1995), retina (Tropepe et al. 2000), optic nerve (Palmer et al. 1999), spinal cord (Weiss et al. 1996), and more debatable in the substantia nigra harbouring the dopaminergic neurons that degenerate in PD (Zhao et al. 2003). As indicated, some controversy remains in relation to the substantia nigra since other research groups have not been able to replicate some of these results (Lie et al. 2002; Frielingsdorf et al. 2004). Lie et al. (2002) found no evidence of either newly generated dopaminergic in the adult rat substantia nigra or neurons of any type *in vivo*. However, when cells from this region were removed and grown *in vitro*, they became capable of neuronal production, indicating that this potential may be inhibited by endogenous signals in the adult brain (Lie et al. 2002). Hermann et al. (2006) have shown the presence of multipotent NSCs in the adult mouse tegmentum (midbrain and hindbrain region) with capacity to differentiate *in vitro* into functional neurons, including the dopaminergic phenotype (Hermann et al. 2006). Thus, the potential existence adult NSCs in the substantia nigra cannot be denied until further clarification has taken place. Despite the presence of endogenous NSCs, the self-repairing activity of the adult mammalian brain is poor. This may be explained by microenvironmental factors present in most areas of the adult brain, which inhibit neural differentiation of NSCs, or by a too small number of endogenous NSCs for effective self-repair.

So far, attempts to develop dopaminergic neurons from NSCs from adult tissue have only been moderately successful both *in vitro* and *in vivo*. In one study NSCs from the SVZ were stimulated to become dopaminergic neurons using a protocol for midbrain dopaminergic induction of ESCs (5-stage method involving addition of Shh and FGF8). It was found to be possible to generate neurons displaying some characteristics of immature dopaminergic neurons, however these cells were limited in their capacity to generate mature dopaminergic neurons showing exclusively a midbrain phenotype (Papanikolaou et al. 2008). Similarly, *in vivo* studies in which adult NSCs have been transplanted into rodent models of PD indicate that any behavioral recovery is due to the general neuroprotective effect of the non-neuronal grafted cells, more than the presence of stem cell derived dopaminergic neurons in the grafts (Richardson et al. 2005; Dziewczapolski et al. 2003).

An alternative strategy is to stimulate endogenous NSCs to differentiate into dopaminergic neurons either in the striatum or the substantia nigra. So far attempts to stimulate the development of new neurons in the 6-OHDA-lesioned rats striatum have not been successful. Some studies have shown that TGFα can stimulate neurogenesis and migration to the striatum, but none of these cells were of dopaminergic or other neuronal phenotypes (Cooper and Isacson 2004; de Chevigny et al. 2008). Ideally, stimulation of neurogenesis in the substantia nigra could reconnect the basal ganglia circuitry and hence increase functional recovery in PD. However, although there might be NSCs in the adult substantia nigra (Zhao et al. 2003) it is only a very small pool of cells insufficient to replace the dopaminergic neuron loss during progressive PD. Moreover, even if it is possible to stimulate neurogenesis in the substantia nigra lack of long-distance axonal growth, along the degenerated nigrostriatal projections, remains a very challenging problem.

3.3 Mesenchymal stem cells

From an immunological and ethical prospective it would be ideal if stem cells could be harvested from, for instance, the patient's own bone marrow and then be used to generate neurons for transplantation. The adult bone marrow contains at least two kinds of stem cell populations: hematopoietic stem cells and mesenchymal stem cells (MSCs) also called bone marrow stromal cells. Hematopoietic stem cells continually repopulate the circulation by differentiating into erythroid, myeloid, and lymphoid lineages, whereas MSCs give rise to mesenchymal derivatives, including osteocytes, chondrocytes, adipocytes and myocytes (Pittenger et al. 1999). MSCs are found only in low numbers in the bone marrow (around 1 MSC per 100 mononuclear marrow cells). They can be purified, from other cells in the bone marrow, on the basis of their ability to adhere to plastic surfaces (Reyes et al. 2001). MSCs are like other stem cells capable of self-renewal, but it has been proposed that self-renewal is less crucial for the physiology of mesenchymal tissue as are multipotentiality and phenotypic flexibility, which indicates that commitment and differentiation are reversible in response to environmental cues. MSCs display the ability of interconversion from one cell type to another at a later differentiation stage than that of other multipotent stem cells (Park, Oreffo, and Triffitt 1999; Beresford et al. 1992). One reason for this potential could be that it is necessary for bone modelling and remodelling (Bianchi et al. 2001).

Several studies provide evidence that MSCs can be induced to overcome their mesenchymal fate and break the barrier of germ layer commitment by transdifferentiation into cell types of other germ layers (Krabbe, Zimmer, and Meyer 2005). In fact, it has been proposed that MSCs have a neural predisposition, since they express neural markers such as neuron specific-enolase, neuronal nuclei, nestin, glial acidic fibrillary protein and TH at basal levels (Blondheim et al. 2006). However, both the transdifferentiation potential of MSCs and the indication that these cells should be biological neurons are controversial. Evidence of a "neuronal" MSC is considered weak and what seems to be transdifferentiation may be explained by a stress response causing a rapid disruption of the actin cytoskeleton with cell shrinkage as a result (Neuhuber et al. 2004) or by cell fusion, in which MSCs have fused with other cell types rather than switching lineage identity (Lu, Blesch, and Tuszynski 2004; Terada et al. 2002).

Nevertheless, efforts are still being made to generate functional neuronal cells from MSCs, and at the beginning of the millennium several research groups have reported that it was possible to induce both human, rat and mouse MSCs to differentiate into neuron-like cells *in vitro* (Black and Woodbury 2001; Deng et al. 2001; Kohyama et al. 2001; Sanchez-Ramos et al. 2000; Woodbury et al. 2000; Munoz-Elias, Woodbury, and Black 2003). Moreover, MSCs were found to migrate and differentiate in a neural-like manner, when transplanted into rat (Azizi et al. 1998) or mouse (Kopen, Prockop, and Phinney 1999) brains, suggesting that the cells, at least theoretically, may represent a future source of cells for treatment of neurodegenerative disorders.

If MSCs are going to be used as a cell source for cell therapy of PD it is important to differentiate these cells into functional dopaminergic neurons, which have been investigated by different strategies. Several groups have induced MSCs by adding cocktails of extrinsic factors to the culture medium (Barzilay et al. 2008; Hermann, Maisel, and Storch 2006; Tatard et al. 2007; Trzaska, Kuzhikandathil, and Rameshwar 2007; Trzaska et al. 2009), others by co-culturing of the MSCs with specific cell types (Jiang et al. 2003), or by genetic manipulation of the cells (Dezawa et al. 2004). From a therapeutically point of view the first mentioned strategy has some advantages, since the cells are not transformed or co-cultured with other cell-types making the cell transplantation more safe. In 2007, Trazska et al. found an effective protocol for dopaminergic differentiation of MSCs in which a cocktail of FGF8, Shh and bFGF were added to the medium. About 67% of the cells expressed the dopaminergic marker TH along with other dopaminergic markers. Moreover, the cells secreted dopamine, but without showing further evidence of being functional mature dopaminergic neurons, and hence they were called dopaminergic progenitors (Trzaska, Kuzhikandathil, and Rameshwar 2007). These results were supported by Barzilay et al. (2008), who tested 20 different protocols for dopaminergic induction of MSCs. They found that the most significant upregulation of TH expression was obtained using BDNF either alone or in combination with GDNF, TGF-β3 and retinoic acid. However, as described by Trzaska et al. (2007), the TH-positive cells did not show mature functional dopaminergic neuron characteristics (Barzilay et al. 2008). In 2009, Trzaska et al. investigated potentially factors that could stimulate the dopaminergic maturation of the cells and found that the MSC-derived neuronal cells showed robust upregulation of tropomyosin-receptor-kinase B beginning at day 9 of the induction. One factor which is known to be involved in the maturation of dopaminergic neurons and which binds to this receptor is BDNF (Baquet, Bickford, and Jones 2005). Hence, they added BDNF to the medium after 9 days of induction and found generation of cells that elicited spontaneous post-synaptic current and secreted dopamine in response to Ca^{2+}-dependent depolarization. These findings show that the MSC-derived dopaminergic neurons can mimic the physiology of native neurons. Moreover, BDNF treatment resulted in KCl-induced depolarization and enhanced dopamine release. They also investigated whether the BDNF-treated cells responded to neurotransmitters such as GABA, acetylcholine and glutamate and found that the BDNF-treated cells responded to both acetylcholine and GABA, but not glutamate. However, the way they responded to GABA and the lack of response to glutamate indicates that these cells were still developing and not fully mature (Trzaska et al. 2009).

All the studies mentioned above indicate that generation of dopaminergic neurons from MSCs may be possible, but to candidate as donor cells for PD, it still remains to be elucidated if the cells contain the entire dopaminergic machinery present in functional dopaminergic neurons *in vivo*.

3.4 Induced pluripotent stem cells

For a long time ESCs have been considered the most promising source of cells for future cell replacement therapy in PD. However, ethical concerns regarding the use of human embryos and the possibility of immune rejection due to immunological incompatibility between patient and donor ESCs may limit their use. To overcome these problems scientists have worked on the development of pluripotent stem cells from adult somatic cells, involving genetic changes (reprogramming) of the somatic cell nucleus. Until recently, reprogramming of cells involved cloning of cells by somatic cell nuclear transfer, where the nucleus in an oocyte is replaced with the nucleus from an adult somatic cell (Wilmut et al. 1997) or by fusion of an adult somatic cell with an ESC (Cowan et al. 2005). However, besides being both time consuming and technical difficult this kind of reprogramming still requires the use of human oocytes or ESCs and hence do not solve the ethical problems.

In 2006, Takahashi and Yamanaka reported for the first time that it was possible to reprogram adult mouse fibroblasts to pluripotent stem cells by retroviral transduction with the four transcription factors Oct3/4, Sox2, c-Myc and Klf4, which are highly expressed in ESCs (Takahashi and Yamanaka 2006). The resulting so-called induced pluripotent stem (iPS) cells share several properties with ESCs, including morphology, growth properties and pluripotency, defined by their ability to form teratomas *in vivo* and differentiate into distinct cell types of all three germ layers, but they are not identical to ESCs when it comes to epigenetic status (Deng et al. 2009) and gene expression (Chin et al. 2009). In addition, the original iPS cells failed to generate postnatal chimeras and contribute to the germline (Takahashi and Yamanaka 2006), but refinement of the method for selection of iPS cells has already solved these issues and moreover, the resulting iPS cells are even more similar to ECSs at the epigenetic level (Okita, Ichisaka, and Yamanaka 2007; Maherali et al. 2007; Meissner, Wernig, and Jaenisch 2007). Shortly after these initial studies in mice, iPS cells were derived from human fibroblasts using slightly different combinations of genes (Takahashi et al. 2007; Yu et al. 2007) and since then, iPS cells have been generated from a number of different cell types and species (Masip et al. 2010).

The similarities of iPS cells to ESCs, and the fact that these cells can be generated from the patient's own cells, make them very attractive candidates for cell-based therapy. However, before iPS cells can be used in the clinic there are several issues that need to be resolved. First, it is extremely important to optimize the procedure for reprogramming of the somatic cells. As described above, many groups have generated iPS cells by use of retroviral vectors. Since retrovirus integrates randomly in the DNA it may alter the differentiation potential or even induce malignant transformation of the iPS cells. Moreover, most research groups have used c-Myc as one of the reprogramming factors and since c-Myc is a proto-oncogene, its reactivation could give rise to transgene-derived tumor formation. In one study 20% out of 121 mice derived from an iPS cell line developed tumors. In these tumors, retroviral expression of c-Myc, but not Oct3/4, Sox2, or Klf4 was reactivated (Okita, Ichisaka, and Yamanaka 2007). Hence, recent studies have focused on developing safer reprogramming strategies, for example, by generation of iPS cells without using the c-Myc oncogene. In 2008, Nakagawa et al. generated iPS cell lines from both mouse and human fibroblasts without the use of c-Myc. They found that it was possible to generate cells expressing ESC markers, and that the induction of the fibroblasts to iPS cells was more specific, since a lower number of non-iPS cells were generated. However, efficiency of the generation process was substantially reduced with the omission of c-Myc. They also examined the tumourigenicity in mice derived from these cells and found that omission of the c-Myc retrovirus significantly reduced the risk of tumorigenicity in chimeras (Nakagawa et al. 2008). Other studies have also examined different combinations of transcription factors, and of the original four transcription factors, Oct3/4 is the only one that cannot be replaced by other transcription family members and have been required in every reprogramming strategy in both mouse and human cells. Other strategies have been to generate iPS cells using integration systems such as plasmids (Kaji et al. 2009) and transposons (Woltjen et al. 2009), which allow removal of these systems after reprogramming. Moreover, iPS cells have also been generated without genomic integration using nonintegrative adenoviral vectors (Zhou and Freed 2009; Stadtfeld et al. 2008), repeated plasmid transfection with or without the use of small molecules (Okita et al. 2010; Okita et al. 2008; Yu et al. 2009) and just addition of recombinant proteins (Zhou et al. 2009; Kim et al. 2009). Although, these methods are not yet as efficient as the retroviral approach, they have clearly shown that random DNA mutagenesis is not a requirement for reprogramming and give hope for the development of clinically applicable iPS cells free of viruses and transgenic integration.

Interestingly, a recent publication have shown a method for direct reprogramming of fibroblasts into neurons, avoiding generation of undifferentiated cells and their following differentiation (Vierbuchen et al. 2010). They started from a pool of nineteen neural-lineage specific transcription factors and identified a combination of only three factors (Mash1, Brn2 and Myt1l) that were sufficient to convert mouse fibroblasts into functional neurons in vitro. Such induced neurons clearly have some advantages to iPS cells, since they avoid generation of pluripotent cells that can give rise to tumors. In this study the induced neurons mainly gave rise to GABAergic neurons after differentiation, but their regional identity is still unclear (Vierbuchen et al. 2010). This strategy offers new perspectives to the reprogramming field and future studies need to determine if certain cell types are more useful in generation of specific cells for replacement strategies and if it is necessary to reprogram cells all the way back to pluripotent stem cells.

	Advantages	Disadvantages
ESCs	• Unlimited proliferation capacity • Potential to generate any cell type (pluripotent) • Generation of stem cell banks	• Risk of teratomas (heterogenous composition) • Time demanding/complex differentiation into dopaminergic neurons • Risk of immune rejection • Ethical issues
NSCs	• Restricted differentiation potential (multipotent) • Low risk of tumor formation	• Limited proliferation capacity • Reduced neuronal differentiation capacity following long-term proliferation • Risk of immune rejection • Ethical issues (fetal NSCs)
MSCs	• Easily harvested • Possibility of generating patient specific cells • No ethical concerns	• Differentiation into "truly" functional dopaminergic neuron still uncertain
iPS cells	• Unlimited proliferation • Potential to generate any cell type (pluripotent) • Generation of stem cell banks • Possibility of generating patient specific cells • No risk of immune rejection • No ethical concerns	• Risk of teratoma (heterogenous composition) • Risk of tumor formation (viral transduction) • Time demanding/complex differentiation into dopaminergic neurons • Expensive procedure

Table 1. Overview of advantages and disadvantages of different types of stem cell for cell replacement therapy in Parkinson's disease.

3.4.1 iPS cells and Parkinson's disease

The therapeutic potential of human iPS cells for cell-based therapy of PD relies on efficient differentiation of iPS cells into functional midbrain dopaminergic neurons. Several groups have worked on generation of dopaminergic neurons from iPS cells *in vitro*. In 2008, Wernig et al. showed that mouse fibroblast-derived iPS cells predifferentiated into dopaminergic neurons could integrate into the host striatum of parkinsonian rats and lead to functional improvements (Wernig et al. 2008). However, these cells also led to teratoma formation as seen after transplantation of ESCs – likely due to the presence of undifferentiated cells (Roy et al. 2006). The occurrence of pluripotent cells was reported to be the most likely cause of teratoma formation in the Wernig et al. study, since viral transcripts were not reactivated in the tumors. Furthermore, they showed that eliminating the undifferentiated cells before transplantation (by depletion of SSEA1-positive cells by FACS) could significantly reduce the risk of tumor formation (Wernig et al. 2008). More recent studies have shown as efficient generation of dopaminergic neurons from human iPS cells as from ESCs, which subsequently could survive and integrate in the host striatum of parkinsonian rats (Swistowski et al. 2010; Cai et al. 2010). In one study, functional recovery of the parkinsonian rats was also reported and furthermore, genome-wide microarray comparison between human iPS cells, ESCs and dopaminergic neurons derived from both sources revealed overall similarity (Swistowski et al. 2010).

Interestingly, the iPS cell technology also provides the basis for development new disease models, since they can be generated from patients with specific diseases. Although, iPS cells can be used for both sporadic and genetic diseases, they might be of particular advantage for diseases with a solid genetic background and/or which occur early in development. Some studies have generated iPS cells from patients suffering from sporadic PD (Park et al. 2008; Soldner et al. 2009). Soldner et al. (2009) developed dopaminergic neurons from iPS cells derived from patients with PD as efficiently as iPS cells from healthy individuals and did not report any phenotypic differences, thus the disease derived cells did not show any specific features of PD *in vitro*. The average age of onset of PD is more than 50 years, hence *in vitro* cell culturing periods of weeks or months may be too short for a pathologic phenotype to arise. However, although it takes many years for the pathologic characteristics to become evident, the disease process might be initiated much earlier, and therefore iPS cells offer the possibility of establishing a new type of disease model to investigate such issues. Indeed, it will be very important to investigate if iPS cells derived from patients are more susceptible to develop PD-like features than fetal tissue after grafting in PD patients (see section 2.2.2.3). Recently, differentiation of the patient-derived iPS cells described by Soldner et al. (2009) into dopaminergic neurons were shown to survive and mediate functional effect after transplantation into a rat model of PD (Hargus et al. 2010).

3.5 Stem cells releasing therapeutic molecules ("cell factories")

Instead of acting as a source of cells for neuronal replacement an alternative use of stem cells for transplantation is as so-called "cell factories" releasing neurotrophic and neuroprotective factors. Several neurotrophic factors have been shown to stimulate survival and/or differentiation of nigral dopaminergic neurons *in vitro* and *in vivo*, which is beyond the aim of this chapter to describe in detail but reviewed elsewhere (Evans and Barker 2008; Levy et al. 2005). Among neurtrophic factors, GDNF and some of the GDNF family members have shown the greatest promise as therapeutic agents for PD. Several studies have shown that GDNF can protect against nigrostiatal lesions in animal models. For instance, intravenous administration of MSCs overexpressing GDNF in mice before lesioning with MPTP has been shown to protect dopaminergic neurons in the substantia nigra as well as their striatal fibers (Park, Eglitis, and Mouradian 2001). In agreement with this observation, another study has shown that GDNF-producing mouse NSCs transplanted into the mouse striatum 16 days prior to 6-OHDA lesioning could prevent death of dopaminergic neurons and resulted in a reduced behavioral impairment (Akerud et al. 2001). A similar protective effect was found by overexpressing Neurturin, another member of the GDNF family, in the same NSC line (c17.2 NSCs derived from the mouse cerebellum) (Liu et al. 2007).

NSCs are considered very suitable for *ex vivo* gene delivery, since they can be cultured, differentiated into specific neuronal subtypes, transduced and selected for subsequent transplantation to the brain where they can migrate and extend projections. Human NCSs genetically modified to overexpress GDNF in an inducible way have been shown to express GDNF for up to 3 month in the brains of rodents and aged primates (Behrstock et al. 2006). Furthermore, transplantation of these cells after a partial lesion of the dopamine system resulted in increased host dopamine neuron survival and fiber outgrowth. MSCs are also very suitable as neuroprotective cells through secretion of neurotrophic factors and furthermore, these cells can easily be harvested from the patient's own bone marrow in order to avoid immune rejection. Along this line, Sadan et al. (2009) have recently developed a protocol to induce MSCs into neurotrophic factor-secreting cells, especially producing GDNF and BDNF without genetic modification of the cells.

Another way to overcome problems of host immunoresponses when using allografts, is the development of new materials to encapsulate transplanted cells, thereby serving as a biological shield to prevent immune rejection and eliminate the need for immunosuppression. The encapsulating material should allow inward diffusion of nutrients to the transplanted cells and at the same time permit outward secretion of trophic factors. Besides protection from the host immune system, these capsules have the advantage that they can be removed for safety reasons or for renewal of cells. Several studies have reported successful delivery of GDNF from encapsulated cells (Kishima et al. 2004; Tseng et al. 1997; Sagot et al. 1996; Ahn et al. 2005). Kishima et al. (2004) found a transient recovery in motor function after intraventricular infusion of encapsulated GDNF-producing cells in MPTP lesioned baboons, however no neuroprotection against the toxin was found. The lack of neuroprotective effect may be due to the intraventricular placement of the capsules resulting in inefficient passage of GDNF to the striatum, thus better graft sites should be used. Furthermore, they reported GDNF release and survival of encapsulated cells for more than 1 year after transplantation (Kishima et al. 2004).

Delivery of neurotrophic factors by co-grafted genetically modified stem cells or cell lines may also serve as a useful tool for stimulation of functional integration and protection of grafted dopaminergic neurons from any source. In one study, Ahn et al. (2005) tested such a strategy by co-grafting an encapsulated cell line overexpressing GDNF with human fetal mesencepahlic tissue into 6-OHDA lesioned rats, leading to increased fiber outgrowth in areas between the capsules and the grafts. This result indicates that continuous delivery of GDNF or other important neurotrophic factors via encapsulated genetically modified cells could further optimize neural transplantation as a therapy for PD.

4. Conclusion

Neural transplantation has emerged as a potential therapy for Parkinson's disease (PD). In experimental studies based on animal models and PD patients, various sources and types of donor cells have been investigated for their potential applicability. Clinical studies performed during the 1980s and 1990s, where dopaminergic neurons derived from human fetal brain tissue were transplanted into striatum of patients with PD, provided proof-of-concept that long-lasting therapeutic benefits can be achieved. Subsequent studies, in particular two double-blind placebo-controlled trials, showed variable and mostly disappointing results. They also revealed that some patients develop graft-induced dyskinesias as side effects. Thus, while nigral transplants clearly work well in certain PD patients, the technique needs refinement before it can successfully be applied on a large series of patients. This optimization includes patient selection (age, medical history, response to L-dopa), trial design, origin and preparation of donor cells, immunosuppression, and surgical techniques for successful functional outcome and avoiding unwanted side effects. Hopefully, the TRANSEURO project will provide some of this essential knowledge and as such contribute to the development of a standardized, efficient and safe protocol that can serve as a template for clinical trials, including expected future stem cell-based trials for PD. However, before such a stem cell therapy can be initiated, also a number fundamental biological issues need to be taken into consideration. Embryonic stem cells (ESCs) and the newly developed induced pluripotent stem (iPS) cells seem to have the greatest potential to generate large numbers of dopaminergic neurons, but the use of these cell types is associated with a risk of tumor formation due to potentially remaining undifferentiated cells in the donor cell preparations. Moreover, using ESCs are related to ethical and immunological concerns. IPS cells and mesenchymal stem cells have the prospect of being made patient specific overcoming the risk of immune rejection, and they are not affiliated with ethical problems. So far it has been difficult to generate large numbers of dopaminergic neurons from neural stem cells, but these cells have a more straightforward differentiation pathway to form midbrain specific dopaminergic neurons, and they are not tumorigenic. Independent of the type of stem cell in question, it will be challenging to develop a differentiation protocol leading to "truly" functional dopaminergic projection neurons with midbrain characteristics without still having undifferentiated cells in the preparation.

5. Abbreviations

BDNF, brain-derived neurotrophic factor; DBS, Deep brain stimulation; ESC, embryonic stem cell; FACS, Fluorescence-activated cell sorting; FGF, fibroblast growth factor; GDNF, glial-derived neurotrophic factor; 6-OHDA, 6-hydroxydopamine; iPS, induced pluripotent stem cell; MPTP, 1-methyl-4-phenyl-1,2,3,6-tetrahydropyridine; MSC, mesenchymal stem cell; NSC, neural stem cell; SDIA, stromal cell-derived inducing activity; PD, Parkinson's disease, PET; Positron Emmision Tomography; Shh, sonic hedgehog; SVZ, subventricular zone; TGF, transforming growth factor; UPDRS, unified Parkinson's disease rating scale.

6. References

Ahn, Y. H., J. C. Bensadoun, P. Aebischer, A. D. Zurn, A. Seiger, A. Bjorklund, O. Lindvall, L. Wahlberg, P. Brundin, and G. S. Kaminski Schierle. 2005. Increased fiber outgrowth from xeno-transplanted human embryonic dopaminergic neurons with co-implants of polymer-encapsulated genetically modified cells releasing glial cell line-derived neurotrophic factor. *Brain Res Bull* 66 (2):135-42.

Akerud, P., J. M. Canals, E. Y. Snyder, and E. Arenas. 2001. Neuroprotection through delivery of glial cell line-derived neurotrophic factor by neural stem cells in a mouse model of Parkinson's disease. *J Neurosci* 21 (20):8108-18.

Allen, G. S., R. S. Burns, N. B. Tulipan, and R. A. Parker. 1989. Adrenal medullary transplantation to the caudate nucleus in Parkinson's disease. Initial clinical results in 18 patients. *Arch Neurol* 46 (5):487-91.

Altman, J., and G. D. Das. 1965. Autoradiographic and histological evidence of postnatal hippocampal neurogenesis in rats. *J Comp Neurol* 124 (3):319-35.

Andersson, E. K., D. K. Irvin, J. Ahlsio, and M. Parmar. 2007. Ngn2 and Nurr1 act in synergy to induce midbrain dopaminergic neurons from expanded neural stem and progenitor cells. *Exp Cell Res* 313 (6):1172-80.

Arjona, V., A. Minguez-Castellanos, R. J. Montoro, A. Ortega, F. Escamilla, J. J. Toledo-Aral, R. Pardal, S. Mendez-Ferrer, J. M. Martin, M. Perez, M. J. Katati, E. Valencia, T. Garcia, and J. Lopez-Barneo. 2003. Autotransplantation of human carotid body cell aggregates for treatment of Parkinson's disease. *Neurosurgery* 53 (2):321-8; discussion 328-30.

Azizi, S. A., D. Stokes, B. J. Augelli, C. DiGirolamo, and D. J. Prockop. 1998. Engraftment and migration of human bone marrow stromal cells implanted in the brains of albino rats--similarities to astrocyte grafts. *Proc Natl Acad Sci U S A* 95 (7):3908-13.

Backlund, E. O., P. O. Granberg, B. Hamberger, E. Knutsson, A. Martensson, G. Sedvall, A. Seiger, and L. Olson. 1985. Transplantation of adrenal medullary tissue to striatum in parkinsonism. First clinical trials. *J Neurosurg* 62 (2):169-73.

Baquet, Z. C., P. C. Bickford, and K. R. Jones. 2005. Brain-derived neurotrophic factor is required for the establishment of the proper number of dopaminergic neurons in the substantia nigra pars compacta. *J Neurosci* 25 (26):6251-9.

Barberi, T., P. Klivenyi, N. Y. Calingasan, H. Lee, H. Kawamata, K. Loonam, A. L. Perrier, J. Bruses, M. E. Rubio, N. Topf, V. Tabar, N. L. Harrison, M. F. Beal, M. A. Moore, and L. Studer. 2003. Neural subtype specification of fertilization and nuclear transfer embryonic stem cells and application in parkinsonian mice. *Nat Biotechnol* 21 (10):1200-7.

Barzilay, R., I. Kan, T. Ben-Zur, S. Bulvik, E. Melamed, and D. Offen. 2008. Induction of human mesenchymal stem cells into dopamine-producing cells with different differentiation protocols. *Stem Cells Dev* 17 (3):547-54.

Bayer, S. A., J. W. Yackel, and P. S. Puri. 1982. Neurons in the rat dentate gyrus granular layer substantially increase during juvenile and adult life. *Science* 216 (4548):890-2.

Behrstock, S., A. Ebert, J. McHugh, S. Vosberg, J. Moore, B. Schneider, E. Capowski, D. Hei, J. Kordower, P. Aebischer, and C. N. Svendsen. 2006. Human neural progenitors deliver glial cell line-derived neurotrophic factor to parkinsonian rodents and aged primates. *Gene Ther* 13 (5):379-88.

Ben-Hur, T., M. Idelson, H. Khaner, M. Pera, E. Reinhartz, A. Itzik, and B. E. Reubinoff. 2004. Transplantation of human embryonic stem cell-derived neural progenitors improves behavioral deficit in Parkinsonian rats. *Stem Cells* 22 (7):1246-55.

Beresford, J. N., J. H. Bennett, C. Devlin, P. S. Leboy, and M. E. Owen. 1992. Evidence for an inverse relationship between the differentiation of adipocytic and osteogenic cells in rat marrow stromal cell cultures. *J Cell Sci* 102 (Pt 2):341-51.

Bianchi, G., A. Muraglia, A. Daga, G. Corte, R. Cancedda, and R. Quarto. 2001. Microenvironment and stem properties of bone marrow-derived mesenchymal cells. *Wound Repair Regen* 9 (6):460-6.

Bjorklund, A., S. B. Dunnett, P. Brundin, A. J. Stoessl, C. R. Freed, R. E. Breeze, M. Levivier, M. Peschanski, L. Studer, and R. Barker. 2003. Neural transplantation for the treatment of Parkinson's disease. *Lancet Neurol* 2 (7):437-45.

Bjorklund, A., and U. Stenevi. 1979. Reconstruction of the nigrostriatal dopamine pathway by intracerebral nigral transplants. *Brain Res* 177 (3):555-60.

Bjorklund, L. M., R. Sanchez-Pernaute, S. Chung, T. Andersson, I. Y. Chen, K. S. McNaught, A. L. Brownell, B. G. Jenkins, C. Wahlestedt, K. S. Kim, and O. Isacson. 2002. Embryonic stem cells develop into functional dopaminergic neurons after transplantation in a Parkinson rat model. *Proc Natl Acad Sci U S A* 99 (4):2344-9.

Black, I. B., and D. Woodbury. 2001. Adult rat and human bone marrow stromal stem cells differentiate into neurons. *Blood Cells Mol Dis* 27 (3):632-6.

Blondheim, N. R., Y. S. Levy, T. Ben-Zur, A. Burshtein, T. Cherlow, I. Kan, R. Barzilai, M. Bahat-Stromza, Y. Barhum, S. Bulvik, E. Melamed, and D. Offen. 2006. Human mesenchymal stem cells express neural genes, suggesting a neural predisposition. *Stem Cells Dev* 15 (2):141-64.

Brevig, T., M. Meyer, T. Kristensen, J. Zimmer, and J. Holgersson. 2001. Xenotransplantation for brain repair: reduction of porcine donor tissue immunogenicity by treatment with anti-Gal antibodies and complement. *Transplantation* 72 (2):190-6.

Brundin, P., O. G. Nilsson, R. E. Strecker, O. Lindvall, B. Astedt, and A. Bjorklund. 1986. Behavioural effects of human fetal dopamine neurons grafted in a rat model of Parkinson's disease. *Exp Brain Res* 65 (1):235-40.

Brundin, P., O. Pogarell, P. Hagell, P. Piccini, H. Widner, A. Schrag, A. Kupsch, L. Crabb, P. Odin, B. Gustavii, A. Bjorklund, D. J. Brooks, C. D. Marsden, W. H. Oertel, N. P. Quinn, S. Rehncrona, and O. Lindvall. 2000. Bilateral caudate and putamen grafts of embryonic mesencephalic tissue treated with lazaroids in Parkinson's disease. *Brain* 123 (Pt 7):1380-90.

Cai, J., M. Yang, E. Poremsky, S. Kidd, J. S. Schneider, and L. Iacovitti. 2010. Dopaminergic neurons derived from human induced pluripotent stem cells survive and integrate into 6-OHDA-lesioned rats. *Stem Cells Dev* 19 (7):1017-23.

Carlsson, A., M. Lindqvist, and T. Magnusson. 1957. 3,4-Dihydroxyphenylalanine and 5-hydroxytryptophan as reserpine antagonists. *Nature* 180 (4596):1200.

Carlsson, T., M. Carta, C. Winkler, A. Bjorklund, and D. Kirik. 2007. Serotonin neuron transplants exacerbate L-DOPA-induced dyskinesias in a rat model of Parkinson's disease. *J Neurosci* 27 (30):8011-22.

Carpenter, M. K., M. S. Inokuma, J. Denham, T. Mujtaba, C. P. Chiu, and M. S. Rao. 2001. Enrichment of neurons and neural precursors from human embryonic stem cells. *Exp Neurol* 172 (2):383-97.

Carta, M., T. Carlsson, D. Kirik, and A. Bjorklund. 2007. Dopamine released from 5-HT terminals is the cause of L-DOPA-induced dyskinesia in parkinsonian rats. *Brain* 130 (Pt 7):1819-33.

Carvey, P. M., Z. D. Ling, C. E. Sortwell, M. R. Pitzer, S. O. McGuire, A. Storch, and T. J. Collier. 2001. A clonal line of mesencephalic progenitor cells converted to dopamine neurons by hematopoietic cytokines: a source of cells for transplantation in Parkinson's disease. *Exp Neurol* 171 (1):98-108.

Chin, M. H., M. J. Mason, W. Xie, S. Volinia, M. Singer, C. Peterson, G. Ambartsumyan, O. Aimiuwu, L. Richter, J. Zhang, I. Khvorostov, V. Ott, M. Grunstein, N. Lavon, N. Benvenisty, C. M. Croce, A. T. Clark, T. Baxter, A. D. Pyle, M. A. Teitell, M.

Pelegrini, K. Plath, and W. E. Lowry. 2009. Induced pluripotent stem cells and embryonic stem cells are distinguished by gene expression signatures. *Cell Stem Cell* 5 (1):111-23.

Christophersen, N. S., X. Meijer, J. R. Jorgensen, U. Englund, M. Gronborg, A. Seiger, P. Brundin, and L. U. Wahlberg. 2006. Induction of dopaminergic neurons from growth factor expanded neural stem/progenitor cell cultures derived from human first trimester forebrain. *Brain Res Bull* 70 (4-6):457-66.

Chung, S., E. Hedlund, M. Hwang, D. W. Kim, B. S. Shin, D. Y. Hwang, U. Jung Kang, O. Isacson, and K. S. Kim. 2005. The homeodomain transcription factor Pitx3 facilitates differentiation of mouse embryonic stem cells into AHD2-expressing dopaminergic neurons. *Mol Cell Neurosci* 28 (2):241-52.

Chung, S., B. S. Shin, E. Hedlund, J. Pruszak, A. Ferree, U. J. Kang, O. Isacson, and K. S. Kim. 2006. Genetic selection of sox1GFP-expressing neural precursors removes residual tumorigenic pluripotent stem cells and attenuates tumor formation after transplantation. *J Neurochem* 97 (5):1467-80.

Chung, S., K. C. Sonntag, T. Andersson, L. M. Bjorklund, J. J. Park, D. W. Kim, U. J. Kang, O. Isacson, and K. S. Kim. 2002. Genetic engineering of mouse embryonic stem cells by Nurr1 enhances differentiation and maturation into dopaminergic neurons. *Eur J Neurosci* 16 (10):1829-38.

Cooper, O., and O. Isacson. 2004. Intrastriatal transforming growth factor alpha delivery to a model of Parkinson's disease induces proliferation and migration of endogenous adult neural progenitor cells without differentiation into dopaminergic neurons. *J Neurosci* 24 (41):8924-31.

Cowan, C. A., J. Atienza, D. A. Melton, and K. Eggan. 2005. Nuclear reprogramming of somatic cells after fusion with human embryonic stem cells. *Science* 309 (5739):1369-73.

Curtis, M. A., M. Kam, U. Nannmark, M. F. Anderson, M. Z. Axell, C. Wikkelso, S. Holtas, W. M. van Roon-Mom, T. Bjork-Eriksson, C. Nordborg, J. Frisen, M. Dragunow, R. L. Faull, and P. S. Eriksson. 2007. Human neuroblasts migrate to the olfactory bulb via a lateral ventricular extension. *Science* 315 (5816):1243-9.

de Chevigny, A., O. Cooper, A. Vinuela, C. Reske-Nielsen, D. C. Lagace, A. J. Eisch, and O. Isacson. 2008. Fate mapping and lineage analyses demonstrate the production of a large number of striatal neuroblasts after transforming growth factor alpha and noggin striatal infusions into the dopamine-depleted striatum. *Stem Cells* 26 (9):2349-60.

Deacon, T., J. Schumacher, J. Dinsmore, C. Thomas, P. Palmer, S. Kott, A. Edge, D. Penney, S. Kassissieh, P. Dempsey, and O. Isacson. 1997. Histological evidence of fetal pig neural cell survival after transplantation into a patient with Parkinson's disease. *Nat Med* 3 (3):350-3.

Deng, J., R. Shoemaker, B. Xie, A. Gore, E. M. LeProust, J. Antosiewicz-Bourget, D. Egli, N. Maherali, I. H. Park, J. Yu, G. Q. Daley, K. Eggan, K. Hochedlinger, J. Thomson, W. Wang, Y. Gao, and K. Zhang. 2009. Targeted bisulfite sequencing reveals changes in DNA methylation associated with nuclear reprogramming. *Nat Biotechnol* 27 (4):353-60.

Deng, W., M. Obrocka, I. Fischer, and D. J. Prockop. 2001. In vitro differentiation of human marrow stromal cells into early progenitors of neural cells by conditions that increase intracellular cyclic AMP. *Biochem Biophys Res Commun* 282 (1):148-52.

Dezawa, M., H. Kanno, M. Hoshino, H. Cho, N. Matsumoto, Y. Itokazu, N. Tajima, H. Yamada, H. Sawada, H. Ishikawa, T. Mimura, M. Kitada, Y. Suzuki, and C. Ide. 2004. Specific induction of neuronal cells from bone marrow stromal cells and application for autologous transplantation. *J Clin Invest* 113 (12):1701-10.

Draper, J. S., K. Smith, P. Gokhale, H. D. Moore, E. Maltby, J. Johnson, L. Meisner, T. P. Zwaka, J. A. Thomson, and P. W. Andrews. 2004. Recurrent gain of chromosomes 17q and 12 in cultured human embryonic stem cells. *Nat Biotechnol* 22 (1):53-4.

Drucker-Colin, R., I. Madrazo, F. Ostrosky-Solis, M. Shkurovich, R. Franco, and C. Torres. 1988. Adrenal medullary tissue transplants in the caudate nucleus of Parkinson's patients. *Prog Brain Res* 78:567-74.

Dunnett, S. B., A. Bjorklund, R. H. Schmidt, U. Stenevi, and S. D. Iversen. 1983. Intracerebral grafting of neuronal cell suspensions. IV. Behavioural recovery in rats with unilateral 6-OHDA lesions following implantation of nigral cell suspensions in different forebrain sites. *Acta Physiol Scand Suppl* 522:29-37.

Dunnett, S. B., A. Bjorklund, U. Stenevi, and S. D. Iversen. 1981. Behavioural recovery following transplantation of substantia nigra in rats subjected to 6-OHDA lesions of the nigrostriatal pathway. II. Bilateral lesions. *Brain Res* 229 (2):457-70.

Dziewczapolski, G., D. C. Lie, J. Ray, F. H. Gage, and C. W. Shults. 2003. Survival and differentiation of adult rat-derived neural progenitor cells transplanted to the striatum of hemiparkinsonian rats. *Exp Neurol* 183 (2):653-64.

Espejo, E. F., R. J. Montoro, J. A. Armengol, and J. Lopez-Barneo. 1998. Cellular and functional recovery of Parkinsonian rats after intrastriatal transplantation of carotid body cell aggregates. *Neuron* 20 (2):197-206.

Evans, J. R., and R. A. Barker. 2008. Neurotrophic factors as a therapeutic target for Parkinson's disease. *Expert Opin Ther Targets* 12 (4):437-47.

Fahn, S. 2006. Levodopa in the treatment of Parkinson's disease. *J Neural Transm Suppl* (71):1-15.

Freed, C. R., R. E. Breeze, N. L. Rosenberg, S. A. Schneck, E. Kriek, J. X. Qi, T. Lone, Y. B. Zhang, J. A. Snyder, T. H. Wells, and et al. 1992. Survival of implanted fetal dopamine cells and neurologic improvement 12 to 46 months after transplantation for Parkinson's disease. *N Engl J Med* 327 (22):1549-55.

Freed, C. R., R. E. Breeze, N. L. Rosenberg, S. A. Schneck, T. H. Wells, J. N. Barrett, S. T. Grafton, S. C. Huang, D. Eidelberg, and D. A. Rottenberg. 1990. Transplantation of human fetal dopamine cells for Parkinson's disease. Results at 1 year. *Arch Neurol* 47 (5):505-12.

Freed, C. R., R. E. Breeze, N. L. Rosenberg, S. A. Schneck, T. H. Wells, J. N. Barrett, S. T. Grafton, J. C. Mazziotta, D. Eidelberg, and D. A. Rottenberg. 1990. Therapeutic effects of human fetal dopamine cells transplanted in a patient with Parkinson's disease. *Prog Brain Res* 82:715-21.

Freed, C. R., P. E. Greene, R. E. Breeze, W. Y. Tsai, W. DuMouchel, R. Kao, S. Dillon, H. Winfield, S. Culver, J. Q. Trojanowski, D. Eidelberg, and S. Fahn. 2001. Transplantation of embryonic dopamine neurons for severe Parkinson's disease. *N Engl J Med* 344 (10):710-9.

Freed, W. J., M. Poltorak, and J. B. Becker. 1990. Intracerebral adrenal medulla grafts: a review. *Exp Neurol* 110 (2):139-66.

Freund, T. F., J. P. Bolam, A. Bjorklund, U. Stenevi, S. B. Dunnett, J. F. Powell, and A. D. Smith. 1985. Efferent synaptic connections of grafted dopaminergic neurons reinnervating the host neostriatum: a tyrosine hydroxylase immunocytochemical study. *J Neurosci* 5 (3):603-16.

Frielingsdorf, H., K. Schwarz, P. Brundin, and P. Mohapel. 2004. No evidence for new dopaminergic neurons in the adult mammalian substantia nigra. *Proc Natl Acad Sci U S A* 101 (27):10177-82.

Friling, S., E. Andersson, L. H. Thompson, M. E. Jonsson, J. B. Hebsgaard, E. Nanou, Z. Alekseenko, U. Marklund, S. Kjellander, N. Volakakis, O. Hovatta, A. El Manira, A. Bjorklund, T. Perlmann, and J. Ericson. 2009. Efficient production of mesencephalic dopamine neurons by Lmx1a expression in embryonic stem cells. *Proc Natl Acad Sci U S A* 106 (18):7613-8.

Galpern, W. R., L. H. Burns, T. W. Deacon, J. Dinsmore, and O. Isacson. 1996. Xenotransplantation of porcine fetal ventral mesencephalon in a rat model of Parkinson's disease: functional recovery and graft morphology. *Exp Neurol* 140 (1):1-13.

Goetz, C. G., G. T. Stebbins, 3rd, H. L. Klawans, W. C. Koller, R. G. Grossman, R. A. Bakay, and R. D. Penn. 1991. United Parkinson Foundation Neurotransplantation Registry on adrenal medullary transplants: presurgical, and 1- and 2-year follow-up. *Neurology* 41 (11):1719-22.

Hargus, G., O. Cooper, M. Deleidi, A. Levy, K. Lee, E. Marlow, A. Yow, F. Soldner, D. Hockemeyer, P. J. Hallett, T. Osborn, R. Jaenisch, and O. Isacson. 2010. Differentiated Parkinson patient-derived induced pluripotent stem cells grow in the adult rodent brain and reduce motor asymmetry in Parkinsonian rats. *Proc Natl Acad Sci U S A* 107 (36):15921-6.

Hauser, R. A., and T. A. Zesiewicz. 2007. Advances in the pharmacologic management of early Parkinson disease. *Neurologist* 13 (3):126-32.

Head, J. R., and W. S. Griffin. 1985. Functional capacity of solid tissue transplants in the brain: evidence for immunological privilege. *Proc R Soc Lond B Biol Sci* 224 (1236):375-87.

Hedlund, E., J. Pruszak, T. Lardaro, W. Ludwig, A. Vinuela, K. S. Kim, and O. Isacson. 2008. Embryonic stem cell-derived Pitx3-enhanced green fluorescent protein midbrain dopamine neurons survive enrichment by fluorescence-activated cell sorting and function in an animal model of Parkinson's disease. *Stem Cells* 26 (6):1526-36.

Hermann, A., M. Maisel, and A. Storch. 2006. Epigenetic conversion of human adult bone mesodermal stromal cells into neuroectodermal cell types for replacement therapy of neurodegenerative disorders. *Expert Opin Biol Ther* 6 (7):653-70.

Hermann, A., M. Maisel, F. Wegner, S. Liebau, D. W. Kim, M. Gerlach, J. Schwarz, K. S. Kim, and A. Storch. 2006. Multipotent neural stem cells from the adult tegmentum with dopaminergic potential develop essential properties of functional neurons. *Stem Cells* 24 (4):949-64.

Hitoshi, S., V. Tropepe, M. Ekker, and D. van der Kooy. 2002. Neural stem cell lineages are regionally specified, but not committed, within distinct compartments of the developing brain. *Development* 129 (1):233-44.

Holden, C. 2009. Neuroscience. Fetal cells again? *Science* 326 (5951):358-9.

Horiguchi, S., J. Takahashi, Y. Kishi, A. Morizane, Y. Okamoto, M. Koyanagi, M. Tsuji, K. Tashiro, T. Honjo, S. Fujii, and N. Hashimoto. 2004. Neural precursor cells derived from human embryonic brain retain regional specificity. *J Neurosci Res* 75 (6):817-24.

Hudson, J. L., A. Hoffman, I. Stromberg, B. J. Hoffer, and J. W. Moorhead. 1994. Allogeneic grafts of fetal dopamine neurons: behavioral indices of immunological interactions. *Neurosci Lett* 171 (1-2):32-6.

Huffaker, T. K., B. D. Boss, A. S. Morgan, N. T. Neff, R. E. Strecker, M. S. Spence, and R. Miao. 1989. Xenografting of fetal pig ventral mesencephalon corrects motor asymmetry in the rat model of Parkinson's disease. *Exp Brain Res* 77 (2):329-36.

Hurtig, H., J. Joyce, J. R. Sladek, Jr., and J. Q. Trojanowski. 1989. Postmortem analysis of adrenal-medulla-to-caudate autograft in a patient with Parkinson's disease. *Ann Neurol* 25 (6):607-14.

Iacovitti, L., A. E. Donaldson, C. E. Marshall, S. Suon, and M. Yang. 2007. A protocol for the differentiation of human embryonic stem cells into dopaminergic neurons using only chemically defined human additives: Studies in vitro and in vivo. *Brain Res* 1127 (1):19-25.

Inden, M., D. Kim, Y. Gu, Y. Kitamura, J. Kondo, D. Tsuchiya, T. Taniguchi, S. Shimohama, A. Akaike, S. Sumi, and K. Inoue. 2004. Pharmacological characteristics of rotational behavior in hemiparkinsonian rats transplanted with mouse embryonic stem cell-derived neurons. *J Pharmacol Sci* 96 (1):53-64.

Itakura, T., Y. Uematsu, N. Nakao, E. Nakai, and K. Nakai. 1997. Transplantation of autologous sympathetic ganglion into the brain with Parkinson's disease. Long-term follow-up of 35 cases. *Stereotact Funct Neurosurg* 69 (1-4 Pt 2):112-5.

Jiang, Y., D. Henderson, M. Blackstad, A. Chen, R. F. Miller, and C. M. Verfaillie. 2003. Neuroectodermal differentiation from mouse multipotent adult progenitor cells. *Proc Natl Acad Sci U S A* 100 Suppl 1:11854-60.

Kaji, K., K. Norrby, A. Paca, M. Mileikovsky, P. Mohseni, and K. Woltjen. 2009. Virus-free induction of pluripotency and subsequent excision of reprogramming factors. *Nature* 458 (7239):771-5.

Kawasaki, H., K. Mizuseki, S. Nishikawa, S. Kaneko, Y. Kuwana, S. Nakanishi, S. I. Nishikawa, and Y. Sasai. 2000. Induction of midbrain dopaminergic neurons from ES cells by stromal cell-derived inducing activity. *Neuron* 28 (1):31-40.

Kim, D., C. H. Kim, J. I. Moon, Y. G. Chung, M. Y. Chang, B. S. Han, S. Ko, E. Yang, K. Y. Cha, R. Lanza, and K. S. Kim. 2009. Generation of human induced pluripotent stem cells by direct delivery of reprogramming proteins. *Cell Stem Cell* 4 (6):472-6.

Kim, H. J., M. Sugimori, M. Nakafuku, and C. N. Svendsen. 2007. Control of neurogenesis and tyrosine hydroxylase expression in neural progenitor cells through bHLH proteins and Nurr1. *Exp Neurol* 203 (2):394-405.

Kim, J. H., J. M. Auerbach, J. A. Rodriguez-Gomez, I. Velasco, D. Gavin, N. Lumelsky, S. H. Lee, J. Nguyen, R. Sanchez-Pernaute, K. Bankiewicz, and R. McKay. 2002. Dopamine neurons derived from embryonic stem cells function in an animal model of Parkinson's disease. *Nature* 418 (6893):50-6.

Kishima, H., T. Poyot, J. Bloch, J. Dauguet, F. Conde, F. Dolle, F. Hinnen, W. Pralong, S. Palfi, N. Deglon, P. Aebischer, and P. Hantraye. 2004. Encapsulated GDNF-producing C2C12 cells for Parkinson's disease: a pre-clinical study in chronic MPTP-treated baboons. *Neurobiol Dis* 16 (2):428-39.

Kohyama, J., H. Abe, T. Shimazaki, A. Koizumi, K. Nakashima, S. Gojo, T. Taga, H. Okano, J. Hata, and A. Umezawa. 2001. Brain from bone: efficient "meta-differentiation" of marrow stroma-derived mature osteoblasts to neurons with Noggin or a demethylating agent. *Differentiation* 68 (4-5):235-44.

Kompoliti, K., Y. Chu, K. M. Shannon, and J. H. Kordower. 2007. Neuropathological study 16 years after autologous adrenal medullary transplantation in a Parkinson's disease patient. *Mov Disord* 22 (11):1630-3.

Kopen, G. C., D. J. Prockop, and D. G. Phinney. 1999. Marrow stromal cells migrate throughout forebrain and cerebellum, and they differentiate into astrocytes after injection into neonatal mouse brains. *Proc Natl Acad Sci U S A* 96 (19):10711-6.

Kordower, J. H., Y. Chu, R. A. Hauser, T. B. Freeman, and C. W. Olanow. 2008. Lewy body-like pathology in long-term embryonic nigral transplants in Parkinson's disease. *Nat Med* 14 (5):504-6.

Kordower, J. H., E. Cochran, R. D. Penn, and C. G. Goetz. 1991. Putative chromaffin cell survival and enhanced host-derived TH-fiber innervation following a functional adrenal medulla autograft for Parkinson's disease. *Ann Neurol* 29 (4):405-12.

Kordower, J. H., T. B. Freeman, B. J. Snow, F. J. Vingerhoets, E. J. Mufson, P. R. Sanberg, R. A. Hauser, D. A. Smith, G. M. Nauert, D. P. Perl, and et al. 1995. Neuropathological evidence of graft survival and striatal reinnervation after the transplantation of fetal mesencephalic tissue in a patient with Parkinson's disease. *N Engl J Med* 332 (17):1118-24.

Kordower, J. H., J. M. Rosenstein, T. J. Collier, M. A. Burke, E. Y. Chen, J. M. Li, L. Martel, A. E. Levey, E. J. Mufson, T. B. Freeman, and C. W. Olanow. 1996. Functional fetal nigral grafts in a patient with Parkinson's disease: chemoanatomic, ultrastructural, and metabolic studies. *J Comp Neurol* 370 (2):203-30.

Krabbe, C., E. Courtois, P. Jensen, J. R. Jorgensen, J. Zimmer, A. Martinez-Serrano, and M. Meyer. 2009. Enhanced dopaminergic differentiation of human neural stem cells by synergistic effect of Bcl-xL and reduced oxygen tension. *J Neurochem* 110 (6):1908-20.

Krabbe, C., J. Zimmer, and M. Meyer. 2005. Neural transdifferentiation of mesenchymal stem cells--a critical review. *APMIS* 113 (11-12):831-44.

Lane, E. L., C. Winkler, P. Brundin, and M. A. Cenci. 2006. The impact of graft size on the development of dyskinesia following intrastriatal grafting of embryonic dopamine neurons in the rat. *Neurobiol Dis* 22 (2):334-45.

Lee, S. H., N. Lumelsky, L. Studer, J. M. Auerbach, and R. D. McKay. 2000. Efficient generation of midbrain and hindbrain neurons from mouse embryonic stem cells. *Nat Biotechnol* 18 (6):675-9.

Levy, Y. S., Y. Gilgun-Sherki, E. Melamed, and D. Offen. 2005. Therapeutic potential of neurotrophic factors in neurodegenerative diseases. *BioDrugs* 19 (2):97-127.

Li, J. Y., E. Englund, J. L. Holton, D. Soulet, P. Hagell, A. J. Lees, T. Lashley, N. P. Quinn, S. Rehncrona, A. Bjorklund, H. Widner, T. Revesz, O. Lindvall, and P. Brundin. 2008. Lewy bodies in grafted neurons in subjects with Parkinson's disease suggest host-to-graft disease propagation. *Nat Med* 14 (5):501-3.

Lie, D. C., G. Dziewczapolski, A. R. Willhoite, B. K. Kaspar, C. W. Shults, and F. H. Gage. 2002. The adult substantia nigra contains progenitor cells with neurogenic potential. *J Neurosci* 22 (15):6639-49.

Lindvall, O., E. O. Backlund, L. Farde, G. Sedvall, R. Freedman, B. Hoffer, A. Nobin, A. Seiger, and L. Olson. 1987. Transplantation in Parkinson's disease: two cases of adrenal medullary grafts to the putamen. *Ann Neurol* 22 (4):457-68.

Lindvall, O., P. Brundin, H. Widner, S. Rehncrona, B. Gustavii, R. Frackowiak, K. L. Leenders, G. Sawle, J. C. Rothwell, C. D. Marsden, and et al. 1990. Grafts of fetal dopamine neurons survive and improve motor function in Parkinson's disease. *Science* 247 (4942):574-7.

Lindvall, O., S. Rehncrona, P. Brundin, B. Gustavii, B. Astedt, H. Widner, T. Lindholm, A. Bjorklund, K. L. Leenders, J. C. Rothwell, R. Frackowiak, D. Marsden, B. Johnels, G. Steg, R. Freedman, B. J. Hoffer, A. Seiger, M. Bygdeman, I. Stromberg, and L. Olson. 1989. Human fetal dopamine neurons grafted into the striatum in two patients with severe Parkinson's disease. A detailed account of methodology and a 6-month follow-up. *Arch Neurol* 46 (6):615-31.

Lindvall, O., G. Sawle, H. Widner, J. C. Rothwell, A. Bjorklund, D. Brooks, P. Brundin, R. Frackowiak, C. D. Marsden, P. Odin, and et al. 1994. Evidence for long-term survival and function of dopaminergic grafts in progressive Parkinson's disease. *Ann Neurol* 35 (2):172-80.

Liste, I., E. Garcia-Garcia, and A. Martinez-Serrano. 2004. The generation of dopaminergic neurons by human neural stem cells is enhanced by Bcl-XL, both in vitro and in vivo. *J Neurosci* 24 (48):10786-95.

Liu, W. G., G. Q. Lu, B. Li, and S. D. Chen. 2007. Dopaminergic neuroprotection by neurturin-expressing c17.2 neural stem cells in a rat model of Parkinson's disease. *Parkinsonism Relat Disord* 13 (2):77-88.

Lohle, M., and H. Reichmann. 2010. Clinical neuroprotection in Parkinson's disease - still waiting for the breakthrough. *J Neurol Sci* 289 (1-2):104-14.

Lois, C., and A. Alvarez-Buylla. 1994. Long-distance neuronal migration in the adult mammalian brain. *Science* 264 (5162):1145-8.

Lotharius, J., S. Barg, P. Wiekop, C. Lundberg, H. K. Raymon, and P. Brundin. 2002. Effect of mutant alpha-synuclein on dopamine homeostasis in a new human mesencephalic cell line. *J Biol Chem* 277 (41):38884-94.

Lu, P., A. Blesch, and M. H. Tuszynski. 2004. Induction of bone marrow stromal cells to neurons: differentiation, transdifferentiation, or artifact? *J Neurosci Res* 77 (2):174-91.

Luquin, M. R., R. J. Montoro, J. Guillen, L. Saldise, R. Insausti, J. Del Rio, and J. Lopez-Barneo. 1999. Recovery of chronic parkinsonian monkeys by autotransplants of carotid body cell aggregates into putamen. *Neuron* 22 (4):743-50.

Ma, Y., A. Feigin, V. Dhawan, M. Fukuda, Q. Shi, P. Greene, R. Breeze, S. Fahn, C. Freed, and D. Eidelberg. 2002. Dyskinesia after fetal cell transplantation for parkinsonism: a PET study. *Ann Neurol* 52 (5):628-34.

Madrazo, I., R. Franco-Bourland, F. Ostrosky-Solis, M. Aguilera, C. Cuevas, F. Alvarez, E. Magallon, C. Zamorano, and A. Morelos. 1990. Neural transplantation (auto-adrenal, fetal nigral and fetal adrenal) in Parkinson's disease: the Mexican experience. *Prog Brain Res* 82:593-602.

Maherali, N., R. Sridharan, W. Xie, J. Utikal, S. Eminli, K. Arnold, M. Stadtfeld, R. Yachechko, J. Tchieu, R. Jaenisch, K. Plath, and K. Hochedlinger. 2007. Directly reprogrammed fibroblasts show global epigenetic remodeling and widespread tissue contribution. *Cell Stem Cell* 1 (1):55-70.

Maitra, A., D. E. Arking, N. Shivapurkar, M. Ikeda, V. Stastny, K. Kassauei, G. Sui, D. J. Cutler, Y. Liu, S. N. Brimble, K. Noaksson, J. Hyllner, T. C. Schulz, X. Zeng, W. J. Freed, J. Crook, S. Abraham, A. Colman, P. Sartipy, S. Matsui, M. Carpenter, A. F. Gazdar, M. Rao, and A. Chakravarti. 2005. Genomic alterations in cultured human embryonic stem cells. *Nat Genet* 37 (10):1099-103.

Markakis, E. A., T. D. Palmer, L. Randolph-Moore, P. Rakic, and F. H. Gage. 2004. Novel neuronal phenotypes from neural progenitor cells. *J Neurosci* 24 (12):2886-97.

Masip, M., A. Veiga, J. C. Izpisua Belmonte, and C. Simon. 2010. Reprogramming with defined factors: from induced pluripotency to induced transdifferentiation. *Mol Hum Reprod* 16 (11):856-68.

Meissner, A., M. Wernig, and R. Jaenisch. 2007. Direct reprogramming of genetically unmodified fibroblasts into pluripotent stem cells. *Nat Biotechnol* 25 (10):1177-81.

Mendez, I., R. Sanchez-Pernaute, O. Cooper, A. Vinuela, D. Ferrari, L. Bjorklund, A. Dagher, and O. Isacson. 2005. Cell type analysis of functional fetal dopamine cell suspension transplants in the striatum and substantia nigra of patients with Parkinson's disease. *Brain* 128 (Pt 7):1498-510.

Mendez, I., A. Vinuela, A. Astradsson, K. Mukhida, P. Hallett, H. Robertson, T. Tierney, R. Holness, A. Dagher, J. Q. Trojanowski, and O. Isacson. 2008. Dopamine neurons implanted into people with Parkinson's disease survive without pathology for 14 years. *Nat Med* 14 (5):507-9.

Morizane, A., J. Takahashi, M. Shinoyama, M. Ideguchi, Y. Takagi, H. Fukuda, M. Koyanagi, Y. Sasai, and N. Hashimoto. 2006. Generation of graftable dopaminergic neuron progenitors from mouse ES cells by a combination of coculture and neurosphere methods. *J Neurosci Res* 83 (6):1015-27.

Morley, J. F., and H. I. Hurtig. 2010. Current understanding and management of Parkinson disease: five new things. *Neurology* 75 (18 Suppl 1):S9-15.

Morshead, C. M., B. A. Reynolds, C. G. Craig, M. W. McBurney, W. A. Staines, D. Morassutti, S. Weiss, and D. van der Kooy. 1994. Neural stem cells in the adult mammalian forebrain: a relatively quiescent subpopulation of subependymal cells. *Neuron* 13 (5):1071-82.

Munoz-Elias, G., D. Woodbury, and I. B. Black. 2003. Marrow stromal cells, mitosis, and neuronal differentiation: stem cell and precursor functions. *Stem Cells* 21 (4):437-48.

Nakagawa, M., M. Koyanagi, K. Tanabe, K. Takahashi, T. Ichisaka, T. Aoi, K. Okita, Y. Mochiduki, N. Takizawa, and S. Yamanaka. 2008. Generation of induced pluripotent stem cells without Myc from mouse and human fibroblasts. *Nat Biotechnol* 26 (1):101-6.

Nakao, N., K. Kakishita, Y. Uematsu, T. Yoshimasu, T. Bessho, K. Nakai, Y. Naito, and T. Itakura. 2001. Enhancement of the response to levodopa therapy after intrastriatal transplantation of autologous sympathetic neurons in patients with Parkinson disease. *J Neurosurg* 95 (2):275-84.

Nakao, N., A. Shintani-Mizushima, K. Kakishita, and T. Itakura. 2004. The ability of grafted human sympathetic neurons to synthesize and store dopamine: a potential mechanism for the clinical effect of sympathetic neuron autografts in patients with Parkinson's disease. *Exp Neurol* 188 (1):65-73.

Neuhuber, B., G. Gallo, L. Howard, L. Kostura, A. Mackay, and I. Fischer. 2004. Reevaluation of in vitro differentiation protocols for bone marrow stromal cells: disruption of actin cytoskeleton induces rapid morphological changes and mimics neuronal phenotype. *J Neurosci Res* 77 (2):192-204.

Nishimura, F., M. Yoshikawa, S. Kanda, M. Nonaka, H. Yokota, A. Shiroi, H. Nakase, H. Hirabayashi, Y. Ouji, J. Birumachi, S. Ishizaka, and T. Sakaki. 2003. Potential use of embryonic stem cells for the treatment of mouse parkinsonian models: improved behavior by transplantation of in vitro differentiated dopaminergic neurons from embryonic stem cells. *Stem Cells* 21 (2):171-80.

Okita, K., H. Hong, K. Takahashi, and S. Yamanaka. 2010. Generation of mouse-induced pluripotent stem cells with plasmid vectors. *Nat Protoc* 5 (3):418-28.

Okita, K., T. Ichisaka, and S. Yamanaka. 2007. Generation of germline-competent induced pluripotent stem cells. *Nature* 448 (7151):313-7.

Okita, K., M. Nakagawa, H. Hyenjong, T. Ichisaka, and S. Yamanaka. 2008. Generation of mouse induced pluripotent stem cells without viral vectors. *Science* 322 (5903):949-53.

Olanow, C. W., C. G. Goetz, J. H. Kordower, A. J. Stoessl, V. Sossi, M. F. Brin, K. M. Shannon, G. M. Nauert, D. P. Perl, J. Godbold, and T. B. Freeman. 2003. A double-blind controlled trial of bilateral fetal nigral transplantation in Parkinson's disease. *Ann Neurol* 54 (3):403-14.

Olanow, C. W., O. Rascol, R. Hauser, P. D. Feigin, J. Jankovic, A. Lang, W. Langston, E. Melamed, W. Poewe, F. Stocchi, E. Tolosa, and Adagio Study Investigators. 2009. A double-blind, delayed-start trial of rasagiline in Parkinson's disease. *N Engl J Med* 361 (13):1268-78.

Ostenfeld, T., E. Joly, Y. T. Tai, A. Peters, M. Caldwell, E. Jauniaux, and C. N. Svendsen. 2002. Regional specification of rodent and human neurospheres. *Brain Res Dev Brain Res* 134 (1-2):43-55.

Pahwa, R., S. A. Factor, K. E. Lyons, W. G. Ondo, G. Gronseth, H. Bronte-Stewart, M. Hallett, J. Miyasaki, J. Stevens, W. J. Weiner, and Neurology Quality Standards Subcommittee of the American Academy of. 2006. Practice Parameter: treatment of Parkinson disease with motor fluctuations and dyskinesia (an evidence-based review): report of the Quality Standards Subcommittee of the American Academy of Neurology. *Neurology* 66 (7):983-95.

Palmer, T. D., E. A. Markakis, A. R. Willhoite, F. Safar, and F. H. Gage. 1999. Fibroblast growth factor-2 activates a latent neurogenic program in neural stem cells from diverse regions of the adult CNS. *J Neurosci* 19 (19):8487-97.

Palmer, T. D., J. Ray, and F. H. Gage. 1995. FGF-2-responsive neuronal progenitors reside in proliferative and quiescent regions of the adult rodent brain. *Mol Cell Neurosci* 6 (5):474-86.

Papanikolaou, T., J. B. Lennington, A. Betz, C. Figueiredo, J. D. Salamone, and J. C. Conover. 2008. In vitro generation of dopaminergic neurons from adult subventricular zone neural progenitor cells. *Stem Cells Dev* 17 (1):157-72.

Park, C. H., J. S. Kang, Y. H. Shin, M. Y. Chang, S. Chung, H. C. Koh, M. H. Zhu, S. B. Oh, Y. S. Lee, G. Panagiotakos, V. Tabar, L. Studer, and S. H. Lee. 2006. Acquisition of in vitro and in vivo functionality of Nurr1-induced dopamine neurons. *FASEB J* 20 (14):2553-5.

Park, C. H., Y. K. Minn, J. Y. Lee, D. H. Choi, M. Y. Chang, J. W. Shim, J. Y. Ko, H. C. Koh, M. J. Kang, J. S. Kang, D. J. Rhie, Y. S. Lee, H. Son, S. Y. Moon, K. S. Kim, and S. H. Lee. 2005. In vitro and in vivo analyses of human embryonic stem cell-derived dopamine neurons. *J Neurochem* 92 (5):1265-76.

Park, I. H., N. Arora, H. Huo, N. Maherali, T. Ahfeldt, A. Shimamura, M. W. Lensch, C. Cowan, K. Hochedlinger, and G. Q. Daley. 2008. Disease-specific induced pluripotent stem cells. *Cell* 134 (5):877-86.

Park, K. W., M. A. Eglitis, and M. M. Mouradian. 2001. Protection of nigral neurons by GDNF-engineered marrow cell transplantation. *Neurosci Res* 40 (4):315-23.

Park, S. R., R. O. Oreffo, and J. T. Triffitt. 1999. Interconversion potential of cloned human marrow adipocytes in vitro. *Bone* 24 (6):549-54.

Paul, G., N. S. Christophersen, H. Raymon, C. Kiaer, R. Smith, and P. Brundin. 2007. Tyrosine hydroxylase expression is unstable in a human immortalized mesencephalic cell line--studies in vitro and after intracerebral grafting in vivo. *Mol Cell Neurosci* 34 (3):390-9.

Perlow, M. J., W. J. Freed, B. J. Hoffer, A. Seiger, L. Olson, and R. J. Wyatt. 1979. Brain grafts reduce motor abnormalities produced by destruction of nigrostriatal dopamine system. *Science* 204 (4393):643-7.

Perrier, A. L., V. Tabar, T. Barberi, M. E. Rubio, J. Bruses, N. Topf, N. L. Harrison, and L. Studer. 2004. Derivation of midbrain dopamine neurons from human embryonic stem cells. *Proc Natl Acad Sci U S A* 101 (34):12543-8.

Peschanski, M., G. Defer, J. P. N'Guyen, F. Ricolfi, J. C. Monfort, P. Remy, C. Geny, Y. Samson, P. Hantraye, R. Jeny, and et al. 1994. Bilateral motor improvement and alteration of L-dopa effect in two patients with Parkinson's disease following intrastriatal transplantation of foetal ventral mesencephalon. *Brain* 117 (Pt 3):487-99.

Pittenger, M. F., A. M. Mackay, S. C. Beck, R. K. Jaiswal, R. Douglas, J. D. Mosca, M. A. Moorman, D. W. Simonetti, S. Craig, and D. R. Marshak. 1999. Multilineage potential of adult human mesenchymal stem cells. *Science* 284 (5411):143-7.

Reyes, M., T. Lund, T. Lenvik, D. Aguiar, L. Koodie, and C. M. Verfaillie. 2001. Purification and ex vivo expansion of postnatal human marrow mesodermal progenitor cells. *Blood* 98 (9):2615-25.

Reynolds, B. A., and S. Weiss. 1992. Generation of neurons and astrocytes from isolated cells of the adult mammalian central nervous system. *Science* 255 (5052):1707-10.

Riaz, S. S., S. Theofilopoulos, E. Jauniaux, G. M. Stern, and H. F. Bradford. 2004. The differentiation potential of human foetal neuronal progenitor cells in vitro. *Brain Res Dev Brain Res* 153 (1):39-51.

Richardson, R. M., W. C. Broaddus, K. L. Holloway, and H. L. Fillmore. 2005. Grafts of adult subependymal zone neuronal progenitor cells rescue hemiparkinsonian behavioral decline. *Brain Res* 1032 (1-2):11-22.

Rodriguez-Gomez, J. A., J. Q. Lu, I. Velasco, S. Rivera, S. S. Zoghbi, J. S. Liow, J. L. Musachio, F. T. Chin, H. Toyama, J. Seidel, M. V. Green, P. K. Thanos, M. Ichise, V. W. Pike, R. B. Innis, and R. D. McKay. 2007. Persistent dopamine functions of neurons derived from embryonic stem cells in a rodent model of Parkinson disease. *Stem Cells* 25 (4):918-28.

Roy, N. S., C. Cleren, S. K. Singh, L. Yang, M. F. Beal, and S. A. Goldman. 2006. Functional engraftment of human ES cell-derived dopaminergic neurons enriched by coculture with telomerase-immortalized midbrain astrocytes. *Nat Med* 12 (11):1259-68.

Roybon, L., T. Hjalt, N. S. Christophersen, J. Y. Li, and P. Brundin. 2008. Effects on differentiation of embryonic ventral midbrain progenitors by Lmx1a, Msx1, Ngn2, and Pitx3. *J Neurosci* 28 (14):3644-56.

Sagot, Y., S. A. Tan, J. P. Hammang, P. Aebischer, and A. C. Kato. 1996. GDNF slows loss of motoneurons but not axonal degeneration or premature death of pmn/pmn mice. *J Neurosci* 16 (7):2335-41.

Sanchez-Ramos, J., S. Song, F. Cardozo-Pelaez, C. Hazzi, T. Stedeford, A. Willing, T. B. Freeman, S. Saporta, W. Janssen, N. Patel, D. R. Cooper, and P. R. Sanberg. 2000. Adult bone marrow stromal cells differentiate into neural cells in vitro. *Exp Neurol* 164 (2):247-56.

Sayles, M., M. Jain, and R. A. Barker. 2004. The cellular repair of the brain in Parkinson's disease--past, present and future. *Transpl Immunol* 12 (3-4):321-42.

Schumacher, J. M., S. A. Ellias, E. P. Palmer, H. S. Kott, J. Dinsmore, P. K. Dempsey, A. J. Fischman, C. Thomas, R. G. Feldman, S. Kassissieh, R. Raineri, C. Manhart, D. Penney, J. S. Fink, and O. Isacson. 2000. Transplantation of embryonic porcine mesencephalic tissue in patients with PD. *Neurology* 54 (5):1042-50.

Schwarz, S. C., J. Wittlinger, R. Schober, A. Storch, and J. Schwarz. 2006. Transplantation of human neural precursor cells in the 6-OHDA lesioned rats: effect of immunosuppression with cyclosporine A. *Parkinsonism Relat Disord* 12 (5):302-8.

Shim, J. W., H. C. Koh, M. Y. Chang, E. Roh, C. Y. Choi, Y. J. Oh, H. Son, Y. S. Lee, L. Studer, and S. H. Lee. 2004. Enhanced in vitro midbrain dopamine neuron differentiation, dopaminergic function, neurite outgrowth, and 1-methyl-4-phenylpyridium resistance in mouse embryonic stem cells overexpressing Bcl-XL. *J Neurosci* 24 (4):843-52.

Shinoda, M., J. L. Hudson, I. Stromberg, B. J. Hoffer, J. W. Moorhead, and L. Olson. 1995. Allogeneic grafts of fetal dopamine neurons: immunological reactions following active and adoptive immunizations. *Brain Res* 680 (1-2):180-95.

Shinoda, M., J. L. Hudson, I. Stromberg, B. J. Hoffer, J. W. Moorhead, L. Olson.1996. Microglial cell responses to fetal ventral mesencephalic tissue grafting and to active and adoptive immunizations. *Exp Neurol* 141 (2):173-80.

Soldner, F., D. Hockemeyer, C. Beard, Q. Gao, G. W. Bell, E. G. Cook, G. Hargus, A. Blak, O. Cooper, M. Mitalipova, O. Isacson, and R. Jaenisch. 2009. Parkinson's disease patient-derived induced pluripotent stem cells free of viral reprogramming factors. *Cell* 136 (5):964-77.

Song, T., G. Chen, Y. Wang, G. Mao, and H. Bai. 2008. Chemically defined sequential culture media for TH+ cell derivation from human embryonic stem cells. *Mol Hum Reprod* 14 (11):619-25.

Sonntag, K. C., R. Simantov, K. S. Kim, and O. Isacson. 2004. Temporally induced Nurr1 can induce a non-neuronal dopaminergic cell type in embryonic stem cell differentiation. *Eur J Neurosci* 19 (5):1141-52.

Stadtfeld, M., M. Nagaya, J. Utikal, G. Weir, and K. Hochedlinger. 2008. Induced pluripotent stem cells generated without viral integration. *Science* 322 (5903):945-9.

Storch, A., G. Paul, M. Csete, B. O. Boehm, P. M. Carvey, A. Kupsch, and J. Schwarz. 2001. Long-term proliferation and dopaminergic differentiation of human mesencephalic neural precursor cells. *Exp Neurol* 170 (2):317-25.

Stromberg, I., M. Bygdeman, M. Goldstein, A. Seiger, and L. Olson. 1986. Human fetal substantia nigra grafted to the dopamine-denervated striatum of immunosuppressed rats: evidence for functional reinnervation. *Neurosci Lett* 71 (3):271-6.

Studer, L., M. Csete, S. H. Lee, N. Kabbani, J. Walikonis, B. Wold, and R. McKay. 2000. Enhanced proliferation, survival, and dopaminergic differentiation of CNS precursors in lowered oxygen. *J Neurosci* 20 (19):7377-83.

Studer, L., V. Tabar, and R. D. McKay. 1998. Transplantation of expanded mesencephalic precursors leads to recovery in parkinsonian rats. *Nat Neurosci* 1 (4):290-5.

Svendsen, C. N., M. A. Caldwell, J. Shen, M. G. ter Borg, A. E. Rosser, P. Tyers, S. Karmiol, and S. B. Dunnett. 1997. Long-term survival of human central nervous system progenitor cells transplanted into a rat model of Parkinson's disease. *Exp Neurol* 148 (1):135-46.

Swistowski, A., J. Peng, Q. Liu, P. Mali, M. S. Rao, L. Cheng, and X. Zeng. 2010. Efficient generation of functional dopaminergic neurons from human induced pluripotent stem cells under defined conditions. *Stem Cells* 28 (10):1893-904.

Takahashi, K., K. Tanabe, M. Ohnuki, M. Narita, T. Ichisaka, K. Tomoda, and S. Yamanaka. 2007. Induction of pluripotent stem cells from adult human fibroblasts by defined factors. *Cell* 131 (5):861-72.

Takahashi, K., and S. Yamanaka. 2006. Induction of pluripotent stem cells from mouse embryonic and adult fibroblast cultures by defined factors. *Cell* 126 (4):663-76.

Tatard, V. M., G. D'Ippolito, S. Diabira, A. Valeyev, J. Hackman, M. McCarthy, T. Bouckenooghe, P. Menei, C. N. Montero-Menei, and P. C. Schiller. 2007. Neurotrophin-directed differentiation of human adult marrow stromal cells to dopaminergic-like neurons. *Bone* 40 (2):360-73.

Terada, N., T. Hamazaki, M. Oka, M. Hoki, D. M. Mastalerz, Y. Nakano, E. M. Meyer, L. Morel, B. E. Petersen, and E. W. Scott. 2002. Bone marrow cells adopt the phenotype of other cells by spontaneous cell fusion. *Nature* 416 (6880):542-5.

Tropepe, V., B. L. Coles, B. J. Chiasson, D. J. Horsford, A. J. Elia, R. R. McInnes, and D. van der Kooy. 2000. Retinal stem cells in the adult mammalian eye. *Science* 287 (5460):2032-6.

Trzaska, K. A., C. C. King, K. Y. Li, E. V. Kuzhikandathil, M. C. Nowycky, J. H. Ye, and P. Rameshwar. 2009. Brain-derived neurotrophic factor facilitates maturation of mesenchymal stem cell-derived dopamine progenitors to functional neurons. *J Neurochem* 110 (3):1058-69.

Trzaska, K. A., E. V. Kuzhikandathil, and P. Rameshwar. 2007. Specification of a dopaminergic phenotype from adult human mesenchymal stem cells. *Stem Cells* 25 (11):2797-808.

Tseng, J. L., E. E. Baetge, A. D. Zurn, and P. Aebischer. 1997. GDNF reduces drug-induced rotational behavior after medial forebrain bundle transection by a mechanism not involving striatal dopamine. *J Neurosci* 17 (1):325-33.

Vierbuchen, T., A. Ostermeier, Z. P. Pang, Y. Kokubu, T. C. Sudhof, and M. Wernig. 2010. Direct conversion of fibroblasts to functional neurons by defined factors. *Nature* 463 (7284):1035-41.

Wagner, J., P. Akerud, D. S. Castro, P. C. Holm, J. M. Canals, E. Y. Snyder, T. Perlmann, and E. Arenas. 1999. Induction of a midbrain dopaminergic phenotype in Nurr1-overexpressing neural stem cells by type 1 astrocytes. *Nat Biotechnol* 17 (7):653-9.

Wang, X., Y. Lu, H. Zhang, K. Wang, Q. He, Y. Wang, X. Liu, and L. Li. 2004. Distinct efficacy of pre-differentiated versus intact fetal mesencephalon-derived human neural progenitor cells in alleviating rat model of Parkinson's disease. *Int J Dev Neurosci* 22 (4):175-83.

Weiss, S., C. Dunne, J. Hewson, C. Wohl, M. Wheatley, A. C. Peterson, and B. A. Reynolds. 1996. Multipotent CNS stem cells are present in the adult mammalian spinal cord and ventricular neuroaxis. *J Neurosci* 16 (23):7599-609.

Wernig, M., J. P. Zhao, J. Pruszak, E. Hedlund, D. Fu, F. Soldner, V. Broccoli, M. Constantine-Paton, O. Isacson, and R. Jaenisch. 2008. Neurons derived from reprogrammed fibroblasts functionally integrate into the fetal brain and improve symptoms of rats with Parkinson's disease. *Proc Natl Acad Sci U S A* 105 (15):5856-61.

Wijeyekoon, R., and R. A. Barker. 2009. Cell replacement therapy for Parkinson's disease. *Biochim Biophys Acta* 1792 (7):688-702.

Wilmut, I., A. E. Schnieke, J. McWhir, A. J. Kind, and K. H. Campbell. 1997. Viable offspring derived from fetal and adult mammalian cells. *Nature* 385 (6619):810-3.

Winkler, C., D. Kirik, and A. Bjorklund. 2005. Cell transplantation in Parkinson's disease: how can we make it work? *Trends Neurosci* 28 (2):86-92.

Woltjen, K., I. P. Michael, P. Mohseni, R. Desai, M. Mileikovsky, R. Hamalainen, R. Cowling, W. Wang, P. Liu, M. Gertsenstein, K. Kaji, H. K. Sung, and A. Nagy. 2009. piggyBac transposition reprograms fibroblasts to induced pluripotent stem cells. *Nature* 458 (7239):766-70.

Woodbury, D., E. J. Schwarz, D. J. Prockop, and I. B. Black. 2000. Adult rat and human bone marrow stromal cells differentiate into neurons. *J Neurosci Res* 61 (4):364-70.

Yang, D., Z. J. Zhang, M. Oldenburg, M. Ayala, and S. C. Zhang. 2008. Human embryonic stem cell-derived dopaminergic neurons reverse functional deficit in parkinsonian rats. *Stem Cells* 26 (1):55-63.

Yang, M., A. E. Donaldson, C. E. Marshall, J. Shen, and L. Iacovitti. 2004. Studies on the differentiation of dopaminergic traits in human neural progenitor cells in vitro and in vivo. *Cell Transplant* 13 (5):535-47.

Yu, J., K. Hu, K. Smuga-Otto, S. Tian, R. Stewart, Slukvin, II, and J. A. Thomson. 2009. Human induced pluripotent stem cells free of vector and transgene sequences. *Science* 324 (5928):797-801.

Yu, J., M. A. Vodyanik, K. Smuga-Otto, J. Antosiewicz-Bourget, J. L. Frane, S. Tian, J. Nie, G. A. Jonsdottir, V. Ruotti, R. Stewart, Slukvin, II, and J. A. Thomson. 2007. Induced pluripotent stem cell lines derived from human somatic cells. *Science* 318 (5858):1917-20.

Zeng, X., J. Cai, J. Chen, Y. Luo, Z. B. You, E. Fotter, Y. Wang, B. Harvey, T. Miura, C. Backman, G. J. Chen, M. S. Rao, and W. J. Freed. 2004. Dopaminergic differentiation of human embryonic stem cells. *Stem Cells* 22 (6):925-40.

Zhang, S. C., M. Wernig, I. D. Duncan, O. Brustle, and J. A. Thomson. 2001. In vitro differentiation of transplantable neural precursors from human embryonic stem cells. *Nat Biotechnol* 19 (12):1129-33.

Zhao, M., S. Momma, K. Delfani, M. Carlen, R. M. Cassidy, C. B. Johansson, H. Brismar, O. Shupliakov, J. Frisen, and A. M. Janson. 2003. Evidence for neurogenesis in the adult mammalian substantia nigra. *Proc Natl Acad Sci U S A* 100 (13):7925-30.

Zhou, H., S. Wu, J. Y. Joo, S. Zhu, D. W. Han, T. Lin, S. Trauger, G. Bien, S. Yao, Y. Zhu, G. Siuzdak, H. R. Scholer, L. Duan, and S. Ding. 2009. Generation of induced pluripotent stem cells using recombinant proteins. *Cell Stem Cell* 4 (5):381-4.

Zhou, W., and C. R. Freed. 2009. Adenoviral gene delivery can reprogram human fibroblasts to induced pluripotent stem cells. *Stem Cells* 27 (11):2667-74.

17

Transplantation of Foetal Ventral Mesencephalic Grafts in Parkinson's Disease: A Still Evolving Concept with New Regulatory Challenges

Sven Möllers, Máté Döbrössy and Guido Nikkhah
Department of Stereotactic and Functional Neurosurgery
University Freiburg - Medical Center
Germany

1. Introduction

Several chapters of this book describe the physiology and symptoms of Parkinson's disease (PD) in great detail, nearly 200 years after the typical shaking palsies were first characterised by James Parkinson and further defined by Jean Martin Chacot as "Morbus Parkinson". More recent investigations, starting in the 1950's, identified PD as an age related phenomena, mainly effecting patients over 50 years old (Pollock & Hornabrook, 1966). The incidence of the onset of the disease in a patient is relatively high, as approximately 1 out of 1000 people in the western world might develop typical symptoms of the disease characterised by muscular rigidity or tremor, slow movements or slow mental activity (Lees, Hardy & Revesz, 2009). Once the high impact of this disease on the aging population was identified, research studies were initiated to identify a cure or symptomatic treatment of PD. Only a decade later, in the 60's, the neurotransmitter dopamine, or more precisely the lack of it was pronounced as the main contributory factor in the pathogenesis of PD (Hornykiewicz, 1962, 1966) and initial clinical studies using L-Dopa showed the effectiveness of this drug to reduce the manifestation of classical symptoms of the disease (Boshes et al., 1969; Mones, 1969).

As discussed in detail in previous chapters, the main cause of PD is considered to be a slow but continuously progressive reduction of dopamine within the midbrain region, namely the substantia nigra (SN), caused by a continuous loss of dopamine-producing cells within this region and consequently a lack of dopamine in the receptor target areas, i.e. the putamen and caudate nucleus. While many investigators addressed this issue by performing studies on the administration of L-dopa in animal models or in patients in order to directly overcome the lack of this substance, others focussed on different strategies: Replacement of what is lost by transplanting dopamine producing cells into the diseased tissue or into regions depleted of dopamine, and thereby reversing the loss of function and initiating regeneration of function (Björklund et al., 1982b; Freed, Cannon-Spoor & Wyatt, 1984b).

Transplanting organs and tissues in clinical situations was becoming state of the art from the beginning of the last century on, but transplanting dopaminergic cells into the central nervous system (Figure 1) raised technical difficulties and was first performed in Sweden by

Olson and colleagues in the 1970s using animals (Olson & Seiger, 1972; Perlow, Freed et al., 1979f). In numerous following studies over the next two decades, a wide range of problems, limitations and proof-of-principal concepts were identified and further addressed, leading to the first clinical trial application of dopaminergic cells from autografts in 1982 (Backlund, Granberg et al., 1985a; Olson, Backlund et al., 1985e) up to the first transplantation of allogenic foetal cells in 1987 (O Lindvall et al. 1989f; Madrazo et al. 1988).

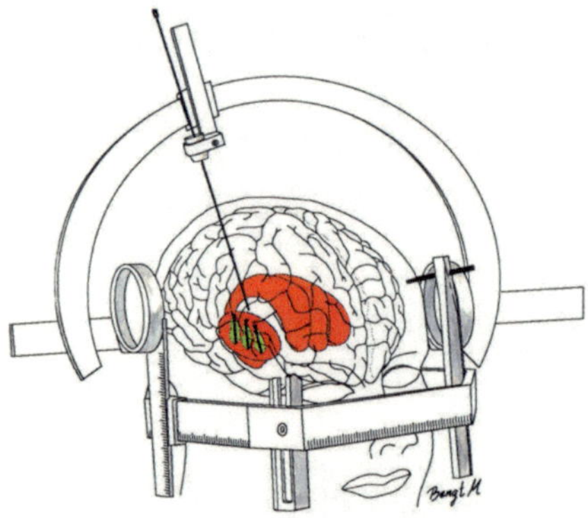

Fig. 1. Example of a stereotactic transplantation of cells
This image shows an example of transplantation of cells into the brain of a patient. Using a stereotactic frame all three axes (X, Y, Z axis) can be adjusted and the cells are then applied accurately into the target area (Nikkhah & Sauer, 1992).

Compared to chemically distinct molecules with defined specifications and characteristics as, for example, therapeutic drugs, it became clear that the transplantation of cells producing the active agents (dopamine, in this case) encompasses numerous unknown, or not well defined, variables during the process of obtaining the source material and converting it into the cells delivered into the brain (Björklund and Lindvall, 2000; Lindvall & Björklund, 2004g).

The concept of using cells as the therapeutic agent is a powerful idea: it potentially represents "true repair" as it purports to replace what has been lost during the progress of the disease. Nevertheless, compared to a classical therapeutic agent, for example a chemical molecule, cells or tissues used commonly have a heterogeneous make-up which makes a direct comparison of effectiveness and mode of action across the traditional and the novel cell therapeutics difficult.

The early pre-clinical studies on cell replacement in Parkinson's disease were confronted with three variables: source, age of tissue, and the mode of preparation. Following initial studies revealing very poor graft survival when transplanting adult CNS tissue into the host adult brain, investigators started using rat foetal ventral mesencephalon (what becomes the substantia nigra) tissue pieces (Hoffer, Freed et al. 1983c; Wyatt et al. 1986), or cell solutions prepared from this tissue (Schmidt, Björklund & Stenevi 1981i), in rodent 6-hydroxydopamine (6-OHDA) lesion models of PD. Both groups realized independently that transplantation of foetal brain tissue or cells can significantly improve on the pathology of the disease, and therefore provided proof of principle on the use of dopaminergic cell transplants almost simultaneously (Figure 2). Still, both groups also showed that size and location of the transplant strongly influence this positive outcome. In addition, later studies added a full variety of new information on the variability of cell transplantation in CNS research. Introduction of the 6-hydroxydopamine lesion model provided a stable and highly reproducible animal model of the disease which could be analyzed in detail by also improved animal behaviour assays (Iversen & Dunnett, 1989e; Klein, Metz et al., 2007c; Kloth, Klein et al., 2006d; Kohn Cordeiro, Jiang et al., 2010b; Nikkhah, Rosenthal et al., 1998h). Having these tools at hand for the last 1-2 decades, recently many groups performing cell therapy research on Parkinson disease realized that small or even no methodological changes in the grafting or housing procedure can result in a great variety of the outcome of the transplantation (Döbrössy et al., 2000; Döbrössy et al., 2010;Nikkhah et al., 1993; Nikkhah, Eberhard, Olsson et al., 1995; Nikkhah, Olsson et al., 1994).

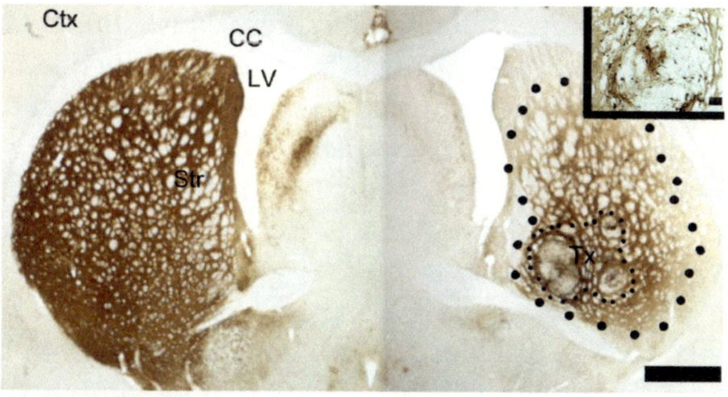

Fig. 2. Cell transplant in the animal model of Parkinson's disease
The picture shows a coronal section of a rat brain stained for Tyrosine Hydroxylase, a key enzyme required for dopamine production and commonly used to identify dopamine neurones and dopamine projections. On the left side is the intact striatum receiving dopamine input from the substantia nigra; on the right is the dopamine depleted striatum that has received rat foetal ventral mesencephalic transplant (within the area delineated by the smaller black dots). The graft tissue has started reinnervating the lesioned striatum and producing dopamine (delineated by larger black dots). The inset is a higher magnification image of a graft with the dopamine neuron cell bodies present. Ctx, cortex; CC, corpus callosum; LV, lateral ventricle; Str, striatum; Tx, transplant. Scale bar = 2 mm; inset = 50μm.

Therefore, graft survival before and after transplantation is a main topic and is being addressed in detail on four levels:

1. The age of the foetal donor tissue regarding its developmental stage not only influences the composition of therapeutic cell types within the graft but also the survival of the graft within the host tissue even though signs of immunological rejection of such grafts generally are very low (Capetian et al., 2011).
2. Modification of the storage or "hibernation" of the donor tissue by controlling storage temperature and the chemical composition of the hibernation medium as well as addition of chemicals and growth supplements can significantly influence the therapeutic strength of the graft as well as (indirectly support) graft survival in the host tissue.
3. The preparation of the foetal tissue for transplantation into the host brain can also have a dramatic influence on the cell quality as well as cell quantity as both mechanical and enzymatic methods are used for preparing grafts. Mechanical dissociation of the tissue is generally performed by cutting of the tissue into small pieces, resulting in severed

and dead cells at the cut surfaces. The disadvantage of the method are countervailed by the still existing "natural" environment for the cells within each tissue piece, an advantage that usually is lost during enzymatic dissociation of foetal tissue where enzymes are used to actively disintegrate the natural environment (the extracellular matrix) of these cells. Here, the main advantage is that less mechanical cell death is being provoked and that single cell suspensions achieved by such methods usually are reproducibly concentrated.

Both methods also directly influence the last main variable in the full treatment process which is:

4. Stereotactic application of therapeutic foetal tissues or cells deeply within the brain. Single cell suspension of a very controlled cell concentration and volume can be injected using much thinner cannulae, while tissue pieces require much larger calibre cannulae with higher risks of damaging the host CNS tissue and much less control of amount of the therapeutic tissue, not even regarding the possible high variability of placement of the graft within the individual host (Nikkhah et al., 2009).

Taken together, the relatively simple concept of replacing lost mature dopaminergic neurons with fetal dopaminergic neuroblasts is technically a highly complex and not yet fully understood process. Nevertheless, numerous groups entered the clinical phases of cell therapy in Parkinson's disease after the strong positive results in the early 80s and the pioneering clinical trials done by Backlund, Madrazo and Lindvall in the mid- and late 80s. These first clinical trials were open-labelled with carefully chosen patients and very low group-sizes. Contrary to most animal data, adrenal autografts containing dopamine producing cells were used in these studies as the need for immunosuppressant after transplantation was eliminated and ethical concerns regarding foetal tissue use were not an issue. The long-term graft survival and functional outcome of adrenal grafts turned out to be poor in the several hundred patients transplanted in numerous trials (Lindvall 1991). In addition, the severity of the side effects of transplanting adrenal medullar tissue into the brain also resulted in high morbidity of patients which was intolerable.

Thereby, in the late 80ies of the last century, researchers proceeded with the initial experimental concept of transplanting foetal dopaminergic CNS tissue as the animal results proved robust data on the efficacy of the grafting method (Björklund et al., 1980a; Björklund et al., 1981c; Nikkhah, Bentlage et al., 1994; Nikkhah, Cunningham, Cenci, McKay et al., 1995). In a number of small open-label clinical trials with 2-6 patients each, the benefit of (allogenic) foetal dopaminergic transplants could be shown ranging from moderate to high, stepwise improved by adapting and further developing the methods of application. These early studies showed that foetal dopaminergic neurons can survive long-term for more then 10 years in patients and are capable of improving the classical symptoms of Parkinson's disease. Most importantly, motivated by these exceptional outcomes, the strong ethical and legal consequences of the use of embryonic and foetal tissue for clinical application were addressed in the creation of clear guidelines restricting the use of these tissues by the applying scientific groups (Boer 1994; Boer 1999). Following these guidelines, more sophisticated double-blinded clinical trials with PD patients were initiated (Freeman et al., 1995d; Olanow et al., 2003).

Nevertheless, it also must be stated that during the last century, some of these studies showed a variation of the therapeutic effect of transplanted foetal tissue and cells in patients suffering on PD, including the development of side effects. The variations of the therapeutic

effects not only differed between study centres, but also within individual study groups of the centres (Brundin et al., 2001; Winkler, Kirik & Björklund, 2005).
The side effects of the cell therapy for PD, which occur beside the mentioned variation of the grafts therapeutic potency, mainly consisted of graft induced dyskinesias (GID), motor fluctuations and abnormal involuntary movements similar to those disturbances induced by L-DOPA medication (LID). Both forms of dyskinesias probably accumulated in some patients and can negatively influence the generally moderate improvement of patients studied in clinical trials, and can be associated to either patient related phenomena or transplantation related concurrency and seems to be wide-spread within the highly diverse clinical study designs analyzed (Hagell & Cenci, 2005). As far as safety issues of the grafts are concerned, animal studies have shown that factors influencing the GID-potential of a foetal nigral tissue graft may include age of the foetus, mode of dissection, time and method of storage, culturing of the cells as well as size and translocation of the graft within the brain (Lane & Smith 2010; Lane et al., 2010).

2. Cell therapies in Parkinson's disease: The new (regulatory) frontier

There are three decades of experience on cell therapy in clinical trials with hundreds of patients having been transplanted with many improving on their disease pattern of PD, yet, many open questions still remain. In particular, since most clinical studies have been conducted independently of one another, there is a marked variability in the individual study protocols that make the general statement about the results highly difficult. This has lead to a desire shared by numerous study centres to generate a single standardized study protocol, based on the experience (positive and negative) of the recent decades that rises to the challenges proposed by clinical cell transplantation into the central nervous system.
One of the reasons explaining the high variability in previous study designs may be due to the lack of legislative basis for tissue engineering or cell therapies in several nations. For many years, this fact was recognized in several European nations as such, but many national legislators were waiting for a common, European legislation on the new fields of genetic engineering, cell therapy and biotech manufacturing to adapt such new legislation into their national regulations. After years of discussion a general regulation was finally adopted within the European Union in 2007, which almost generally defines all products from genetically engineered or biotechnologically produced material, tissue or cells as a medicinal drug. This regulation is in force since the 30th December 2008. (Regulation (EC) No 1394/2007 of 13 November 2007).

2.1 What does EC 1394/2007 mean for the field of cell therapies in the central nervous system, particularly for the treatment of PD?

The main subject of the regulation EC 1394/2007 is the definition of advanced therapeutic medicinal products (ATMP), their production processes as well as their marketing as an approved drug.
The ATMP include gene therapy, somatic cell therapy, tissue engineered products and "combined advanced therapy medicinal products" which are cell and tissue products that contain medical devices or other products as an integral part of it. As a new EU pharmaceutical legislation for Regenerative Medicine, the Regulation 1394/2007/EU (ATMP-Regulation) is valid for all Member States of the EU. The rules set out herein are to be used by all Member States and shall be converted into national law. To meet the special

characteristics of cell and tissue-based products, the ATMP-Regulation provides several additions and modifications of existing European laws and calls for new support measures and initiatives on part of the (national) authorities. It should be stated that products classified as ATMP follow the principles of existing legislation on medicines, including marketing authorisation, demonstration of quality, safety and efficacy as well as post-authorisation vigilance. A centralised application and approval procedure is mandatory and supported by pooling of Community expertise, harmonisation of requirements & evaluation as well as uniform and direct access to market once the products is approved. For this reason, it should be evaluated at a very early stage of the development of a cell-based therapy, whether the future cell product falls within the definition of an ATMP and would therefore be developed and produced according to the recognized rules of GCP and GMP. For this purpose, a Committee for Advanced Therapies (CAT) has been established that supports the Committee for Human Medicinal Products (CHMP) on this classification for each application (Figure 3).

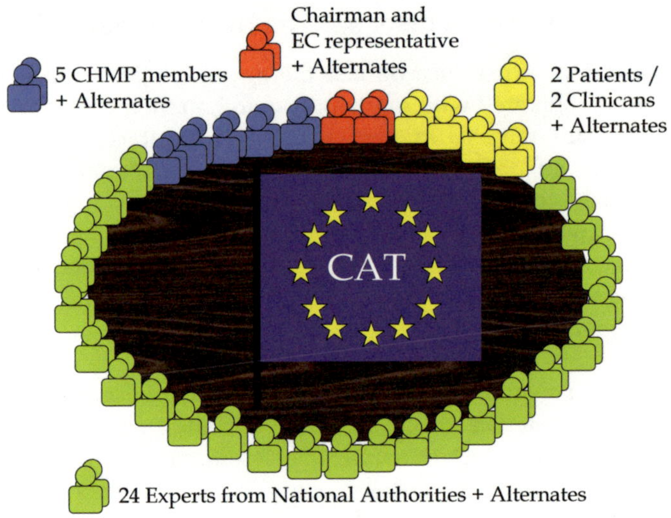

Fig. 3. Committee for Advanced Therapies (CAT)
The CAT is a multidisciplinary committee composed of experts and interest groups from all European Countries. Each member state is sending one expert representative and alternate. The main working task of the committee is to assess the quality, safety and efficacy of an ATMP. It also contributes greatly to certification of quality and non-clinical data of small and medium-sized enterprises, scientific advices for ATMP development, elaboration of any documents related to the fulfilment of the objectives of *Regulation (EC) No 1394/2007* and related activities as requested by the CHMP or the EC.
Modified from first EMEA Workshop on Advanced Therapy Medicinal Products (ATMPs), presentation No.3, 3/04/2009, London (UK)

This CAT is composed of multidisciplinary experts of the scientific field of advanced therapies. The main responsibility of the CAT is to prepare a draft opinion on each ATMP application submitted to the European Medicines Agency (EMA), before the Committee for Medicinal Products for Human Use (CHMP) adopts a final opinion on the granting, variation, suspension or revocation of a marketing authorisation for the medicine concerned (from EMA webpage). It is also participating in Agency procedures for the certification of quality and non-clinical data for small and medium-sized enterprises developing advanced-therapy medicinal products, and participating in Agency procedures for the provision of scientific recommendations on the classification of advanced-therapy medicinal products in accordance with Article 17 of Regulation (EC) No 1394/2007. Despite several other tasks, this committee is also advising, at the request of the CHMP, on any medicinal product which may require, for the evaluation of its quality, safety or efficacy, expertise in ATMPs.

2.2 How to define the PD cell therapy an ATMP?

A PD cell therapy can be considered an ATMP by definition when it is a "tissue engineered product that contains or consists of engineered cells or tissues, and is presented as having properties for, or is used in or administered to human beings with a view to regenerating, repairing or replacing a human tissue. The cells or tissues may be viable or non-viable. It may also contain additional substances, such as cellular products, bio-molecules, biomaterials, chemical substances, scaffolds or matrices." (Regulation (EC) No 1394/2007) By this definition, cell therapy comes under the ATMP regulations if the cells used are engineered. The term "engineered" is defined for cells or tissues as that which have been subject to substantial manipulation, so that biological characteristics, physiological functions or structural properties relevant for the intended regeneration, repair or replacement are achieved. Also, the cells or tissues are considered ATMP if they are "not intended to be used for the same essential function or functions in the recipient as in the donor". Any cell or tissue preparation that has been substantially manipulated can thereby be considered an ATMP. "Not substantially manipulated" also has been defined as cutting, grinding, shaping, and centrifugation, soaking in antibiotic or antimicrobial solutions, sterilization, irradiation, cell separation, concentration or purification, filtering, lyophilisation, freezing, cryo-preservation, vitrification.

It should be noted that the full process from harvesting of the tissue up to the therapeutic application of the cell therapy needs to be analyzed and considered by the regulatory bodies to decide if a cell therapy becomes an ATMP or not. That decision or definition may have a significant influence on the therapeutic approach and its implementation in clinical practice, as each ATMP is to follow the defined standards of good manufacturing and good clinical practice as within the EU being defined in additional regulations.

2.3 A cell therapy for PD becomes ATMP: What are the implications for the clinical practice?

Some cell therapies may be excluded from the ATMP regulation if they fulfil the criteria of the so-called "hospital-exemption", a paragraph included in most former national health acts. This exemption should allow an application of the therapy which is "prepared on a non-routine basis according to specific quality standards, and used within the same Member State in a hospital under the exclusive professional responsibility of a medical practitioner, in order to comply with an individual medical prescription for a custom-made product for an individual patient."(Regulation (EC) No 1394/2007). Thereby, some cell therapy approaches might be applied without the full consideration of the EMA, but generally a standard cell therapy approach is too complex to be realized by one medical practitioner only.

This is true for some of the cell therapies clinically applied in the late 90's of the last century. As an example, CNS tissue was dissected from young human foetuses, minced, enzymatically dissociated in combination with DNAse and finally transplanted stereotactically into the brain of PD-patients (Figure 4).

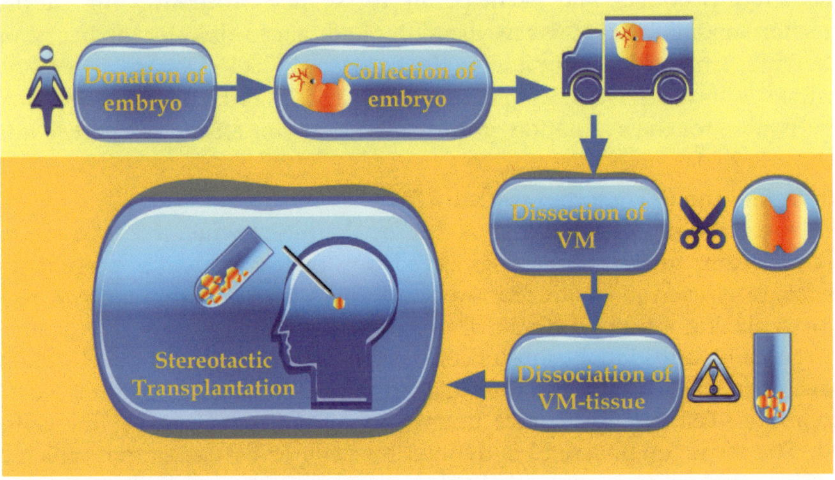

Fig. 4. Flow-Sheet of a possible cell therapy for Parkinson's Disease
This flow sheet shows schematically the conventional process steps for the production of the cell preparation for the previously mentioned clinical studies.
A foetus is donated by a woman and transported in medium to the hospital (yellow). In the clinic (orange), under responsibility of the practitioner, the CNS is taken from the foetus and the ventral mesencephalon (VM) dissected mechanically. Foetal dopaminergic cells are obtained by enzymatic dissociation, washed and injected into the brain by stereotactic guided transplantation.

This relatively easy concept of a cell therapeutic approach might now be translated into the "new language" after the ATMP-regulation became active. "Easy concept" in this case is generally spoken compared to possible modern or future approaches using for example iPS cells, which have been genetically engineered, cultured in humid incubators or bioreactors for days and further manipulated using growth factors and hydrogels, while the classical and most applied concept of cell therapy for Parkinson's disease generally was mostly composed of cells and tissue fragments, dissected from foetal brain tissue without further cell culture but rather direct transplantation into the brain of a patient.
As to date - to our knowledge - there is no application sent to the EMA regarding this cell therapy approach. There might likely be applications in the near future as the data of the earlier clinical trials are promising but need further refinement which can be achieved via additional pre-clinical studies. These investigations will be confronted with defined expressions like good laboratory practice (GLP), good manufacturing practice (GMP) and good clinical practice (GCP), generally considered good professional practice (GxP) as the ATMP regulation is defining such cell therapies as medicinal products, whose production are further defined commonly in numerous regulations and directives.

3. Translating the regulations into (practical) clinical research

In general, a new clinical trial in Parkinson's disease in the EU using the cell therapy approach which likely becomes the status of an ATMP, would have to be conducted following the Clinical Trial Directive (Directive 2001/20/EC) as well as the GCP Directive (Directive 2005/28/EC). While these directives are individually to be implemented at a national level for each Member State and can thereby be interpreted variably, the content for EU wide clinical studies is directly applicable. For the example of cell therapy as a clinical study, the manufacture of test material ("the cells") and the production of scientific data on the safety of the test material are particularly relevant. The GCP-Directive provides, inter alia, that relevant data from preclinical experiments should be planned and conducted by following the standards of good laboratory practice (Directive 2004/10/EC), which means in particular for university facilities a major hurdle as GLP accredited laboratories are rare at such institutes and preclinical data at the university level is usually achieved from via basic research. The logical background to the requirement that certain pre-clinical data shall be generated to the standards of GLP is based on the fact that safety issues of the treatment have been generated by reproducible and fully traceable experiments. GLP also means that the data obtained is reliable and understandable for the authorities; that the data will be archived and regularly monitored; and that audits of the laboratory by the authorities are able to demonstrate sustained and continuous improvement. All aspects of a treatment or manufacturing processes that could result in harm to the patient should therefore be carried out with the best possible method to precisely reduce the risk of the patient. In the field of cell therapy, where the cells are considered an implantable drug, the risks considered are aspects of biocompatibility, toxicity, formulation and use of additives or their removal.

Nevertheless, it is our experience that regulatory authorities generally do follow and control upon the principles defined in these GCP and GLP directives. The future clinical trial application on the cell therapy approach for Parkinson's disease using the mentioned set up of enzymatically dissociated primary foetal cells needs to include experimental data generated according to these principles, for example. In addition, it might also be important for the clinical trial group to include a strategy paper on the requirements for the cell therapy approach once the projects leaves the research phases and is about to enter the therapy phase as at this stage GMP principles are to be followed upon as on the EU level this is directed by Regulation (EC) No 1394/2007.

3.1 PD cell therapy according to GLP and GMP

We pointed out that new clinical cell therapy approaches for PD very likely are to be conducted following the international principles of GLP and GMP, and maybe implemented in slightly varied national versions. As both GLP/ GMP were originally developed on an industrial level for decades to ensure product quality (and safety), such industrial standards are likely to be difficult to implement into a historically evolved research institution as most universities hospitals are like. Even though these research institutions generally conduct research in a "good" way, most likely recognized and approved by high ranking, peer reviewed journals and experts in the specific field of science, this "good" way is different to the requirements of GLP and GMP. We highlight the most crucial elements of both GLP and GMP for the example of cell therapy mentioned above and we will try to provide information on the possible implications of these principles for a university hospital set-up. Both GMP/ GLP share a main common feature: A handbook or manual. This collection of written documents should describe all aspects of the quality management and quality assurance of the proposed cell therapy, and ensure that all activities needed to conduct the safety studies, or the manufacture of the test equipment is shown in clear instructions (standard operation procedures or SOPs) and will be documented in writing. In fact, both manuals have a large amount of common ground as quality is managed similar; but because of their different application areas strong differences stand out. The specific requirements of the manuals are described in the various directives and should be available separately for both the GLP studies as well as GMP manufacturing. It is easily predictable even from this requirement that modern studies of cell therapy now in addition to the clinical study plan, other, more comprehensive documentation are required.

As mentioned, both manuals need to define the quality management system. In principle, this management describes who is authorizing the work (Chapter "Management"), where the work is being done (Chapter "Application area"), who is performing the work (Chapter "Personnel"), what equipment and material will be used (Chapter "Equipment", "Substances", "Purchase and Storage") and how the quality is being maintained (Chapter "Document control", "Quality Assurance"). These possible subdivisions of the term "quality" have been established internationally and this can be found for Europe in the EN ISO 9000 / 9001. Following these requirements, an organization or, as in the example of cell therapy, the clinical facility, can officially be certified to present to the outside the implementation of a quality management system. Especially for the later production according to GMP, the implementation of this process is very important because the regulatory agencies will require an efficient quality management system for the manufacturing license (Regulation (EC) No 1394/2007).

A clinical director therefore requires the implementation of a quality system "by the book" (EN ISO 9001) as it is required for GLP and GMP. However, the clinical director must stand behind that decision and also self-identify himself as a model to implement the benefits of an effective quality management system. He must accompany objectives defined by the development of the system, reclaim reports on a regular basis, arrange and identify corrective measures and ensure that agreements are kept up to date. It is not enough here to employ appropriate quality personnel essential to obtain a certification; quality must be understood and experienced as such, otherwise the implementation of the system is condemned to failure from the start.

Once the clinical director identified and implemented such quality measures as a crucial part of clinical cell therapy according to the regulations, he now will be confronted with the details of GLP and GMP.

3.2 The good practice in the lab: An introduction to quality assurance

As mentioned above, now that it is required to have a quality management system in place, it also is required to produce quality. For example, in both GLP and GMP, it needs to be ensured that cell therapy for the animal safety studies or for the clinical study is being performed under aseptic conditions. While for a specialist in cell culture or the surgeon in the operating room this situation is clearly understood and naturally carried out using corresponding measures consistently, the proof of sterility at medicinal drug manufacturing under GLP and GMP conditions is mandatory. In addition, of course, working environments have to be clean and need to fulfil the prescribed requirements for the manufacturing of ATMP sufficiently.

In the given example, all high risk steps of the preparation of the cell product (opening vials, pipetting, etc) must therefore be carried out in a so-called "class A in Class B environment" according to the Directive 2003/94/EC and further defined in EudraLex Volume 4. In general, it means that a conventional safety cabinet (Class A) is installed in a category B clean room (EudraLex Volume 4, Annex I). For the class B clean room, strictly defined requirements are in place, which vary significantly from the usual requirements of the operating room. For example, it must be a separated room with restricted access and specifically trained staff. The trained staff of the class B clean room must include a Head of Production and a Head of Quality assurance with separated and defined responsibilities. It should also include a Qualified Person who ensures that each lot was produced and tested in accordance with the guidelines and the specifications set within the QM-Handbook. The responsibilities of and legal requirements for a qualified persons are also defined within national/international directives and regulations and usually include a minimum of 2 years work experience with all processes and within the technical requirements (e.g. class B clean room). Aseptic working conditions of the environment should be ensured by performing online particle counts on volumetric air sampling as well as microbiological monitoring using methods such as settle plates or surface sampling during production. Surface sampling includes the active personnel, which fingers should be tested for microbes after each critical process step and less then 5 microbes / 25cm^2 in class B environment or >1/25cm^2 inside the class A workbench should be identified (EudraLex, Volume 4, Annex I). It should also be noted that culture and evaluation of the microbiological sampling plates also need to be performed according to the GLP regulations; for example the incubator should be qualified and monitored constantly.

Although these examples cited might be considered as common sense, the actual implementation into a regulatory acceptable level is a very serious and work-intensive task. The authorities' want these investigations not only being performed and analyzed, but definitely want to have ensured that all tests or production processes can be performed reproducibly within the acceptable specifications. On the industrial side, from where the regulations originate from, these requirements under GMP conditions are usually implemented through activities such as qualification and validation. In consideration of the aseptic work environment mentioned in this paragraph, in the academic research environment one would ensure quality by qualifying the class A work bench, for example. This type of qualification is, according to the GMP regulations, being performed by the implementation steps of design qualification (what kind of class A bench is needed and how to purchase), installation qualification (verification of complete delivery and installation according to the specifications), operational qualification (writing of SOP and test of functionality) and finally performance qualification (is the work bench fully capable of specification delivery for production).

This qualification process, using the bench as the example, shows that a large number of documents and tests must be written and performed on a single device, contributing significantly to the manufacturing effort. It is generally not sufficient to order a laboratory work bench from a supplier and use the device directly to produce a cell therapy product. The qualification of the workbench is rather to ensure that optimal aseptic work environment can actually be made possible from a technical point of view and that the equipment is ideal for the production process. The necessary evidence here is carried out as part of the validation, a definition for which there also are continuously evolving industrial standards available (aka ISO norms) that should be followed upon as part of GMP, as well as GLP. For example, the aseptic preparation within the bench it needs to be proven that aseptic conditions actually are achieved before manufacturing begins. This can for example be performed by a cleaning validation, which provides the proof on the basis of scientific methods that both the optimum cleaning procedure, the best method as well as the most suitable chemicals were used to scientifically exclude risks to the cell product by exposure to microbes or to the cleaning procedure itself. It is conceivable to prepare an aseptic work surface to roughly prepare or cut the tissue for later cell preparation steps. In this case, however, it should be proven by scientific evidence that no risk is transmitted by the surface to the tissue or indirectly to the patient by chemical residues left over after the cleaning process, a simple fact but overlooked easily and actually technically difficult to prove.

Using as an example the need for aseptic work environment leading up to clinical treatment, it becomes clear that the preparation for cell therapy under either GLP or GMP purposes is labour intensive, including the generation of several SOPs, performing of several validation tests and filling out forms to collect the data. The validation activities thereby need to be planned very carefully as the clinical director never wants only to focus on single issues of the process but on all aspects of the full manufacturing process. For planning validations in a good practice environment, a so-called validation master plan should thereby be discussed and generated before any validation is actually being performed. This plan is (yet) not mandatory in the regulations, but is one of the first documents a regulator officer will ask for during an audit. It provides information of how the clinical department operates, who is in control of the different validation activities, and how the manufacturing, quality control and personnel are being managed. Main integral part of the validation master plan generally is the previously mentioned qualification procedure, but it also includes activities performed to generate general risk analysis documentation, validation approaches to deal with identified risks and timelines to finish the validation activities.

Finally, it is clear that in addition to the head of production, the Quality Assurance Manager and the Qualified Person, a validation expert should also be present in addition to seamlessly link the areas of manufacturing and quality assurance of the product by adapted validation activities. It also becomes clear that once the proposed cell therapy is defined as a medicinal product by the authorities, the principle investigator of the cell therapy - used to research standards - now is confronted with multiple legal requirements that for newcomers might become irritating and frustrating. A high number of needs are to be fulfilled, not only requiring a tremendous piece of work time to be invested to "get the paper work done", but also technical and personal requirements need to be put in place, most likely coming along with a substantial amount of financial demand. If one considers the usually small numbers of "products" the principle investigator will need to address small clinical trials, these high risk investments will not easily find the internal support needed. Nevertheless, in the long-term, once implemented into a working system, this newly implemented system will lead to less hassles and burdens to carry out additional cell therapy studies and significantly promote the standardisation in multicenter trials.

4. Standardizing new cell therapies for PD: The TRANSEURO project

As discussed in the introduction of this chapter, in recent decades several clinical studies using cell therapy in PD were investigated often producing large differences in the outcome (Winkler, Kirik & Björklund 2005h). In many cases it was found that the protocols needed to conduct the therapy varied significantly in many places and a generalized statement about the efficiency of the studies was difficult to reach. In parallel, the legislation has only recently clearly and very significantly changed so that the implementation of studies on cell therapy for small clinical facilities and centres quickly reaches the limits of feasibility, when all the national and international laws and guidelines need to be considered.

With the desire of reducing the inconsistencies and variations across centres, a consortium of European based leading clinical and research centres implicated in cell therapy recently have been awarded European Union funding aimed at addressing critical questions in the context of cell therapy in PD, particularly concerning patient selection, tissue preparation, cell delivery, immunosuppression, and off-state dyskinesia. A key objective of the TRANEURO project funded by the FP7 European Commission Health programme is to generate standardized protocols that can serve as a template for all future clinical trials in the cell therapy field including stem cell-based therapies for PD. As part of an international multi-centre clinical study, both preclinical and clinical standards are being defined across the centres in order to generate the best practice approaches investigating the feasibility and clinical efficacy of foetal cell therapy in PD (see also TransEuro homepage http://www.transeuro.org.uk/). Furthermore, the stringent regulatory requirements to implement the standards of GMP and GCP will be addressed by close cooperation between the various centres in particular through joint protocol development and the intensive exchange between the project managers of the different areas to combine synergies to effectively take-on the numerous technical and regulatory hurdles together. By using modern communication media such as web meetings, online training classes, an international project management, but also classic laboratory visits, all elements for manufacturing and the clinical treatment of patients are developed and established, to conserve resources and optimize the expected outcome.

The legislature has certainly imposed very high standards of patients' safety in clinical trials, but as illustrated in the previous examples, such standards hereby reached a high level that can only be met with great difficulty by classical research institutions alone. The declared goal of the TRANSEURO consortium is to achieve successful cell therapy for patients suffering from PD, but at the same time to provide the feasibility of implementing a therapy at regulatory acceptable level. It is the authors' opinion that the enhancement of the regulations during the last years is a double-edged sword with a potential to become a sharp "weapon". On one hand it maximizes patient and promotes the standardization of innovative procedures. On the other side, it creates a substantial challenge, both for personal and financial resources, to meet the new regulatory processes and requirements especially for university and other academic institutions.

5. Conclusion

Cell transplantation for PD-patients is a promising therapy, based on the previous pre-clinical and clinical research. The use of foetal tissue as proposed in the TRANSEURO project holds a number of (ethical) concerns and technical handicaps, but is an ideal candidate to merge basic science and industrial standards to achieve an efficient therapy. This may set the basis of future cell therapeutically approaches with considerably more complex processes and thereby noticeable higher regulatory demands. The worldwide effort working with embryonic stem cells and with induced pluripotent stem cells (iPS) might in the near future generate alternative candidate cells for clinical therapy in PD. However, complicated manufacturing processes involving gene manipulation, advanced cell culture techniques and risk of tumorigenicity will benefit greatly from the currently planned

TransEuro clinical trial, as this will set the stage for the potential and risks of clinical cell therapy in PD for the near future.

6. Acknowledgement

The authors are partially funded by the European Commission under the 7th Framework Programme - HEALTH - Collaborative Project Transeuro (Contract n°242003) - www.transeuro.org.uk

7. References

Backlund, E O, P O Granberg, B Hamberger, E Knutsson, A Mårtensson, G Sedvall, A Seiger, and L Olson. 1985a. "Transplantation of adrenal medullary tissue to striatum in parkinsonism. First clinical trials." *Journal of Neurosurgery* 62 (2) (February): 169-173. doi:10.3171/jns.1985.62.2.0169.

Björklund, A, SB Dunnett, U Stenevi, M E Lewis, and S D Iversen. 1980a. "Reinnervation of the denervated striatum by substantia nigra transplants: functional consequences as revealed by pharmacological and sensorimotor testing." *Brain Research* 199 (2) (October 20): 307-333.

Björklund, A, and O Lindvall. 2000. "Cell replacement therapies for central nervous system disorders." *Nature Neuroscience* 3 (6) (June): 537-544. doi:10.1038/75705.

Björklund, A, U Stenevi, SB Dunnett, and F H Gage. 1982b. "Cross-species neural grafting in a rat model of Parkinson's disease." *Nature* 298 (5875) (August 12): 652-654.

Björklund, A, U Stenevi, SB Dunnett, and S D Iversen. 1981c. "Functional reactivation of the deafferented neostriatum by nigral transplants." *Nature* 289 (5797) (February 5): 497-499.

Boer, GJ. 1994. "Ethical guidelines for the use of human embryonic or fetal tissue for experimental and clinical neurotransplantation and research. Network of European CNS Transplantation and Restoration (NECTAR)." *Journal of Neurology* 242 (1) (December): 1-13.

Boer GJ. 1999. "Ethical issues in neurografting of human embryonic cells." *Theoretical Medicine and Bioethics* 20 (5) (September): 461-475.

Boshes, B, E R Blonsky, J Arbit, and K Klein. 1969. "Effect of L-dopa on individual symptoms of parkinsonism." *Transactions of the American Neurological Association* 94: 229-231.

Brundin P, S Dunnett, A Björklund, Nikkhah G. 2001. "Transplanted dopaminergic neurons: more or less?" *Nature Medicine.* (May) 7(5): 512-513.

Capetian, P, M Döbrössy, C Winkler , M Prinz, GNikkhah. 2011. "To be or not to be accepted: the role of immunogenicity of neural stem cells following transplantation into the brain in animal and human studies." *Seminars in Immunopathology.* [Epub ahead of print]

Cordeiro, Karina Kohn, Wei Jiang, Anna Papazoglou, Sérgio Bernardo Tenório, M Döbrössy, and Guido Nikkhah. 2010b. "Graft-mediated functional recovery on a skilled forelimb use paradigm in a rodent model of Parkinson's disease is dependent on reward contingency." *Behavioural Brain Research* 212 (2) (October 15): 187-195. doi:10.1016/j.bbr.2010.04.012.

Directive 2001/20/EC of 4 April 2001, of the European Parliament and of the Council on the approximation of the laws, regulations and administrative provisions of the Member States relating to implementation of good clinical practice in the conduct of clinical trials on medicinal products for human use

Directive 2003/94/EC, of 8 October 2003, of the European Parliament and of the Council laying down the principles of good manufacturing practice in respect of medicinal products for human use and investigational medicinal products for human use

Directive 2004/10/EC, of 11 February 2004, of the European Parliament and of the Council on the harmonisation of laws, regulations and administrative provisions relating to the application of the principles of good laboratory practice and the verification of their applications for tests on chemical substances (codified version).

Directive 2005/28/EC, of 8 April 2005, of the European Parliament and of the Council laying down principles and detailed guidelines for good clinical practice as regards investigational medicinal products for human use, as well as the requirements for authorisation of the manufacturing or importation of such products

Döbrössy, MD, M Le Moal, M F Montaron, and N Abrous. 2000. "Influence of environment on the efficacy of intrastriatal dopaminergic grafts." *Experimental Neurology* 165 (1) (September): 172-183. doi:10.1006/exnr.2000.7462.

Döbrössy M, M Busse, T Piroth, A Rosser, S Dunnett, G Nikkhah. 2010. "Neurorehabilitation with neural transplantation." *Neurorehabilitation and Neural Repair.* (Oct) 24(8): 692-701

EN ISO 9001, 2000, *Quality Management Systems - Requirements*, International Organization for Standardization

EudraLex, Volume 4, *The Rules Governing Medicinal Products in the European Union, EU Guidelines to Good Manufacturing Practice Medicinal Products for Human and Veterinary Use*, Dec. 2010

Freed, WJ, H E Cannon-Spoor, and R J Wyatt. 1984b. "Embryonic brain grafts in an animal model of Parkinson's disease. Criteria for human application." *Applied Neurophysiology* 47 (1-2): 16-22.

Freeman, T B, C W Olanow, R A Hauser, G M Nauert, DA Smith, C V Borlongan, P R Sanberg, D A Holt, J H Kordower, and F J Vingerhoets. 1995d. "Bilateral fetal nigral transplantation into the postcommissural putamen in Parkinson's disease." *Annals of Neurology* 38 (3) (September): 379-388. doi:10.1002/ana.410380307.

Hagell, Peter, and M Angela Cenci. 2005. "Dyskinesias and dopamine cell replacement in Parkinson's disease: a clinical perspective." *Brain Research Bulletin* 68 (1-2) (December 15): 4-15. doi:10.1016/j.brainresbull.2004.10.013.

Hoffer, B, W Freed, L Olson, and R J Wyatt. 1983c. "Transplantation of dopamine-containing tissues to the central nervous system." *Clinical Neurosurgery* 31: 404-416.

Hornykiewicz. 1962. "[Dopamine (3-hydroxytyramine) in the central nervous system and its relation to the Parkinson syndrome in man]." *Deutsche Medizinische Wochenschrift (1946)* 87 (September 7): 1807-1810. doi:10.1055/s-0028-1114024.

Hornykiewicz, O. 1966. "Dopamine (3-hydroxytyramine) and brain function." *Pharmacological Reviews* 18 (2) (June): 925-964.

Iversen, S D, and SB Dunnett. 1989e. "Functional compensation afforded by grafts of foetal neurones." *Progress in Neuro-Psychopharmacology & Biological Psychiatry* 13 (3-4): 453-467.

Klein, A, Gerlinde A Metz, Anna Papazoglou, and Guido Nikkhah. 2007c. "Differential effects on forelimb grasping behavior induced by fetal dopaminergic grafts in hemiparkinsonian rats." *Neurobiology of Disease* 27 (1) (July): 24-35. doi:10.1016/j.nbd.2007.03.010.

Kloth, Verena, A Klein, David Loettrich, and Guido Nikkhah. 2006d. "Colour-coded pellets increase the sensitivity of the staircase test to differentiate skilled forelimb performances of control and 6-hydroxydopamine lesioned rats." *Brain Research Bulletin* 70 (1) (June 15): 68-80. doi:10.1016/j.brainresbull.2006.04.006.

Lane, EL, and GA Smith. 2010. "Understanding graft-induced dyskinesia." *Regenerative Medicine* 5 (5) (September): 787-797. doi:10.2217/rme.10.42.

Lane, E, Anders Björklund, S Dunnett, and Christian Winkler. 2010. "Unravelling the mechanisms underlying graft-induced dyskinesia." *Progress Brain Research.* 184: 295-309.

Lees, Andrew J, John Hardy, and Tamas Revesz. 2009. "Parkinson's disease." *Lancet* 373 (9680) (June 13): 2055-2066. doi:10.1016/S0140-6736(09)60492-X.

Lindvall, O. 1991. "Transplants in Parkinson's disease." *European Neurology* 31 Suppl 1: 17-27.

Lindvall, O, S Rehncrona, P Brundin, B Gustavii, B Astedt, H Widner, T Lindholm, et al. 1989f. "Human fetal dopamine neurons grafted into the striatum in two patients with severe Parkinson's disease. A detailed account of methodology and a 6-month follow-up." *Archives of Neurology* 46 (6) (June): 615-631.

Lindvall, Olle, and Anders Björklund. 2004g. "Cell therapy in Parkinson's disease." *NeuroRx: The Journal of the American Society for Experimental NeuroTherapeutics* 1 (4) (October): 382-393.

Madrazo, I, V León, C Torres, M C Aguilera, G Varela, F Alvarez, A Fraga, R Drucker-Colín, F Ostrosky, and M Skurovich. 1988. "Transplantation of fetal substantia nigra and adrenal medulla to the caudate nucleus in two patients with Parkinson's disease." *The New England Journal of Medicine* 318 (1) (January 7): 51. doi:10.1056/NEJM198801073180115.

Mones, R J. 1969. "An evaluation of L-dopa in Parkinson patients." *Transactions of the American Neurological Association* 94: 307-309.

Nikkhah, G, H Sauer. 1992. "Transplantation von Gehirnzellen - Vision oder Realität?" Deutsches Ärzteblatt. 89 (3A): 106-114

Nikkhah, G, C Bentlage, M G Cunningham, and A Björklund. 1994. "Intranigral fetal dopamine grafts induce behavioral compensation in the rat Parkinson model." *The Journal of Neuroscience: The Official Journal of the Society for Neuroscience* 14 (6) (June): 3449-3461.

Nikkhah, G, M G Cunningham, M A Cenci, R D McKay, and A Björklund. 1995. "Dopaminergic microtransplants into the substantia nigra of neonatal rats with bilateral 6-OHDA lesions. I. Evidence for anatomical reconstruction of the nigrostriatal pathway." *The Journal of Neuroscience: The Official Journal of the Society for Neuroscience* 15 (5 Pt 1) (May): 3548-3561.

Nikkhah, G, W M Duan, U Knappe, A Jödicke, and A Björklund. 1993. "Restoration of complex sensorimotor behavior and skilled forelimb use by a modified nigral cell suspension transplantation approach in the rat Parkinson model." *Neuroscience,* 56 (1) (September): 33-43.

Nikkhah, G, M Olsson, J Eberhard, C Bentlage, M G Cunningham, and A Björklund. 1994. "A microtransplantation approach for cell suspension grafting in the rat Parkinson model: a detailed account of the methodology." *Neuroscience,* 63 (1) (November): 57-72.

Nikkhah, G, J Eberhard, M Olsson, and A Björklund. 1995. "Preservation of fetal ventral mesencephalic cells by cool storage: in-vitro viability and TH-positive neuron survival after microtransplantation to the striatum." *Brain Research,* 687 (1-2) (July 31): 22-34.

Nikkhah, G, C Rosenthal, H J Hedrich, and M Samii. 1998h. "Differences in acquisition and full performance in skilled forelimb use as measured by the 'staircase test' in five rat strains." *Behavioural Brain Research* 92 (1) (April): 85-95.

Nikkhah G, C Rosenthal, G Falkenstein, A Roedter, A Papazoglou, A Brandis. 2009. "Microtransplantation of dopaminergic cell suspensions: further characterization and optimization of grafting parameters." *Cell Transplantation,* 18(2): 119-133.

Olanow, C Warren, Christopher G Goetz, Jeffrey H Kordower, A Jon Stoessl, Vesna Sossi, Mitchell F Brin, Kathleen M Shannon, et al. 2003. "A double-blind controlled trial of bilateral fetal nigral transplantation in Parkinson's disease." *Annals of Neurology* 54 (3) (September): 403-414. doi:10.1002/ana.10720.

Olson, L, E O Backlund, W Freed, M Herrera-Marschitz, B Hoffer, A Seiger, and I Strömberg. 1985e. "Transplantation of monoamine-producing cell systems in oculo and intracranially: experiments in search of a treatment for Parkinson's Disease." *Annals of the New York Academy of Sciences* 457: 105-126.

Olson, L, and A Seiger. 1972. "Brain tissue transplanted to the anterior chamber of the eye. 1. Fluorescence histochemistry of immature catecholamine and 5-hydroxytryptamine neurons reinnervating the rat iris." *Zeitschrift Für Zellforschung Und Mikroskopische Anatomie (Vienna, Austria: 1948)* 135 (2): 175-194.

Perlow, M J, WJ Freed, BJ Hoffer, A Seiger, L Olson, and R J Wyatt. 1979f. "Brain grafts reduce motor abnormalities produced by destruction of nigrostriatal dopamine system." *Science (New York, N.Y.)* 204 (4393) (May 11): 643-647.

Pollock, M, and RW Hornabrook. 1966. "The prevalence, natural history and dementia of Parkinson's disease." *Brain* 89 (3): 429-448.

Regulation (EC) No 1394/2007 of the European Parliament and of the Council of 13 November 2007 on advanced therapy medicinal products and amending Directive 2001/83/EC and Regulation (EC) No 726/2004,

Schmidt, R H, A Björklund, and U Stenevi. 1981i. "Intracerebral grafting of dissociated CNS tissue suspensions: a new approach for neuronal transplantation to deep brain sites." *Brain Research* 218 (1-2) (August 10): 347-356.

Winkler, Christian, Deniz Kirik, and Anders Björklund. 2005h. "Cell transplantation in Parkinson's disease: how can we make it work?" *Trends in Neurosciences* 28 (2) (February): 86-92. doi:10.1016/j.tins.2004.12.006.

Wyatt, R J, J M Morihisa, R K Nakamura, and WJ Freed. 1986. "Transplanting tissue into the brain for function: use in a model of Parkinson's disease." *Research Publications - Association for Research in Nervous and Mental Disease* 64: 199-208.